BEHAVIOR ANALYSIS

Also Available

Handbook of Applied Behavior Analysis, Second Edition
Edited by Wayne W. Fisher, Cathleen C. Piazza,
and Henry S. Roane

Behavior Analysis

TRANSLATIONAL PERSPECTIVES AND CLINICAL PRACTICE

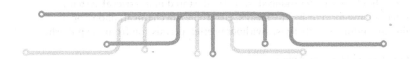

Edited by
Henry S. Roane
Andrew R. Craig
Valdeep Saini
Joel E. Ringdahl

THE GUILFORD PRESS
New York   London

Library of Congress Cataloging-in-Publication Data
Names: Roane, Henry S., editor.
Title: Behavior analysis : translational perspectives and clinical practice
  / edited by Henry S. Roane, Andrew R. Craig, Valdeep Saini, Joel E.
  Ringdahl.
Description: New York, NY : The Guilford Press, 2024. | Includes
  bibliographical references and index. |
Identifiers: LCCN 2023021509 | ISBN 9781462553488 (paperback) |
  ISBN 9781462553495 (cloth)
Subjects: LCSH: Behaviorism (Psychology) | Behavioral assessment. |
  Ethics—Research.
Classification: LCC BF199 .B34 2024 | DDC 150.19/43—dc23/eng/20230928
LC record available at *https://lccn.loc.gov/2023021509*

About the Editors

Henry S. Roane, PhD, BCBA-D, is the Liptak Professor of Child Development, Executive Director of the Golisano Center for Special Needs, and Chief of the Division of Development, Behavior, and Genetics at the State University of New York Upstate Medical University. He serves on the editorial boards of several journals in the fields of behavior analysis, school psychology, and pediatrics. Dr. Roane has coauthored over 100 research articles and chapters on the assessment and treatment of behavior problems and related subjects, and is coeditor of books including *Behavior Analysis: Translational Perspectives and Clinical Practice* and *Handbook of Applied Behavior Analysis, Second Edition.* He is a Fellow of the Association for Behavior Analysis International (ABAI), a member of the Society for Pediatric Research, and a recipient of the ABAI Nathan H. Azrin Distinguished Contribution to Applied Behavior Analysis Award from Division 25 of the American Psychological Association (APA).

Andrew R. Craig, PhD, is Assistant Professor of Pediatrics, Behavior Analysis Studies, and Neuroscience and Physiology; Director for Research in the Golisano Center for Special Needs; and Chair of the Behavior Analysis Studies Program at the State University of New York Upstate Medical University. Dr. Craig is Associate Editor for the *Journal of the Experimental Analysis of Behavior* and *Behavior Analysis: Research and Practice,* Guest Associate Editor for the *Journal of Applied Behavior Analysis,* and an ad hoc editor or reviewer for several other journals. He serves in leadership positions in Division 25 of the APA and the Society for the Quantitative Analyses of Behavior. He is a recipient of the B. F. Skinner Foundation New Researcher Award from APA Division 25 and the Joseph V. Brady Significant Research Contribution Award from the Society for the Experimental Analysis of Behavior.

Valdeep Saini, PhD, BCBA-D, is Associate Professor in the Department of Applied Disability Studies at Brock University in St. Catharines, Ontario, Canada. His primary research interest is the translation of basic behavioral sciences to areas of societal importance. Dr. Saini's approach prioritizes improving the longevity of behavioral interventions by integrating the findings of laboratory research into clinical applications of behavior therapy. This research is executed in both laboratory settings and clinical contexts. He has published over 40 peer-reviewed papers in more than 10 different behavioral and/or psychology journals.

Joel E. Ringdahl, PhD, BCBA, is Professor in the Department of Communication Sciences and Special Education at the University of Georgia. Dr. Ringdahl has served as Associate Editor or Editor-in-Chief of various behavior-analysis-focused journals. He has coauthored over 70 research articles and chapters on the assessment and treatment of behavior disorders in children with intellectual and developmental disabilities and has served as a grant reviewer on these topics for the National Institutes of Health and the National Science Foundation.

Contributors

Charlene N. Agnew, PhD, Proud Moments ABA, New York, New York

Francisco Arcediano, PhD, Department of Psychology, Oakland University, Rochester, Michigan

Kevin M. Ayres, PhD, Department of Communication Sciences and Special Education, The University of Georgia, Athens, Georgia

Jordan Belisle, PhD, Department of Psychology, Missouri State University, Springfield, Missouri

Zebulon K. Bell, PhD, Department of Psychology, Louisiana State University of Alexandria, Alexandria, Louisiana

Alec M. Bernstein, PhD, Department of Pediatrics, Children's Mercy Kansas City, Kansas City, Missouri

Alison M. Betz, PhD, ABA Technologies, Melbourne, Florida

Adam Brewer, PhD, Department of Education and Educational Psychology, Western Connecticut State University, Danbury, Connecticut

Katherine R. Brown, PhD, Department of Psychology, Utah State University, Logan, Utah

Nathan A. Call, PhD, Department of Pediatrics, Marcus Autism Center, Emory University School of Medicine, Atlanta, Georgia

Sarah Cowie, PhD, School of Psychology, University of Auckland, Auckland, New Zealand

Alison D. Cox, PhD, Department of Applied Disability Studies, Brock University, St. Catharines, Ontario, Canada

Andrew R. Craig, PhD, Departments of Pediatrics, Behavior Analysis Studies, and Neuroscience and Physiology, State University of New York Upstate Medical Center, Syracuse, New York

Nicole M. DeRosa, PsyD, Kelberman: The Center of Excellence for Autism, Utica, New York

Martha Escobar, PhD, Department of Psychology, Oakland University, Rochester, Michigan

Tara A. Fahmie, PhD, Munroe-Meyer Institute, University of Nebraska Medical Center, Omaha Nebraska

Terry S. Falcomata, PhD, Department of Special Education, The University of Texas at Austin, Austin, Texas

Rafaela M. Fontes, PhD, Fralin Biomedical Research Institute, Virginia Tech, Roanoke, Virginia

Adam E. Fox, PhD, Psychology Department, St. Lawrence University, Canton, New York

Jonathan E. Friedel, PhD, Department of Psychology, Georgia Southern University, Statesboro, Georgia

Dana M. Gadaire, PsyD, Department of Pediatrics and Communicable Diseases, University of Michigan Health, Ann Arbor, Michigan

Shawn Gilroy, PhD, Department of Psychology, Louisiana State University, Baton Rouge, Louisiana

Stephanie Gomes-Ng, PhD, School of Social Science and Public Policy, Auckland University of Technology, Auckland, New Zealand

Brian D. Greer, PhD, Department of Pediatrics, Robert Wood Johnson Medical School, New Brunswick, New Jersey

Jeremy M. Haynes, PhD, Department of Psychology, Temple University, Philadelphia, Pennsylvania

Richelle Hurtado, PhD, Vanderbilt University Medical Center, Nashville, Tennessee

Einar T. Ingvarsson, PhD, Virginia Institute of Autism, Charlottesville, Virginia

David P. Jarmolowicz, PhD (deceased), Department of Applied Behavioral Science, The University of Kansas, Lawrence, Kansas

Corina Jimenez-Gomez, PhD, Department of Psychology, University of Florida, Gainesville, Florida

Michael E. Kelley, PhD, Department of Psychiatry, University of Michigan Medical School, Ann Arbor, Michigan

David Kuhn, PhD, Milestones Behavioral Services, Orange, Connecticut

Stephanie C. Kuhn, PhD, Department of Education, Western Connecticut State University, Danbury, Connecticut

Elizabeth G. E. Kyonka, PhD, Department of Psychology, California State University, East Bay, Hayward, California

Kennon A. Lattal, PhD, Department of Psychology, West Virginia University, Morgantown, West Virginia

Robert S. LeComte, MA, Department of Applied Behavioral Science, The University of Kansas, Lawrence, Kansas

Yanerys Leon, PhD, Department of Psychology, University of Miami, Coral Gables, Florida

Dorothea C. Lerman, PhD, Department of Psychology, University of Houston Clear Lake, Houston, Texas

Karen M. Lionello-DeNolf, PhD, Department of Psychology, Assumption University, Worcester, Massachusetts

Gregory J. Madden, PhD, Department of Psychology, Utah State University, Logan, Utah

Jennifer J. McComas, PhD, Department of Educational Psychology, University of Minnesota, Minneapolis, Minnesota

Rusty W. Nall, PhD, Department of Psychology, Jacksonville State University, Jacksonville, Alabama

Allen Neuringer, PhD, Department of Psychology, Reed College, Portland, Oregon

Amy L. Odum, PhD, Department of Psychology, Utah State University, Logan, Utah

Anna Ingeborg Petursdottir, PhD, Department of Psychology, Texas Christian University, Fort Worth, Texas

Carol Pilgrim, PhD, Department of Psychology, University of North Carolina Wilmington, Wilmington, North Carolina

Christopher A. Podlesnik, PhD, Department of Psychology, University of Florida, Gainesville, Florida

Derek D. Reed, PhD, Institutes for Behavior Resources, Baltimore, Maryland

Catalina N. Rey, PhD, Munroe-Meyer Institute, University of Nebraska Medical Center, Omaha, Nebraska

Joel E. Ringdahl, PhD, Department of Communication Sciences and Special Education, University of Georgia, Athens, Georgia

Carolyn M. Ritchey, MS, Department of Psychology, Auburn University, Auburn, Alabama

Henry S. Roane, PhD, Departments of Pediatrics and Psychiatry, State University of New York Upstate Medical Center, Syracuse, New York

Valdeep Saini, PhD, Department of Applied Disability Studies, Brock University, St. Catharines, Ontario, Canada

Kelly M. Schieltz, PhD, Stead Family Department of Pediatrics, University of Iowa, Iowa City, Iowa

Michael W. Schlund, PhD, Department of Psychology, Georgia State University, Atlanta, Georgia

Rebecca A. Sharp, PhD, School of Psychology, University of Auckland, Auckland, New Zealand

Shrinidhi Subramaniam, PhD, Department of Psychology and Child Development, California State University, Stanislaus, Turlock, California

William E. Sullivan, PhD, Department of Pediatrics, State University of New York Upstate Medical Center, Syracuse, New York

Jonathan Tarbox, PhD, Department of Psychology, University of Southern California, Los Angeles, California

Eric A. Thrailkill, PhD, Department of Psychological Science, The University of Vermont, Burlington, Vermont

Maria G. Valdovinos, PhD, Department of Psychology and Neuroscience, Drake University, Des Moines, Iowa

Victoria R. Verdun, PhD, Department of Pediatrics, Marcus Autism Center, Emory University School of Medicine, Atlanta, Georgia

Craige Wrenn, PhD, Department of Pharmaceutical Science, Drake University, Des Moines, Iowa

Amanda N. Zangrillo, PsyD, Munroe-Meyer Institute, University of Nebraska Medical Center, Omaha, Nebraska

Preface

TRANSLATIONAL PERSPECTIVES
ON APPLIED BEHAVIOR ANALYSIS

> And as we continue to improve our understanding of the basic science
> on which applications increasingly depend, material benefits of this
> and other kinds are secured for the future.
> —HENRY TAUBE, Nobel banquet, 1983

Mastery of basic principles and foundational knowledge is a critical element for health care professionals. For example, although most physicians do not practice laboratory biology on a regular basis, knowledge of cellular physiology is a key component of diagnosing and treating many diseases. Beyond medicine, other disciplines require students to acquire foundational knowledge in the natural sciences. Civil engineers apply basic principles of physics to build skyscrapers, and chefs leverage an understanding of basic chemistry when preparing foods.

B. F. Skinner (1938) characterized behavioral science as a component of natural science. Inasmuch, training in behavior analysis parallels training in other disciplines rooted in the natural sciences. In 2022, the Behavior Analyst Certification Board® (BACB) updated education and eligibility guidelines to include an increased focus on training in foundational knowledge (e.g., basic skills, underlying principles) as well as application of that knowledge. The new eligibility guidelines introduced, for the first time, a requirement that training programs provide coursework related to basic behavior analysis (also referred to as the experimental analysis of behavior [EAB]). Thus, like the physician must have core knowledge of biology, chemistry, and other basic sciences, so too must behavior analysts have knowledge of the natural science of behavior. The current text is our attempt to bridge this gap by offering readers foundational knowledge examined through the lenses of both EAB and applied behavior analysis (ABA).

Throughout this volume, many of the research paradigms and methodologies across EAB and ABA are presented within the "bench-to-bedside" approach of translational research described by the National Institutes of Health. This approach to scientific inquiry is notable due to its focus on linking basic research findings to clinical interventions, with the function of progressing treatments more quickly to consumers. This translational approach to behavior analysis is evinced by each chapter introducing a core principle and describing this principle with equivalent coverage of basic (EAB) and applied (ABA) findings. For the majority of chapters, we have been fortunate to include at least two authors: one with expertise in EAB and the other with expertise in ABA. We hope that this relatively novel approach to tackling behavior-analytic content will give the reader a unique perspective from both disciplines across chapters.

The first few chapters of the text introduce underlying core tenets of behaviorism, as well as core characteristics and methods that define the field of behavior analysis. First, the fields of EAB and ABA are described. Quantitative analyses of behavior also are summarized, as these approaches to understanding behavior process recently have found much utility in translational research in behavior analysis. Next, particular "nuts and bolts" of behavior-analytic research methods and data collection are presented across three chapters wherein the authors discuss similarities and differences in methods that are used across EAB and ABA.

The next several chapters of the book introduce the reader to some of the foundational principles of behavior analysis, with coverage from both the EAB and ABA perspectives. Included within are chapters on classical conditioning, reinforcement, extinction, and verbal behavior, among others. This content is common throughout behavior-analytic texts, but our hope with this volume is that the reader will acquire knowledge about the more nuanced way that ABA and EAB diverge and converge in their treatments of these topics.

The final chapters of the book cover topics for which ample basic, applied, and translational research has been conducted. These chapters will give the reader insight into broader applications of multiple behavior principles, as well as demonstrate the manner by which EAB and ABA researchers and clinicians might collaborate to solve societal problems. The text concludes with a chapter on ethics, which includes content related to ethical issues in research and in clinical practice, and the ethical use of nonhuman animals and special populations in research.

This book is the first comprehensive text detailing a translational approach to topics within the field of behavior analysis by directly bridging EAB and ABA. The contributors are leading experts in EAB, ABA, translational research, and clinical practice. This book is appropriate for upper-level undergraduate students, graduate students, researchers, and practitioners in psychology, education, or behavior analysis. It is applicable to courses in psychology, education, or behavior analysis on topics related to EAB, ABA, and applied learning theory and practice. In most cases, this book would be considered the primary textbook for courses. We hope the reader will find it as informative and useful as it was enjoyable for us to edit.

HENRY S. ROANE
ANDREW R. CRAIG
VALDEEP SAINI
JOEL E. RINGDAHL

REFERENCE

Skinner, B. F. (1938). *The behavior of organisms: An experimental analysis*. Appleton-Century.

Acknowledgments

We would like to acknowledge the central role filled by often-marginalized populations, such as individuals with intellectual and developmental disabilities and their families, that allow for advancements in the science and practice of behavior analysis to take place. As a group of editors, scientists, and practitioners, we recognize the crucial contributions made by these individuals. We would also like to acknowledge the many human and nonhuman animal subjects who have contributed countless data points to our collective research. Finally, we would like to acknowledge the various scholars who provided anonymous feedback on the proposal for this project.

Contents

PART IV. OPERANT CONDITIONING

PART V. ADVANCED TOPICS IN TRANSLATIONAL RESEARCH

PART I

BASIC PRINCIPLES
OF BEHAVIOR ANALYSIS

CHAPTER 1

Translational Science in Behavior Analysis
SOME OBSERVATIONS AND A CASE HISTORY

Carol Pilgrim
Richelle Hurtado

Translational research is hot. Indeed, calls for an emphasis on translational approaches and translational science are widely in evidence not only within behavior analysis but also throughout science and medicine more broadly (e.g., Austin, 2018, 2021; Fort et al., 2017). We find the term *translational* increasingly in the titles of scholarly books (e.g., this one) and journals (e.g., *American Journal of Translational Research, Journal of Clinical and Translational Science*), as well as in the chapters and articles that appear within them; in characterizations of research agendas (e.g., of academic job candidates, or in grants submitted for federal funding); in graduate curriculum listings (e.g., as individual course titles or even as program tracks); in branches of key science agencies (e.g., the National Center for Advancing Translational Sciences, of the National Institute of Health); and in named honors and positions within our major professional organizations (e.g., the Scientific Translation Award of the Society for the Advancement of Behavior Analysis; the Society for the Experimental Analysis of Behavior Don Hake Translational Research Award of Division 25 of the American Psychological Association; the Editor for Translational Research of the *Journal of the Experimental Analysis of Behavior*; and the Associate Editor for Translational Research of the *Journal of Applied Behavior Analysis*). The collective message is clear that translation is viewed as important and that it is highly valued in our scientific endeavors. Also clear in such messaging, however, is the tacit recognition that special support may be required to ensure the adoption and implementation of translational approaches, while the continued appeals for translational work may be seen as indicative of concern about its relative overall frequency. One suggestion is that the naturally occurring contingencies of science have not always been sufficient for fostering attention to translation, and that the often-assumed "trickle down" of understanding from the proverbial "bench" of the basic experimental laboratory to the "bedside" of a patient or client in need is not automatic.

As for what is implied when we speak of translational research and why it might be important, certainly much has been written on the topic, with respect to both science in general (e.g., Stokes, 2011; Woolf, 2008; Zerhouni, 2005) and behavior analysis in particular (e.g., Critchfield, 2011; Mace & Critchfield, 2010). It is the latter, of course, that is of special interest for this text, and it is a thesis of this chapter that translational work is perhaps uniquely essential to our field, along dimensions that not only include but also extend traditional characterizations of translation. To begin to illustrate the point for present purposes, Figure 1.1 depicts the field of behavior analysis as a continuum of three primary domains of endeavor (adapted from Moore, 2008; and see Moore & Cooper, 2003). In broad strokes, where the experimental analysis of behavior entails highly controlled basic laboratory research designed to address questions about fundamental principles of behavior, applied behavior analysis is characterized by research designed to address questions about effective interventions with socially significant behavioral targets. The third domain, applied behavior-analytic service provision, focuses on the professional delivery of principled applications designed to facilitate meaningful behavior change for an individual or social group. Importantly, there is overlap in the domains rather than firm boundaries between them, and underlying all three is a unifying conceptual foundation—the comprehensive worldview known as behaviorism (although "behaviorism" today may take any of several forms; e.g., Skinner, 1953; Baum, 1994; Hayes et al., 2001).

Figure 1.2 adds to the representation an indicator of that province of behavior analysis that has received greatest emphasis in discussions of translational efforts for our field. The bolded bracket highlights the interplay between basic laboratory and applied research. One key premise in such considerations is that new discoveries made possible in the laboratory, where relevant variables can be tightly managed, should next be evaluated for their potential in understanding and working effectively with significant behavioral targets (rather than key pecks or lever presses) under more naturally occurring conditions, such as a clinic or school or home. An implicit assumption is that once applied research has demonstrated validity, an empirically generated finding or concept will be adopted and disseminated among practitioners, although this outcome rarely receives explicit attention. The more astute discussions of translation also underscore the importance of basic laboratory scientists taking inspiration for at least some of their experimental questions and directions from important behavioral effects observed during applied

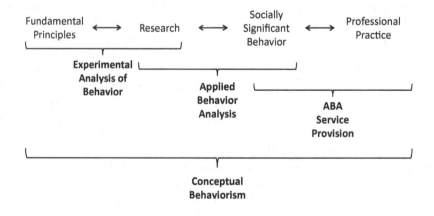

FIGURE 1.1. The domains of behavior analysis.

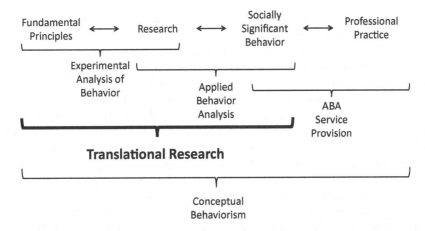

FIGURE 1.2. Translational research and the domains of behavior analysis.

analyses, so that their research might be informed by, and thereby speak more directly to, issues of social relevance. Thus, a reciprocal, bidirectional, and progressive exchange between basic laboratory and applied research is envisioned, with benefits accruing for each domain independently, and for the field of behavior analysis more generally. The importance of this sort of translational chemistry can hardly be overestimated, and emphasis on it is not surprising. Still, even a brief scan of Figure 1.2 reveals that portions of the defining content of our field fall outside of the highlighted intersection. It might even be argued that much of the truly influential work in behavior analysis could be characterized in terms of translations between and among any number of the *foci* depicted, and that consideration of the full range of intersections possible within our multifaceted field deserves greater attention in our approach to translational efforts. A case history from the realm of stimulus equivalence is used here to illustrate these points, as well as some of the benefits of integrating basic, applied, and conceptual behavior analysis and its practice.

Laying the Foundations

Behavior-analytic work on equivalence constitutes a particularly apt example to consider in the present context, even from its very beginnings. In contrast to many topics explored in basic experimental labs, the origin story of equivalence research places us firmly in the sphere of practical need, with its focus on reading comprehension. The two inaugural studies in equivalence research (Sidman, 1971; Sidman & Cresson, 1973; see also Sidman, 1994) involved three young men (ages 17–19) with severe intellectual and developmental disabilities who lived in a state facility. Despite extensive teaching histories, the young men had developed no reading skills whatsoever. All three could match dictated names with pictures, and could produce names for most of the pictures, but could not match either dictated names or pictures with the corresponding written words, nor could they produce names for the written words. Subsequent to these reading-skill assessments, a single teaching step was provided. The young men were taught, painstakingly via differential reinforcement, to choose the appropriate one of 20 written words in response to its dictated counterpart. Though unexpected by the researchers (Sidman, 1994, 2007), the now-familiar result of that limited training was that all three students also demonstrated significant improvements in reading comprehension, as indicated by accurately matching written words and pictures, and in oral reading, as indicated by their production of the appropriate spoken name for each written word. These momentous matches were truly heard round the (behavior-analytic) world, potent harbingers of a vibrant experimental, applied, and conceptual analysis that continues to this day (e.g., Pilgrim, 2020). In Sidman's (1994) words, "So it really looked as though we had a tiger by the tail: new performances emerging that we had not specifically taught, of a type that was important in everyday life, and that our background had not prepared us to consider. We were off on a long-term adventure" (p. 60). With a few additional replications under their belt (e.g., Sidman et al., 1974), it was time for this beginning program of study to shift to the laboratory, where important control conditions and methodological refinements could be implemented, and generality could be explored more thoroughly.

But let's consider what's happened in this brief portion of the research program with respect to translation. The arrows of Figure 1.3 (with domain brackets omitted, for clarity of presentation) trace the influence of stumbling blocks in teaching reading comprehension (i.e., professional practice involving socially significant behavior) on the content of an applied analysis of a teaching approach (e.g., Sidman, 1971; Sidman & Cresson, 1973). Results of the applied analysis, in turn, gave rise to questions about the fundamental principles that might be responsible for the emergent performances obtained, inspiring the design of a series of laboratory experiments (i.e., experimental analysis) to investigate their determinants (e.g., Sidman et al., 1982; Sidman & Tailby, 1982). Indeed, with their seminal experimental work, Sidman and Tailby ensured that the adventure, and the translation, would continue and expand.

Figure 1.4 illustrates the basics of Sidman and Tailby's (1982) experimental arrangement with a schematic format that has since become standard for describing equivalence work. Four stimulus sets (designated as A, B, C, and D, where each set included three stimuli) were used instead of three (i.e., spoken words, pictures, and written words) as in the earlier studies. All stimuli were selected to be abstract from the perspective of the 5- to

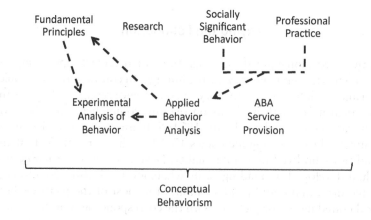

FIGURE 1.3. Mapping translations: Early work in stimulus equivalence.

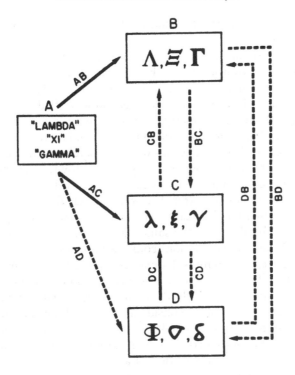

FIGURE 1.4. Trained and tested relations. From Sidman and Tailby (1982). Reprinted with permission of John Wiley & Sons, Inc.

7-year-old typically developing children who served as participants, and the relations established between stimuli were unfamiliar and/or arbitrary (i.e., physically dissimilar; designated by the researchers), ruling out the possibility that they might have been acquired extra-experimentally. The matching procedure (technically, match-to-sample) employed in the original reading research was used again for teaching and testing. Where the previous work was based on two sets of trained (or baseline) matching relations (i.e., spoken word to picture, and spoken word to written word), the solid arrows in Figure 1.4 indicate that three conditional discriminations (AB, AC, and DC) were taught directly, via differential reinforcement. Arrows always point from a set of sample stimuli to an array of comparison stimuli presented on a given trial, such that during training, selecting the first B stimulus listed here, after presentation of the first A stimulus listed, would produce reinforcers; selecting the second B stimulus after presentation of the second A stimulus would do so, and so on, for each of the arrows. Dashed arrows in Figure 1.4 indicate the six new sets of conditional relations that were tested after the first three were taught. The important distinction between these probed relations and the trained ones (shown with solid arrows) was that no programmed consequences were provided for responses on the test trials. Six of the eight children in this study demonstrated all of the tested relations outlined here, and on subsequent naming tests (not included on the figure), they spoke the A-stimulus label for each of the related B, C, and D stimuli. In short, based on a minimum of training, three groups of four physically dissimilar stimuli proved to be functionally interchangeable in any combination, yielding a cohesive and generative stimulus-control repertoire that could not have been predicted in terms of known principles of behavior.

It is difficult to overstate the impact of these provocative results, or the extent to which they have inspired translation. To begin, they provided the springboard for the introduction of a powerful new conceptualization of stimulus classes viewed as behavioral analogues of mathematical equivalence relations and identified in terms of equivalence-set properties (i.e., reflexivity, symmetry, and transitivity; see Sidman & Tailby, 1982, Table 1, p. 6, for their elegant presentation of the model). Figure 1.5 illustrates the operational definitions of equivalence properties within a match-to-sample paradigm. Positive outcomes on all of the trial types denoted by dashed arrows, after the training denoted by solid arrows, would constitute a demonstration of equivalence-class formation, where the members of each stimulus class (for this example, A1, B1, and C1; A2, B2, and C2; and A3, B3, and C3) function identically, whether as sample or comparison stimulus, in relation to any other stimulus from the same class. (More concretely, for the Figure 1.5 example, a total of 27 individual relations could result from teaching only six.)

This defining conceptual analysis (Sidman & Tailby, 1982; Sidman et al., 1982) laid the foundation for translation to important forms of complex human performance often deemed cognitive in nature, especially those involving verbal behavior and semantics. Viewed through an equivalence lens, consideration of such performances could then be translated back into systematically related laboratory investigations, providing for exploration and analysis of phenomena commonly held to be outside the auspices of behavior analysis. Furthermore, Sidman's replication of an extended and strikingly coherent pattern of untrained performances, under conditions of tight experimental control, made the potential for applications of the equivalence arrangement immediately apparent, and translations into teaching procedures targeting a range of functional skills and populations quickly began in earnest. Indeed, demonstrating a reliable laboratory model for the production and description of emergent repertoires was critical in its own right, allowing for further experimental analysis of generativity and the variables controlling it (topics frequently posited as challenges for a reinforcement-based account). These early findings

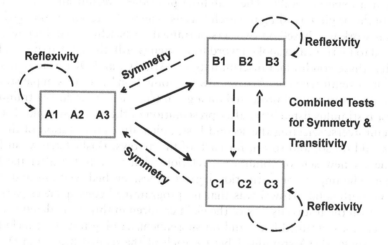

FIGURE 1.5. Defining properties of equivalence as reflected in match-to-sample training and testing, where each alphanumeric designation reflects a unique stimulus.

of Sidman and colleagues were similarly translated into additional experimental questions about the generality of equivalence outcomes and the necessary and sufficient conditions for producing them. Such research, in turn, carried implications for understanding the basic behavioral principles that might be at play and inspired development of varied theoretical treatments of the origins of equivalence and other relational responding. It might reasonably be argued that few investigations have had as great an impact as a translational nexus, at least within behavior analysis.

In Figure 1.6, the translational sequelae just outlined are added to our developing template. Results from the seminal experimental analysis led to a new conceptualization, which promoted behavior-analytic consideration of critical higher-order performances of great significance (e.g., verbal behavior, cognition, generativity). These considerations were translated in turn into new experimental questions. Demonstration of emergent and systematic patterns of stimulus control based on minimal training translated into a range of applied analyses of equivalence approaches and into teaching practices in clinics and classrooms (e.g., Pilgrim, 2020). The laboratory findings gave rise to further questions about controlling variables and generality, translating into additional experimental analyses, challenges for the adequacy of existing fundamental principles (e.g., Catania, 1998; Sidman, 1994), and explication of behavioral theory with sweeping scope (e.g., Sidman, 1994, 2000; Horne & Lowe, 1996; Hayes et al., 2001). The adventure had indeed begun!

A Case History

A little closer to home, while the research programs painted earlier with broad brush were unfolding, work in our own lab also reflected an ongoing interchange of influences from varied quarters. Because a continuing role for translation might be more clearly operationalized with specific examples, we will consider here a series of four studies from our lab, with an eye toward highlighting benefits that can follow from integration across

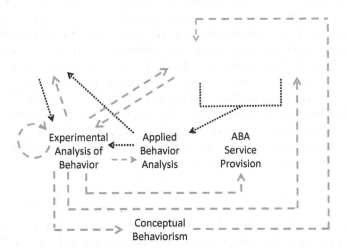

FIGURE 1.6. Cumulative translations, post Sidman and Tailby (1982). Original interchanges are indicated by dotted arrows; added interchanges are indicated by dashed arrows.

domains. Methodological details of the work are included only to the extent necessary to frame its development.

This particular research story launches from a purely practical starting point. Like many other researchers, we had eagerly embarked on investigations of equivalence with young children, hoping to avoid at least some of the complicating histories that adults bring to an experiment and to involve participants who might teach us the most about early occurrences of equivalence outcomes. Such studies often begin by teaching arbitrary conditional discriminations, first one and then others, in a match-to-sample format (when presented with sample stimulus A1, selection of comparison stimulus B1 from an array results in a reinforcer delivery; given sample A2, selecting B2 from the array is reinforced, etc.). Once established, these trained conditional discriminations make possible the critical emergent performances of interest. There was just one catch. Many of the typically developing children in our studies failed to acquire the conditional discriminations when targeted with differential reinforcement contingencies alone. In fact, a compilation of data across all of our experiments involving children at the time made clear that even with a programmed teaching sequence in place (Pilgrim et al., 2000), there was considerable variability in the number of sessions required to meet mastery (see also, e.g., Augustson & Dougher, 1991; Zygmont et al., 1992), especially among the least advanced children who might stand to benefit most from equivalence-based instructional approaches. This seemed a potentially significant challenge if equivalence approaches were to achieve their promise in applications and practice, especially with young children and individuals with intellectual or developmental disabilities.

These practical concerns did not exist in a vacuum, of course. Of particular relevance in this case was their consideration in light of Sidman's (1994, 2000) theoretical position on the origins of equivalence. Leaving debate about the implications and relative merits of his position to a more appropriate venue, the important point for present purposes is that this conceptual treatment suggested a path forward. The argument, in a nutshell, was that "equivalence is a direct outcome of reinforcement *contingencies*" [note the emphasis on contingencies plural, as in *any* n-term contingency] and that "equivalence relations consist of . . . all positive elements that participate in the contingency" (Sidman, 2000, p. 128), suggesting that an optimally arranged contingency could result in an equivalence relation including not only the antecedent stimuli but also the response and the reinforcer. Given the much more straightforward task of establishing three-term contingencies with children, rather than the four-term conditional discriminations typically arranged in equivalence work, and given successful laboratory evidence of reinforcers functioning as equivalence-class members (e.g., Dube et al., 1987, 1989; Varella & de Souza, 2014), Sidman's position suggested an intriguing and inherently empirical question. Would it be possible to generate equivalence classes through simple discrimination training if reinforcers were set up as class members? Inspired, then, by practical matters as well as conceptual ones, we were back to the lab.

Study 1

The approach involved teaching children a series of nine simple discriminations in a discrete-trial procedure. For purposes of experimental control, abstract line drawings served as S+ and S− stimuli, with their functions arbitrarily designated. On each trial, one S+ and two S− stimuli were presented in three of the four corners of a computer screen. Figure 1.7 presents a schematic of one such discrimination training trial, with stimulus

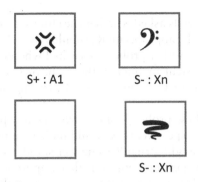

S+ : A1   S- : Xn

S- : Xn

FIGURE 1.7. Schematic of a discrimination training trial from Study 1. Stimulus labels are added here for descriptive purposes; they did not appear on actual trial presentations.

labels added to clarify exposition. A mouse click on the S+ produced as a consequence one of three auditory–visual compounds particular to the S+ (i.e., the consequences were class-specific), where each compound comprised a different computer-generated jingle presented together with its own geometric display. A mouse click on either S– produced a buzzer, and the S– stimuli presented on any given trial were unique for each S+. The nine discriminations were trained individually, and their presentation was intermixed as training progressed. Table 1.1 outlines the three-term contingencies that were arranged, where each alphanumeric label (e.g., A1, B1, C1) specifies one of the nine different S+ stimuli. The S– stimuli presented together with an S+ are represented in parentheses, and the consequence produced by correct selection of the S+ is indicated following the arrow. The critical feature of the training was that one auditory–visual compound (hereafter, Reinforcer 1, or R1) was presented as the consequence for correct selections when A1, B1, or C1 served as S+ on a trial; a second auditory–visual compound (i.e., Reinforcer 2, or R2) followed correct selections of A2, B2, or C2; and a third compound (i.e., Reinforcer 3, or R3) followed correct selections of A3, B3, or C3. Even with nine different S+ stimuli incorporated in the final intermixed baseline (see Table 1.1), the children quickly acquired and then maintained these simple discriminations.

Foundations thus established, the pressing question of interest was whether they would prove sufficient for demonstration of generative equivalence outcomes. More specifically, would we see evidence for the four-member equivalence classes (i.e., A1B1C1R1; A2B2C2R2; A3B3C3R3) that could possibly follow from our training? The next step then, was to include conditional discrimination probe tests within the mixed training

TABLE 1.1. Simple Discrimination Training with Class-Specific Consequences

A discriminations	B discriminations	C discriminations
A1 (*Xn*, *Xn*) → R1	B1 (*Xn*, *Xn*) → R1	C1 (*Xn*, *Xn*) → R1
A2 (*Xn*, *Xn*) → R2	B2 (*Xn*, *Xn*) → R2	C2 (*Xn*, *Xn*) → R2
A3 (*Xn*, *Xn*) → R3	B3 (*Xn*, *Xn*) → R3	C3 (*Xn*, *Xn*) → R3

Note. Each *X* indicates a unique line S– drawing; *n* denotes a numerical identifier omitted here to prevent confusion with class designations.

baseline. In essence, probe trials asked whether the children would match A, B, or C stimuli presented as samples to the appropriate R stimulus (R1, R2, or R3) when presented as comparisons, and vice versa. Other probe trials asked whether A, B, or C samples would be matched in a class-consistent manner to the A, B, or C comparisons (e.g., matching an A1 sample to an A1, B1, or C1 comparison, depending on the probe type), and vice versa, in any combination.

Positive responses to these probe questions would carry potentially important implications. From a practical perspective, they would indicate a promising teaching arrangement for participants who might struggle to master standard conditional discrimination training but could otherwise benefit from equivalence approaches. From a theoretical perspective, they would provide some support for the position that a range of contingencies can produce equivalence relations inclusive of all contingency elements. From an applied perspective, consider that teaching nine quickly acquired simple discriminations could possibly result in a total of 48 emergent conditional relations (i.e., for those interested in the specifics, 12 reflexive relations involving the A, B, C, and R stimuli; and three relations each for AR, RA, BR, RB, CR, RC, AB, BA, AC, CA, BC, and CB probes, where the first letter of each pair demotes the sample stimulus set and the second letter denotes the comparison stimulus set), suggesting a greatly enhanced degree of generativity relative to standard training arrangements. As for the results, more than 50 children (ages 4 to 12), though not all, have confirmed the general patterns described here, across a number of studies in our lab (e.g., Boye, 2008; Leuck, 2017; Hurtado, 2020, 2021). Indeed, this basic training and testing protocol has become a standard platform for us when investigating a broad range of questions about equivalence with children, even as it has inspired questions about critical controlling variables within the protocol (e.g., Sheehan, 2018; Shepherd, 2019). Figure 1.8 highlights the influences that gave rise to the study described here (i.e., practical, conceptual, and applied), as well as the return implications for domains within and outside of experimental analysis. The Study 1 intersections are

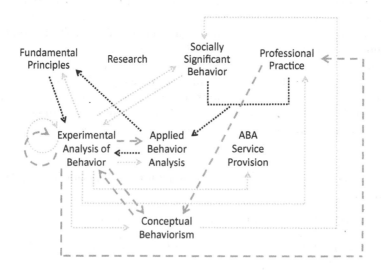

FIGURE 1.8. Cumulative translations, Study 1. Original interchanges indicated by dotted arrows; added interchanges indicated by dashed arrows.

superimposed on the foundational work described previously, for a cumulative view of the unfolding translations.

Study 2

Following one of those connections, we next explored the possibility that the abstract relations among line drawings created in the lab might be reimagined so as to have potential societal relevance. In this case (Yonkers, 2012), participants were four 5- to 7-year-old children with academic delays who earned low scores on an arithmetic pretest and had been identified by their teachers as needing help with math. Once again, we taught a series of nine simple discriminations, where each involved one S+ and two S− stimuli, and correct selections produced a compound auditory–visual consequence specific to the S+. The critical change to the procedures involved the nature of the stimuli. Rather than the abstract line drawings used previously, simple numeric stimuli were chosen on the basis of each child's skill level. To illustrate, for two children, the S+ stimuli included numerals (A stimuli: 4, 7, and 10) and addition problems (B stimuli: 3 + 1, 6 + 1, and 9 + 1; and C stimuli: 2 + 2, 5 + 2, and 8 + 2). For each S+, the two S− stimuli included the same number or addition problem rotated to either a 90-degree orientation (such that it appeared sideways in the display) or a 180-degree orientation (such that it appeared upside down). To illustrate, Figure 1.9 presents a schematic of a numeral discrimination training trial. The compound consequence that followed selection of an S+ entailed simultaneous presentation of a printed and a spoken number word (i.e., either *four, seven,* or *ten*), as appropriate to the S+. Table 1.2 presents the stimulus sets. As in the previous study, all four children learned the nine trained discriminations, individually and then intermixed, usually within the minimum number of sessions required to meet mastery criteria.

In another variation from the first study, design of the test procedures required periodic assessments to ensure that patterns of class-consistent responses were the result of the experimental training, as opposed to regular classroom instruction. Furthermore, the specifics of the compound consequences used here suggested the potential for three five-member equivalence classes to emerge, where each class could include a numeral, a +1 addition problem, a +2 addition problem, a spoken word, and a written word (i.e., A1B1C1R1r1; A2B2C2R2r2; A3B3C3R3r3; where R and r represent different components of the consequence compound). Such classes were again evaluated through conditional

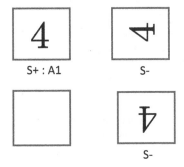

FIGURE 1.9. Schematic of a discrimination training trial from Study 2. Stimulus labels are added here for descriptive purposes; they did not appear on actual trial presentations.

TABLE 1.2. Math Skills Stimulus Sets

A numerals	B + 1 stimuli	C + 2 stimuli	Consequences
4	3 + 1	2 + 2	"Four," FOUR
7	6 + 1	5 + 2	"Seven," SEVEN
10	9 + 1	8 + 2	"Ten," TEN

discrimination probe trials, which asked, for example, whether 4, 3 + 1, 2 + 2, *four,* and FOUR (and likewise for the seven and 10 stimulus groups) would be matched to each other in any combination of sample and comparison array. All told, training nine simple discriminations with compound class-specific consequences had laid the foundation for 75 individual stimulus relations to emerge (i.e., again, for fellow equivalence geeks, 15 potential reflexive relations involving the A, B, C, R, and r stimuli; and three relations each for Rr, rR, AR, RA, Ar, rA, BR, RB, Br, rB, CR, RC, Cr, rC, AB, BA, AC, CA, BC, and CB conditional discrimination probes). What's more, this would be an emergent repertoire of educational significance for the children involved (i.e., the beginnings of simple arithmetic skills). As for results, three of the four children in this proof-of-concept extension demonstrated the emergent relations of interest that could be tested. This successful application replicated and thus strengthened the previous laboratory findings, as well as their conceptual implications; it illustrated the feasibility of similarly structured equivalence-based programming for practical educational purposes and for populations with delays; and it suggested an interesting further question related to the strategic use of compound stimuli in generating large equivalence classes, as with the compound consequences used here. These new translations are added in Figure 1.10.

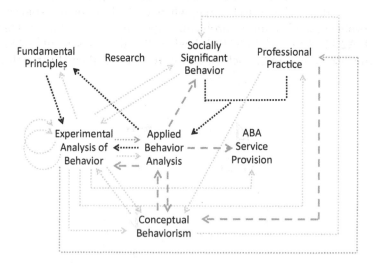

FIGURE 1.10. Cumulative translations, Study 2. Previous interchanges are indicated by dotted arrows; new interchanges are indicated by dashed arrows.

Study 3

The math skills study had illustrated clearly that distinct components of the class-consistent compound consequences (i.e., the spoken and written number words) came to function independently as equivalence-class members (see also Varella & de Souza, 2014). Conceptually, this finding had a bearing on the position that one outcome of a reinforcement contingency is an equivalence relation inclusive of all elements that comprise the contingency. The spoken and written words used in Study 2 were equally defining of each of the three-term contingencies arranged in training. It was also the case that both laboratory (e.g., Markam & Dougher, 1993) and applied (e.g., Stromer & Mackay, 1992, 1993) equivalence work utilizing standard conditional discrimination training had shown that components of compounds presented as sample stimuli can function as separable class members. A return to the lab seemed called for then, to investigate whether presenting compound discriminative stimuli in three-term contingency training with class-specific compound consequences might yield expanded equivalence outcomes with even greater potential (Williams, 2016).

The general training setup will be familiar by now. Class-consistent compound consequences were arranged for S+ selections on simple discrimination trials, as in the two previous studies. In this case, however, we sought to teach six discriminations, where each of the six S+ stimuli was a unique compound made up of two abstract line drawings arranged side by side. To illustrate, Figure 1.11 presents a schematic of an A1B1 discrimination training trial. Selecting the S+ compound produced two class-specific picture tokens, delivered simultaneously (e.g., a smiley face token and a thumbs-up token were presented for correct selections of an A1B1 or C1D1 compound), while selecting any S– compound produced a token marked with an "X." Table 1.3 outlines the training contingencies that were arranged. For each trained discrimination, the S+ compound is identified first, the S– stimuli are included in parentheses, and the consequence produced by correct selection of the S+ is indicated following the arrow. As Table 1.3 and Figure 1.11 illustrate, the two S– stimuli presented with a given S+ were also compounds, designed such that discrimination mastery would require control by both elements of the S+. Each of the S– compounds included one of the S+ components (e.g., for an AB discrimination, either the A or the B line drawing), as well as a second component unique to that particular S– (e.g., for an AB discrimination, either a W or X line drawing, where

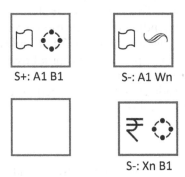

S+: A1 B1   S-: A1 Wn

S-: Xn B1

FIGURE 1.11. Schematic of a discrimination training trial from Study 3. Stimulus labels are added here for descriptive purposes; they did not appear on actual trial presentations.

TABLE 1.3. Simple Discrimination Training with Compound Discriminative Stimuli and Compound Class-Specific Consequences

AB-compound discriminations	CD-compound discriminations
A1B1 (A1Wn, XnB1) → R1r1	C1D1 (C1Yn, ZnD1) → R1r1
A2B2 (A2Wn, XnB2) → R2r2	C2D2 (C2Yn, ZnD2) → R2r2
A3B3 (A3Wn, XnB3) → R3r3	C3D3 (C3Yn, ZnD3) → R3r3

Note. Each Wn, Xn, Yn, and Zn designation denotes a unique S– line drawing; n denotes a numerical identifier omitted here to prevent confusion with class designations.

X and Y stimuli were always S–). With this composition, both of the S+ elements were necessary to the three-term contingency. If contingencies produce equivalence relations involving all defining elements, this added twist to the procedure suggested that teaching only six simple discriminations might create six-member equivalence classes (e.g., A1B1C1D1R1r1; A2B2C2D2R2r2; A3B3C3D3R3r3).

A variety of probe-trial types was needed to evaluate all of the emergent relations made possible by this novel training arrangement. We tested for untrained conditional discriminations involving the compounds used in training (e.g., would A1B1 be matched to C1D1, rather than C2D2 or C3D3, or to R1r1 rather than R2r2 or R3r3?), untrained conditional discriminations involving compounds not used in training (e.g., would B1C1 be matched to A1D1, rather than A2D2 or A3D3?), untrained conditional discriminations involving individual elements used in training (e.g., would A1 be matched to B1, C1, D1, R1, or r1, and vice versa, depending on the comparison array?), and untrained simple discriminations involving compounds not used in training (would B2C2 be selected rather than B2C1 or B2C3, or C3R3 rather than C3R1 or C3R2?). Class-consistent responses on all possible probe types would represent more than 100 different emergent conditional relations involving individual stimulus elements, plus more than 100 different emergent conditional relations involving untrained compounds, plus more than 100 different emergent discriminative compounds, collectively representing quite a yield for so little direct training.

Two of the four children in this study (typically developing and ranging in age from 7 to 10 years) completed all training and testing phases. Both demonstrated emergent performances on the probe trials sampled from each of the categories just described, all with unfamiliar abstract line drawings. This laboratory analysis had thus addressed a question of interest for basic research, extending the delineation of procedures sufficient to create predictable and impressively generative patterns of stimulus control, while simultaneously holding direct relevance for important conceptual treatments and offering promise for ever-more efficient teaching arrangements by which to establish socially significant targets. Figure 1.12 reflects the additional interconnections that followed from this study, in the context of those already established.

Study 4

An opportunity to explore one of the linkages from Study 3 became possible given a very real need in our local community. Many migrant Spanish-speaking families had recently moved to the area, and their young children were often placed in standard public classrooms or Head Start programs. With few or no English language skills, this

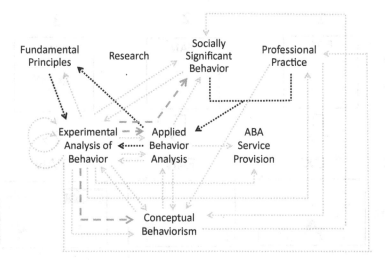

FIGURE 1.12. Cumulative translations, Study 3. Previous interchanges are indicated by dotted arrows; new interchanges are indicated by dashed arrows.

created a far from optimal introduction to a new educational system. We wondered if the laboratory procedures that had proved successful in generating so many relations among abstract line drawings could be adapted to facilitate some basic vocabulary acquisition, and another feasibility study was designed (La Cruz Montilla, 2018). The participants were seven preschoolers who spoke Spanish only and were nonreaders in any language. Drawing directly from the previous laboratory work, training targeted a series of six simple discriminations involving compound S+, S−, and consequence stimuli. In this case, however, the stimuli used to compose the compounds included spoken and printed English words and their pictorial representations.

Each S+ compound included a written English word presented above a corresponding picture (e.g., the printed word, FAN, and a drawing of a fan). Two unique S− compounds appeared with each S+, as usual. For one S−, the printed word from the S+ was presented together with the picture of a familiar but unrelated item from the training set (e.g., the printed word, FAN, and a drawing of a fox); for the other S−, a different printed word from the training set was presented together with the picture from the S+ (e.g., the printed word, FOX, and the drawing of the fan). Selection of the S+ thus required control by both the word and the picture elements. Three S+ compounds were taught in each phase, with the training sets composed so as to require control by both onset and rime of the written words (e.g., FOX, FAN, and PAN) across training trials. Selecting the S+ on any given trial produced a compound class-specific consequence. The experimenter would name the S+ orally, in English, while presenting a picture card with six different images (e.g., drawings, cartoons, photographs) of the S+ word (e.g., saying, "FAN," while showing a card with pictures of six different fans), displayed in two rows of three. Each training contingency thus involved a printed English word, a corresponding picture, a spoken English word, and six additional picture exemplars. Figure 1.13 illustrates a possible arrangement of three S+ compounds from one training set, along with the class-specific consequences produced when the S+ was selected.

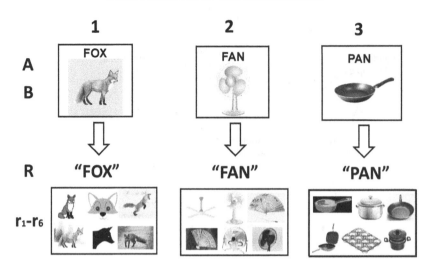

FIGURE 1.13. Illustration of S+ and consequence compounds for one training set.

By the view that reinforcement contingencies produce equivalence relations among all elements of the contingency, this simple discrimination training for each stimulus set provided a foundation for the potential emergence of three equivalence classes, each composed of at least nine members (i.e., A B R r_1 r_2 r_3 r_4 r_5 r_6, for each of the three classes). The possibility of even larger classes was suggested by the design of the picture cards arranged as consequences. Might inclusion of such feature classes facilitate generalization of the equivalence relation to novel images never presented during the simple discrimination training (see also, e.g., Fields et al., 1991)? Of note then, for present considerations, this applied investigation, designed to address practical needs (i.e., in vocabulary acquisition), simultaneously allowed for further exploration of experimental and conceptual analyses (i.e., of equivalence), while also raising new questions about implications for basic principles (e.g., stimulus generalization).

A large battery of probe trial types was required to sample the more than 500 possible emergent relations for each training set. These included simple discrimination probes with untrained compounds (e.g., Would a printed word presented together with an image from the corresponding consequence card be selected, rather than the same word presented with images from the other cards?); conditional discrimination probes with individual elements from the compounds (e.g., Would a printed word be matched to an image from the corresponding picture card? Would a spoken word lead to selection of the corresponding written word, or to the selection of an image from the corresponding picture card?); conditional discrimination probes with individual elements and novel pictures not included in training (providing for even more emergent relations); and also naming probes, where the child was asked "What is it?" for printed words as well as pictures, both novel and from training. Given the nature of the stimuli involved, it was also necessary to repeat assessments throughout the study, to ensure that any change in probe performance occurred when and only when the relevant training steps had been mastered, rather than as a result of classroom instruction, for example. All seven children exposed to these procedures demonstrated the emergent relations indicative of class formation involving the written English words, the pictures trained as components of discriminative compounds, the pictures presented as consequences, and the novel exemplars, all in a pattern specific to their training. The outcomes were replicated with the two participants who received training with additional word sets, and all five participants presented with the relevant probes demonstrated emergent naming as well.

These findings suggest ties forward to several distinct domains. To start, the work demonstrated the feasibility of a three-term-contingency equivalence-based approach to vocabulary instruction, indicating considerable potential for incorporation into regular school classrooms. A related point of emphasis here is that as steps are taken in approximating actual practice (e.g., in school systems, organizations or business, community programs), critical new issues in translation arise. Careful attention is demanded to design approaches that are well-matched to the needs of a particular practice setting (e.g., in this case, choosing target words from the preschool's curriculum), and that ensure cultural sensitivity and respect for all involved (e.g., the culture of the children and their families, as well as those of the classrooms and the schools in which the study was conducted; Conners & Capell, 2020), optimally as supported by social validity measures (e.g., endorsement by parents and teachers). Improvements based on social validity findings can also suggest procedural changes, which must then be evaluated in turn.

Along a more specific dimension of the present results, the striking number of emergent relations produced by the simple discrimination training speaks again to applied analysis and practice goals, where engineering flexible repertoires in young learners could stand in stark contrast to the "rote pairings" that behavior analysts are often caricatured as promoting. The breadth of the repertoire established also carries further implications for conceptual analyses of equivalence and how best to define it (e.g., the new relations demonstrated go far beyond reflexivity, symmetry, and transitivity; see, e.g., Pilgrim, 2016), as well as of generativity, perhaps more broadly, all of which may have bearing on how best to consider foundational principles related to emergent outcomes (e.g., Is equivalence a behavioral "primitive" [e.g., Sidman, 2000] or a higher-order unit born of simpler processes [e.g., Horne & Lowe, 1996; Hayes et al., 2001]?). And, as always, the questions calling for additional experimental analysis (e.g., about critical controlling variables; about limits on the number of compound elements that can be added) are many. Figure 1.14 adds these new arms to the cumulative history.

To Sum

The adventure continues, of course, but the point for present purposes has no doubt been characterized sufficiently. Even a quick comparison of Figure 1.14 with our starting point in Figure 1.2 reveals the heart of the matter. Translational science can be a many-splendored thing. Indeed, a key theme explored through this case history has focused on benefits that accrue when our work is informed, purposefully and systematically, by relevant issues across the domains of the field. And while useful as illustration, the intertwining of domains represented for the present series of experiments is hardly unique. In advocating for a translational approach, then, restricting the targets of our advice to any subset of the many domain connections available would appear to sell the enterprise short. If we are to realize the full power of translational science, the rich coherence of behavior analysis as a field provides a fitting framework.

A broad consideration of translation options would certainly reflect continuity with seminal foundations that helped to establish, define, and inspire our field. By way of

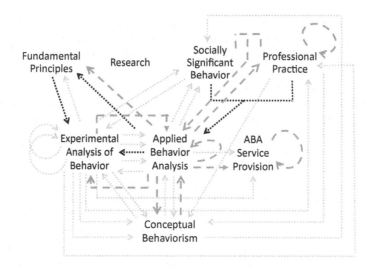

FIGURE 1.14. Cumulative translations, Study 4. Previous interchanges are indicated by dotted arrows; new interchanges are indicated by dashed arrows.

example, Skinner's *Science and Human Behavior* (1953) provided a treatise on fundamental principles elucidated by careful laboratory analyses, their role in accounting for significant patterns of human endeavor ranging from the personal to the cultural, and their implications for impacting meaningful behavior change across those levels. Similarly, in the inaugural issue of its namesake journal, Baer et al. (1968) defined *applied behavior analysis* partly in terms of "conceptual systems" that highlight "relevance to principle" (p. 96), so as to best function as a discipline rather than a "collection of tricks," and in terms of generality, along many dimensions, but especially regarding widespread practical change. These and many other examples underscore an essential role for integration across domains, both for the continued success of behavior analysis as a whole and for each of its constituent components. It is of some concern, then, that in an era of increasing specialization, there seems a tendency for behavior analysts to identify with and work within a single domain of the field. To do otherwise is challenging, to be sure. Voluminous literatures and sophisticated skill sets now characterize each area of conceptual, experimental, and applied analysis, and service provision. A perhaps even greater obstacle lies in the tendency for current graduate training to focus a program or an individual student's work within a single domain, with little emphasis on integration across areas, even if the curriculum provides a requisite course in each. These hardly seem optimal conditions for cross-domain connections, despite their role in past successes. Indeed, the current state of the field provides important context in occasioning calls for translational science. Where integration was once assumed and expected, it now requires differential attention.

To be clear, not every individual experiment need reflect nor proffer immediate cross-domain links. And when one does, any connection has the potential to yield advances. In fact, a few of the relation types considered earlier are represented in our literatures relatively often. It might even be suggested that some of the separate components highlighted in this discussion are implied dimensions of either experimental or applied research. We

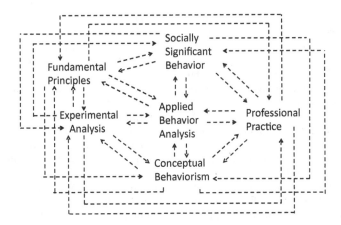

FIGURE 1.15. Translational opportunities in behavior analysis.

believe there is value, however, in making explicit the types of variables controlling our own behavior as scientists and as behavior analysts. In developing programs of study, drawing inspiration from multiple and varied angles can help produce novel juxtapositions that give rise to just the sorts of creative, productive analyses and interventions we seek, thereby improving both our science and our practice. Figure 1.15 summarizes the argument with a final representation of translational options in behavior analysis. Its guidance for us all suggests starting with one's own primary domain, then following an arrow—any arrow. Who knows what might emerge?

ACKNOWLEDGMENTS

We wish to thank our sisters from the University of North Carolina, Wilmington (UNCW) Equivalence Lab for their essential contributions to this work. Portions of this chapter were presented by the first author as part of addresses delivered to the Berkshire Association for Behavior Analysis and Therapy (2018), the North Carolina Association of Behavior Analysis (2018), the Maryland Association of Behavior Analysis (2018), and the California Association for Behavior Analysis (2017).

REFERENCES

Augustson, K. G., & Dougher, M. J. (1991). Teaching conditional discrimination to young children: Some methodological successes and failures. *Experimental Analysis of Human Behavior Bulletin, 9*(2), 21–24.

Austin, C. P. (2018). Translating translation. *Nature Reviews Drug Discovery, 17*(7), 455–456.

Austin, C. P. (2021). Translational misconceptions. *Nature Reviews Drug Discovery, 20*(7), 489–490.

Baer, D. M., Wolf, M. M., & Risley, T. R. (1968). Some current dimensions of applied behavior analysis. *Journal of Applied Behavior Analysis, 1*(1), 91–97.

Baum, W. M. (1994). *Understanding behaviorism: Science, behavior, and culture.* HarperCollins College Division.

Boye, J. (2008). *Can simple discrimination training produce emergent conditional discriminations and equivalence class formation in young children?* Unpublished master's thesis, University of North Carolina, Wilmington.

Catania, A. C. (1998). *Learning* (4th ed.). Prentice Hall.

Conners, B. M., & Capell, S. T. (Eds.). (2020). *Multiculturalism and diversity in applied behavior analysis: Bridging theory and application.* Routledge.

Critchfield, T. S. (2011). Translational contributions of the experimental analysis of behavior. *Behavior Analyst, 34*(1), 3–17.

Dube, W. V., McIlvane, W. J., Mackay, H. A., & Stoddard, L. T. (1987). Stimulus class membership established via stimulus–reinforcer relations. *Journal of the Experimental Analysis of Behavior, 47*(2), 159–175.

Dube, W. V., McIlvane, W. J., Maguire, R. W., Mackay, H. A., & Stoddard, L. T. (1989). Stimulus class formation and stimulus–reinforcer relations. *Journal of the Experimental Analysis of Behavior, 51*(1), 65–76.

Fields, L., Reeve, K. F., Adams, B. J., & Verhave, T. (1991). Stimulus generalization and equivalence classes: A model for natural categories. *Journal of the Experimental Analysis of Behavior, 55*(3), 305–312.

Fort, D. G., Herr, T. M., Shaw, P. L., Gutzman, K. E., & Starren, J. B. (2017). Mapping the evolving definitions of translational research. *Journal of Clinical and Translational Science, 1*(1), 60–66.

Hayes, S. C., Barnes-Holmes, D., & Roche, B. (Eds.). (2001). *Relational frame theory: A post-Skinnerian account of human language and cognition.* Plenum Press.

Horne, P. J., & Lowe, C. F. (1996). On the origins of naming and other symbolic behavior. *Journal of the Experimental Analysis of Behavior, 65*(1), 185–241.

Hurtado, R. (2020). *Compound class-specific consequences and equivalence-class formation: Does the composition of the compound matter?* Unpublished master's thesis, University of North Carolina, Wilmington.

Hurtado, R. (2021). *Further analysis of mixed-compound consequences and their role in equivalence-class formation* (Publication No. 28863949). Doctoral dissertation, University of North Carolina, Wilmington.

La Cruz Montilla, A. (2018). *Simple discrimination training with compound stimuli and class-specific consequences—An application of a stimulus equivalence approach to early reading skills.* Unpublished master's thesis, University of North Carolina, Wilmington.

Leuck, A. (2017). *Will stimulus classes established by simple discrimination training meet the formal definitions of stimulus equivalence.* Unpublished master's thesis, University of North Carolina, Wilmington.

Mace, F. C., & Critchfield, T. S. (2010). Translational research in behavior analysis: Historical traditions and imperative for the future. *Journal of the Experimental Analysis of Behavior, 93*(3), 293–312.

Markham, M. R., & Dougher, M. J. (1993). Compound stimuli in emergent stimulus relations: Extending the scope of stimulus equivalence. *Journal of the Experimental Analysis of Behavior, 60*(3), 529–542.

Moore, J. (2008). *Conceptual foundations of radical behaviorism.* Sloan.

Moore, J., & Cooper, J. O. (2003). Some proposed relations among the domains of behavior analysis. *Behavior Analyst, 26*(1), 69–84.

Pilgrim, C. (2016). Considering definitions of stimulus equivalence. *European Journal of Behavior Analysis, 17*(1), 105–114.

Pilgrim, C. (2020). Equivalence-based instruction. In J. O. Cooper, T. E. Heron, & W. L. Heward (Eds.), *Applied behavior analysis* (3rd ed., pp. 452–496). Pearson.

Pilgrim, C., Jackson, J., & Galizio, M. (2000). Acquisition of arbitrary conditional discriminations by young normally developing children. *Journal of the Experimental Analysis of Behavior, 73*(2), 177–193.

Sheehan, C. (2018). *An evaluation of training and testing procedures designed to facilitate the emergence of early probe performances following simple discrimination training in young children.* Unpublished master's thesis, University of North Carolina, Wilmington.

Shepherd, A. (2019). *An analysis of the impact of identity training with consequence images on the emergence of equivalence classes based on class-specific consequences.* Unpublished master's thesis, University of North Carolina, Wilmington.

Sidman, M. (1971). Reading and auditory-visual equivalences. *Journal of Speech and Hearing Research, 14*(1), 5–13.

Sidman, M. (1994). *Equivalence relations and behavior: A research story.* Authors Cooperative.

Sidman, M. (2000). Equivalence relations and the reinforcement contingency. *Journal of the Experimental Analysis of Behavior, 74*(1), 127–146.

Sidman, M. (2007). The analysis of behavior: What's in it for us? *Journal of the Experimental Analysis of Behavior, 87*(2), 309–316.

Sidman, M., & Cresson, O. (1973). Reading and crossmodal transfer of stimulus equivalences in severe retardation. *American Journal of Mental Deficiency, 77*(5), 515–523.

Sidman, M., Cresson, O., Jr., & Willson-Morris, M. (1974). Acquisition of matching to sample via mediated transfer. *Journal of the Experimental Analysis of Behavior, 22*(2), 261–273.

Sidman, M., Rauzin, R., Lazar, R., Cunningham, S., Tailby, W., & Carrigan, P. (1982). A search for symmetry in the conditional discriminations of rhesus monkeys, baboons, and children. *Journal of the Experimental Analysis of Behavior, 37*(1), 23–44.

Sidman, M., & Tailby, W. (1982). Conditional discrimination vs. matching to sample: An expansion of the testing paradigm. *Journal of the Experimental Analysis of Behavior, 37*(1), 5–22.

Skinner, B. F. (1953). *Science and human behavior.* Simon & Schuster.

Stokes, D. E. (2011). *Pasteur's quadrant: Basic science and technological innovation.* Brookings Institution Press.

Stromer, R., & Mackay, H. A. (1992). Spelling and emergent picture-printed word relations established with delayed identity matching to complex samples. *Journal of Applied Behavior Analysis, 25*(4), 893–904.

Stromer, R., & Mackay, H. A. (1993). Delayed identity matching to complex samples: Teaching students with mental retardation spelling and the prerequisites for equivalence class-es. *Research in Developmental Disabilities, 14*(1), 19–38.

Varella, A. A., & de Souza, D. G. (2014). Emergence of auditory–visual relations from a visual–visual baseline with auditory-specific consequences in individuals with autism. *Journal of the Experimental Analysis of Behavior, 102*(1), 139–149.

Williams, B. (2016). *Simple discrimination training and class expansion with compound stimuli and compound class-specific reinforcer.* Unpublished master's thesis, University of North Carolina, Wilmington.

Woolf, S. H. (2008). The meaning of translational research and why it matters. *Journal of the American Medical Association, 299*(2), 211–213.

Yonkers, K. M. (2012). *Simple discrimination training in studying stimulus equivalence and math skills acquisition in developmentally-delayed children.* Unpublished master's thesis, University of North Carolina, Wilmington.

Zerhouni, E. A. (2005). Translational and clinical science—time for a new vision. *New England Journal of Medicine, 353*(15), 1621–1623.

Zygmont, D. M., Lazar, R. M., Dube, W. V., & McIlvane, W. J. (1992). Teaching arbitrary matching via sample stimulus-control shaping to young children and mentally retarded individuals: A methodological note. *Journal of the Experimental Analysis of Behavior, 57*(1), 109–117.

CHAPTER 2

Quantitative Approaches to Translational Research in Behavior Analysis

Adam E. Fox

In some ways, the quantitative analysis of behavior (QAB) has always been about translation and application.[1] Take, for example, the matching law and its iterations (Baum, 1974; Herrnstein, 1961, 1974; Jensen & Neuringer, 2009; Killeen, 1972). The matching law is a quantitative description of how and why an organism engages in one behavior at the expense of other options in the environment. Any student of behavior, no matter their specific research or clinical interest, is interested in the answer to this question. All operant behavior is choice, whether the alternatives are measured or not, and the determinants of choice are imperative to prediction and control. In its most basic form, the matching law is simply a ratio equation in which relative rates of behavior "match" relative rates of reinforcement in the environment. However, theoretically, conceptually, and practically, it has profound implications that can reach beyond the experimental analysis of behavior into applied behavior analysis, clinical practice, and neuroscience. For example, consider harmful substance use. In the laboratory, basic application of the matching law helps us understand how drug reinforcers may compete with non-drug reinforcers and how behavior is allocated across parametric manipulations of each type of reinforcer; in applied and clinical settings, how alternative reinforcement may help reduce drug seeking and administering; and finally, how pharmacological and neurobiological manipulations might increase choice for non-drug reinforcers when drug reinforcers are concurrently available (Anderson et al., 2002; Holtyn et al., 2014; Hutsell et al., 2015; Jarvis et al., 2019; Jimenez-Gomez & Shahan, 2008; Koffarnus & Woods, 2008; Quick et al., 2011; Silverman et al., 2016).

There is translational value in understanding choice behavior across such a diverse range of settings using one simple mathematical principle of behavior. This is just the tip

---

[1] Indeed, there is evidence from the early history of the Society for the Quantitative Analyses of Behavior (SQAB) that mathematical modeling of behavior always had implications for applied and translational application (Commons, 2001)—such a focus has been even more apparent in recent years, even as many of us in the field may readily admit to model fitting being "a genuine thrill" (Nevin, 2008, p. 123) in and of itself.

of the iceberg—similar examples will be discussed in this chapter, ranging from impulsive choice to time perception, to extinction learning and relapse phenomena. An introduction to using mathematical terms to approach translational questions in behavior science is the focus. Formal equations have been left out to aid in accessibility and readability, but such treatments using equations are available (Critchfield & Reed, 2009; Jacobs et al., 2013; Marr, 1989; Mazur, 2006). First, though, let's turn our attention to what is likely at the top of "mind" for anyone without much formal training in QAB: Why quantitative models? Why math (ugh . . . I *hate* math)? Why now?

Why Quantitative Models for Translation?

If I were to guess, most applied behavior scientists and clinicians who read this book will not be "dog earing" this chapter for a careful read and regular revisit. In fact, while there has been a growing interest and trend toward more quantitative modeling within the experimental analysis of behavior (EAB) (Mazur, 2006; Nevin, 2008), there has been substantial skepticism within the applied wing of the science and practice of behavior analysis (Critchfield & Reed, 2009; Cullen, 1981) and even within EAB itself (Catania, 2012; Moore, 2008). While traditional principles of behavior (e.g., reinforcement, punishment, extinction) derived from the basic laboratory have been readily and effectively applied in translational and clinical work, mathematical models, which have increasingly come to define EAB (Critchfield & Reed, 2009; Mazur, 2006), have been met with greater resistance in contemporary behavior analysis.

So, let's define the value of thinking about mathematical models for applied and translational purposes. First, quantitative models describe and predict behavior better and more precisely than visual analyses and verbal descriptions. As Mazur (2006) put it, mathematical models are "better than mere words" (p. 278), because when we use mathematics to describe behavior, we can quantify and observe differences between interventions, theories, and predictions of behavior. In other words, we can quantify functional relations between independent variables and behavior, making description and prediction of behavioral processes clearer, more objective, and more effective, which, one might argue, is the primary concern of any behavior analyst.

A very straightforward example of this is how delayed reinforcement impacts behavior. If we use words to describe how delay impacts the value or efficacy of a reinforcer, we might say simply that "delays degrade a reinforcer's effectiveness," or "delays reduce a reinforcer's value." However, we have not said how, even if we can relate verbally that relatively short delays reduce a reinforcer's efficacy more than relatively longer delays, and we can cite the relevant basic research to support such a claim (e.g., Reilly & Lattal, 2004). We have left the precise relationship between the delay and behavior ambiguous, not only within subject but also in comparisons between subjects and across populations. If we fit a hyperbolic model to behavior as a function of the delay, as Reilly and Lattal did, we can compare the steepness parameter of the function (typically k) both within subject (comparing fixed-interval [FI] and variable-interval [VI]) and between subjects (between pigeons). Reilly and Lattal found that response rates decreased hyperbolically for pigeons exposed to increasing delays to reinforcement in both VI and FI schedules, and that response rates were well characterized by the model across pigeons. Now we can say in precise quantifiable terms how delay impacted behavior (hyperbolically with a steepness of k) and relative to other conditions and subjects (differences in k). Furthermore, the impact of delay on behavior has been shown to have serious clinical implications, allowing for further extrapolation and translation from the model to human behavior—something that we will return to later in the chapter—and it has inspired translational work employing delays to increase sustainable behavior (Fox, Buchanan, et al., 2019).

If you are convinced that models can be of use in communicating functional relations within behavior analysis, it should also be clear that the same is true for communicating outside of behavior analysis. The jargon within our field, and the difficulties it presents in communicating with other scientific and lay audiences, has been well documented (Critchfield, 2017; Critchfield et al., 2017; Lindsley, 1991; but cf. Kazdin & Cole, 1981). Furthermore, visual analyses and verbal descriptions of data and functional relations are viewed with a great deal of skepticism outside of behavior analysis and are not readily accepted. Thus, to increase the impact of behavior-analytic work, acquire grants, publish widely, and, in short, communicate outside the field, we must, at least sometimes, use a more widely accepted approach (Fox, 2018; Huitema, 1986; Madden, 2013). Mathematics may make for a very nice approach, indeed. Mathematics is used across the natural sciences (Marr, 1989) and has the added benefit of being more precise and descriptive within and across spoken languages as well. Where verbal descriptions are often imprecise and unwieldy, mathematics is precise, parsimonious, and can often "say" things that words cannot (Critchfield & Reed, 2009; Mazur, 2006). In the earlier example on how delay impacts reinforcer value, k is more informative and is more widely interpretable than any verbal explanation of the functional relation. As Killeen (1999, p. 276) put it, "Models are go-betweens: They go between the data and our sense of understanding."

What Is a Quantitative Model? How Do I Choose the Right One?

If there is value in a quantitative analysis, a "modeling of behavior," if you will, then what does the appropriate model look like? How will you know when you've found the right one? How must it be applied? Doesn't this get confusing?

Let me put this as clearly as possible: Stop worrying about it so much. There is no "right" or "correct" model. Take, for example, the study of timing behavior, a field notorious for its many models (e.g., the pacemaker–accumulator model; Gibbon, 1991, 1992) and their varying quantifiable predictions. None of them is right. What matters is utility. Again, from Killeen (1999): "If you think models are about the truth . . . then you are in trouble. There is no best model, any more than there is a best car model . . . even though each of us may have our favorites. It all depends on what you do with the model" (p. 275). Models are a tool for quantifying functional relations and communicating about them. "Models of phenomena are not causes of phenomena" (p. 276). In translational and applied science, models can help quantify functional relations, clarify behavioral principles, parse the effectiveness of certain interventions within and across subjects, and help predict and control behavior in sharper ways than verbalizations can (Mazur, 2006). It is not the model, it is what you do with it.

And you can do quite a lot with models. As the earlier example on delayed reinforcement illustrates, a researcher or clinician can quantify functional relations for comparison and translational purposes, which may elucidate controlling variables in meaningful, sometimes nonintuitive ways. This is accomplished by using the "free parameters" of the model, the parts of the model that change to fit a particular dataset. Free parameters can be thought of as dependent measures that are derived from the raw dependent measures obtained across a range of independent variable measures. The simplest and most familiar example of this is a line. If you fit a line to a series of data points, there are two free parameters that can change to assist with that fit: the slope and the intercept. Most everyone has experience with this type of a model from as early as grade school, and it is a good example, because most models have such free parameters. Some of the most famous models in all of behavior analysis are even simpler than a line (in terms of free parameters). For example, as mentioned earlier, the most basic form of the hyperbolic model applied to delay discounting behavior has just one free parameter, k. As in fitting the slope and intercept to a straight line, the k parameter changes to fit the hyperbolic "steepness" or "slope" of delay discounting data. Larger values of k indicate a steeper discounting function (i.e., behavior is more "impulsive"). Figure 2.1 shows four examples of how different k values result in functions of different relative "steepness" for

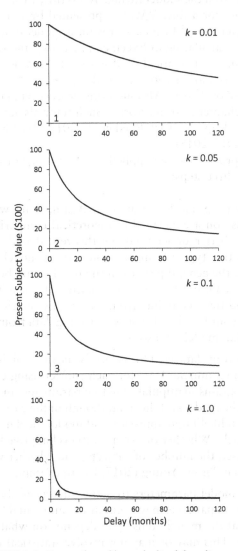

FIGURE 2.1. Examples of hyperbolic delay discounting.

four hypothetical subjects. The examples are arranged from least impulsive (1) to most impulsive (4). As k becomes larger, the function becomes steeper. At a 120-month delay, the reinforcer has retained nearly half of its value for the first individual, but that halving of value is reduced to approximately 18, 10, and 1 month for individuals two, three, and four, respectively. Thus, in this case, it is easy to not just visualize the differences in how delay affected reward value for these subjects but to quantify that difference, just as by comparing the slope parameter for different lines, we can quantify differences in steepness across a range of scenarios using k.

All of this notwithstanding, getting from a dataset to a model to fitting the model and ultimately using the output can be challenging, especially for newcomers. So, let's briefly review the model fitting process. Basic model fitting uses a regression-based approach: minimizing the distance on a graph between the raw data points and the predicted data points (the fit) obtained from the model fitting. To do this, variance accounted for (VAC) must be maximized (e.g., for a line, VAC is represented by R^2). Greater values of VAC indicate a relatively better model fit (i.e., you want a model that has high VAC). Doing this by hand, or even by calculating in Excel, can be tricky and tedious. Luckily, we live in an age where applying mathematical models to data is easier than ever. Most of the work has been done for us and the tools we need (e.g., Excel Solver, SPSS, R) are readily available, and in the case of R, free. Although this process will get attention presently, it is not the focus of this chapter to be a tutorial. Such tutorials across a range of scenarios are available (DeHart & Kaplan, 2019; Reed et al., 2012; Reed & Dixon, 2009; Reed & Kaplan, 2011; Young, 2017, 2018).

The model fitting process can be applied across a range of translational scenarios, but in general there are three steps:

1. Find a model appropriate for your data. Again, don't worry about getting the "correct" model. Unless you are engaged in theoretical comparisons between different models or you want to better understand the theoretical underpinnings of a model's behavioral predictions, this typically means you want a model that approximates the "shape" of your data or the general pattern in the relationship between the independent and dependent variables. Often, this is just a matter of consulting the literature. For example, if you have indifference points from a delay discounting task, then the hyperbolic model is probably your best bet. If you have timing data from a peak procedure, you probably want a Gaussian model, and so on.

2. Fit the model to your dataset. This typically means "solving" for the free parameters in your model by maximizing VAC for each subject using computational software (e.g., R). To do this, programs manipulate the free parameters in the model to minimize the difference between the model and the data, though in the case of multilevel modeling, you may use a maximum likelihood approach and model the data at the group and individual level simultaneously. Whether or not a multilevel approach is warranted depends on the size of your dataset, the number of subjects, and whether you have repeated measures (or "hierarchical data"); see Young (2017) for an example.

3. Use the derived model parameters to make inferences about the functional relations that interest you. Comparisons may occur at the individual level, the group level, or some combination. What the model "tells" you depends on what your independent and dependent variables are. This may or may not involve statistical tests, again, depending on your methodological approach.

For example, *k* from a hyperbolic modeling of delay discounting data can inform you about the functional relationship between delay and reward value within and across individuals for different commodities. You may find that most individuals value food less than money as the delay to the receipt of those reinforcers is increased, but that the extent to which the delay devalues those reinforcers varies wildly across individuals. These findings have theoretical and clinical implications for understanding the behavioral process, predicting future behavior, and changing future behavior to some clinical end (e.g., Bickel et al., 1999; Odum, 2011a, 2011b; Perry et al., 2005; Rung et al., 2019)—for example, identifying which of the individuals may be more at risk for harmful substance use. Similarly, we have used a simple two-parameter Guassian function to describe and quantify pigeon behavior in a peak procedure timing task (Fox & Kyonka, 2013, 2015, 2016). A Guassian model is essentially a "bell curve" function with "peak" (highest point) and "width" (or standard deviation) free parameters. When fit to timing data from the peak procedure, the peak parameter is a measure of timing accuracy, in this case, when the pigeon expected food to be delivered, and the width parameter is a measure of timing precision, in this case, variability in when the pigeon expected food to be delivered. Using these parameters, we compared timing behavior within and between subjects across a range of conditions designed to assess variables implicated in timing behavior. It is also possible to translate such modeling to human operant work (Subramaniam & Kyonka, 2022) and to clinical populations (Buhusi & Meck, 2005).

The Broader Landscape

Finally, a note about the broader implications of adopting a quantitative modeling approach to research and practice. Behavior analysis is not happening in a bubble, though it may sometimes seem so at our annual conferences and in the pages of our journals. We must pay attention to the broader landscape in which our science is participating—not only in psychology and neuroscience more generally, but also in the social, political, and cultural systems in which we live. For example, statistical analyses are a form of mathematical modeling that have been a part of behavior science for decades (typically some form of linear regression, e.g., analysis of variance [ANOVA]). Although traditional approaches are not without their limitations (Branch, 1999, 2014), newer approaches that combine traditional QAB model fitting with multilevel ("hierarchical" or "mixed") modeling are powerful and bring back into focus variability at the individual subject level (Boisgontier & Cheval, 2016; Bolker et al., 2009; Fox, 2018; Kirkpatrick et al., 2018; Young, 2017, 2018), a thought that should warm the heart of any of us trained in behavior analysis. In addition, statistical modeling can be useful even at the single-subject level (e.g., reversal designs) to help compare the effectiveness of an intervention within and across subjects (Huitema & McKean, 2000). Taking such approaches is not akin to defecting to the dark side, it is simply employing a tool that exists to diversify your approach and communicate your results. Thus, understanding and applying mathematical models of behavior is important for not only a small group of QAB researchers but also any student of behavior wishing to interpret findings, communicate findings, publish research, and compete for grant funding across behavior science. Moreover, it may be fundamental if we wish to shape the political and cultural contexts in which we live.

Applying Quantitative Models: Getting Started

A Simple Example

In translating a mathematical model to new settings and scenarios, it is helpful to start with a straightforward example of how models are fit to data and what the result might provide. The earlier hyperbolic discounting model (k) was a preview of this. Here we consider learning rate—a basic behavioral process that may be of interest to the basic, translational, and applied researcher/clinician alike. For example, one might be interested in the rate at which a functional communication response (FCR) is acquired across different settings, different individuals, or under different intervention preparations. For simplicity, let's assume that during baseline there were no FCRs across three individuals. After the intervention is applied, rates of FCRs increase for all three individuals A, B, and C, shown in Figure 2.2. The data points represent the number of responses per session, and the overlaid lines represent the best-fitting sigmoid function. A *sigmoid* is an "S" shaped function that is often used to quantify learning rate or response rate when the function ramps upward in an "S"-like pattern (e.g., Fox & Kyonka, 2013; Peartree et al., 2012). A straightforward sigmoid model has three free parameters: the midpoint parameter (the time/session at which responding reached half of its maximum), the slope parameter (the steepness or speed of response acquisition in this case), and the asymptote parameter (the maximum response rate). VAC can also be taken into consideration as a measure of the extent to which the sigmoid is a good model for the data in question.

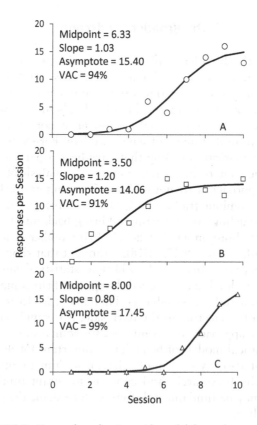

FIGURE 2.2. Examples of a sigmoid model fit to three subjects.

In Figure 2.2, the sigmoid clearly fits the data well for all three individuals, with greater than 90% VAC observed across them, and no systematic deviations from the model are detected upon visual inspection. Visual analysis might suggest that all three individuals acquired the response, with individual C perhaps a bit later. The quantitative modeling output offers some additional insight. For example, the midpoint parameter suggests that acquisition occurred in at least half as many sessions for individual B compared to individuals A and C; the slope parameter suggests that once the response was increasing in frequency, it did so at roughly the same rate (but most steeply for individual C); finally the asymptote parameter suggests that 15 responses per session was roughly the maximum across individuals, but that for individual C, the maximum may not yet have been observed in the obtained data. The analysis, although generic here, may also allow for very straightforward comparisons within and across different research scenarios—for example, comparing acquisition in the nonhuman basic research lab, applied research lab, and clinical setting. You can replace "A," "B," and "C" in Figure 2.2 with pretty much any scenario you can devise. By using the model, you have "normalized" the analysis across such scenarios by using the same model parameters as outcome variables. The analysis also makes communicating about the results and running formal statistical analyses more straightforward. For example, if you have enough subjects, you can run a statistical analysis comparing the midpoint parameter between two different contexts. Do subjects acquire the response at significantly different rates across contexts? In behavior analysis, though, we are often interested in single-subject designs with few subjects. Thus, a different modeling approach may be warranted.

A Single-Subject Scenario

Quantitative analyses are not limited to large datasets or to work involving many subjects. Model fitting may be useful for comparing the impact of an independent variable manipulation within subject (e.g., in a reversal design) using a linear regression modeling strategy. The approach outlined here may also be used in basic laboratory work, again making within- and cross-setting translational comparisons more quantitative in nature. A regression-based approach also makes the analysis more consistent with common practices outside of behavior analysis (e.g., ANOVA) and contrasts it with common traditional approaches to quantifying single-subject data within behavior analysis that come with significant drawbacks and are as obscure to those outside of behavior analysis as visual analyses are (e.g., percent nonoverlapping data [PND] analyses; Salzberg et al., 1987; Schlosser et al., 2008; Scruggs et al., 1987; Scruggs & Mastropieri, 2013; Wolery et al., 2010).

Figure 2.3 shows the model fit to a simple ABAB reversal design. The data points represent the dependent variable of interest, and the dashed lines represent the best-fitting model. Visual analysis suggests a clear effect during the first A to B transition in terms of level. The impact is less clear upon the return to the A condition, though there is a reduction in level that eventually appears to resemble the first A condition. Finally, there is a clear upward trend in the final A to B transition. Thus, the visual analysis would likely indicate that the dependent measure was somewhat higher in the B compared to A condition, but that the change in the dependent variable was not always immediate. The model offers a corresponding outcome that may help bolster the visual analysis and make communicating the results more effective: a significant level change during the first A to B transition ($p = .001$); a modest level ($p = .07$) and slope ($p = .09$) change during the B to A transition, with the level change as an increase, supporting the lack of immediacy

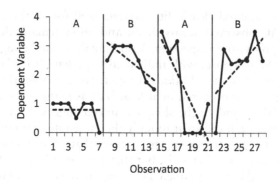

FIGURE 2.3. Example of single-subject linear regression modeling.

in the transition; and a significant level ($p = .02$) and slope ($p < .001$) change during the final transition, again highlighting the manipulation's effect on increasing the dependent measure.

Developed by Huitema and McKean (2000), the model is linear, with "dummy" variables to allow the model to "break" at each phase/condition change point, essentially fitting a linear model for each phase of the design. It includes regression coefficients, and corresponding p values, if one is so inclined, for the level and slope change at each transition. Thus, the model quantifies behavior change at each transition. It can be used in conjunction with visual analysis to quantify and statistically analyze these changes, using a statistical modeling approach to bolster a visual and/or PND analysis and make results more familiar to an outside audience (e.g., Fox, Buchanan, et al., 2019).

The modeling is not perfect, and it does not always correspond to a sophisticated visual analysis. There may be important considerations that the model simply cannot account for (e.g., the clinical relevance and value of a behavior change whether it is statistically significant or not). In addition, a behavior analyst might respond that they see everything the modeling has offered, plus much more. That may well be true, but training sophisticated visual analysis skills has proven difficult (e.g., Fisher et al., 2003; Kazdin, 2019; O'Grady et al., 2018; Wolfe et al., 2016; Wolfe & Slocum, 2015), with considerable within- and between-subject variability. Also, remember that modeling is a tool. It is not meant to replace critical thinking or to necessarily supplant other forms of analysis. Using this kind of modeling in a translational context improves the likelihood that the work will make connections with basic work, applied work, and a much broader scientific audience, particularly outside of behavior analysis, where visual analyses are not taken very seriously.

Direct Translational Applications of Quantitative Models

Preclinical Approaches

Now we move to increase the complexity of our model fitting approach. Using mathematical models to describe behavior for translational or comparative purposes (e.g., Daniels et al., 2015) or to study preclinical animal models of psychoneurological disorders is common (e.g., Balci et al., 2008; Deane et al., 2017; DeCoteau & Fox, 2022; Fox et al., 2017; Hand et al., 2006; Karson & Balcı, 2021). Such a practice has the advantage of describing behavioral phenotypes quantitatively in a manner that can be translated to work with human clinical populations. In other words, the same models can be used to characterize behavior in the basic lab with rats and mice, the human operant lab, the clinic, and the home. Thus, models provide a framework for identifying important similarities and differences in behavioral phenotypes across organisms and settings, and for understanding how behavioral abnormalities observed in the lab translate to clinical settings and populations. They also aid with predicting how interventions will translate from the lab to the clinic, and, generally, integrating work across the basic–translational–applied spectrum (Mazur, 2006). In this section, several examples of how this may be accomplished are reviewed with varying depth.

Animal Models of Psychoneurological Disorders

Environmentally induced models of psychoneurological disorders are one way that etiology and phenotype may be studied experimentally for translational purposes. Models with high face and construct validity have particular value for understanding a disorder and testing possible intervention strategies for treating it. One timely and relevant example of such a model is the valproic acid (VPA) rat model of autism spectrum disorder (ASD). ASD is prevalent (~1.7% of children in developed countries; Christensen et al., 2019) and expensive to treat ($268 billion estimated annually in societal costs; Leigh & Du, 2015; Rogge & Janssen, 2019). It has no known single etiology, and there is a great deal of heterogeneity in symptoms.

The VPA rat model is induced by exposing rat pups to VPA *in utero*. The model has high face and construct validity, because *in utero* VPA exposure in humans is a risk factor for ASD and rat pups exposed to VPA *in utero* have analogous behavioral abnormalities to those observed in humans diagnosed with ASD (e.g., increased repetitive behaviors, reduced social interaction; Bambini-Junior et al., 2014; Banji et al., 2011; Chomiak et al., 2013; Favre et al., 2013; Fontes-Dutra et al., 2019; Markram et al., 2008; Schneider et al., 2006; Schneider & Przewłocki, 2005). The VPA model has translational promise, because researchers can study the etiology and phenotype of the model experimentally, and the results can be compared with and translated to the human ASD clinical population. Note that the preclinical animal research does not have to occur before the clinical work. The research can be multidirectional, with applied work informing basic and translational approaches, and vice versa. Furthermore, it can be easily extended to other preclinical models of ASD, such as genetically modified models (e.g., "knockout" gene models). Thus, mathematical modeling of behavior allows for a quantitative framework from which to better understand and contextualize this work in a multidirectional fashion.

For example, timing behavior is often measured using a temporal bisection task in which organisms learn a relatively short and a relatively long anchor duration, and responding in relation to them is measured. In these tasks, a basic sigmoid function may be used to describe behavior in rat models of ASD (e.g., DeCoteau & Fox, 2022; Poulin & Fox, 2021) and in humans diagnosed with ASD (e.g., Allman et al., 2011), revealing striking similarities not only with the basic structure of behavior but with possible abnormalities in timing behavior often observed in the clinical population. Figure 2.4 shows temporal bisection data from the *CNTNAP2* gene knockout rat model of ASD (A) (Poulin & Fox, 2021) and from the VPA rat model of ASD (B) (DeCoteau & Fox, 2022). These general patterns of behavior are strikingly similar to those observed in a temporal bisection task with children diagnosed with ASD (Allman et al., 2011). Despite the differences in species, the type of ASD animal model, and the fact that the tasks were

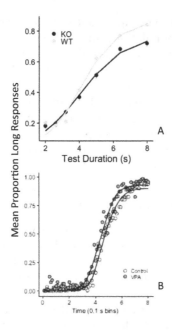

FIGURE 2.4. Examples of sigmoid model fit to autism spectrum disorder timing data from (A) Poulin and Fox (2021) and (B) DeCoteau and Fox (2021). Panel A reprinted with permission from Elsevier. Panel B reprinted with permission from Springer Nature. KO, "knockout" ASD model; WT, "wild type" control (A); VPA, valproic acid (B).

different (Panel A and the Allman et al. [2011] data are from a discrete trial temporal bisection task [Church & Deluty, 1977]; Panel B is from a free operant temporal bisection task [Platt & Davis, 1983]), the results are remarkable for at least two reasons. First, the sigmoid is clearly an excellent fit to the data—eloquently quantifying the functional relation between time and behavior in all three examples. Second, the modeling indicates important similarities: a shift of the function leftward for the ASD groups, and a flattening of the function at the relatively longer durations relative to control subjects. This suggests that in both humans diagnosed with ASD and these rat models of ASD, timing may be faster (leftward shift) and less precise at relatively longer durations (flatter and lower asymptotes) in ASD.

The implication of this work is that time perception may be fundamentally altered in ASD. Research with both animal models and human clinical populations suggest this is the case. It is easy to imagine what the next steps in such work might be: interventions aimed at improving timing of behavior and discrimination of duration. Mathematical models of behavior like the one employed in these examples provide a framework for translating the work from lab to clinic and back again.

Behavioral and Human Operant Models

Translational preclinical work using mathematical modeling is not limited to rodent models of psychoneurological disorders. Models may also be applied to study and translate behavioral phenomena with particular clinical or theoretical importance. Such an approach might be straightforward, such as Baum's early extension of the matching law to a human operant setting (Baum, 1975), or more complex, such as comparative work across scholarly fields or species.

Figure 2.5 shows how Daniels and colleagues (2015) used the same quantitative modeling approach to compare rat, pigeon, and human performance on an FI temporal bisection task (Platt & Davis, 1983). Procedurally, for a random half of all trials in the task, the reinforcer is arranged on the short FI, and for the other half on the long FI. Once a reinforcer is earned, there is typically an intertrial interval before the next trial begins. In the task, subjects "switch" from a relatively short FI option to a relatively long FI option during trials in which the reinforcer is arranged on the latter. These are the trials of interest from a timing perspective, because time is the dominant controlling variable determining the switch. Thus the "switch point" is the primary timing dependent measure, and as a trial progresses the subject is more likely to switch from responding on the short FI to responding on the long FI. In their study, after baseline performance was established, the reinforcer magnitude was increased on the longer of the two FIs in the task. Doing this resulted in a consistent change in the behavior of rats and pigeons,

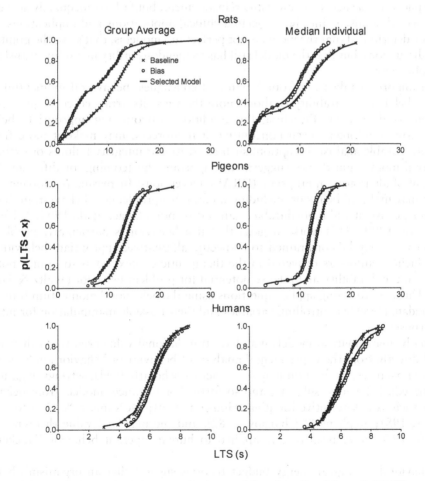

FIGURE 2.5. Comparative quantitative modeling from Daniels et al. (2015).

but the opposite effect in humans (in Figure 2.5, the "bias" data are shifted left for the rats and pigeons, but right for the humans). In this case, the reinforcer magnitude manipulation resulted in earlier switching for the rats and pigeons but later switching for the humans, highlighting a possibly important species difference that may inform future translational work investigating timing behavior.

Similar analyses can be conducted using a quantitative model as the starting point. Behavioral momentum theory is a quantitative model of behavioral persistence that was established and extended in the basic laboratory (Nevin, 1974; Nevin et al., 1983; Nevin & Shahan, 2011). The model suggests that behavioral persistence is a function of the overall reinforcer density experienced in a context (i.e., all reinforcement; Pavlovian association between reinforcement density and context). It has a range of possible implications for clinically relevant behavior, including how to treat persistent problem behavior (e.g., Mace et al., 2010; Mace & Nevin, 2017). Nevin and colleagues (2017) used behavioral momentum theory to investigate its application across a range of clinically relevant relapse phenomena in a powerful demonstration of how one mathematical model can be used to synthesize and analyze a large body of existing work and make predictions about the model's value for future work. They suggest that the theory accounts well for relapse phenomena such as renewal and reinstatement, but fails to adequately account for resurgence while discussing the associated clinical applications and implications. In the end, they determined that the model is not perfect (no model is, that's not the point!—see earlier discussion), but that the model still has tremendous utility in guiding translational and applied work.

An important takeaway from Nevin and colleagues' behavioral momentum work is that a behavior's durability is about more than just its arranged consequences, it is also context dependent. Enriching the conditions surrounding appropriate behavior by increasing reinforcers, even noncontingent reinforcers, may make it more frequent and more durable against disruption, such as treatment integrity failures or extinction. Behavioral momentum theory suggests an important shortcoming for differential reinforcement of alternative/appropriate (DRA) interventions: Increasing reinforcement in a context may make all behavior, including undesirable/problematic behavior, in that context more persistent and more durable against disruption (Mace et al., 1990, 2010; Mace & Belfiore, 1990). This work suggests that if a behavior is particularly problematic, reinforcement may be constrained to a specific alternative, appropriate behavior only, thus reducing reinforcers delivered in the therapeutic context so as to limit a potential increase in the durability and relapse potential for problem behavior (Waltz & Follette, 2009). Thus, approaching applied questions using the behavioral momentum framework can elucidate possible controlling variables and their possible manipulation for intervention purposes.

Finally, mathematical models may have translational value even when they are not derived directly from the experimental analysis of behavior or behavior analysis. Under such circumstances, translation may occur across scholarly fields, settings (e.g., natural or contrived), behaviors, subjects, and so forth. For instance, models from behavioral ecology such as risk-sensitive foraging (Houston, 1991; McNamara & Houston, 1992; Stephens, 1981; Stephens & Charnov, 1982), and the marginal value theorem (MVT; Charnov, 1976) have been readily applied to human operant behavior (Hackenberg, 1998).

Behavioral ecological energy budget theories suggest that an organism's behavior can be constrained under negative and positive budgets, which result in straightforward behavioral predictions. Under a negative budget, the organism's energy reserves plus its mean rate of daily energy gain will not be enough to survive the night. The model predicts the animal should choose riskier options that may have a higher payoff but could pay off with much less. The animal needs to "hit" the higher payoff to survive, and the only way to do it is to make riskier decisions. For example, by pursuing a larger prey that may be more difficult to catch, the animal increases chances for survival in an all-or-none gambit. Under a positive budget, the organism's energy reserves plus its mean rate of daily energy gain is enough to survive the night, and the model predicts the animal should be risk-averse, opting for options that have a more modest, certain outcome. The animal needs some, but not a lot, to survive. Thus, it should choose some smaller amount it can obtain with greater certainty, for example, choosing to forage for berries.

These models have been extended to the nonhuman operant lab (Hastjarjo et al., 1990) and to the human operant lab, where, instead of food outcomes, subjects make choices about monetary outcomes (i.e., "earnings budgets"; Pietras & Hackenberg, 2001). With remarkable consistency, earnings budget models adequately predict human risky-choice behavior in the operant laboratory across a range of independent variable manipulations such as budget reserves, rate of gain, outcome variability, response cost, and even cooperative behavior (Bennett & Pietras, 2021; Jimenez & Pietras, 2018; Pietras et al., 2008; Searcy & Pietras, 2011). This work may help us understand why people make seemingly "desperate" decisions in natural settings. One only needs to take into account the "budget" constraining behavior. Perhaps the risky, desperate choice was the one necessary for survival and was predicted by the model.

The energy budget framework outlined has even been extended to men's Division 1 college basketball (Fox & Kyonka, 2011; data from 2009–2010 games involve an Associated Press top 25 teams between Nov. 8 and Feb. 18 for a total of 201 games and 23,048 shots). In basketball, there are two possible shot types: a 2-point shot or a 3-point shot. Since 2-point shots were more likely to be made and resulted in a less variable outcome, they were considered the risk-averse choice. The score of the game was considered the budget: If a team was down by 2 or fewer points or in the lead, it was considered to be in a positive budget; if a team was down by 3 or more, it was considered to be in a negative budget. Data were analyzed as a function of time left in the game (analogous to a foraging day). Consistent with the model's predictions, as time left in the game decreased, teams in a negative budget were more likely to attempt the riskier 3-point shot, as shown in Figure 2.6. Shot selection for teams in a positive budget did not change as time in the game decreased, again suggesting that in times of relative desperation, organisms are more likely to make the risky choices necessary to "survive" in accordance with an energy budget modeling framework.

Similarly, the MVT framework has been used to study behavior in nonhuman and human operant laboratories, using a time-based diminishing returns procedure. Briefly, MVT is a mathematical prediction for when organisms should "give up" foraging at one patch because the rate of gain becomes so low that incurring the costs of traveling to a new, richer patch is worth it (Charnov, 1976). For example, an animal foraging a patch of berries may first consume the easy-to-reach ones but then find that effort and time increase for harder-to-reach ones. At some point, it becomes optimal to give up and leave the hard-to-reach ones to travel to a new patch, where presumably, there are more easy-to-reach ones.

In operant preparations, these scenarios are sometimes modeled by providing organisms with a choice between concurrent progressive and fixed-time or -interval schedules

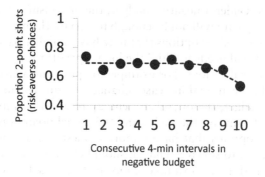

FIGURE 2.6. Risky choice in NCAA men's basketball: Example using an energy budget model framework. Dashed line represents best-fitting bilinear model.

of reinforcement. The progressive schedule starts out at 0 seconds and increases by some amount after every consecutive choice (i.e., diminishing returns). The fixed schedule is relatively long, but resets the progressive schedule back to 0 seconds. In this scenario, the progressive schedule is the current "foraging patch" that offers diminishing returns for staying put. The fixed schedule is the travel time to a new "patch." Depending on the durations arranged on the two schedules, there is some number of consecutive progressive schedule choices that results in the optimal amount of reinforcement. For example, if a progressive-time 4 seconds, fixed-time 60 seconds schedule is arranged, the optimal number of choices on the progressive schedule is five. The consecutive choices on the PT schedule result in reinforcement delays of 0, 4, 8, 12, and 16 seconds. At that point, it becomes optimal to defect to the fixed-time schedule to reset the progressive schedule to 0 seconds. In this way, reinforcement is maximized.

Pigeons (Hackenberg & Hineline, 1992) and humans (Hackenberg & Axtell, 1993; Jacobs & Hackenberg, 1996) readily learn the optimal "switch point" in these tasks using food and money as reinforcers, respectively, in the operant laboratory. The paradigm has been directly translated to research on rule-governed behavior and response-cost punishment (Fox & Kyonka, 2017; Fox & Pietras, 2013; Hackenberg & Joker, 1994; Nergaard & Couto, 2021). It has also helped to inform applied work related to rule-following behavior (e.g., Otalvaro et al., 2020; Sauter et al., 2020). Such a sweeping translation of models designed to explain foraging behavior by nonhumans in natural settings is an impressive testament to the power of quantitative treatments of behavior.

Direct Translation to Clinical and Applied Settings

Although it was impossible to avoid up to this point, we now turn our attention directly to the applied application of quantitative models: using mathematical models to describe and predict behavior in natural settings, often with clinical objectives. As has been previously suggested, perhaps two of the best examples of this are the treatment of choice behavior as a function of reinforcement and delay by the matching law and hyperbolic delay discounting (also see Critchfield & Reed, 2009; Jacobs et al., 2013; Waltz & Follette, 2009). These models have been translated across the research spectrum. Behavioral economics will also be considered as a broader research area related to discounting.

The Matching Law

In its simplest form, the matching law is a quantitative description of how behavior is allocated between two options. It predicts that the time spent engaging in a behavior relative to other behaviors (typically one other behavior in the laboratory) is equal to the rate of reinforcement available for that behavior relative to other sources of reinforcement. In other words, relative rates or time spent engaging in a behavior "matches" the relative reinforcement earned for that behavior (Baum, 1974; Herrnstein, 1974). Figure 2.7 shows this relationship, using the log form of the equation for simplicity. As reinforcement ratios move in favor of one of the two alternatives, the matching law predicts that response ratios will move in direct proportion. For example, if reinforcement is arranged so that alternative 1 is reinforced twice as often as alternative 2, all else being equal, responding should occur twice as often on alternative 1 as on alternative 2.

The matching law was established in the nonhuman operant laboratory (e.g., Baum, 1974; Herrnstein, 1961, 1974; Jensen & Neuringer, 2009) and extended to human operant work (e.g., Baum, 1975), applied settings (e.g., Borrero et al., 2010; Carr & McDowell, 1980), and even to professional sports (Cox et al., 2017; Critchfield et al., 2014; Critchfield & Stilling, 2015; Seniuk et al., 2015; Stilling & Critchfield, 2010). It is nothing short of astonishing that in as complex a scenario as a professional sports game, the simple matching law can so accurately describe and predict the most fundamental behaviors of the game, such as play calls in American football.

The clinical implications of the model are easily ascertained. All behavior is choice behavior, and clinical and applied psychologists have an interest in increasing choices for healthy, adaptive behavior and decreasing choices for unhealthy, maladaptive behavior. Harmful substance use (procuring and using a drug) comes at the expense of adaptive alternatives (procuring and attending a job or to a family). Self-injurious behavior or classroom outbursts for an elementary-age child come at the expense of adaptive alternatives (on task behavior, coursework, skill development, etc.). The matching law tells us that it is a fool's errand to focus only on the problem behavior and the reinforcement arranged in the environment for it. In fact, the matching law tells us that we don't even need to change the reinforcement available for problem behavior at all, and that a good clinical approach is to focus on appropriate behavior and its available reinforcers as well (McDowell, 1988; Waltz & Follette, 2009).

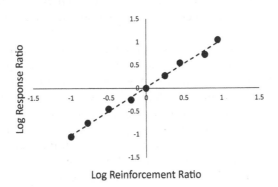

FIGURE 2.7. Example matching law model fit.

Take self-injurious behavior (SIB) as an example. Early applications of the matching law to SIB date back four decades (Carr & McDowell, 1980; McDowell, 1982, 1988). The premise is straightforward, and many applications of differential reinforcement of alternative behavior (DRA) take advantage of the matching law, whether those administering the treatment realize it or not. Clinicians may first identify the reinforcer for SIB (e.g., through a functional analysis; Iwata et al., 1994). Suppose SIB is maintained by attention. The matching law offers several possible avenues for reducing SIB. First, therapy may be targeted at decreasing attention (i.e., reinforcement) for SIB. This is an obvious starting point, and the matching law predicts that reducing reinforcement for SIB will increase the relative reinforcement for other, one would hope, appropriate behaviors in the environment, and that they will increase while SIB decreases. This may be impossible or difficult, however (e.g., all sources of attention cannot be controlled, as in a classroom or at-home scenario, or in the case of "automatically" reinforced SIB). The matching law offers an important alternative: Therapy may be targeted at increasing reinforcers for any alternative, appropriate behavior. This has the result of reducing the relative rate of reinforcement for SIB, thus increasing appropriate behavior and decreasing SIB, without ever altering the reinforcer for SIB. Of course, methods that accomplish both (e.g., place SIB on extinction and increase reinforcement for alternatives) may be even more effective, because the behavior–reinforcement ratios according to the matching law will swing even more in the clinician's and client's favor.

The matching law's predictions may have even more obvious value when treating harmful substance use. It is nearly impossible for the clinician to remove or even degrade the value of a drug reinforcer. Even obvious negative health outcomes and information campaigns do little to control drug seeking and self-administering. In other words, knowing about or directly experiencing the negative outcomes of substance use may do little to alter drug procurement and use behaviors. Enter the matching law. One need not worry about preventing the reinforcer for substance use, one can focus exclusively on the reinforcers available for alternative, appropriate behaviors. By richly reinforcing alternative behaviors, drug seeking and self-administering will decrease proportionally according to the matching law. Such reinforcers may include direct benefits, such as in contingency management programs (e.g., Petry et al., 2000), or more natural reinforcers such as the benefits of a steady job and social support system (e.g., Holtyn et al., 2014; Silverman et al., 2001). Of course, targeting both the neurobiological mechanism of a drug (i.e., reducing its subjective reinforcement value via some pharmacological means) and reinforcement for appropriate alternative behavior (e.g., increasing social support for drug abstinence) may be even more effective than targeting one behavior alone (e.g., Jarvis et al., 2019).

A more nuanced understanding of an individual's behavior may also be elucidated using more complex versions of the matching law incorporating bias and sensitivity parameters (Baum, 1974, 1975), which may suggest the most advantageous types of intervention. For example, if an individual is less sensitive to changes in reinforcement rate, the best intervention may involve very large increases in reinforcement rate. Large changes to reinforcer availability might be clinically impractical in the long term, but they can eventually be thinned. On the other hand, if an individual is more sensitive to changes in reinforcement rate, the appropriate clinical approach may involve less substantial changes in reinforcement rate that are more practical and sustainable. Future work may be aimed at extending the matching framework to more clinically relevant behaviors and behavior modification approaches to improving people's lives.

Hyperbolic Delay Discounting

Hyperbolic delay discounting describes in quantitative terms how a delay to obtain some reinforcer degrades its current subjective value. In other words, when you have to wait for something, it is worth less to you now than if it had been available immediately. The hallmark characteristic of the model is that relatively short delays degrade reinforcer value more steeply than relatively long delays (Madden & Johnson, 2010), as shown in Figure 2.1. Importantly, for individuals with relatively steep functions (i.e., more impulsive; Individual 4 in Figure 2.1), preference may "reverse" from the larger, later adaptive reinforcer to the smaller, sooner maladaptive reinforcer, as time to the decision point decreases (e.g., Ainslie & Herrnstein, 1981; Green, Fristoe, et al., 1994; Green & Estle, 2003). For example, the night before getting up early to exercise, one may genuinely prefer exercise, but when the alarm goes off at 5:00 A.M., hitting snooze and skipping exercise becomes more likely: Preference has reversed. Preference reversals are more likely to occur for more impulsive individuals, because at the choice point, the value of the smaller, sooner reinforcer has increased steeply in relative value, but the relative value of the larger, later outcome has not increased much, and the model predicts it will not until the larger, later reinforcer becomes more temporally proximate. Such outcomes and predictions have obvious clinical relevance. In this example, a clinically relevant question is how to reduce "snoozing" and increase getting out of bed and going for a run.

Hyperbolic delay discounting is somewhat of a success story in modern translational research within behavior analysis (see also Jacobs et al., 2013). Perhaps more than any other behavioral phenomenon, it has been studied and extended from the basic laboratory to natural settings, to clinical settings, and everywhere in between. Experimental work began in the nonhuman and human operant laboratory (e.g., Green et al., 1999; Green, Fry, et al., 1994; Kirby & Maraković, 1995; Myerson & Green, 1995; Vanderveldt et al., 2016), where researchers engaged in developing the model and considering quantitative alternatives, but was quickly translated to an array of clinical contexts (e.g., to understand cigarette smoking; Bickel et al., 1999).

Individual discounting rates are often quantified by fitting the hyperbolic model to the subjective present value of a reinforcer across a range of delays (indifference points). As noted previously, the simplest form of the model has one free parameter, k, which is an index of individual discounting rate. Larger values of k indicate a steeper discounting function (i.e., more "impulsive"). Individual discounting rates vary widely but are relatively stable within subjects across contexts. This has led some to posit that discounting rate is a stable phenomenon with trait-like properties (Odum, 2011b, 2011a). Steep discounting (i.e., large k estimates) is implicated in a wide range of psychoneurological disorders and behavior problems, from attention-deficit/hyperactivity disorder (ADHD) to harmful substance use, to texting while driving, suggesting that it may be an underlying factor undergirding a wide range of behavioral maladies (Bickel et al., 2012, 2019; Bickel & Mueller, 2009). Hence, understanding discounting at individual and group levels may have profound clinical relevance, especially if it can be changed, because this work suggests that reducing steep discounting may come with a reduction in other maladaptive behaviors (though the causal link between steep discounting and behavioral problems remains unclear; i.e., some other behavioral mechanism may cause steep discounting and other maladaptive behavior).

A growing body of preclinical and clinical work suggests that there may be multiple avenues for reducing steep discounting (for reviews, see Rung et al., 2019; Rung &

Madden, 2018; Smith et al., 2019). For example, working memory training (Bickel et al., 2011), commitment responses (Rachlin, 2016; Rachlin & Green, 1972) and episodic future thinking (EFT), thinking in specific ways about where one will be and what they will be doing in the future (Daniel et al., 2013; Peters & Büchel, 2010; Stein et al., 2017), have been shown to reduce discounting rates. In preclinical rat models, extended, forced exposure to delayed reinforcement has been shown to result in robust reductions in discounting across an array of scenarios (e.g., Bailey et al., 2018; Fox, Visser, et al., 2019; Marshall et al., 2014; Panfil et al., 2020; Peterson & Kirkpatrick, 2016; Renda et al., 2018; Renda & Madden, 2016; Stein et al., 2013, 2015). Similar work has shown that experiencing delays may reduce impulsive choice in children with developmental disabilities (e.g., Binder et al., 2000; Dixon & Cummings, 2001). Quantitative modeling in these research domains has been used mostly for descriptive purposes, but it could be used for translational purposes.

The implications for this work are clear, and future translational work may be aimed at extending preclinical work in the nonhuman laboratory to the human operant laboratory and/or applied/natural settings. Does experiencing repeated delays reduce impulsive choice in adult humans? Can conducting brief waiting exercises with children reduce future impulsive choice? To what extent does EFT work to reduce impulsive choice across a range of clinical diagnoses? Many questions remain, but a quantitative foundation for the work has been established and has proven fruitful for a great deal of productive and multidirectional research and practice.

Behavioral Economics

Delay discounting may be considered a subarea of behavioral economics (Francisco et al., 2009) that assumes organisms are not rational decision makers (as is typically assumed in economic models), and seeks to understand behavioral decision making through an economic model lens. Behavioral economic models enjoy broad popular appeal (e.g., the popular book *Nudge*; Thaler & Sunstein, 2009), and are seemingly complimentary to a behavior-analytic framework for studying behavior (Hursh, 1980, 1984; Hursh & Roma, 2016; Reed et al., 2013). While the field of behavioral economics is broad, the focus here is on one model that may be of particular relevance for translational behavior analysis: demand functions. Although beyond the scope of this chapter, more thorough treatments of behavioral economics and their application within behavior analysis are available (e.g., Reed et al., 2013), with equations if one is so inclined (e.g., Hursh & Roma, 2016).

Demand functions are mathematical models of how some reinforced behavior is affected by the "cost" or "price" of the reinforcer. For example, how does increasing the number of lever presses ("cost") to obtain a food reinforcer impact response rate for a food-restricted rat in an operant chamber? How does increasing the number of questions about his day my 4-year-old has to answer to access the iPad affect the rate and probability of question answering?

The extent to which behavior is maintained across increasing "costs" is considered "demand." Reinforcers that have higher demand will more readily maintain behavior as the cost increases (often referred to as "inelastic" demand, because behavior is maintained). Reinforcers that have lower demand result in decreases in behavior as the cost increases (often referred to as "elastic" demand, because behavior is not maintained).

Most reinforcers enjoy inelastic demand up to a certain cost point, at which demand becomes elastic, producing positively decelerating curves when consumption (i.e., the number of reinforcers earned) is plotted as a function of cost (Hursh, 1980, 1984). That cost point at which the transition from inelastic to elastic demand occurs, sometimes called *P-max*, differs across reinforcers and individuals. Reinforcers that are inelastic up to a higher cost–effort point for an individual are more likely to be efficacious reinforcers in the long term as cost or time to acquire the reinforcer increases (Reed et al., 2013). For example, access to the iPad has much higher demand (i.e., is more inelastic) than access to Legos for my 4-year-old; thus, he will answer more of my "dad questions" when he is reinforced with iPad access compared to Lego access. In the context of a demand function, the iPad reinforcer has a greater *P-max* value than the Legos reinforcer. If I want my son to engage in more behavior, I should use the iPad reinforcer.

Comparing demand functions for different reinforcers may have significant applied and translational value. For example, schedule thinning or leaning is often used in behavioral interventions to reduce the response effort and intrusiveness involved in administering an intervention and, at the same time, maintain behavior. For example, one might increase the number of appropriate academic target responses required to obtain attention in a classroom setting. Thus, reinforcers with greater demand are likely to maintain target response rates as the schedule is thinned relative to reinforcers with lower demand. For example, in research conducted with horses, aimed at reducing problem behavior, researchers have employed differential reinforcement of other behavior (DRO) schedules, and have increased the DRO interval to make it practical for horse owners and trainers to implement on their own (e.g., from 15 seconds to 2 or 3 minutes; Fox et al., 2012; Fox & Belding, 2015). Under such circumstances, a demand analysis may indicate that while equally effective at short DRO intervals, small bits of apple or carrot may be more inelastic as the delay increases compared to small bits of hay; that is, they enjoy a higher *P-max* value in the context of the demand function. Though the necessary research has not been conducted, it is valuable, because it would suggest that employing apples or carrots will result in a maintenance of the behavior change over longer DRO intervals and may also be more resistant to treatment integrity failures. Similar circumstances have been reported in other contexts, for example, in developmental disabilities (see Roane et al., 2001). Importantly, typical preference assessments may not indicate relative demand between reinforcers. Several reinforcers may be identified as preferred but may have very different demand functions as cost increases, effecting treatment in the long term. My son loves both the iPad and Legos. They both function as reinforcers, but the iPad enjoys greater demand and is more inelastic as a reinforcer as I increase the cost associated with obtaining it.

The examples in this section suggest that mathematical models can provide an important and productive framework by which to study behavior translationally. Models describe behavior, yes, but also make important predictions about what to expect under certain environmental conditions and how to better control behavior. How do specific genes impact behavior in psychoneurological disorders? How and why does a child's problem behavior persist? When are people more or less likely to make risky choices? What is the probability of a behavior in a sporting event? How do we reduce maladaptive choice? What is the best reinforcer for a behavioral intervention? In all cases, work from the nonhuman literature is readily translated to human and clinical settings using quantitative models as an underlying, unifying scaffold. Future translational work can be improved by extending the modeling framework across these scenarios.

Limitations and Future Directions

The goal of this chapter has been to introduce quantitative modeling to the interested reader using an approachable translational framework. I can't help but think, however, that many readers will simply return to life after this, i.e., life without mathematical models. There is good reason to believe that. I must first admit, excellent lines of translational work can occur without a unifying mathematical principle undergirding it (e.g., research on rich-to-lean transitions and their applied significance; Castillo et al., 2018; Jessel et al., 2020; Jessel & Ingvarsson, 2017; Perone & Courtney, 1992; Toegel & Perone, 2022; Wade-Galuska et al., 2005; Williams et al., 2011), though this alone cannot be reason to discard a quantitative approach given the value outlined here and elsewhere. Models can be beneficial, helpful, unifying, and informative, even if they are not always necessary. They aid in our understanding and can help us translate basic work to applied work, but may also get in the way, particularly for those untrained in and unfamiliar with mathematical modeling (something we must work to change given their growing use and application).

Efforts to increase exposure to, and training with, quantitative analyses and mathematical models will go a long way in reducing their intimidation and increasing their accessibility and use. This is particularly important in terms of bridging the basic-applied research gap as quantitative modeling becomes more and more prominent in the experimental analysis of behavior. Doing so starts in advanced coursework at the undergraduate level, but is likely most important in graduate training programs. For example, in an advanced undergraduate course I teach, we cover the Rescorla and Wagner (1972) model, the matching law, and hyperbolic delay discounting, including application of the equations themselves in some instances. Such a strategy familiarizes students with mathematical treatments of behavior. Although students generally start out with a groan when I put an equation on the slide, some are in awe that seemingly complex behavior can be described so adequately and across such a diverse range of scenarios using fairly simple equations. At the graduate level, a single course, or even part of a course, devoted to quantitative modeling will help improve understanding and application of models. Importantly, if aspiring basic and applied scientists can take these courses together, all the better. They will be treated with an expansive understanding from multiple ends of the research spectrum. Courses that incorporate statistical modeling, especially multilevel approaches, are even better. The future of modeling, even the present, one might argue, is in employing quantitative models using a multilevel approach (e.g., Boisgontier & Cheval, 2016; Fox, 2018; Kirkpatrick et al., 2018; Young, 2017, 2018). A student of behavior is put at a distinct disadvantage if not, however briefly, exposed to such techniques and applications. Such training also makes quantitative modeling a bit less scary, introduces basic scientists to applications, and applied scientists to basic science, which can go a long way in getting folks across the research spectrum talking and collaborating.

The future success of the field may well depend on such collaborations. Translational quantitative modeling work offers a productive avenue for basic research to impact applied and clinical work (and vice versa), to earn increasingly competitive extramural funding, and to impact cultural behavioral trends and public policy. Any time we quantify behavior, modeling is possible, and it can enrich our understanding and ability to communicate our work. The end goal of this work is to use modeling as a tool to provide insight into the functional relations that control behavior, so that we in turn may make better, more quantified predictions about behavior with precision and complexity that we simply cannot conjure verbally. This work will be more likely to be accepted, valued, and held up as an example in contexts outside of behavior analysis, while simultaneously improving our work inside of behavior analysis. After all, the quantitative analysis of behavior has always been about translation, and the work continues.

AUTHOR NOTE

This chapter is dedicated to David P. Jarmolowicz, whose passion for behavior analysis, quantitative analyses, translational research, science, and life inspired so many of us.

REFERENCES

Ainslie, G., & Herrnstein, R. J. (1981). Preference reversal and delayed reinforcement. *Animal Learning and Behavior, 9*(4), 476–482.

Allman, M. J., DeLeon, I. G., & Wearden, J. H. (2011). Psychophysical assessment of timing in individuals with autism. *American Journal on Intellectual and Developmental Disabilities, 116*(2), 165–178.

Anderson, K. G., Velkey, A. J., & Woolverton, W. L. (2002). The generalized matching law as a predictor of choice between cocaine and food in rhesus monkeys. *Psychopharmacology, 163*(3–4), 319–326.

Bailey, C., Peterson, J. R., Schnegelsiepen, A., Stuebing, S. L., & Kirkpatrick, K. (2018). Durability and generalizability of time-based intervention effects on impulsive choice in rats. *Behavioural Processes, 152*, 54–62.

Balci, F., Papachristos, E. B., Gallistel, C. R., Brunner, D., Gibson, J., & Shumyatsky, G. P. (2008). Interval timing in genetically modified mice: A simple paradigm. *Genes, Brain and Behavior, 7*(3), 373–384.

Bambini-Junior, V., Zanatta, G., Nunes, G. D. F., de Melo, G. M., Michels, M., Fontes-Dutra, M., . . . Gottfried, C. (2014). Resveratrol prevents social deficits in animal model of autism induced by valproic acid. *Neuroscience Letters, 583*, 176–181.

Banji, D., Banji, O. J. F., Abbagoni, S., Hayath, S., Kambam, S., & Chiluka, V. L. (2011). Amelioration of behavioral aberrations and oxidative markers by green tea extract in valproate induced autism in animals. *Brain Research, 1410*, 141–151.

Baum, W. M. (1974). On two types of deviation from the Matching Law: Bias and undermatching. *Journal of the Experimental Analysis of Behavior, 22*(1), 231–242.

Baum, W. M. (1975). Time allocation in human

vigilance. *Journal of the Experimental Analysis of Behavior, 23*(1), 45–53.

Bennett, J. A., & Pietras, C. J. (2021). Human choices respond to added costs according to the energy budget rule. *Learning and Motivation, 75*, Article 101745.

Bickel, W. K., Athamneh, L. N., Basso, J. C., Mellis, A. M., DeHart, W. B., Craft, W. H., & Pope, D. (2019). Excessive discounting of delayed reinforcers as a trans-disease process: Update on the state of the science. *Current Opinion in Psychology, 30*, 59–64.

Bickel, W. K., Jarmolowicz, D. P., Mueller, E. T., Koffarnus, M. N., & Gatchalian, K. M. (2012). Excessive discounting of delayed reinforcers as a trans-disease process contributing to addiction and other disease-related vulnerabilities: Emerging evidence. *Pharmacology and Therapeutics, 134*(3), 287–297.

Bickel, W. K., & Mueller, E. T. (2009). Toward the study of trans-disease processes: A novel approach with special reference to the study of co-morbidity. *Journal of Dual Diagnosis, 5*(2), 131–138.

Bickel, W. K., Odum, A. L., & Madden, G. J. (1999). Impulsivity and cigarette smoking: Delay discounting in current, never, and ex-smokers. *Psychopharmacology, 146*(4), 447–454.

Bickel, W. K., Yi, R., Landes, R. D., Hill, P. F., & Baxter, C. (2011). Remember the future: Working memory training decreases delay discounting among stimulant addicts. *Biological Psychiatry, 69*(3), 260–265.

Binder, L. M., Dixon, M. R., & Ghezzi, P. M. (2000). A procedure to teach self-control to children with attention deficit hyperactivity disorder. *Journal of Applied Behavior Analysis, 33*(2), 233–237.

Boisgontier, M. P., & Cheval, B. (2016). The

ANOVA to mixed model transition. *Neuroscience and Biobehavioral Reviews, 68,* 1004–1005.

Bolker, B. M., Brooks, M. E., Clark, C. J., Geange, S. W., Poulsen, J. R., Stevens, M. H. H., & White, J.-S. S. (2009). Generalized linear mixed models: A practical guide for ecology and evolution. *Trends in Ecology and Evolution, 24*(3), 127–135.

Borrero, C. S. W., Vollmer, T. R., Borrero, J. C., Bourret, J. C., Sloman, K. N., Samaha, A. L., & Dallery, J. (2010). Concurrent reinforcement schedules for problem behavior and appropriate behavior: Experimental applications of the Matching Law. *Journal of the Experimental Analysis of Behavior, 93*(3), 455–469.

Branch, M. N. (1999). Statistical inference in behavior analysis: Some things significance testing does and does not do. *Behavior Analyst, 22*(2), 87–92.

Branch, M. N. (2014). Malignant side effects of null-hypothesis significance testing. *Theory and Psychology, 24*(2), 256–277.

Buhusi, C. V., & Meck, W. H. (2005). What makes us tick?: Functional and neural mechanisms of interval timing. *Nature Reviews Neuroscience, 6*(10), 755–765.

Carr, E. G., & McDowell, J. J. (1980). Social control of self-injurious behavior of organic etiology. *Behavior Therapy, 11*(3), 402–409.

Castillo, M. I., Clark, D. R., Schaller, E. A., Donaldson, J. M., DeLeon, I. G., & Kahng, S. (2018). Descriptive assessment of problem behavior during transitions of children with intellectual and developmental disabilities. *Journal of Applied Behavior Analysis, 51*(1), 99–117.

Catania, A. C. (2012). The flight from experimental analysis. *European Journal of Behavior Analysis, 13*(2), 165–176.

Charnov, E. L. (1976). Optimal foraging, the marginal value theorem. *Theoretical Population Biology, 9*(2), 129–136.

Chomiak, T., Turner, N., & Hu, B. (2013). What we have learned about autism spectrum disorder from valproic acid. *Pathology Research International, 2013,* Article 712758.

Christensen, D. L., Maenner, M. J., Bilder, D., Constantino, J. N., Daniels, J., Durkin, M. S., . . . Dietz, P. (2019). Prevalence and characteristics of autism spectrum disorder among children aged 4 years—Early Autism and Developmental Disabilities Monitoring Network, seven sites, United States, 2010, 2012, and 2014. *Morbidity and Mortality Weekly Report. Surveillance Summaries (Washington, DC: 2002), 68*(2), 1–19.

Church, R. M., & Deluty, M. Z. (1977). Bisection of temporal intervals. *Journal of Experimental Psychology: Animal Behavior Processes, 3*(3), 216–228.

Commons, M. L. (2001). A short history of the Society for Quantitative Analyses of Behavior. *Behavior Analyst Today, 2*(3), 275–279.

Cox, D. J., Sosine, J., & Dallery, J. (2017). Application of the matching law to pitch selection in professional baseball. *Journal of Applied Behavior Analysis, 50*(2), 393–406.

Critchfield, T. S. (2017). Visuwords®: A handy online tool for estimating what nonexperts may think when hearing behavior analysis jargon. *Behavior Analysis in Practice, 10*(3), 318–322.

Critchfield, T. S., Doepke, K. J., Kimberly Epting, L., Becirevic, A., Reed, D. D., Fienup, D. M., . . . Ecott, C. L. (2017). Normative emotional responses to behavior analysis jargon or how not to use words to win friends and influence people. *Behavior Analysis in Practice, 10*(2), 97–106.

Critchfield, T. S., Meeks, E., & Stilling, S. T. (2014). Explanatory flexibility of the Matching Law: Situational bias interactions in football play selection. *Psychological Record, 64*(3), 371–380.

Critchfield, T. S., & Reed, D. D. (2009). What are we doing when we translate from quantitative models? *Behavior Analyst, 32*(2), 339–362.

Critchfield, T. S., & Stilling, S. T. (2015). A matching law analysis of risk tolerance and gain–loss framing in football play selection. *Behavior Analysis: Research and Practice, 15*(2), 112–121.

Cullen, C. (1981). The flight to the laboratory. *Behavior Analyst, 4*(1), 81–83.

Daniel, T. O., Stanton, C. M., & Epstein, L. H. (2013). The future is now: Reducing impulsivity and energy intake using episodic future thinking. *Psychological Science, 24*(11), 2339–2342.

Daniels, C. W., Fox, A. E., Kyonka, E. G., & Sanabria, F. (2015). Biasing temporal judgments in rats, pigeons, and humans. *International Journal of Comparative Psychology, 28*(1).

Deane, A. R., Millar, J., Bilkey, D. K., & Ward, R. D. (2017). Maternal immune activation in rats produces temporal perception impairments in adult offspring analogous to those observed in schizophrenia. *PLOS One, 12*(11), Article e0187719.

DeCoteau, W. E., & Fox, A. E. (2022). Timing and intertemporal choice behavior in the valproic acid rat model of autism spectrum disorder. *Journal of Autism and Developmental Disorders, 52,* 2414–2429.

DeHart, W. B., & Kaplan, B. A. (2019). Applying mixed-effects modeling to single-subject designs: An introduction. *Journal of the Experimental Analysis of Behavior, 111*(2), 192–206.

Dixon, M. R., & Cummings, A. (2001). Self-control in children with autism: Response allocation during delays to reinforcement. *Journal of Applied Behavior Analysis, 34*(4), 491–495.

Favre, M. R., Barkat, T. R., Lamendola, D., Khazen, G., Markram, H., & Markram, K. (2013). General developmental health in the VPA-rat model of autism. *Frontiers in Behavioral Neuroscience, 7,* Article 88.

Fisher, W. W., Kelley, M. E., & Lomas, J. E. (2003). Visual aids and structured criteria for improving visual inspection and interpretation of single-case designs. *Journal of Applied Behavior Analysis, 36*(3), 387–406.

Fontes-Dutra, M., Nunes, G. D.-F., Santos-Terra, J., Souza-Nunes, W., Bauer-Negrini, G., Hirsch, M. M., . . . Bambini-Junior, V. (2019). Abnormal empathy-like pro-social behaviour in the valproic acid model of autism spectrum disorder. *Behavioural Brain Research, 364,* 11–18.

Fox, A. E. (2018). The future is upon us. *Behavior Analysis: Research and Practice, 18*(2), 144–150.

Fox, A. E., Bailey, S. R., Hall, E. G., & St. Peter, C. C. (2012). Reduction of biting and chewing of horses using differential reinforcement of other behavior. *Behavioural Processes, 91*(1), 125–128.

Fox, A. E., & Belding, D. L. (2015). Reducing pawing in horses using positive reinforcement. *Journal of Applied Behavior Analysis, 48*(4), 936–940.

Fox, A. E., Buchanan, I., Roussard, Q., Hurley, K., Thalheim, I., & Joyce, J. M. (2019). Using delays to decrease paper consumption in food service and laboratory settings. *Psychological Record, 59,* 215–223.

Fox, A. E., Caramia, S. R., Haskell, M. M., Ramey, A. L., & Singha, D. (2017). Stimulus control in two rodent models of attention-deficit/hyperactivity disorder. *Behavioural Processes, 135,* 16–24.

Fox, A. E., & Kyonka, E. G. E. (2011, May). *NCAA basketball and optimal foraging theory.* Presented at the annual meeting of the Society for the Quantitative Analysis of Behavior, Denver, CO.

Fox, A. E., & Kyonka, E. G. (2013). Pigeon responding in fixed-interval and response-initiated fixed-interval schedules. *Journal of the Experimental Analysis of Behavior, 100*(2), 187–197.

Fox, A. E., & Kyonka, E. G. (2015). Timing in response-initiated fixed intervals. *Journal of the Experimental Analysis of Behavior, 103*(2), 375–392.

Fox, A. E., & Kyonka, E. G. (2016). Effects of signaling on temporal control of behavior in response-initiated fixed intervals. *Journal of the Experimental Analysis of Behavior, 106*(3), 210–224.

Fox, A. E., & Kyonka, E. G. E. (2017). Searching for the variables that control human rule-governed "insensitivity." *Journal of the Experimental Analysis of Behavior, 108*(2), 236–254.

Fox, A. E., & Pietras, C. J. (2013). The effects of response-cost punishment on instructional control during a choice task. *Journal of the Experimental Analysis of Behavior, 99*(3), 346–361.

Fox, A. E., Visser, E. J., & Nicholson, A. M. (2019). Interventions aimed at changing impulsive choice in rats: Effects of immediate and relatively long delay to reward training. *Behavioural Processes, 158,* 126–136.

Francisco, M. T., Madden, G. J., & Borrero, J. (2009). Behavioral economics: Principles, procedures, and utility for applied behavior analysis. *Behavior Analyst Today, 10*(2), 277–294.

Gibbon, J. (1991). Origins of scalar timing. *Learning and Motivation, 22*(1–2), 3–38.

Gibbon, J. (1992). Ubiquity of scalar timing with a Poisson clock. *Journal of Mathematical Psychology, 36*(2), 283–293.

Green, L., & Estle, S. J. (2003). Preference reversals with food and water reinforcers in rats. *Journal of the Experimental Analysis of Behavior, 79*(2), 233–242.

Green, L., Fristoe, N., & Myerson, J. (1994). Temporal discounting and preference reversals in choice between delayed outcomes. *Psychonomic Bulletin and Review, 1*(3), 383–389.

Green, L., Fry, A. F., & Myerson, J. (1994). Discounting of delayed rewards: A life-span comparison. *Psychological Science, 5*(1), 33–36.

Green, L., Myerson, J., & Ostaszewski, P. (1999).

Discounting of delayed rewards across the life span: Age differences in individual discounting functions. *Behavioural Processes, 46*(1), 89–96.

Hackenberg, T. D. (1998). Laboratory methods in human behavioral ecology. In K. A. Lattal & M. Perone (Eds.), *Handbook of research methods in human operant behavior* (pp. 541–577). Springer.

Hackenberg, T. D., & Axtell, S. A. M. (1993). Humans' choices in situations of time-based diminishing returns. *Journal of the Experimental Analysis of Behavior, 59*(3), 445–470.

Hackenberg, T. D., & Hineline, P. N. (1992). Choice in situations of time-based diminishing returns: Immediate versus delayed consequences of action. *Journal of the Experimental Analysis of Behavior, 57*(1), 67–80.

Hackenberg, T. D., & Joker, V. R. (1994). Instructional versus schedule control of humans' choices in situations of diminishing returns. *Journal of the Experimental Analysis of Behavior, 62*(3), 367–383.

Hand, D. J., Fox, A. T., & Reilly, M. P. (2006). Response acquisition with delayed reinforcement in a rodent model of attention-deficit/hyperactivity disorder (ADHD). *Behavioural Brain Research, 175*(2), 337–342.

Hastjarjo, T., Silberberg, A., & Hursh, S. R. (1990). Risky choice as a function of amount and variance in food supply. *Journal of the Experimental Analysis of Behavior, 53*(1), 155–161.

Herrnstein, R. J. (1961). Relative and absolute strength of response as a function of frequency of reinforcement. *Journal of the Experimental Analysis of Behavior, 4*(3), 267–272.

Herrnstein, R. J. (1974). Formal properties of the matching law. *Journal of the Experimental Analysis of Behavior, 21*(1), 159–164.

Holtyn, A. F., Koffarnus, M. N., DeFulio, A., Sigurdsson, S. O., Strain, E. C., Schwartz, R. P., . . . Silverman, K. (2014). The therapeutic workplace to promote treatment engagement and drug abstinence in out-of-treatment injection drug users: A randomized controlled trial. *Preventive Medicine, 68*, 62–70.

Houston, A. I. (1991). Risk-sensitive foraging theory and operant psychology. *Journal of the Experimental Analysis of Behavior, 56*(3), 585–589.

Huitema, B. E. (1986). Statistical analysis and single-subject designs: Some misunderstandings. In A. Poling & R. W. Fuqua (Eds.), *Research methods in applied behavior analysis* (pp. 209–232). Springer.

Huitema, B. E., & McKean, J. W. (2000). Design specification issues in time-series intervention models. *Educational and Psychological Measurement, 60*(1), 38–58.

Hursh, S. R. (1980). Economic concepts for the analysis of behavior. *Journal of the Experimental Analysis of Behavior, 34*(2), 219–238.

Hursh, S. R. (1984). Behavioral economics. *Journal of the Experimental Analysis of Behavior, 42*(3), 435–452.

Hursh, S. R., & Roma, P. G. (2016). Behavioral economics and the analysis of consumption and choice. *Managerial and Decision Economics, 37*(4–5), 224–238.

Hutsell, B. A., Negus, S. S., & Banks, M. L. (2015). A generalized matching law analysis of cocaine vs. food choice in rhesus monkeys: Effects of candidate "agonist-based" medications on sensitivity to reinforcement. *Drug and Alcohol Dependence, 146*, 52–60.

Iwata, B. A., Dorsey, M. F., Slifer, K. J., Bauman, K. E., & Richman, G. S. (1994). Toward a functional analysis of self-injury. *Journal of Applied Behavior Analysis, 27*(2), 197–209.

Jacobs, E. A., Borrero, J. C., & Vollmer, T. R. (2013). Translational applications of quantitative choice models. In G. J. Madden, W. V. Dube, T. D. Hackenberg, G. P. Hanley, & K. A. Lattal (Eds.), *APA handbook of behavior analysis: Vol. 2. Translating principles into practice* (pp. 165–190). American Psychological Association.

Jacobs, E. A., & Hackenberg, T. D. (1996). Humans' choices in situations of time-based diminishing returns: Effects of fixed-interval duration and progressive-interval step size. *Journal of the Experimental Analysis of Behavior, 65*(1), 5–19.

Jarvis, B. P., Holtyn, A. F., DeFulio, A., Koffarnus, M. N., Leoutsakos, J.-M. S., Umbricht, A., . . . Silverman, K. (2019). The effects of extended-release injectable naltrexone and incentives for opiate abstinence in heroin-dependent adults in a model therapeutic workplace: A randomized trial. *Drug and Alcohol Dependence, 197*, 220–227.

Jensen, G., & Neuringer, A. (2009). Barycentric extension of generalized matching. *Journal of the Experimental Analysis of Behavior, 92*(2), 139–159.

Jessel, J., & Ingvarsson, E. T. (2017). Using rich-to-lean transitions following errors during discrete-trial instruction. *European Journal of Behavior Analysis, 18*(2), 291–306.

Jessel, J., Ma, S., Spartinos, J., & Villanueva, A. (2020). Transitioning from rich to lean reinforcement as a form of error correction. *Journal of Applied Behavior Analysis, 53*(4), 2108–2125.

Jimenez, S., & Pietras, C. (2018). An investigation of the probability of reciprocation in a risk-reduction model of sharing. *Behavioural Processes, 157,* 583–589.

Jimenez-Gomez, C., & Shahan, T. A. (2008). Matching law analysis of rats' alcohol self-administration in a free-operant choice procedure. *Behavioural Pharmacology, 19*(4), 353–356.

Karson, A., & Balcı, F. (2021). Timing behavior in genetic murine models of neurological and psychiatric diseases. *Experimental Brain Research, 239*(3), 699–717.

Kazdin, A. E. (2019). Single-case experimental designs. Evaluating interventions in research and clinical practice. *Behaviour Research and Therapy, 117,* 3–17.

Kazdin, A. E., & Cole, P. M. (1981). Attitudes and labeling biases toward behavior modification: The effects of labels, content, and jargon. *Behavior Therapy, 12*(1), 56–68.

Killeen, P. (1972). The Matching Law. *Journal of the Experimental Analysis of Behavior, 17*(3), 489–495.

Killeen, P. R. (1999). Modeling. *Journal of the Experimental Analysis of Behavior, 71*(2), 275–280.

Kirby, K. N., & Maraković, N. N. (1995). Modeling myopic decisions: Evidence for hyperbolic delay-discounting within subjects and amounts. *Organizational Behavior and Human Decision Processes, 64*(1), 22–30.

Kirkpatrick, K., Marshall, A. T., Steele, C. C., & Peterson, J. R. (2018). Resurrecting the individual in behavioral analysis: Using mixed effects models to address nonsystematic discounting data. *Behavior Analysis: Research and Practice, 18*(3), 219–238.

Koffarnus, M. N., & Woods, J. H. (2008). Quantification of drug choice with the generalized matching law in rhesus monkeys. *Journal of the Experimental Analysis of Behavior, 89*(2), 209–224.

Leigh, J. P., & Du, J. (2015). Brief report: Forecasting the economic burden of autism in 2015 and 2025 in the United States. *Journal of Autism and Developmental Disorders, 45*(12), 4135–4139.

Lindsley, O. R. (1991). From technical jargon to plain English for application. *Journal of Applied Behavior Analysis, 24*(3), 449–458.

Mace, F. C., & Belfiore, P. (1990). Behavioral momentum in the treatment of escape-motiva-tion stereotypy. *Journal of Applied Behavior Analysis, 23*(4), 507–514.

Mace, F. C., Lalli, J. S., Shea, M. C., Lalli, E. P., West, B. J., Roberts, M., & Nevin, J. A. (1990). The momentum of human behavior in natural settings. *Journal of the Experimental Analysis of Behavior, 54*(3), 163–172.

Mace, F. C., McComas, J. J., Mauro, B. C., Progar, P. R., Taylor, B., Ervin, R., & Zangrillo, A. N. (2010). Differential reinforcement of alternative behavior increases resistance to extinction: Clinical demonstration, animal modeling, and clinical test of one solution. *Journal of the Experimental Analysis of Behavior, 93*(3), 349–367.

Mace, F. C., & Nevin, J. A. (2017). Maintenance, generalization, and treatment relapse: A behavioral momentum analysis. *Education and Treatment of Children, 40*(1), 27–42.

Madden, G. J. (2013). Go forth and be variable. *Behavior Analyst, 36*(1), 137–143.

Madden, G. J., & Johnson, P. S. (2010). A delay-discounting primer. In G. J. Madden & W. K. Bickel (Eds.), *Impulsivity: The behavioral and neurological science of discounting* (pp. 11–37). American Psychological Association.

Markram, K., Rinaldi, T., Mendola, D. L., Sandi, C., & Markram, H. (2008). Abnormal fear conditioning and amygdala processing in an animal model of autism. *Neuropsychopharmacology, 33*(4), 901–912.

Marr, M. J. (1989). Some remarks on the quantitative analysis of behavior. *Behavior Analyst, 12*(2), 143–151.

Marshall, A. T., Smith, A. P., & Kirkpatrick, K. (2014). Mechanisms of impulsive choice: I. Individual differences in interval timing and reward processing. *Journal of the Experimental Analysis of Behavior, 102*(1), 86–101.

Mazur, J. E. (2006). Mathematical models and the experimental analysis of behavior. *Journal of the Experimental Analysis of Behavior, 85*(2), 275–291.

McDowell, J. J. (1982). The importance of Herrnstein's mathematical statement of the law of effect for behavior therapy. *American Psychologist, 37*(7), 771–779.

McDowell, J. J. (1988). Matching theory in natural human environments. *Behavior Analyst, 11*(2), 95–109.

McNamara, J., & Houston, A. (1992). Risk-sensitive foraging: A review of the theory. *Bulletin of Mathematical Biology, 54*(2–3), 355–378.

Moore, J. (2008). A critical appraisal of contemporary approaches in the quantitative analysis of behavior. *Psychological Record, 58*(4), 641–664.

Myerson, J., & Green, L. (1995). Discounting of delayed rewards: Models of individual choice. *Journal of the Experimental Analysis of Behavior, 64*(3), 263–276.

Nergaard, S. K., & Couto, K. C. (2021). Effects of reinforcement and response-cost history on instructional control. *Journal of the Experimental Analysis of Behavior, 115*(3), 679–701.

Nevin, J. A. (1974). Response strength in multiple schedules. *Journal of the Experimental Analysis of Behavior, 21*(3), 389–408.

Nevin, J. A. (2008). Control, prediction, order, and the joys of research. *Journal of the Experimental Analysis of Behavior, 89*(1), 119–123.

Nevin, J. A., Craig, A. R., Cunningham, P. J., Podlesnik, C. A., Shahan, T. A., & Sweeney, M. M. (2017). Quantitative models of persistence and relapse from the perspective of behavioral momentum theory: Fits and misfits. *Behavioural Processes, 141*, 92–99.

Nevin, J. A., Mandell, C., & Atak, J. R. (1983). The analysis of behavioral momentum. *Journal of the Experimental Analysis of Behavior, 39*(1), 49–59.

Nevin, J. A., & Shahan, T. A. (2011). Behavioral momentum theory: Equations and applications. *Journal of Applied Behavior Analysis, 44*(4), 877–895.

Odum, A. L. (2011a). Delay discounting: I'm a k, you're a k. *Journal of the Experimental Analysis of Behavior, 96*(3), 427–439.

Odum, A. L. (2011b). Delay discounting: Trait variable? *Behavioural Processes, 87*(1), 1–9.

O'Grady, A. C., Reeve, S. A., Reeve, K. F., Vladescu, J. C., & Lake, C. M. (2018). Evaluation of computer-based training to teach adults visual analysis skills of baseline-treatment graphs. *Behavior Analysis in Practice, 11*(3), 254–266.

Otalvaro, P. A., Krebs, C. A., Brewer, A. T., Leon, Y., & Steifman, J. S. (2020). Reducing excessive questions in adults at adult-day training centers using differential-reinforcement-of-low rates. *Journal of Applied Behavior Analysis, 53*, 545–553.

Panfil, K., Bailey, C., Davis, I., Mains, A., & Kirkpatrick, K. (2020). A time-based intervention to treat impulsivity in male and female rats. *Behavioural Brain Research, 379*(3), Article 112316.

Peartree, N. A., Sanabria, F., Thiel, K. J., Weber, S. M., Cheung, T. H. C., & Neisewander, J. L. (2012). A new criterion for acquisition of nico-tine self-administration in rats. *Drug and Alcohol Dependence, 124*(1–2), 63–69.

Perone, M., & Courtney, K. (1992). Fixed-ratio pausing: Joint effects of past reinforcer magnitude and stimuli correlated with upcoming magnitude. *Journal of the Experimental Analysis of Behavior, 57*(1), 33–46.

Perry, J. L., Larson, E. B., German, J. P., Madden, G. J., & Carroll, M. E. (2005). Impulsivity (delay discounting) as a predictor of acquisition of IV cocaine self-administration in female rats. *Psychopharmacology, 178*(2–3), 193–201.

Peters, J., & Büchel, C. (2010). Episodic future thinking reduces reward delay discounting through an enhancement of prefrontal–mediotemporal interactions. *Neuron, 66*(1), 138–148.

Peterson, J. R., & Kirkpatrick, K. (2016). The effects of a time-based intervention on experienced middle-aged rats. *Behavioural Processes, 133*, 44–51.

Petry, N. M., Martin, B., Cooney, J. L., & Kranzler, H. R. (2000). Give them prizes and they will come: Contingency management for treatment of alcohol dependence. *Journal of Consulting and Clinical Psychology, 68*(2), 250–257.

Pietras, C. J., & Hackenberg, T. D. (2001). Risk-sensitive choice in humans as a function of an earnings budget. *Journal of the Experimental Analysis of Behavior, 76*(1), 1–19.

Pietras, C. J., Searcy, G. D., Huitema, B. E., & Brandt, A. E. (2008). Effects of monetary reserves and rate of gain on human risky choice under budget constraints. *Behavioural Processes, 78*(3), 358–373.

Platt, J. R., & Davis, E. R. (1983). Bisection of temporal intervals by pigeons. *Journal of Experimental Psychology: Animal Behavior Processes, 9*(2), 160–170.

Poulin, C. J., & Fox, A. E. (2021). Preliminary evidence for timing abnormalities in the CNTNAP2 knockout rat. *Behavioural Processes, 190*, Article 104449.

Quick, S. L., Pyszczynski, A. D., Colston, K. A., & Shahan, T. A. (2011). Loss of alternative non-drug reinforcement induces relapse of cocaine-seeking in rats: Role of dopamine D1 receptors. *Neuropsychopharmacology, 36*(5), 1015–1020.

Rachlin, H. (2016). Self-control based on soft commitment. *Behavior Analyst, 39*(2), 259–268.

Rachlin, H., & Green, L. (1972). Commitment,

choice and self-control. *Journal of the Experimental Analysis of Behavior, 17*(1), 15–22.

Reed, D. D., & Dixon, M. (2009). Using Microsoft Office Excel 2007 to conduct generalized matching analyses. *Journal of Applied Behavior Analysis, 42*(4), 867–875.

Reed, D. D., & Kaplan, B. A. (2011). The Matching Law: A tutorial for practitioners. *Behavior Analysis in Practice, 4*(2), 15–24.

Reed, D. D., Kaplan, B. A., & Brewer, A. T. (2012). A tutorial on the use of Excel 2010 and Excel for Mac 2011 for conducting delay-discounting analyses. *Journal of Applied Behavior Analysis, 45*(2), 375–386.

Reed, D. D., Niileksela, C. R., & Kaplan, B. A. (2013). Behavioral economics: A tutorial for behavior analysts in practice. *Behavior Analysis in Practice, 6*(1), 34–54.

Reilly, M. P., & Lattal, K. A. (2004). Within-session delay-of-reinforcement gradients. *Journal of the Experimental Analysis of Behavior, 82*(1), 21–35.

Renda, C. R., & Madden, G. J. (2016). Impulsive choice and pre-exposure to delays: III. Four-month test–retest outcomes in male Wistar rats. *Behavioural Processes, 126*, 108–112.

Renda, C. R., Rung, J. M., Hinnenkamp, J. E., Lenzini, S. N., & Madden, G. J. (2018). Impulsive choice and pre-exposure to delays: IV. Effects of delay-and immediacy-exposure training relative to maturational changes in impulsivity. *Journal of the Experimental Analysis of Behavior, 109*(3), 587–599.

Rescorla, R. A., & Wagner, A. R. (1972). A theory of Pavlovian conditioning: Variations in the effectiveness of reinforcement. In A. H. Black & W. G. Prokasy (Eds.), *Classical conditioning II* (pp. 64–69). Appleton-Century-Crofts.

Roane, H. S., Lerman, D. C., & Vorndran, C. M. (2001). Assessing reinforcers under progressive schedule requirements. *Journal of Applied Behavior Analysis, 34*(2), 145–167.

Rogge, N., & Janssen, J. (2019). The economic costs of autism spectrum disorder: A literature review. *Journal of Autism and Developmental Disorders, 49*, 2873–2900.

Rung, J. M., & Madden, G. J. (2018). Experimental reductions of delay discounting and impulsive choice: A systematic review and meta-analysis. *Journal of Experimental Psychology: General, 147*(9), 1349–1381.

Rung, J. M., Peck, S., Hinnenkamp, J. E., Preston, E., & Madden, G. J. (2019). Changing delay discounting and impulsive choice: Implications for addictions, prevention, and human

health. *Perspectives on Behavior Science, 42,* 397–417.

Salzberg, C. L., Strain, P. S., & Baer, D. M. (1987). Meta-analysis for single-subject research: When does it clarify, when does it obscure? *Remedial and Special Education, 8*(2), 43–48.

Sauter, J. A., Stocco, C. S., Luczynski, K. C., & Moline, A. D. (2020). Temporary, inconsistent, and null effects of a moral story and instruction on honesty. *Journal of Applied Behavior Analysis, 53,* 134–146.

Schlosser, R. W., Lee, D. L., & Wendt, O. (2008). Application of the percentage of non-overlapping data (PND) in systematic reviews and meta-analyses: A systematic review of reporting characteristics. *Evidence-Based Communication Assessment and Intervention, 2*(3), 163–187.

Schneider, T., & Przewłocki, R. (2005). Behavioral alterations in rats prenatally exposed to valproic acid: Animal model of autism. *Neuropsychopharmacology, 30*(1), 80–89.

Schneider, T., Turczak, J., & Przewłocki, R. (2006). Environmental enrichment reverses behavioral alterations in rats prenatally exposed to valproic acid: Issues for a therapeutic approach in autism. *Neuropsychopharmacology, 31*(1), 36–46.

Scruggs, T. E., & Mastropieri, M. A. (2013). PND at 25: Past, present, and future trends in summarizing single-subject research. *Remedial and Special Education, 34*(1), 9–19.

Scruggs, T. E., Mastropieri, M. A., & Casto, G. (1987). The quantitative synthesis of single-subject research: Methodology and validation. *Remedial and Special Education, 8*(2), 24–33.

Searcy, G. D., & Pietras, C. J. (2011). Optimal risky choice in humans: Effects of amount of variability. *Behavioural Processes, 87*(1), 88–99.

Seniuk, H. A., Williams, W. L., Reed, D. D., & Wright, J. W. (2015). An examination of matching with multiple response alternatives in professional hockey. *Behavior Analysis: Research and Practice, 15*(3–4), 152–160.

Silverman, K., Holtyn, A. F., & Morrison, R. (2016). The therapeutic utility of employment in treating drug addiction: Science to application. *Translational Issues in Psychological Science, 2*(2), 203–212.

Silverman, K., Svikis, D., Robles, E., Stitzer, M. L., & Bigelow, G. E. (2001). A reinforcement-based therapeutic workplace for the treatment of drug abuse: Six-month abstinence outcomes. *Experimental and Clinical Psychopharmacology, 9*(1), 14–23.

Smith, T., Panfil, K., Bailey, C., & Kirkpatrick, K. (2019). Cognitive and behavioral training interventions to promote self-control. *Journal of Experimental Psychology: Animal Learning and Cognition, 45*(3), 259–279.

Stein, J. S., Johnson, P. S., Renda, C. R., Smits, R. R., Liston, K. J., Shahan, T. A., & Madden, G. J. (2013). Early and prolonged exposure to reward delay: Effects on impulsive choice and alcohol self-administration in male rats. *Experimental and Clinical Psychopharmacology, 21*(2), 172–180.

Stein, J. S., Renda, C. R., Hinnenkamp, J. E., & Madden, G. J. (2015). Impulsive choice, alcohol consumption, and pre-exposure to delayed rewards: II. Potential mechanisms. *Journal of the Experimental Analysis of Behavior, 103*(1), 33–49.

Stein, J. S., Sze, Y. Y., Athamneh, L., Koffarnus, M. N., Epstein, L. H., & Bickel, W. K. (2017). Think fast: Rapid assessment of the effects of episodic future thinking on delay discounting in overweight/obese participants. *Journal of Behavioral Medicine, 40*(5), 832–838.

Stephens, D. W. (1981). The logic of risk-sensitive foraging preferences. *Animal Behaviour, 29*(2), 628–629.

Stephens, D. W., & Charnov, E. L. (1982). Optimal foraging: Some simple stochastic models. *Behavioral Ecology and Sociobiology, 10*(4), 251–263.

Stilling, S. T., & Critchfield, T. S. (2010). The matching relation and situation-specific bias modulation in professional football play selection. *Journal of the Experimental Analysis of Behavior, 93*(3), 435–454.

Subramaniam, S., & Kyonka, E. G. E. (2022). Human temporal learning with mixed signals. *Behavioural Processes, 195*, Article 104568.

Thaler, R. H., & Sunstein, C. R. (2009). *Nudge: Improving decisions about health, wealth, and happiness* (rev. and expanded ed.). Penguin Books.

Toegel, F., & Perone, M. (2022). Effects of advance notice on transition-related pausing in pigeons. *Journal of the Experimental Analysis of Behavior, 117*, 3–19.

Vanderveldt, A., Oliveira, L., & Green, L. (2016). Delay discounting: Pigeon, rat, human—Does it matter? *Journal of Experimental Psychology: Animal Learning and Cognition, 42*(2), 141–162.

Wade-Galuska, T., Perone, M., & Wirth, O. (2005). Effects of past and upcoming response-force requirements on fixed-ratio pausing. *Behavioural Processes, 68*(1), 91–95.

Waltz, T. J., & Follette, W. C. (2009). Molar functional relations and clinical behavior analysis: Implications for assessment and treatment. *Behavior Analyst, 32*(1), 51–68.

Williams, D. C., Saunders, K. J., & Perone, M. (2011). Extended pausing by humans on multiple fixed-ratio schedules with varied reinforcer magnitude and response requirements. *Journal of the Experimental Analysis of Behavior, 95*(2), 203–220.

Wolery, M., Busick, M., Reichow, B., & Barton, E. E. (2010). Comparison of overlap methods for quantitatively synthesizing single-subject data. *Journal of Special Education, 44*(1), 18–28.

Wolfe, K., Seaman, M. A., & Drasgow, E. (2016). Interrater agreement on the visual analysis of individual tiers and functional relations in multiple baseline designs. *Behavior Modification, 40*(6), 852–873.

Wolfe, K., & Slocum, T. A. (2015). A comparison of two approaches to training visual analysis of AB graphs. *Journal of Applied Behavior Analysis, 48*(2), 472–477.

Young, M. E. (2017). Discounting: A practical guide to multilevel analysis of indifference data. *Journal of the Experimental Analysis of Behavior, 108*(1), 97–112.

Young, M. E. (2018). Discounting: A practical guide to multilevel analysis of choice data. *Journal of the Experimental Analysis of Behavior, 109*(2), 293–312.

PART II

EXPERIMENTAL METHODOLOGY

CHAPTER 3

Single-Case Experimental Designs

Kevin M. Ayres

Sidman's publication *Tactics of Scientific Research* (1960) is frequently cited as one of the first textbooks in single-case experimental design (SCED). Researchers in multiple disciplines beyond behavior analysis use these designs, including, education, special education, social work, nursing, athletic training, and speech pathology. The designs lend themselves well to human service fields, where evaluation of intervention at the individual level is important. This chapter describes the underlying logic and design features that make SCED a compelling option for drawing causal conclusions, especially in situations where a researcher does not have access to a large enough pool of participants to satisfy requirements for statistical power or where the phenomenon under investigation may benefits from a more nuanced level of analysis that monitors change closely over time. Regardless of why a researcher chooses an SCED in place of, or to augment, a group design, SCED includes several variations that offer researchers rigorous options to control for threats to internal validity.

In contrast to group design and group design logic, participants in an SCED study serve as their own control. In other words, the behavior of each participant in an SCED study is measured in two or more conditions and is only compared to their own behavior in another condition. Sometimes referred to as *baseline logic* (Ledford & Gast, 2018), this practice allows flexibility within a study and can help account for many differences between participants including skills repertoire and reinforcement history, among others. Generally considered an inductive rather than deductive approach to answering research questions (Plavnik & Ferreri, 2013), SCED relies heavily on replication within and across subjects. The designs discussed later in this chapter reflect this emphasis on repeated demonstration of effect at different points in time (Horner et al. 2005).

Underlying Assumptions and Logic

If you have taken coursework dedicated to SCED, then this chapter will serve as a review. If you have not taken coursework related to SCED, this chapter will provide a basic survey of the most common designs, the types of questions for which they are suited, and general information about how researchers tend to write their research reports. This chapter is organized around the typical layout of an SCED research report. This provides the opportunity to discuss relevant aspects of design features and reporting standards as they relate to different report sections (e.g., participants, measurement) and key considerations for ensuring high quality and control for threats to internal validity. The section specific to design types goes into as much detail as is feasible in a single chapter and describes the most common SCEDs and how they control for threats to internal validity, as well as any special considerations with those designs. The design section starts with a discussion of simple AB designs as a building block for more rigorous evaluations and begins to describe the process of visual analysis. The chapter concludes with a discussion of data analysis. While visual analysis has served as the benchmark standard for evaluation of causal relations in SCED, significant new work has made quantitative statistical analysis and synthesis possible (see Kratochwill et al., 2021).

Throughout the chapter, readers will have opportunities to examine graphs relevant to the different designs. The graphs have been crafted to represent "ideal" cases and showcase standard practice in graphing conventions, as well as data presentation. Most textbooks dedicated to single-case designs contain more comprehensive and extensive examples of graphs (both of contrived data and published data) to help readers learn to discriminate effects from noneffects with different SCED. For the purpose of this chapter, and to provide an introduction to SCEDs, we will look at very simple graphs of contrived data to highlight key features.

Introductions

The introductions of most SCED reports differ little, if at all, from reports on group designs. Usually, the researcher frames a rationale regarding some significant problem in society or gap in the scientific literature. They synthesize relevant studies related to the phenomena, citing current and seminal work to build the case that their study can make a contribution to scientific knowledge. In doing so, they incorporate both other SCEDs, as well as relevant group designs. Applied studies may draw on basic or translational work, and vice versa, to provide a cogent rationale for their investigation. The introduction usually concludes with a statement of the research question(s).

While generally not a design used in a traditional hypothesis-testing manner, SCED research questions generally take one of two forms. The first form, perhaps analogous to a two-tailed hypothesis, sets up the question to suggest that the participant's responding could increase or decrease: "What effect do signaled reinforcement delays have on participant responding?" In a more exploratory sense, perhaps in an area of work where there are fewer studies exploring the same phenomena, the two-tailed approach leaves open some possibility that the experimental manipulation could cause acceleration, deceleration, or no change at all in responding. In contrast to a more one-tailed type approach: "Do signaled delays to reinforcement result in decreased response rates?" A one-tailed type route represents a more conservative approach to posing the question and, in the earlier case, also suggests what aspect of responding one expects to observe. Following the posing of the research question, the report moves into the method section.

Method

Participants and Participant Description

While basic researchers typically have more control than applied researchers over participant homogeneity, SCED provides an opportunity for researchers to consider populations that are more diverse on general demographic-type characteristics. As described by Wolery and Ezell (1983) for participants in SCED, the most important aspect of a participant's description and characteristics revolves around their baseline level performance and the reason for that level of responding. In applied studies, this might include information from a functional analysis to describe the maintaining reinforcers for some target problem behavior, whereas in basic experiments, this would include information about the species, experimental history/naiveté, or aspects of current access to reinforcement (e.g., 80% of free feeding weight).

Basic researchers are often able to secure the precise participant types they want. Many applied researchers have participant pools more influenced by convenience. Either way, thorough descriptions benefit research consumers and other researchers, because they communicate something about the extent to which one might expect results to generalize (i.e., have external validity). Moreover, good descriptions can assist in contextualizing idiosyncratic results (e.g., if one participant's responding did not replicate another's, and further examination of their characteristics reveals, perhaps, they have more experimental experience—basic, or they had entry level skills not understood to be related to the dependent variable—applied).

Related to internal validity, good descriptions of participants also allow the researcher to communicate about potential selection bias by clearly discussing recruitment procedures, as well as inclusion–exclusion criteria. Additionally, the participant section would include descriptions of any participant attrition. This becomes a concern if an insufficient number of participants complete the experimental protocol, thus limiting opportunities to evaluate effects, or if some pattern of attrition emerges that relates to the experiment. For example, participants in the final legs of a multiple baseline drop out because of treatment delays.

Settings and Arrangements

After a thorough participant description, typical SCED reports describe the settings and arrangements of the baseline and experimental conditions. This usually includes a physical description of the location. For example, participants sat in a 5m × 5m office that included a desk and an iMac computer running a customized software package. A researcher sat behind them and to the side. The room contained a camera oriented toward their face mounted on the ceiling. The purpose of all of this, as with the participant description, is to facilitate replication. Often, this area of a report also includes information about any materials (short of the procedures that might be incorporated into a computer program). This part of most reports likely has less bearing on explaining attempts to guard against threats to internal validity but has greater relation to external validity and replication.

Measurement and Reliability

Whereas basic and translational research often rely on automated data collection, applied researchers usually rely on human observers coding videos or live observation. Regardless of research domain, clear descriptions of dependent variables and the means of measuring them are critical. Identifying the dimension (i.e., repeatability, temporal extent, or temporal locus) steers the researcher to identify an appropriate measurement system.

To guard against instrumentation threats and to bolster confidence in data accuracy, researchers using single-case designs generally aim to collect interrater reliability in a minimum of 30% of sessions for each participant in each condition (and for each primary data collector if more than one individual collects primary data; Ledford & Gast, 2018). There are several means by which to compute reliability dependent on the nature of the dependent variable. Generally, the reliability is reported in terms of percentage agreement. In some instances, to mitigate inflation of agreement by chance correspondence of the observations, researchers report kappa (Kratochwill et al., 2010). Scoring and evaluating reliability during the course of the study rather than post hoc allows researchers to address low reliability immediately (e.g., retrain observers).

Researchers report reliability data in their measurement section. The way they report it varies, but in general they provide the range and mean for each dependent variable, ideally broken down by research participant. Depending on the nature of the dependent measure and data source, the usual standard threshold of agreement is 80% agreement or 0.6 kappa (Kratochwill et al., 2013). As noted by Kennedy (2005), these standards for level of reliability are arbitrary and may be insufficient at detecting instrumentation threats. In instances where researchers have a permanent product (e.g., a written response), one would anticipate higher reliability than in a study where the dependent variable focuses on speech production during live observation. In situations where interobserver agreement is below the minimum acceptable level, the researchers should provide some indication for the discrepancy and what they did to address it.

The Independent Variable

SCED studies involve the active manipulation of the independent variable by the researchers. Describing the parameters and procedures before and after the manipulation is critical for potential replication. Information about experimental sessions typically begins with a set of general procedures that are common across conditions (e.g., session length) and then are followed by an explicit, step-by-step outline of what the researchers (or other active nonparticipants—therapists, teachers, parents) did in the course of the session in relation to the participant responding. Each condition (e.g., baseline, intervention) has its own section of the study description, in which researchers provide detailed descriptions.

To assure themselves, as well as consumers of their work, that the procedures were implemented as described in all conditions, researchers should report procedural fidelity data. Researchers should be sensitive to errors of commission (e.g., extra prompting) and omission (i.e., failing to reinforce a response meeting definition; DiGennaro Reed & Codding, 2014; Kodak et al., 2022). Like reliability, collecting procedural fidelity across at least 30% of sessions in each condition (and for each interventionist) is important for building confidence that the experiment shows what the researchers intended. Moreover, when collected and analyzed during the experiment, fidelity data can help alert researchers to any issues with treatment integrity, so they can make appropriate adjustments. Also, like reliability, procedural fidelity data are often reported as a percentage. Researchers usually describe their procedures for gathering procedural fidelity alongside their description of reliability and report the data there in a manner like reports of reliability (i.e., mean, range, and explanation of any instances in which fidelity is lower than acceptable).

Research Designs

The components of SCED described earlier are common to all contemporary research using single-case designs in behavior analysis. This section provides brief overviews of the most common designs, the types of questions for which they are best suited, and a summary of how they guard against or detect different threats to internal validity. Example graphs illustrate the means of data presentation and analysis to help put the design in context. Each of these designs builds on baseline logic in various ways and use simple A-B comparisons as their foundation. The sequencing and repetition of these A-B contrasts fundamentally differentiate each design.

Figure 3.1 shows a simple AB design. The researcher has collected data in the absence of treatment for self-injurious behavior (SIB). They begin intervention and SIB decreases. This correlation might indicate positive treatment effects. However, with just one demonstrated change in the dependent variable, one must consider other alternatives. For example, did the participant happen to begin a new medication on the exact same day

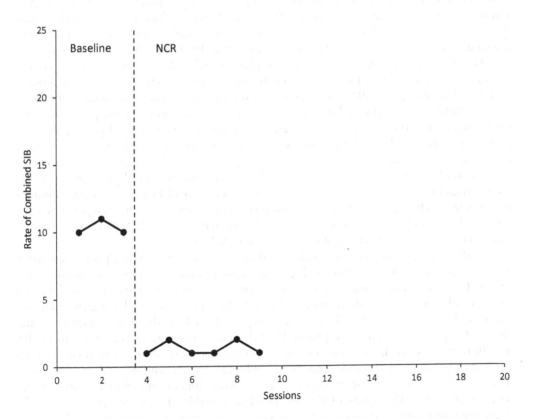

FIGURE 3.1. Hypothetical A-B graph. NCR, noncontingent reinforcement.

behavioral treatment began? Perhaps not likely, but not impossible. An AB design begins to suggest that there might be a relation (a correlation), but the researcher needs replication. A withdrawal design can provide that.

Withdrawal and Reversal Designs

On a graph, withdrawal and reversal designs often look very similar and frequently the terms are used interchangeably. Delving into the differences is beyond the scope of this chapter but readers might refer to Leitenberg (1973), who originally drew the distinction, and Wine et al. (2015), who provide an argument against a distinction. These designs are powerful tools for answering questions related to free-operant responding and situations where behavior has a reasonable probability of returning to prior levels of responding once intervention is withdrawn. In human experiments, researchers do not frequently use this design to evaluate instructional type interventions whereby participants learn a particular skill (e.g., reading) that is unlikely to degrade with removal of instruction. Other SCEDs are more suited to these sorts of questions.

Researchers sometimes refer to withdrawal or reversal designs as ABAB designs, because of the specific sequence and repetition of the baseline (A) and treatment (B) conditions. Regardless of how researchers refer to the design, the basic elements involve establishing steady-state responding in the first phase prior to moving to the second phase. The term *condition* refers to the experimental condition (e.g., baseline, intervention), and *phase* refers to the time frame in the experiment that typically corresponds to the conditions but not always (this distinction will be described later in multielement designs).

The stability of the data path in the first phase should allow the researcher to predict the value of the next data point if the researcher makes no changes in the independent variable. This usually involves collection of three or more consecutive data points with low variability. More data, following that same pattern, would make the prediction easier. In Figure 3.2, the gray boxes represent where the researcher would predict the data path to go if they made no changes in the independent variable. This hypothetical prediction acts, in some ways, like a null hypothesis. For example, if the data are 10 responses per minute, 11 responses per minute, and 10 responses per minute, the researcher would likely predict the next data point would fall between 10 and 11 responses per minute if they made no change; therefore, they can introduce a change in the independent variable. If the data changes, in correlation to the change in the independent variable, the researcher may have a demonstration of experimental effect.

With this example, the researcher makes a change, and participant responding decreases to 1 response per minute, 2 responses per minute, 1 response per minute, and finally 1 response per minute. At this point, the researcher can look at their data and make another prediction about where the next data point would be if they made no changes. Then they would make a change (typically back to the prior condition, what they had in place during the first phase). If, at this point, the data increase back to 11, 10, and 10 responses per minute, the researcher's confidence regarding the relation between their manipulation of the independent variable and the dependent variable increases. They now have two demonstrations of effect, at two points in time, that also correspond to their change in the status of the independent variable. The logic here rests on the decreasing probability that some other factor (history threat, maturation, etc., has influenced the data. The threshold, however, to assert experimental control or a functional relation (i.e., causation) requires at least one more demonstration of effect. At this point,

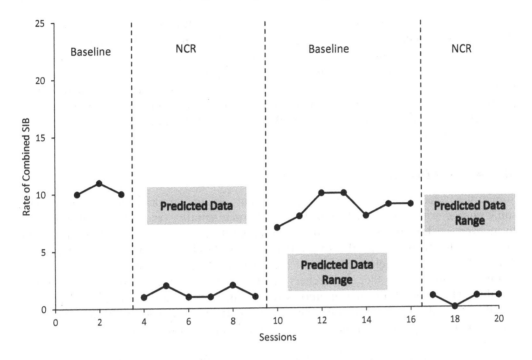

FIGURE 3.2. Data from a hypothetical withdrawal design. The gray boxes represent where one would predict data from the previous condition would be if the conditions did not change. NCR, noncontingent reinforcement.

the researcher is in the second A phase (i.e., A-B-A) and, if the data are steady, will make the same prediction they have been making, followed by a change.

Researchers generally regard this design as the most powerful demonstration of experimental control. The dependent variable only changes when the independent variable changes. The design has built in intrasubject replication and allows for detection of history and maturation threats by the returning to baseline and reintroduction of intervention. If something outside of the experiment was influencing the dependent variable, then the data likely would not return to baseline levels of responding when intervention is withdrawn. Further strengthening confidence that the lone factor responsible for this change involves the manipulation of the independent variable comes when the intervention is reintroduced and similar levels of responding in this fourth phase mirror the second.

Extensions

When researchers want to make comparisons of more than one independent variable to a baseline, they can extend this design while maintaining the same logic. Where an A-B-A-B represents the comparison of a baseline (A) to treatment (B), an A-B-A-B-C-B-C represents that same comparison but adds another by contrasting B to C. In the analysis and evaluation of these graphs, researchers generally only compare adjacent conditions (A to B, B to C, but not A to C) and like conditions (i.e., A to A) to draw conclusions. This recognizes the potential influence that, in this example, B might have on C. Therefore, the researcher would compare A1 (i.e., the first A phase) to B1 and A2, but they would not typically make a comparison of the A phases to C1 or C2. Like a regular withdrawal, the same safeguards for internal validity are in place, but the researcher needs to concern themselves with the sequence issue mentioned previously. If they had additional participants, and the logic of the treatments permits, adding those additional participants and counterbalancing the treatment order would potentially help reveal sequence threats (i.e., A-C-A-C-B-C-B).

Multielement Designs

Sometimes referred to as alternating treatment designs, multielement designs share some characteristics with A-B-A-B designs. Fundamentally, researchers may use them to answer similar questions related to free-operant responding or in situations where behavior is likely to be amenable to reverting to prior levels of responding. Different from A-B-A-B designs, multielement designs do not rely on steady-state responding prior to changing conditions. In fact, researchers rapidly alternate conditions irrespective of data stability. This type of alternation allows rapid data collection on multiple independent variables in a short period of time. This comes with the drawback that the rapid alternations may hamper discrimination of the condition, resulting in significant carryover between conditions.

Figure 3.3 depicts a hypothetical, two-condition alternating treatments design contrasting two reinforcer arrangements and their effect on SIB. The fact that the differential reinforcement of alternative (DRA) condition drops and then rises again is not as important as the consistency of the differences between the two lines (i.e., lack of overlap).

This design can be combined with other designs to respond to multifaceted questions. The data paths do not differentiate; sometimes researchers change their design approach and use an A-B-A-B design, as these tend to promote greater discrimination as a function of more consecutive sessions in a single condition before alternating. With a multielement, sometimes adding very salient discriminative stimuli to the sessions enhances discrimination.

Ideally, Figure 3.4 would have condition labels above the associated phases but, to continue from the previous figure and to avoid crowding the top of the figure, I have relied on different shaped data points and a legend to the side. In the first phase, researchers collected baseline data. They followed this with a multielement design. They could have included alternations of baseline sessions within this phase, but sometimes fewer conditions in a comparison phase permit better discrimination. Because of the overlap between the data paths, the hypothetical researchers returned to baseline and began an A-B-A-B style comparison. By doing this, they mitigate some of the multitreatment interference threat that could have contributed to the undifferentiated data paths during the comparison phase. By running out an A-B-A-B with both independent variables, the researchers can identify successful treatments more clearly.

In applied settings, researchers often use multielement designs to set up functional analyses to identify the reinforcers maintaining a client's problem behavior. These provide a powerful tool in those contexts but are adaptable to a range of scenarios where the researcher can quickly move back and forth between conditions. The sequence or order of the conditions is frequently planned with some sort of rule in mind so as to prevent several of the same conditions from occurring in a row. For example, if a researcher

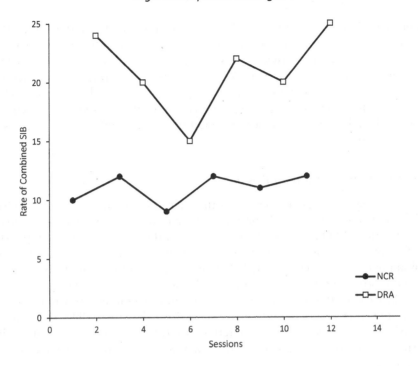

FIGURE 3.3. A hypothetical multielement study. NCR, noncontingent reinforcement; DRA, differential reinforcement of alternative behavior.

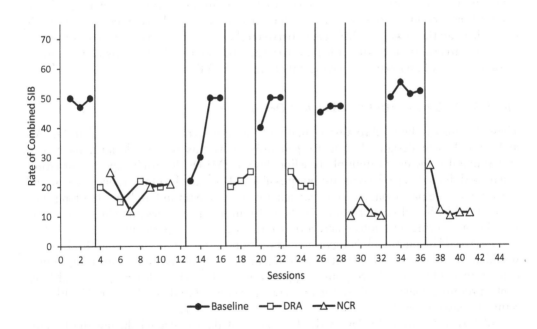

FIGURE 3.4. Hypothetical data with a multielement design in the second phase combined with a withdrawal design. NCR, noncontingent reinforcement; DRA, differential reinforcement of alternative behavior.

implements a study with conditions A, B, C, and D, they might randomize within each block or series, so that the participant is exposed to each condition once before being exposed to another condition twice. They might generate a sequence of C-A-D-B and then in the next series randomly select A-B-D-C. The randomization assists with reducing the likelihood that some pattern develops as a function of the sequence. There are other occasions, however, where the sequence is specifically set and remains constant to capitalize on changing motivation across conditions (i.e., establishing operations; Hammond et al., 2013).

Adapted Alternating Treatment Designs

Sindelar et al. (1985) proposed a version of the alternating treatments design (referred to as *multielement* earlier) that would permit such an evaluation. With adapted alternating treatment design (AATD), the researcher has to identify two behaviors of approximately equal difficulty (e.g., same number of steps, same number and type of discriminations) and then apply one treatment to one behavior (e.g., video modeling to making a sandwich) and the other treatment to the other behavior (e.g., *in vivo* modeling to popping popcorn). Cariveau et al. (2021) provide an overview of techniques researchers have used to identify appropriate targets and equate their difficulty. Regardless of method used, once identified, researchers usually counterbalance this order (i.e., reverse it) with a second participant and try to get at least three or four participants so they can see if the results replicate.

To begin the experiment, the researchers start baseline similar to what is described for a withdrawal, and then apply both interventions to their respective responses. This application would continue until one response reaches mastery criteria, then typically run out until the second response reaches mastery or some a priori decision point to stop. The researcher can then evaluate differences between the treatments based on acquisition rate and errors to criterion, among others. Carriveau and Fetzner (2022) provided a comprehensive review of analyzing experimental control in AATDs.

Multiple-Probe and Multiple-Baseline Designs

These designs can be used to answer many of the same types of questions that A-B-A-B and multielement designs do but are generally viewed as weaker designs. Baer et al. (1968) detailed the use of multiple-baseline designs (MBDs) for use in specific situations where withdrawal-type designs are not possible. MBDs tend to take longer to run and, if using multiple participants, some participants may remain in baseline for a long time, increasing likelihood of attrition. MBDs and multiple-probe designs (MPDs) are well suited to answering questions where a return to baseline level performance is unlikely or to do so would be unethical. For example, if teaching letter sounds to young children, one would not desire to punish correct responding in a return to baseline. While programmed extinction might result in response suppression, skills such as learning to read likely contact reinforcement outside of the experimental context and are therefore less likely to return to baseline levels.

MBDs differ from MPDs in the frequency of data collected during the baseline phase. When Horner and Baer (1978) introduced MPD, their aim was to examine the gradual increase in acquisition of chained behaviors (e.g., Steps 1–3, then Steps 4–6, and finally Steps 7–10). Contemporary applications have expanded beyond this. Both designs are set up in tiers whereby the introduction of intervention is staggered so that while the first tier experiences the independent variable manipulation, the other tiers do not. The graph depicted in Figure 3.5 shows a hypothetical MBD across participants used to evaluate the effects of a token economy on work engagement. Notice that the researcher reports three baseline data points for the first participant, nine for the second, and 16 for the third. This "stagger" of baseline lengths prior to intervention provides basic control for history and maturation threats. If the data accelerated in the Participant 3's baseline, then that should alert the researcher to a possible history threat. Perhaps the Participant 3 observed what Participant 1 was doing and responded to that. Regardless, the stability

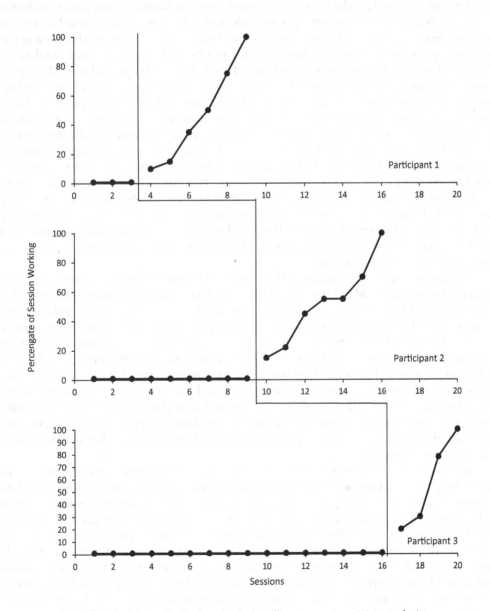

FIGURE 3.5. A hypothetical multiple-baseline, across-participants design.

of these baselines prior to intervention and the change only after intervention is in place, provides the researcher the ability to demonstrate experimental control.

Ideally, baseline lengths of the first tier would be at least three data points to demonstrate stability. Second and third tiers would reflect the same number of data points as in the baseline of the first tier, plus at least as many data points as the preceding tier required to reach some set criterion indicating meaningful behavior change. This demonstrates that responding during the second and third tiers will not change just because of repeated exposure to the baseline conditions.

Returning to the distinction between MBD and MPD, summarily, in a multiple baseline data are collected on the tiers not receiving intervention every time data is collected on the tier receiving intervention. In a multiple probe, the data collection in baseline on tiers not receiving intervention is simply less frequent. Figure 3.6 shows the same hypothetical experiment as Figure 3.5 but arranged as a multiple probe. The gaps in data on the second and third tiers indicate that researchers did not collect data during those time spans. This approach is most often taken for one of two reasons. First, the researchers may be evaluating some sort of instructional procedure and repeated exposure in baseline (i.e., every session) to stimuli with which the participant is unfamiliar or to which the participant cannot respond correctly, which may result in either an inhibitive testing threat (i.e., the participant just stops responding because they have contacted extinction so many times) or a facilitative testing threat in which, over time, they start to respond correctly by chance through repeated exposures. The other reason a researcher might resort to an MPD is just pragmatic. MPDs are less time and labor intensive (i.e., fewer sessions). This, however, exposes the researcher to risk in that they lose the opportunity to detect history threats when not collecting data. Note, each tier still has a different number of data points. This, again, helps to demonstrate that repeated exposure to baseline alone will not result in change.

Researchers generally arrange MBD and MPD across behaviors, participants, or settings. In situations where the researcher can identify three or more behaviors of a participant that might be sensitive to the independent variable, they may run the experiment across behaviors. For example, if using strategic incremental rehearsal (e.g., Finn et al., 2023) to teach letter identification, the researcher might create groups of five letters and implement with one set of letters receiving intervention on the first tier while the other two remain in baseline. Once the participant masters the first set of letters, they introduce intervention on the second set while the third set remains in baseline. When the participant masters the second set, the researcher applies intervention to the third set. While this provides a good opportunity for intrasubject replication of effects, having additional participants exposed to the same intervention in a similar manner would enhance the experiment.

In some cases, a researcher's treatment might be very narrowly tailored, and a single participant might not have multiple behaviors for which the intervention would be appropriate. For example, chances are, a researcher evaluating an intervention to teach toileting to young children could only apply the treatment to that single behavior and therefore would recruit at least three total participants (more participants are always better, as this guards against attrition). In this case, the researcher runs the multiple baseline across participants. In other situations, a researcher might have an intervention that would be appropriately evaluated across settings. For example, in a school context, a researcher might want to evaluate some group contingency such as the Good Behavior Game (introduced by Schmidt & Ulrich, 1969) on classroom behavior. They could use a

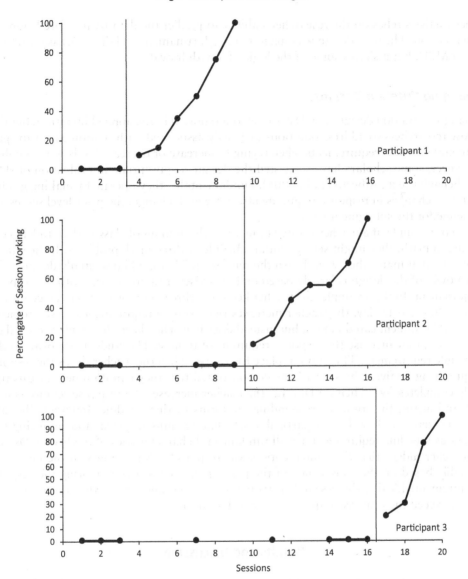

FIGURE 3.6. Similar hypothetical data to Figure 3.5 but shown in the context of a multiple-probe design across participants.

withdrawal design but might encounter resistance from classroom teachers if the teachers observe positive effects. The researcher can identify three or more classroom contexts for the same group of participants (perhaps an elementary-age cohort that travels to three different classes together). They can then evaluate the effects of the Good Behavior Game on reading time, art class, and lunchtime.

Together, MPD and MBD provide researchers a way to answer specific questions, especially those related to some form of skill acquisition, when other designs are not possible or desirable. Stability in baseline before introducing treatment on any tier is critical, since analysis relies on the researcher's ability to predict the data path before beginning intervention. The next design was suggested by Hartmann and Hall (1976) as a variation of an MPD, but it shares some of the logic of a withdrawal.

Changing Criterion Designs

Changing criterion designs (CCDs) are seldom reported in the applied literature, but they allow researchers to address questions primarily associated with reinforcement (or punishment) schedule requirements when trying to increase or decrease levels of responding. However, some scholars have suggested the design is appropriate in evaluation of shaping behavior (e.g., Alberto et al., 2006). Fundamentally, they operate by making gradual stepwise changes in response requirements. After each change, the prior level serves as a baseline for the subsequent level.

For example, if a teacher wanted to increase the amount of classwork a student completed in math, they might set the initial schedule at three math problems. If the student achieved that many, they would earn the reinforcer. They could potentially do more, but the power of the design is largely based on how closely responding fits with the response requirement. In this example, the teacher keeps the three math problems in place for four days. On the fifth day, the teacher increases the response requirement to five problems. Again, the student can do more, but instead does five. They keep this in place for 3 days. On Day 7, they increase the response requirement to nine. The student conforms to that schedule requirement. This stays in place for 2 days. Then the teacher drops the response requirement to five. The student has demonstrated that they can do nine, but this time only completes five. Then on Day 12, the teacher increases the response requirement to 10, and again, the student's responding conforms to the schedule. Intentionally varying the step size, how long a particular schedule remains in place, and returning to a previous schedule requirement are all fundamental characteristics of quality CCDs. The researcher judges that their intervention was responsible for changes in the dependent variable based on the consistency of the participant's responses mirroring the response requirement. Ideally, the researcher arranges the experiment such that the participant could exceed the response requirement (but does not).

Results and Discussion

One unique characteristic of SCED is that the research consumer sees all the data the researcher sees to draw their conclusions. Researchers have traditionally relied on visual analysis as the primary means to evaluate their data in SCED studies. This involves, as discussed throughout, observing changes in the dependent variable only when they have manipulated the independent variable. Researchers look for six basic data features (Horner et al., 2005): changes in level, trend, variability, overlap, immediacy of change, and similarity of like conditions. These features are examined around the condition change line (ABAB, MPD, MBD) or in sequential contrast (multielement, CCD). At least one, level, trend, or variability should show changes between adjacent conditions or sequential contrast. And then the researcher should observe low overlap between adjacent conditions and immediacy of effects (more overlap or delayed changes indicating less powerful effects). Finally, they look to see consistency of effects across like conditions:

B1 to B2 in a withdrawal, consistent changes from baseline to intervention in MBD and MPD, and low overlap in multielement and AATDs.

Contemporary researchers have begun to conduct some quantitative analysis of their data beyond simple means and medians. While attempts at quantifying changes and statistically analyzing them have gone on for a long time, greater consensus and acceptability has begun to emerge among researchers. Discussion of all the reasons and arguments surrounding different means of quantifying SCED studies is beyond the scope of this chapter, but the general discussion has provided opportunities for researchers to look at their data more critically and consider alternatives for analysis (for some examples and discussion, see Kratochwill et al., 2021).

Despite the growing interest in quantitative analysis (i.e., effect sizes), these procedures are still generally considered secondary and corroborative of determinations regarding a functional relation. Some statistical tests exist to evaluate whether a result is likely due to chance, but these are largely absent from the published empirical studies. Rather, researchers display graphs for each participant and discuss those participants' data and any differences in outcomes between one participant and another. They then summarize limitations related to their design, data, and experiment to situate their findings humbly within the context of related work.

After a researcher reports their results, they conclude with a section designed to contextualize the results in the larger scope of science. They normally return to their research questions and discuss how their findings answer those questions, and what those answers mean relative to other published work (e.g., corroborate, refute, extend). Also, researchers discuss the limitations of their study and highlight for readers issues that arose during the study that might temper any conclusions one draws from the data. This also may suggest changes in procedures or design that would strengthen a potential replication.

SCEDs provide valuable opportunities to ask questions in contexts or situations that are not amenable to group designs. Researchers operating in client-centered environments can evaluate the effects of their treatment and draw causal conclusions. They can also capitalize on this inductive approach to reasoning and contribute to the larger body of research. Rigorous SCED can inform the scientific community about phenomena that group designs and other research traditions cannot. The unique and dynamic nature of these designs and the flexibility they afford researchers make them invaluable.

REFERENCES

Alberto, P., Troutman, A. C., & Axe, J. B. (2006). *Applied behavior analysis for teachers* (pp. 1–474). Pearson Merrill Prentice Hall.

Baer, D. M., Wolf, M. M., & Risley, T. R. (1968). Some current dimensions of applied behavior analysis. *Journal of Applied Behavior Analysis, 1*(1), 91–97.

Cariveau, T., Batchelder, S., Ball, S., & La Cruz Montilla, A. (2021). Review of methods to equate target sets in the adapted alternating treatments design. *Behavior Modification, 45*(5), 695–714.

Cariveau, T., & Fetzner, D. (2022). Experimental control in the adapted alternating treatments design: A review of procedures and outcomes. *Behavioral Interventions, 37*(3), 805–818.

DiGennaro Reed, F. D., & Codding, R. S. (2014). Advancements in procedural fidelity assessment and intervention: Introduction to the special issue. *Journal of Behavioral Education, 23*(1), 1–18.

Finn, C. E., Ardoin, S. P., & Ayres, K. M. (2023). Effects of incremental rehearsal on sight word and letter acquisition among students with autism and cognitive impairment. *Journal of Applied School Psychology, 39*(2), 179–200.

Hammond, J. L., Iwata, B. A., Rooker, G. W., Fritz, J. N., & Bloom, S. E. (2013). Effects of fixed versus random condition sequencing during multielement functional analyses. *Journal of Applied Behavior Analysis, 46*(1), 22–30.

Hartmann, D. P., & Hall, R. V. (1976). The changing criterion design. *Journal of Applied Behavior Analysis, 9*(4), 527–532.

Horner, R. D., & Baer, D. M. (1978). Multiple-probe technique: A variation on the multiple baseline. *Journal of Applied Behavioral Analysis, 11*(1), 189–196.

Horner, R. H., Carr, E. G., Halle, J., McGee, G., Odom, S., & Wolery, M. (2005). The use of single-subject research to identify evidence-based practice in special education. *Exceptional Children, 71*(2), 165–179.

Kennedy, C. H. (2005). *Single-case designs for educational research*. Allyn & Bacon.

Kodak, T., Bergmann, S., & Waite, M. (2022). Strengthening the procedural fidelity research-to-practice loop in animal behavior. *Journal of the Experimental Analysis of Behavior, 118*, 215–236.

Kratochwill, T. R., Hitchcock, J., Horner, R. H., Levin, J. R., Odom, S. L., Rindskopf, D. M., & Shadish, W. R. (2010). *Single-case designs technical documentation*. What Works Clearinghouse.

Kratochwill, T. R., Hitchcock, J. H., Horner, R. H., Levin, J. R., Odom, S. L., Rindskopf, D. M., & Shadish, W. R. (2013). Single-case intervention research design standards. *Remedial and Special Education, 34*(1), 26–38.

Kratochwill, T. R., Horner, R. H., Levin, J. R., Machalicek, W., Ferron, J., & Johnson, A. (2021). Single-case design standards: An update and proposed upgrades. *Journal of School Psychology, 89*, 91–105.

Ledford, J. R., & Gast, D. L. (Eds.). (2018). *Single case research methodology*. Routledge.

Leitenberg, H. (1973). The use of single-case methodology in psychotherapy research. *Journal of Abnormal Psychology, 82*, 87–101.

Plavnick, J. B., & Ferreri, S. J. (2013). Single-case experimental designs in educational research: A methodology for causal analyses in teaching and learning. *Educational Psychology Review, 25*(4), 549–569.

Schmidt, G. W., & Ulrich, R. E. (1969). Effects of group contingent events upon classroom noise. *Journal of Applied Behavior Analysis, 2*, 171–179.

Sidman, M. (1960). *Tactics in scientific research*. Basic Books.

Sindelar, P. T., Rosenberg, M. S., & Wilson, R. J. (1985). An adapted alternating treatments design for instructional research. *Education and Treatment of Children, 8*, 67–76.

Wine, B., Freeman, T. R., & King, A. (2015). Withdrawal versus reversal: A necessary distinction? *Behavioral Interventions, 30*(1), 87–93.

Wolery, M., & Ezell, H. K. (1993). Subject descriptions and single-subject research. *Journal of Learning Disabilities, 26*(10), 642–647.

CHAPTER 4

Hybrid Experimental Designs
COMBINING SINGLE-SUBJECT AND GROUP-BASED METHODS

Jonathan E. Friedel
Jeremy M. Haynes
Katherine R. Brown
Amy L. Odum

Behavior analysts traditionally have relied on single-subject research designs, in which each participant serves as their own control (Sidman, 1960). Therefore, one might ask: Why is there a chapter advocating for between-group designs in a book about behavior analysis? Simply, there are some research questions that are difficult or impossible to answer with single-subject designs. Despite the focus in the experimental analysis of behavior on reversal designs, learning is not a reversible process. Behavior is like a river: just as one cannot touch the same water twice because the same flow will never pass again, one cannot observe behavior in the exact same state twice. The organism will be different or changed based on experience. As an example, behavior change techniques to reduce or eliminate a behavior do not cause unlearning or forgetting (Bouton et al., 2021), so behavior cannot return to the state it was in prior to the learning process. Under the right conditions, behavior can be very durable. Sometimes the remarkable durability of learned behavior is desirable, such as when we ride a bicycle gracefully after years without practice; however, sometimes the remarkable durability of learned behavior is undesirable, such as when a child readily resumes screaming in the absence of their communication device. Although learning is not reversible, we can learn more functional behaviors over time, even as the old behavior remains forever in our repertoire, ready to reemerge should conditions warrant.

Despite the irreversibility of learning, behavior analysis was founded on the central notion that behavior should be directly observed[1] and analyzed at the individual level. The flagship *Journal of the Experimental Analysis of Behavior* was founded in 1958 to provide an outlet "for the original publication of experiments relevant to the behavior of

---

[1] See Kyonka and Subramaniam (Chapter 5, this volume) for measurement considerations.

individual organisms," which is still its mission today. A mere decade later, the *Journal of Applied Behavior Analysis* was launched to extend this mission, with a particular focus on "the analysis of behavior to problems of social importance." Indeed, there are major benefits to single-subject design, in which each participant serves as their own control (Sidman, 1960). The focus on the individual ensures outcomes that are beneficial and practical at the personal level, which is especially useful when the population under study is heterogenous and/or small (Horner et al., 2016). Furthermore, single-subject design is particularly useful in clinical settings, in which the purpose of the investigation is to directly benefit the client.

Despite the enduring value of single-subject research designs, there are several advantages to adopting group-based designs in behavior analysis. Throughout this chapter, we discuss when group-based designs may be considered in lieu of or as a complement to single-subject designs. In addition to contemplating group-based designs for methodological purposes, incorporating group-based designs may have a number of other benefits (Davison, 1999; Fisher & Lerman, 2014). Foremost of these, a wide array of inferential statistical analyses has been developed to analyze data from group-based studies, and statistics remain the most common way to communicate scientific findings. For example, 80% of psychology journals require inferential statistics for submission (Hubbard et al., 2016). Without group-based designs, behavior analysts are limited in our ability to broadly communicate findings. Poorly informed consumers of research readily conflate single-subject design experiments with anecdotal or case-study observations, as well as assume that the absence of statistical analysis equates to an inferior science. Incorporating group-based designs may also help address common criticisms of single-subject methodology such as the file drawer problem (Hagopian, 2020; Laraway et al., 2019; Tincani & Travers, 2019) and difficulty with replication (Tincani & Travers, 2019) of behavior analytic interventions across different populations of people, both of which we discuss later in this chapter.

As strongly as behavior analysts advocate for single-subject designs, they are also at times notably averse to group-based designs (Sidman, 1960). Behavior analysts have argued eloquently that behavior is a phenomenon of the individual. Experimental designs that rely on comparisons across groups seem at odds with the focus on the behavior of individuals. The core component of a group-based experimental design is always a comparison of aggregated data obtained from one group to aggregated data obtained from another (or more than one) group. Branch (1999) warns against using "the aggregate as the unit of analysis" (p. 90). Group-based experimental designs, like any other research methodology, are merely a tool, and researchers are wise to be aware of any tool that might be helpful in their research. There are some behavioral phenomena that, by their very nature, only exist as differences between individuals. For example, effects of biological sex, genetics, birth order, cultural background, addiction history, and other factors can only be studied between individuals.

Our goal in this chapter is to describe group-based experimental designs as they may be useful for a behavior analyst. We do not intend to convince behavior analysts to abandon irreplaceable single-subject experimental designs. Nor do we wish to "put lipstick on a pig" and argue that group-based experimental designs are better for studying behavioral phenomena than single-subject experimental designs. We outline research questions for which group-based experimental designs can be used simultaneously with single-subject experimental designs. For clarity, we refer to single-subject designs that also have group-based design components as "hybrid experimental designs." We also point out some of the potential weaknesses and issues related to internal validity of group and hybrid experimental designs, especially as they apply to behavioral research. Finally, we briefly touch on some of the data analysis practices, including some statistical techniques, for behavioral experiments employing group designs.

Single-Subject, Group-Based, and Hybrid Experimental Designs

A Brief History of Group-Based Designs

In 1935, R. A. Fisher published one of the most influential scientific books: *The Design of Experiments*. Fisher outlined several formalized experimental designs so that researchers could "add to natural knowledge by experimentation" (p. 3). The experimental designs described by Fisher were the starting point for the modern treatment of *design of experiments,* which as a term refers to the systematic design of an experiment in an effort to produce efficient analysis of data. Specifically, Fisher wrote, "I propose to consider a number of different types of experimentation, with especial reference to their logical structure, and to show that when the appropriate precautions are taken to make this structure complete, entirely valid inferences may be drawn from them" (p. 7). Fisher argued that careful design and execution of experiments would further knowledge by allowing clear answers to questions of interest. He also believed proper experimental design was the only way to develop knowledge from the limited sample of data that any scientist could collect. Behavior analysts will find much in common with the logic and conceptual goals outlined by Fisher in terms of finding knowledge about natural processes.[2]

Many behavior analysts would likely agree with Fisher's desire to use experimentation to develop knowledge about natural processes; however, they are also likely to find little of practical value in terms of experimental design in Fisher's seminal work. The experimental designs outlined by Fisher were all group-based experimental designs aimed at maximizing any differences between groups, so that the difference could be detected statistically (assuming there is a real difference between those groups). The search for orderly functional relations between the environment and behavior (Sidman, 1960) are, at best, difficult with Fisher's experimental designs. Additionally, Fisher's book contains the first reference to a formalized "null-hypothesis" (in essence, that there is no effect to be detected; Fisher, 1935, p. 15) that is at the core of significance testing, the dominant data-analytic approach in a variety of scientific fields. The formalized methods that have developed around the "design of experiments" all follow from Fisher's initial efforts. Null-hypothesis significance testing has largely been rejected as the principal method of data analysis among behavior analysts (Ator, 1999; Branch, 2014; Branch, 1999; Perone, 1999). Thus, it is not surprising that a behavior analyst would not find much practical use for the experimental designs outlined by Fisher.

Experimental and Observational Group-Based Studies

Group-based studies may be experimental or observational, depending on how the levels of the independent variable (IV) occur between subjects. For a study design to be

---

[2]Despite the importance of Fisher's work in statistics and other areas, we recognize that he held problematic ideas about genetics (as was not uncommon among scientists in his time; see Bodmer et al., 2021).

classified as an experiment, the researchers must have the ability to manipulate some IV to determine the effects on a dependent variable (DV). Some group-based studies are only observational in nature, in that the researcher does not have active control of the IV of interest (e.g., Cox & Reid, 2000). For example, Sloman et al. (2005) observed caregiver–child interactions to identify the frequency of problem behavior surrounding caregiver reprimands. In this example, there was no manipulation of the IV variable (reprimands). Many epidemiological studies, by their very nature, are observational. For example, studies examining the unsupported claim that vaccines are causal factors in autism do not manipulate vaccine delivery to detect changes in the rates of autism diagnoses (for a brief review, see Dudley et al., 2018).

Considering the variety of subject-level variables that are outside the control of an experimenter (especially in the applied realm; e.g., Cox & Virues-Ortega, 2016, 2022), it is not unreasonable that a behavior analyst would want to be aware of observational experimental designs. Hybrid designs may have features of single-subject experimental designs and group-based *observational* designs. Although some variables within the study can be manipulated, other variables can only be observed, and any effects of those variables on behavior must be inferred. For example, a researcher may have the ability to control the delivery of an intervention (e.g., using a multiple baseline design) but may not have the ability to control the client's diagnosis or medications (e.g., Cox & Virues-Ortega, 2016). Even though some of the variables may be outside of the control of the experimenter, the hybrid design would still be experimental in nature.

When the distinction is necessary, we refer to variables related to features of the organism (age, sex, species, etc.) that the experimenter is likely unable to control outside of the laboratory as "subject variables." We hope this distinction will be helpful in describing how experimental controls for subject variables are developed (see below).

Threats to Internal Validity and Group-Based Experimental Designs

There are different types of group-based experimental designs. Most relevant to behavior analysts, group-based experimental designs may also include repeated measurements of the same phenomena within the groups (e.g., hybrid designs). Rather than focus on specific types of group-based experimental designs, we wish to focus on the general methods of group-based experimental designs and how they relate to determining functional relations between IVs and behavior (i.e., controlling threats to internal validity). Practically, it is not possible within the scope of a single chapter to outline the various types of group-based experimental designs. Multiple books are devoted to the topic for the interested (e.g., Cox & Reid, 2000; Mukerjee & Wu, 2006; Webster & Sell, 2007). It is our hope that this section will be a resource to identify some of the key components in the event a researcher wishes to create a hybrid experimental design. Thus, our focus is on how components of group-based experimental designs can be used as experimental controls.

Biased Groups

One potential problem with a study that includes group-based components is that group membership may confound the effects of the IV on the DV. The general concern with grouping and bias is that there is the potential for unintended and uncontrolled relations between a confounding variable and group membership. For example, Matthews et al. (1977) described an experiment in which group-based analyses were conducted for a group of participants for whom operant behaviors (button and key presses) were shaped and a group of participants for whom the operant behavior was demonstrated by the experimenter. However, participants were assigned to the demonstration group if the shaping process went too slowly. Thus, the grouping by "demonstration" was also confounded with a failure to rapidly learn via the shaping process. The authors attributed an insensitivity to the schedules of reinforcement to the demonstration of the operant behavior by the experimenter. However, a possible alternative explanation is that the group was insensitive to the contingencies the experimenters arranged, which was demonstrated first as a failure to learn by shaping and then via changes in schedules of reinforcement.

As another example of group membership confounded with another variable, it is well established that cigarette smokers are more likely to steeply discount delayed outcomes compared to nonsmokers (Bickel et al., 1999; DeHart et al., 2020; Friedel et al., 2014, 2016). Nonsmokers also tend to obtain higher levels of education than cigarette smokers (Jaroni et al., 2004). If a study is designed to compare the degree of discounting across levels of education, then a researcher may end up with a sample that incidentally has more smokers across some groups than across others based on the distribution of people who do and do not smoke cigarettes across the levels of education. A researcher may conclude that there is a higher degree of delay discounting in Group A than Group B because of the level of education, but the effect could have been caused by the unaccounted-for differences in smoking status. Experimental design textbooks that espouse group design research will quickly focus on the importance of random assignment of participants to groups to reduce the likelihood that a confounding variable covaries with group membership.

As an experimental control, random assignment is designed to decrease the likelihood that a third variable associated with specific subjects confounds the relation between the independent and DVs (for a discussion of random assignment as it relates to behavior analysis, see Jacobs, 2019). Imagine a scenario in which the researcher is unaware there is a single, binary confounding variable. If 20 subjects need to be divided into two equal groups, then there are 184,756 possible ways to arrange those 20 subjects into two groups. Thus, there is only a 1 in 184,756 chance ($p = .000005$) that all of the subjects with one level of the variable end up in group A and all of the subjects with the second level of the variable end up in group B. In any sample, if the subjects are randomly assigned to groups, we expect the different levels of the confounding variable to be spread evenly across the groups.

An important consideration with random assignment is that it is often not possible to randomly assign participants to different groups (i.e., observational research). Research questions about subject-level variables (e.g., preexisting populations of people) often make random assignment impossible. For example, when examining autism spectrum disorder (ASD) treatments, those recruited for that study from a clinic do not represent a random sample of autistic people/people with ASD (e.g., geographic location, socioeconomic status [SES], ethnicity; Pickard & Ingersoll, 2016). As another example, school-based research on the Good Behavior Game (for review, see Embry, 2002) operates on preexisting groups of participants (e.g., classes, schools, districts; Leflot et al., 2010). If a research question relies on a preexisting subject variable, then we no longer have a fully random assignment. For other questions, it might be technically possible but (more importantly) unethical to randomly assign people to certain groups. For example, we cannot assign people to be cigarette smokers or nonsmokers. When participants or nonhuman animal subjects cannot be randomly assigned, there are two main controls that can be used for hybrid designs to combine single-subject experimental designs with observational group-based experimental designs: stratified assignment and matched-pairs designs.

Stratified assignment is a common tool that researchers use when accounting for potential confounds that depend on features of the subjects. With stratified assignment, the subpopulations are identified by relevant subject variables or features (e.g., cigarette smoking status, ASD diagnosis), and then participants from each subpopulation are randomly sampled and randomly assigned to each of the experimental groups. With this technique, the researcher can be assured that an equal number of participants from each level of the subject variable have been randomly assigned to the different experimental groups. With stratified sampling and then random assignment, if a known or unanticipated confound exists, then the confound will not inadvertently covary with group assignment. For example, if a research question is related to weight loss or gain in rats, it is important to know the sex of the rats, because male and female rats have different growth curves (e.g., Charles River, 2021). Male rats could be randomly assigned to the experimental groups and then female rats could be randomly assigned to the experimental groups to make sure that sex is balanced across the groups. We are currently unaware of any hybrid experimental designs that have included a stratified sampling technique in the applied analysis of behavior.

Another common design used to address situations in which random assignment is difficult or impossible is a matched-pairs design. In a matched-pairs design, two subjects are matched together as a pair based on similar levels of a subject variable or presumed confound. After the pairs are established, the first subject in a pair is randomly assigned to one group, then the second subject is assigned to the other group. Thus, there is an even distribution of the pairs across the groups. (If there are J experimental groups, then the researcher would need matched sets of J subjects.) Matched-pairs designs are typically taught in research methodology and statistics courses to be most appropriate when subjects in a study have some preexisting relationship that cannot be avoided (cf. Cozby & Bates, 2011; McBride, 2018). For example, in any study of monozygotic twins, the siblings have—at the very least—overlapping genetics that may lead the siblings to have more similar behavior than two random people selected from the population. Within behavior analysis, a common matched-pairs technique is to take sets of subjects that were otherwise randomly sampled from the population and match them based on some shared feature prior to randomly assigning the subjects within that set to different groups. For example, Edlund (1972) examined the effects of putative candy reinforcers on IQ test performance in children. Edlund matched 11 pairs of children based on similar baseline IQ scores, age, sex, and reported enjoyment of candy, then randomly assigned one child from each pair to either the experimental group or the control group. In another example of a matched-pairs design, Peterson et al. (2016) compared two different treatments for pediatric feeding disorders. They employed a single-subject design within a matched-pairs design by randomly assigning recruited children to treatment in pairs (one child in the dyad received applied behavior analysis [ABA] and the other received a sequential oral sensory approach). With matched-pairs designs, the researcher is ensuring that the subject variable or potential confound will be similar across the groups. For that reason, matched designs can be particularly helpful if the final sample size and resulting group sizes are relatively small or if it will be particularly difficult or unlikely for random assignment to lead to an even distribution of potentially confounding covariates across the groups. In both cases, a matched-pairs design ensures similar levels of the subject variable across the groups.

A tactic that is used frequently in behavior-analytic hybrid designs is to match subjects based on some measure of behavior, then randomly assign those sets of subjects. For example, Shahan et al. (2020) examined the effects of decreases in rate of reinforcement on resurgence in rats using a hybrid design. For the group-based portion of the hybrid design, 50 male and 42 female rats were assigned to one of five groups. Within each sex, the rats were matched such that rates of lever pressing for food were not meaningfully different in the final three sessions prior to the experimental manipulation. After the matched sets were identified, rats from each set were randomly assigned to groups associated with differential decreases in the rate of reinforcement. In other respects, the experimental design was a more typical single-subject design with comparisons of a subject's own behavior to itself (e.g., periods of variable-interval reinforcement, extinction). As another example, Hoerger and Mace (2006) paired 15 children with attention-deficit/hyperactivity disorder (ADHD) to 15 gender- and age-matched children without ADHD based on a computerized test to measure self-control (although that study did not include a single-subject experimental design component). Group-based designs with subjects matched on some behavioral measure are good examples of studies that effectively employ hybrid experimental designs.

Attrition, History, and Maturation

Attrition, history, and maturation are threats to internal validity that have historically been less of a concern for single-subject experimental designs. *Attrition* refers to subjects not completing the entire experiment, *history* (as used in terms of traditional descriptions of threats to internal validity) refers to variables that occur outside of the control of the experimenter, and *maturation* refers to changes in the DV that are related to the natural growth of the subject (Thye, 2007). Single-subject experimental designs have robust methods to account for these threats to internal validity. If an individual subject does not complete the experiment (e.g., participant moves away, rat becomes ill), their data will be left unanalyzed or limited conclusions will be drawn. Because the behavior during a baseline condition serves as the control for the behavior in the experimental condition, a single missing subject does not affect the behavior of the other subjects (assuming the research does not involve some inherently social component). The standard methods for transitioning between baseline and experimental conditions (e.g., reversal designs, multiple baselines; see Johnston & Pennypacker, 2009; Sidman, 1960) are all designed to account for history variables that coincidentally co-occur with experimental manipulations. The same methods to account for history variables also tend to account for maturation effects. For example, if there is an irreversible change in behavior due to a child maturing, then such a change would be detected when behavior fails to return to a baseline level in a reversal design.

Attrition is a threat to the internal validity of a hybrid experimental design if there are specific differences across the groups in the study. In the case of attrition, subjects may be likely to stop participating because the intervention associated with their assigned group is not effective for them or is simply undesirable. For example, Halpern et al. (2015) examined the effectiveness of contingency management reward-based payment schedules (i.e., those characterized by providing monetary incentives for drug-negative samples) and contingency management with deposit-based payment schedules (i.e., those that require an initial deposit of money that is earned back with drug-negative samples). Across both types of schedules, the average amount of money a participant could expect to take home at the end of the study was similar, so one group did not earn more money than another group. For the reward-based contingency management, 90.0% of participants completed the full study, but for the deposit-based contingency management, only 13.7% of participants completed the study. When examining the effectiveness by the number of people who were successfully abstinent from smoking cigarettes, reward-based programs were more effective, because these programs were more widely accepted. However, after accounting for the differential attrition, Halpern et al. reported that deposit-based contingency management had higher rates of abstinence overall. Thus, the loss of participants can affect the outcome of a study if the IV and the attrition covary.

There are special concerns in hybrid designs related to history and maturation effects, although these concerns are also common in single-subject and group-based designs. In hybrid and group-based designs, a history effect exists if a potential confound happens to occur in relation to only one specific group. For example, students in classroom A experienced something unrelated to the study that students in classroom B did not experience. Differential maturation across groups is of greater concern in hybrid designs in which there is no random assignment and the subjects are different ages. A proper hybrid experimental design (e.g., random assignment with a multiple baseline) will decrease the likelihood of these threats to internal validity. A behavior analyst should be aware of these threats in case there is an alternative explanation for the obtained pattern of results.

Regression

Regression to the mean refers to the fact that, all else being equal, a measurement of a behavior that is an extreme value is likely to be less extreme when measured again (Thye, 2007). At the most basic level, all measurements of any phenomenon include some degree of random measurement error. With well-designed studies, the standard deviation of the measurement error can be reduced (differences in thousands of key pecks across sessions to hundreds of key pecks), but we can never perfectly measure a phenomenon. In other words, if there is no change in the environment, then we expect the average rate of behavior to remain unchanged, but we do not expect the *exact* same number of responses each session. Thus, if nothing in the environment changes and a very high response rate is recorded for one session, then we expect the number of responses to be closer to the typical baseline response rate on the next session. As a threat to internal validity, regression to the mean is critically important in hybrid designs if subjects are assigned to groups based on their performance on some measure of behavior during baseline (i.e., a nonrandom assignment). However, it should also be noted that regression to the mean is less of a concern with long-term, repeated measurements, because the average variation in scores (i.e., random error) should be zero over time.

Figure 4.1 displays how regression to the mean can be a concern for a hybrid experimental design. Imagine an experiment in which low-performing students are assigned to some treatment designed to increase performance. Panel A of Figure 4.1 displays how students would be identified to be included in the treatment. Panel B displays posttest scores for the low-performance group only, with the high performers not given a posttest. If the goal of the experiment is to increase the performance of the low performers,

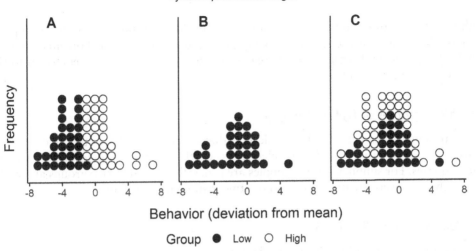

FIGURE 4.1. Regression to the mean as a threat to internal validity. Measures of some behavior in some hypothetical experiment in which subjects were assigned to low- and high-performing groups prior to the intervention (Panel A). Panel B shows what appears to be an increase in the low-performing group. Panel C demonstrates there is no fundamental changes in behavior pretreatment and posttreatment, because after the second measurement, low performers tended to have higher scores and high performers tended to have lower scores.

then it would be reasonable for posttests to be administered only to the low performers and not high performers. Based on Panel B, it appears that overall performance of the low performers increased as the scores tended to shift upward. As mentioned in the previous paragraph, we should not expect measures of behavior to be exactly the same across successive measurements. Panel C shows posttest scores for all of the students originally tested; the scores for the low-performance group are the same in Panels B and C, and the overall distribution of scores is the same in Panels A and C. The "effective" treatment for low performers did tend to be associated with increased scores for many students. However, the students originally designated as high performers tended to have decreased scores. Due to random measurement error or other sources of variability, and with no relation to the IV, the measures for the students' performance have changed. In this case, the correct interpretation is that the distribution of scores was different on the second measurement because of regression to the mean, and that the treatment was not effective.

Regression to the mean is a particular concern if subjects are assigned to groups based on the relative levels of the DV. Regression to the mean may be less of a concern in a hybrid design that includes a large number of measurements of behavior across each condition of the experiment. For example, Kolokotroni et al. (2014) examined the effects of chronic nicotine administration and subsequent withdrawal on discounting of delayed food in rats. Their analysis focused on dichotomizing the rats into groups of high impulsivity (high degree of discounting) and low impulsivity (low degree of discounting) based on behavior prior to the administration of nicotine. The authors reported that the low-impulsivity group had *increases* in the degree of discounting when nicotine was withdrawn, whereas the high-impulsivity group had *decreases* in the degree of discounting when nicotine was withdrawn. It is possible that this transient effect—the high-impulsivity group appearing less impulsive and the low-impulsivity group appearing more impulsive—was due in part to a regression to the mean. Kolokotroni et al. used a hybrid experimental design, so it is reasonable to question whether regression to the mean was a confound in this study.

Notable Examples of Hybrid Designs

There are some special cases of hybrid designs that we also describe. In the following sections, we describe randomized controlled trials, waitlist controls, crossover designs, and Latin squares. For simplicity, the examples are generally limited to two groups and an IV with only two levels (treatment and no treatment/standard/placebo).

Randomized Controlled Trials

Perhaps the most well-known group design is the randomized controlled trial (also referred to as a randomized clinical trial [RCT]). RCTs are often considered the "gold standard" in research (Concato et al., 2000; Feinstein, 1984; for rejoinder, see Smith & Pell, 2003). In this design, participants are randomized into groups, one of which is the control group, who receives either placebo, no treatment, or standard treatment, depending on the study design, and the other is the experimental group, whose participants are exposed to the IV of interest (e.g., the treatment; Kendall, 2003). If statistically significant differences are observed between groups, this finding suggests a causal relationship between the independent and dependent variables (Kendall, 2003). For example, Dallery et al. (2017) conducted an RCT hybridized with single-subject design components to examine the effects of online-based contingency management to reduce cigarette smoking. With the contingency management group, participants received financial incentives for providing video recordings of reduced carbon monoxide readings (which are elevated when smoking cigarettes). The control group received financial incentives for submitting samples in the same manner but were not required to have reduced carbon monoxide readings. After the random assignment, participants submitted carbon monoxide readings for 7 weeks, with repeated opportunities for monetary incentives. Dallery and colleagues reported that the contingency management group had higher rates of abstinence from cigarette smoking. With the RCT design, the only difference between the groups was whether the participant was required to submit evidence of abstinence to receive the monetary incentive. Therefore, the authors concluded that requiring participants to submit reduced carbon monoxide readings caused a decrease in cigarette smoking.

In an effort to standardize and clearly communicate RCT methodology and findings, researchers across many fields have developed a set of evidence-based reporting recommendations known as the Consolidated Standards of Reporting Trials (CONSORT; see *www.consort-statement.org*). The CONSORT statement is a 25-item checklist and flow diagram that promotes transparency and adequate reporting of RCTs. For example, the CONSORT statement requires researchers to provide important information such as eligibility criteria, sample size, and adequate intervention information to allow future replication. Including the appropriate information suggested by the CONSORT statement conveys much of the information related to whether the RCT was well designed. Although it is not a requirement that an RCT follow the CONSORT guidelines, researchers who disregard the guidelines do so at their own peril by inadvertently suggesting their RCT was not well designed.

Waitlist Control Design

In a waitlist control design, one group of participants initially receives no treatment or a "standard" treatment and, during a second phase of the experiment, receive the treatment of interest (thus, they are on a "waitlist" to receive the treatment). A second group receives the treatment of interest during both phases of the experiment. This arrangement allows a comparison of treatment effectiveness across groups (during the initial phase), and all subjects receive the treatment at some point in the experiment (allowing for single-subject comparisons; see Kinser & Robins, 2013). For example, Levin et al. (2014) randomly assigned participants to either a 3-week intervention or a 3-week waitlist control. Participants assigned to the intervention completed a web-based acceptance and commitment therapy (ACT) program over a 3-week period, whereas participants assigned to waitlist control waited 3 weeks before completing the ACT program. A waitlist control is like a multiple baseline design in that the participants in the intervention group receive the treatment according to an ABB design, and participants in the waitlist control group receive the treatment according to an AAB design (Baer et al., 1968). Waitlist control groups are beneficial in that they allow provision of an intervention to all participants in a study, while also allowing the researcher to maintain the randomization required for an RCT.

Crossover Design

In crossover designs, participants in one group initially receive either placebo, no treatment, or standard treatment, and then receive the treatment of interest, while the second group initially receives the treatment of interest and then receives either placebo, no treatment, or standard treatment (Grizzle, 1965). In a traditional crossover design, the change of the IV for each group occurs at the same time, so the groups "cross over" one another as the IV switches levels between the groups. Benefits of the crossover design are that all of the participants experience all of the experimental conditions, and order effects can be detected if they are of interest. In one example of a crossover design, Johnson and Idol-Maestas (1986) determined whether access to tutoring sessions functioned as a reinforcer for on-task behavior for two pairs of children that typically had low rates of on-task behavior. Initially, both pairs of children were exposed first to a baseline condition, then a condition in which feedback on performance was given, and then a reinforcer-sampling condition in which students were given free access to the tutoring sessions. In the next phase of the experiment, which included the experimental manipulation, the first pair of children was only given access to the tutoring sessions based on meeting a criterion for on-task behavior, whereas the second pair of children was given daily access to the tutors regardless of behavior. After this condition was complete, the contingencies switched: The first pair was given daily access to the tutors regardless of behavior, and the second pair was given access to the tutoring sessions based on meeting a criterion for on-task behavior (i.e., the pairs "crossed over"). In both groups, requiring on-task behavior to gain access to tutoring maintained high rates of on-task behavior. Johnson and Idol-Maestas were also able to demonstrate that there was an order effect: Free access to tutors only maintained high rates of on-task behavior in the students who had first experienced a requirement to be on-task to gain access to the tutoring, but when students had free access to tutors first, this condition did not maintain a high rate of on-task behavior. A crossover design is a two-group case of a broader set of experimental designs referred to as Latin squares (described next).

TABLE 4.1. Example of a 3 × 3 Latin Square Design

Subject	Condition Order		
	1	2	3
1	A	B	C
2	B	C	A
3	C	A	B

Latin Squares

Latin squares are experimental designs used to counterbalance conditions both within and across subjects to control variation due to the order in which sequential treatments are applied (Richardson, 2018). For example, behavioral pharmacologists often employ Latin squares to counterbalance the order in which individual subjects (e.g., rats) or groups of subjects receive different doses of a drug (e.g., Richards et al., 1999). Formally, a Latin square is an n by m grid in which a symbol (historically Latin letters) occurs only once in each column, as well as only once in each row. Table 4.1 is a Latin square design for treatments A, B, and C in which there are three subjects (rows) and three phases of the experiment (columns). In this design, treatments A, B, and C occur once per subject (rows) and once in each condition order (columns), and blocking occurs on rows and columns. Thus, each treatment is administered once as the first, second, and third treatment.

Single-subject designs that use Latin squares for counterbalancing can account for some of the influence of the temporal order in which a treatment occurs. However, Latin square designs do not control for carryover effects that may occur in sequentially applied treatments (Bugelski, 1949). For example, in Table 4.1, if treatment A influences the efficacy of treatment B, then it will become more difficult to estimate the true effect of treatment B without including more subjects that receive treatment B first (as in the second row). The confounding of order effects can be overcome by increasing the number of subjects and expanding the Latin square, and ensuring that each treatment is preceded by every other treatment. Increasing the number of subjects may not be feasible in terms of the number of subjects required for such a design if there are a large number of conditions.

The Analysis of Data from Hybrid Experimental Designs

Visual Analysis

Behavior-analytic research has often been the search for large and orderly effects of IVs on behavior. The search for large effects is the function of two main factors. In ABA, meaningful change for the client is a foundational tenet of the field (e.g., Baer et al., 1968). The second factor in the search for large effects is that both experimental and applied analyses of behavior have relied on visual analysis. If there is a high degree of variability in the data or a relatively small effect, then visual analysis can be complex, and a decision about the effects of the IV on behavior can be difficult (see Kratochwill et al., 2010, for visual analysis standards and how to apply these to discern if a study meets evidence standards). If, however, there is little variability in the data, or a relatively large effect, then discerning effects via visual analysis can be easy because there are clear and obvious differences in behavior across the different levels of the IV. As in many other fields, behavior analysis has informally adopted the "interocular trauma test" (Edwards et al., 1963) as a method for interpreting the results of an experiment with clear behavior change, that is, "you know what the data mean when the conclusion hits you between the eyes" (p. 217). In other words, clear conclusions tend to be associated with relatively large effects.

Behavior analysts have a long, rich tradition of visual presentation of data (e.g., Ferster & Skinner, 1957). The inclusion of visual presentations of data from group-based experimental designs is often an aid to supplement the statistical analysis of those data. Therefore, graphical displays in group-based designs are often focused on clearly displaying information that pertains to the statistical analysis (e.g., means, standard errors, confidence intervals). Focusing on presenting summary measures alone, however, can make the identification of functional relations within single subjects difficult (Sidman, 1960). However, visually presenting summary statistics is not the only way to present data from group-based experimental designs.

Tufte (1983) and Leland (2005) both make strong cases that there are no standard methods of visually presenting different types of data. Rather, visual presentation should rely on methods that allow "for reasoning about quantitative information" (Tufte, 1983, p. 12). When displaying differences across groups, researchers may conventionally present points or bars indicating the mean with positive and negative measures of error. However, researchers can also present individual subject data. For example, Galizio et al. (2020) reported a study of the resurgence of response variability in humans. In that study, the authors grouped the data based on whether response variability (as measured with U-value) was consistent with resurgence, extinction without resurgence, or nonsystematic responding. The left panel of Figure 4.2 displays the individual subject data as displayed in Galizio et al. The right panel displays only the group means and 95% confidence intervals of those same data. If someone is interested in the data path of a single subject, it is possible—although difficult—to call out details of that subject in the left panel. The individual differences in how extinction decreased the degree of variability and the return of response variability during the resurgence test are visible. For Group A, there is a pattern of resurgence (high response variability in baseline, low variability in extinction, then a return to previous levels in the testing condition), but for Group B, there is a pattern of possibly extinction-induced variability. Based on the means, it is not possible to determine what behavior the subjects were emitting in the nonsystematic group (Group C). In other words, if we consider only the bottom-right panel (Group C summary), it is not possible to answer whether the subjects in the group respond in a within-group consistent pattern or if the group is a random collection of participants with vastly different patterns of behavior who were "lumped together" because they could not be easily categorized into the other two groups. This example from Galizio et al. is meant to demonstrate how the uncritical display of summary statistics, common in some group-based design research, can hide or obfuscate the relations that typically interests behavior analysts.

Statistical Analysis

As we discussed at the beginning of the chapter, there is a long history of using some form of statistical analysis to interpret data obtained from a group-based experimental design. Statistical analyses are employed in group-based research as a method of handling subject-to-subject variability that is inherent when comparing observations from different individuals rather than the same individuals, as in single-subject designs (Ator, 1999). This is not to say that statistical analyses should be used over other means of handling variability such as experimental control. In fact, experimental control should be prioritized in group-based designs just as in single-subject designs because of the increased amount of subject-to-subject variability in comparisons of the behavior of different individuals. Just as there is an array of group-based experimental designs, so, too, is there an array of statistical analyses. In this section, we highlight some of the chief concerns related to conducting statistical analyses with group-based or hybrid experimental designs.

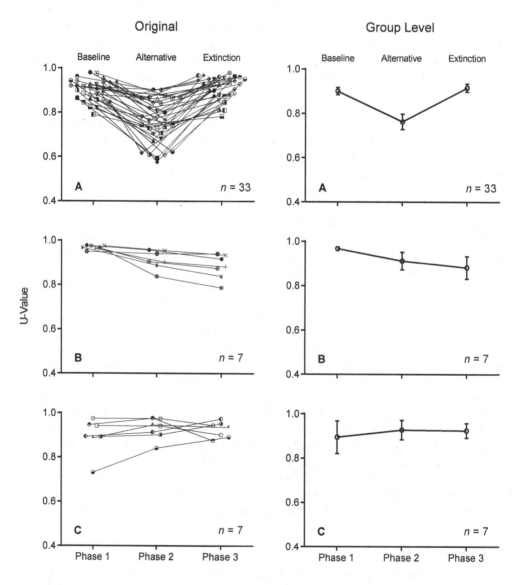

FIGURE 4.2. Example of individual- and group-level data presentation. Original data (left) and summary data (right) replotted from Galizio et al. (2020). Left panel Copyright © 2020 Society for the Experimental Analysis of Behavior. Reprinted with permission.

With the simplest two-group design, a *t*-test is usually a sufficient analytic plan to compare the mean level of behavior across groups.[3] With a between-groups *t*-test (i.e., independent samples), the *p*-value indicates the likelihood of the empirically obtained difference under the assumption that there is no actual difference between the groups (i.e., the null hypothesis). With a statistically significant *p*-value, the researcher must make a leap in logic that if the obtained data were unlikely under the null hypothesis, then the research hypothesis (i.e., the alternative hypothesis) is likely to be true (although this leap in logic is invalid, it is still commonly believed to be a correct inference; for reviews see Branch, 1999, 2014; Wasserstein & Lazar, 2016; Wasserstein et al., 2019).

If there are three or more groups, then an analysis of variance (ANOVA) is the appropriate statistical analysis with the same goal of attempting to determine if the means of the groups are dissimilar from each other (Cohen, 2008; Oehlert, 2010). With multiple groups, an important post hoc follow-up is to determine specifically how the means of each group are similar or dissimilar from the other groups. Post hoc pairwise comparisons are typically some form of a *t*-test with a correction to maintain the familywise Type I error (i.e., false-positive) rate constant, because multiple comparisons are being conducted. Most statistical packages (e.g., SPSS) automatically conduct the familywise correction for multiple comparisons. For a more thorough introduction for considerations of conducting statistical analysis of behavior analytic data, we recommend Huitema (1986).

When conducting any statistical analysis, it is important to ensure that the features of the data appropriately match the analytical technique being used. First, it is important to consider whether the data are normally (i.e., bell-shaped) or non-normally distributed. Panel A of Figure 4.3 displays a normal distribution with a mean of zero and a non-normal χ^2 distribution with two degrees of freedom. There are formal statistical tests (e.g., Shapiro–Wilk test) or alternative visual methods to determine if data are normally distributed. Panel B of the figure displays a quantile–quantile plot (Q-Q plot), which is a visual method to determine if data are normally distributed. In a Q-Q plot, the distribution of the obtained values is plotted against the predicted distribution of the data if the data points were normally distributed. Typically, on a Q-Q plot, a line is provided that indicates how perfectly normal data would be distributed. If the pattern on the Q-Q plot deviates from that line by a "large" amount, then the data are not normally distributed (for a more thorough discussion of assessing normality using Q-Q plots, see Oehlert, 2010). The data from the normal distribution closely follow the line in the Q-Q plot, whereas there is a clear pattern of deviations in the data from the non-normal χ^2 distribution. If the data follow a normal distribution using visual inspection, researchers can proceed with parametric statistical analyses such as a *t*-test or an ANOVA. If the data do not follow a normal distribution, it is sometimes possible to transform the data so that the assumptions of normality will be met. When transforming data, the goal is to express the data differently, without changing the overall pattern of the data (Oehlert, 2010). As an example, calculating the log of a dataset (i.e., a log transformation) is a common method to make heavily skewed data more normal. If a transformation is not possible, nonparametric statistical analyses should be considered. For discussions determining the

---

[3]For brevity, we focus on typical frequentist, parametric statistical tests. Additionally, we recognize that much of the distinction between "two"-variables and "three-plus"-variables statistical methods is moot if we include our independent variables as predictors in the general linear model perspective.

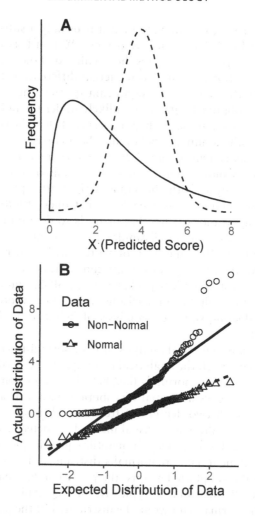

FIGURE 4.3. Normal and non-normal distributions and a Q-Q plot of normal and non-normal data. Panel A is a frequency distribution curve for the normal distribution and a non-normal distribution (χ^2 distribution). Panel B is a Q-Q plot that shows the distribution of the obtained data points against where the values should be if they are normally distributed. If the data points follow the straight line, then the obtained data match the normal distribution.

normality of data see Oehlert (2010), or for nonparametric statistical analyses for behavior analysis, see Davison (1999) or Craig and Fisher (2019).

For many statistical tests, researchers should also check for homogeneity of variance (referred to as homoscedasticity in regression). Homogeneity of variance is an assumption of parametric statistical analyses in which the variance or spread of each group is approximately equal. Heterogeneous variances can occur if a treatment (e.g., the administration of a drug) causes increased variability in the behavior of interest relative to a control condition. Levene's test for homogeneity of variance can be used to decide whether one can assume homogeneous variances (Oehlert, 2010). When using Levene's test, the null hypothesis is to assume homogeneous variances. Therefore, a p-value less than .05 would be evidence that the variances of two (or more) groups are different. Levene's test is provided in many statistical packages (e.g., SPSS). Many statistical packages can also correct for heterogeneous variances; therefore, when conducting parametric statistical analyses, researchers should check for heterogeneity of variance and proceed with the necessary corrections if violations of this assumption are apparent.

Finally, it is important that observations in a statistical analysis are independent of one another. This assumption is difficult to test; however, the design of an experiment allows researchers to identify when this assumption may be violated. For example, observations collected from the same individual can be assumed to be nonindependent, whereas observations collected from different individuals, sampled using appropriate randomization techniques, can be assumed to be independent. When using hybrid experimental designs, we can assume that observations collected between subjects are independent, whereas observations collected within subjects are not independent. To account for this kind of structure in the data, researchers need to specify which observations are from the same individual in their statistical analysis. For data with complex data structures (e.g., nested datasets), we recommend using mixed-effects modeling (also referred to as multilevel modeling) to address issues associated with the nonindependence of observations (Hox et al., 2017).

The Importance of Replication

Behavior analysts consider replication a key component of their science, owing to powerful texts such as Sidman's (1960) *Tactics of Scientific Research* (Locey, 2020). However, more recently, psychology has experienced a replication crisis, a finding that represents a serious issue to psychology as a science (Open Science Collaboration, 2015); that is, results from many published papers in psychological journals are not reproducible, especially in areas that rely more heavily on group-based experimental designs and less on designs that require repeated measurements (e.g., single-subject, pre–post, hybrid designs). The replication crisis has been attributed to several factors, including questionable research practices, inadequate training in statistics, and publication bias. As discussed in the previous section, behavior analysts rarely rely solely on statistical methods for analyzing their data. Behavior analysts have long relied on replication as the core component of single-subject experimental designs. Visual analysis, sometimes with supplemental statistical analysis, in combination with rigorous within-experiment replication, have been core components of protecting behavior analysis from a replication crisis. However, as Hantula (2019) and Tincani and Travers (2019) have discussed, some of the causes associated with failures to replicate (e.g., selective publication of studies, lack of published studies with no effect) can still occur within behavior analysis. This point is particularly important considering that "No similar efforts [to systematically replicate studies] have been mounted in ABA, leaving the credibility of published scientific findings open to question" (Tincani & Travers, 2019, p. 64). With the introduction of a new methodology such as a group-based experimental design, improperly controlled hybrid experimental designs can exacerbate issues associated with reproducibility. To properly employ a group-based design, and to increase the likelihood that a result will be reproducible, researchers should consider power analysis as an important step in designing an experiment with between-subject manipulations.

Statistical Power

In the pursuit of using inferential statistics to identify IVs that have orderly effects on behavior, researchers must consider the level of power they have to identify those orderly effects. Conceptually, the power of a study refers to a researcher's ability to detect an effect when it does in fact exist; that is, given that an effect exists (e.g., a between-group difference), *power* refers to our likelihood of detecting that effect (Kyonka, 2019). Power is often associated with statistical hypothesis testing; however, as Kyonka eloquently described, power also reflects the degree of experimental control that a researcher exerts. For example, maintaining nonhuman animals (e.g., rats) at a lower body weight via food restriction is a commonly used method to motivate the subject to engage in a particular task (Toth & Gardiner, 2000). Failing to control the degree of food restriction could lead to greater individual differences in performance on the task (e.g., rate of lever pressing). Increases in individual differences will in turn lead to greater variability, thus decreasing our ability to determine whether an IV influences performance on the task (i.e., lowering our power). Thus, higher experimental control reduces variability, which allows researchers to draw more accurate conclusions from their data. Therefore, although we focus on power primarily in terms of how it can be used to estimate a priori (beforehand) sample sizes for a statistical test to detect a true effect, we also emphasize that power should be considered more broadly as encompassing the rigor with which researchers can detect effects of scientific importance with their experimental design.

A priori statistical power analyses (i.e., occurring prior to recruiting subjects for the experiment) are commonly used to estimate the appropriate number of subjects required to detect an effect (Kyonka, 2019). Including too many or too few subjects can lead to wasted resources (e.g., time and money; Lenth, 2001) and may contribute to issues associated with reproducibility in science (Anderson & Maxwell, 2017; Kyonka, 2019). Lower power, often associated with too few subjects, is associated with a lower probability of detecting a real effect (Type II error) and inflated effect size estimates if an effect is detected (Button et al., 2013). Thus, if a study that is underpowered and has a statistically significant result is repeated, the new study is more likely to have a different pattern of results (e.g., Open Science Collaboration, 2015). Higher power is associated with more subjects and a higher probability of detecting a statistically significant effect, but not necessarily a scientifically important effect; that is, including too many subjects in a study (i.e., an overpowered study) will allow a researcher to detect statistical significance; however, the researcher is also more likely to detect extremely small effects. Additionally, it is unreasonable and potentially unethical to use more subjects for a research question than are necessary (National Research Council, 2011; Russell & Burch, 1959). Thus, selecting the appropriate sample size for a study is important for ensuring that the study is appropriately powered, allowing the researcher to draw valid scientific conclusions from their data.

Several programs are available to conduct a priori power analyses. G*Power (Faul et al., 2009), a freely available program to conduct power analyses, is widely used to estimate sample-size requirements, in addition to other power analyses (e.g., post hoc power analyses). G*Power is a point-and-click software; however, other free programs such as R (R Core Team, 2021) are available to conduct power analyses. Regardless of the program used, a priori power analyses require (at minimum) estimates of effect size, significance level (α), and desired power ($1 - \beta$). Conventionally, significance levels are often set to .05, and power is often set to .80; however, estimates of effect size generally require calculating effect sizes from previous research. The measure of effect size (e.g., Cohen's *d* or *f*) for the power analysis depends on the statistical test that will be used and may require transformation between effect sizes (Cohen, 1988). For the sake of brevity, we direct the reader to Lakens (2013) and others (e.g., Cohen, 1988) for detailed description on how to calculate effect sizes. In addition, there are multiple resources for transforming between effect sizes as well that the reader can review (e.g., Lenhard & Lenhard, 2016). Finally, there are also widely accepted standard resources (Cohen, 1988) for how to estimate an effect size for a power analysis when there is no clear prior effect size in the literature. Kyonka (2019) provides a tutorial on how to estimate an effect size that is both statistically and functionally appropriate for a behavior analyst.

Limitations of Statistical Testing

Unfortunately, in many fields, there is an expectation that statistical analyses will always be conducted and that they provide a robust analysis of experimental data (for discussion, see Huitema, 1986). As we mentioned earlier, there are well-argued critiques of inferential statistical testing for science in general and in behavior analysis in particular (Ator, 1999; Branch, 1999, 2014; Perone, 1999). We only highlight some of the arguments against null-hypothesis significance testing (NHST) as they relate to hybrid experimental designs. The basic statistical analyses such as *t*-tests and ANOVAs described in the Statistical Analysis section are examples of NHST.

One pernicious side effect of NHST is the conflation of statistical significance with the size of an effect (see Branch, 2014, as this relates to behavior analysis). In NHST, statistical significance only provides information on the likelihood of obtaining the pattern of data if the null hypothesis is assumed to be true. Statistical significance is a function of several variables, including but not limited to, effect size and sample size. Based on how most statistical tests are performed, an IV associated with a small effect size may not be statistically significant in a small sample. However, that same small effect may be statistically significant with an extremely large sample. Thus, a statistically significant result may be a small effect that is of little pragmatic value. Relying on *p*-values without considering effect sizes is one contributing factor to issues with scientific reproducibility in psychology (Open Science Collaboration, 2015). The math that drives statistical significance testing does not provide information about whether a purported effect is a correct interpretation or meaningful in terms of how behavior is actually affected. There is also concern with the increasing reliance on inferential statistical testing that behavior analysts will abandon the search for orderly effects of the environment on behavior (see Locey, 2020). In some cases, only large effects may be meaningful (e.g., a reduction of potentially fatal self-injurious behavior) and in other cases even small effects might be meaningful (e.g., an increase in eye contact with parents).

For hybrid experimental design research, there is no practical reason for behavior analysts to stop searching for meaningful and orderly effects of IVs on behavior even if statistical analysis is part of the research. If an IV that requires study through a group-based methodology produces a large effect on behavior, then that effect will be detectable with both visual analysis and with an inferential statistical analysis. As Branch (2014) points out, behavioral science is not about cataloging statistically significant effects; behavioral science is about finding and describing orderly functional relations between the environment and behavior. Statistical analyses may aid in the search for orderly functional relations, but those analyses should not be the only tool a researcher uses.

Conclusion

As behavior is emitted by an organism, it flows like a river. Some IVs may lead to transient changes in behavior; reinforcers make the river swell, and removal of the reinforcers allow the river to recede to its natural level. Single-subject designs are well suited to study the effects of such IVs. Other IVs cause irreversible changes in behavior. For example, a behavioral cusp (Rosales-Ruiz & Baer, 1997) is like a dam breaking, carving out land as new paths for the flow of the river. Single-subject designs may be helpful when studying these sorts of variables (e.g., a multiple baseline). In other cases, an appropriate research methodology may require a hybridization of single-subject and group-based designs. Although group-based designs are frequently not ideal tools to study the behavior of individual organisms, they are sometimes useful or necessary. We hope the reader finds this chapter helpful in considering the utility of group-based design in their behavior-analytic research.

REFERENCES

Anderson, S. F., & Maxwell, S. E. (2017). Addressing the "replication crisis": Using original studies to design replication studies with appropriate statistical power. *Multivariate Behavioral Research, 52*(3), 305–324.

Ator, N. A. (1999). Statistical inference in behavior analysis: Environmental determinants? *Behavior Analyst, 22*(2), 93–97.

Baer, D. M., Wolf, M. M., & Risley, T. R. (1968). Some current dimensions of applied behavior analysis. *Journal of Applied Behavior Analysis, 1*(1), 91–97.

Bickel, W. K., Odum, A. L., & Madden, G. J. (1999). Impulsivity and cigarette smoking: Delay discounting in current, never, and ex-smokers. *Psychopharmacology, 146*(4), 447–454.

Bodmer, W., Bailey, R. A., Charlesworth, B., Eyre-Walker, A., Farewell, V., Mead, A., & Senn, S. (2021). The outstanding scientist, R. A. Fisher: His views on eugenics and race. *Heredity, 126*(4), 565–576.

Bouton, M. E., Maren, S., & McNally, G. P. (2021). Behavioral and neurobiological mechanisms of Pavlovian and instrumental extinction learning. *Physiological Reviews, 101*(2), 611–681.

Branch, M. N. (1999). Statistical inference in behavior analysis: Some things significance testing does and does not do. *Behavior Analyst, 22*(2), 87–92.

Branch, M. (2014). Malignant side effects of null-hypothesis significance testing. *Theory and Psychology, 24*(2), 256–277.

Bugelski, B. R. (1949). A note on Grant's discussion of the Latin square principle in the design of experiment. *Psychological Bulletin, 46*(1), 49–50.

Button, K. S., Ioannidis, J. P., Mokrysz, C., Nosek, B. A., Flint, J., Robinson, E. S., & Munafo, M. R. (2013). Power failure: Why small sample size undermines the reliability of neuroscience. *Nature Reviews Neuroscience, 14*(5), 365–376.

Charles River. (2021). Long–Evans rat. Retrieved June 20, 2021, from *www.criver.com/products-services/find-model/long-evans-rat?region=3611*.

Cohen, B. H. (2008). *Explaining psychological statistics* (4th ed.). Wiley.

Cohen, J. (1988). *Statistical power analysis for the behavioral sciences* (2nd ed.). Erlbaum.

Concato, J., Shah, N., & Horwitz, R. I. (2000). Randomized, controlled trials, observational studies, and the hierarchy of research designs. *New England Journal of Medicine, 342*(25), 1887–1892.

Cox, A. D., & Virues-Ortega, J. (2016). Interactions between behavior function and psychotropic medication. *Journal of Applied Behavior Analysis, 49*(1), 85–104.

Cox, A. D., & Virues-Ortega, J. (2022). Long-term functional stability of problem behavior exposed to psychotropic medications. *Journal of Applied Behavior Analysis, 55*, 214–229.

Cox, D. R., & Reid, N. (2000). *The theory of the design of experiments.* Chapman & Hall/CRC.

Cozby, P. C., & Bates, S. C. (2011). *Methods in behavioral research* (11th ed.). McGraw-Hill.

Craig, A. R., & Fisher, W. W. (2019). Randomization tests as alternative analysis methods for behavior-analytic data. *Journal of the Experimental Analysis of Behavior, 111*(2), 309–328.

Dallery, J., Raiff, B. R., Kim, S. J., Marsch, L. A., Stitzer, M., & Grabinski, M. J. (2017). Nationwide access to an internet-based contingency management intervention to promote smoking cessation: A randomized controlled trial. *Addiction, 112*(5), 875–883.

Davison, M. (1999). Statistical inference in behavior analysis: Having my cake and eating it? *Behavior Analyst, 22*(2), 99–103.

DeHart, W. B., Friedel, J. E., Berry, M., Frye, C. C. J., Galizio, A., & Odum, A. L. (2020). Comparison of delay discounting of different outcomes in cigarette smokers, smokeless tobacco users, e-cigarette users, and non-tobacco users. *Journal of the Experimental Analysis of Behavior, 114*(2), 203–215.

Dudley, M. Z., Salmon, D. A., Halsey, N. A., Orenstein, W. A., Limaye, R. J., O'Leary, S. T., & Omer, S. B. (2018). Do vaccines cause autism? In *The clinician's vaccine safety resource guide* (pp. 197–204). Springer.

Edlund, C. V. (1972). The effect on the test behavior of children, as reflected in the I.Q. scores, when reinforced after each correct response. *Journal of Applied Behavior Analysis, 5*(3), 317–319.

Edwards, W., Lindman, H., & Savage, L. J. (1963). Bayesian statistical inference for psychological research. *Psychological Review, 70*(3), 193–242.

Embry, D. D. (2002). The good behavior game: A best practice candidate as a universal behavioral vaccine. *Clinical Child and Family Psychology Review, 5*(4), 273–297.

Faul, F., Erdfelder, E., Buchner, A., & Lang, A.-G. (2009). Statistical power analyses using G*Power 3.1: Tests for correlation and regression analyses. *Behavior Research Methods, 41*, 1149–1160.

Feinstein, A. R. (1984). Current problems and future challenges in randomized clinical trials. *Circulation, 70*(5), 767–774.

Ferster, C., & Skinner, B. (1957). *Schedules of reinforcement.* Appleton-Century-Crofts.

Fisher, R. A. (1935). *The design of experiments.* Oliver & Boyd.

Fisher, W. W., & Lerman, D. C. (2014). It has been said that, "There are three degrees of falsehoods: Lies, damn lies, and statistics." *Journal of School Psychology, 52*(2), 243–248.

Friedel, J. E., DeHart, W. B., Frye, C. C., Rung, J. M., & Odum, A. L. (2016). Discounting of qualitatively different delayed health outcomes in current and never smokers. *Experimental and Clinical Psychopharmacology, 24*(1), 18–29.

Friedel, J. E., DeHart, W. B., Madden, G. J., & Odum, A. L. (2014). Impulsivity and cigarette smoking: Discounting of monetary and consumable outcomes in current and non-smokers. *Psychopharmacology, 231*(23), 4517–4526.

Galizio, A., Friedel, J. E., & Odum, A. L. (2020). An investigation of resurgence of reinforced behavioral variability in humans. *Journal of the Experimental Analysis of Behavior, 114*(3), 381–393.

Grizzle, J. E. (1965). The two-period change-over design and its use in clinical trials. *Biometrics, 21*(2), 467–480.

Hagopian, L. P. (2020). The consecutive controlled case series: Design, data-analytics, and reporting methods supporting the study of generality. *Journal of Applied Behavior Analysis, 53*(2), 596–619.

Halpern, S. D., French, B., Small, D. S., Saulsgiver, K., Harhay, M. O., Audrain-McGovern, J., . . . Volpp, K. G. (2015). Randomized trial of four financial-incentive programs for smoking cessation. *New England Journal of Medicine, 372*(22), 2108–2117.

Hantula, D. A. (2019). Editorial: Replication and reliability in behavior science and behavior analysis: A call for a conversation. *Perspectives on Behavior Science, 42*(1), 1–11.

Hoerger, M. L., & Mace, F. C. (2006). A computerized test of self-control predicts classroom behavior. *Journal of Applied Behavior Analysis, 39*(2), 147–159.

Horner, R. H., Carr, E. G., Halle, J., McGee, G., Odom, S., & Wolery, M. (2016). The use of single-subject research to identify evidence-based practice in special education. *Exceptional Children, 71*(2), 165–179.

Hox, J. J., Moerbeek, M., & van de Schoot, R. (2017). *Multilevel analysis: Techniques and applications.* Routledge.

Hubbard, R., Parsa, R. A., & Luthy, M. R. (2016). The spread of statistical significance testing in psychology. *Theory and Psychology, 7*(4), 545–554.

Huitema, B. E. (1986). Statistical analysis and single-subject designs: Some misunderstandings. In A. D. Poling & R. W. Fuqua (Eds.), *Research methods in applied behavior analysis* (pp. 209–232). Plenum Press.

Jacobs, K. W. (2019). Replicability and randomization test logic in behavior analysis. *Journal of the Experimental Analysis of Behavior, 111*(2), 329–341.

Jaroni, J. L., Wright, S. M., Lerman, C., & Epstein, L. H. (2004). Relationship between education and delay discounting in smokers. *Addictive Behaviors, 29*(6), 1171–1175.

Johnson, L. J., & Idol-Maestas, L. (1986). Peer-tutoring as a reinforcer for appropriate tutee behavior. *Journal of Special Education Technology, 7*(4), 14–21.

Johnston, J. M., & Pennypacker, H. S. (2009). *Strategies and tactics of behavioral research* (3rd ed.). Routledge.

Kendall, J. M. (2003). Designing a research project: Randomised controlled trials and their principles. *Emergency Medicine Journal, 20*(2), 164–168.

Kinser, P. A., & Robins, J. L. (2013). Control group design: Enhancing rigor in research of mind-body therapies for depression. *Evidence-Based Complementary and Alternative Medicine, 2013*, Article 140467.

Kolokotroni, K. Z., Rodgers, R. J., & Harrison, A. A. (2014). Trait differences in response to chronic nicotine and nicotine withdrawal in rats. *Psychopharmacology, 231*(3), 567–580.

Kratochwill, T. R., Hitchcock, J., Horner, R. H., Levin, J. R., Odom, S. L., Rindskopf, D. M., & Shadish, W. R. (2010). *Single-case designs technical documentation*. What Works Clearinghouse.

Kyonka, E. G. E. (2019). Tutorial: Small-N power analysis. *Perspectives on Behavior Science, 42*(1), 133–152.

Lakens, D. (2013). Calculating and reporting effect sizes to facilitate cumulative science: A practical primer for t-tests and ANOVAs. *Frontiers in Psychology, 4*, Article 863.

Laraway, S., Snycerski, S., Pradhan, S., & Huitema, B. E. (2019). An overview of scientific reproducibility: Consideration of relevant issues for behavior science/analysis. *Perspectives on Behavior Science, 42*(1), 33–57.

Leflot, G., van Lier, P. A., Onghena, P., & Colpin, H. (2010). The role of teacher behavior management in the development of disruptive behaviors: An intervention study with the good behavior game. *Journal of Abnormal Child Psychology, 38*(6), 869–882.

Leland, W. (2005). *The grammar of graphics*. Springer.

Lenhard, W., & Lenhard, A. (2016). Calculation of effect sizes. Retrieved June 2021, from *www.psychometrica.de/effect_size.html*.

Lenth, R. V. (2001). Some practical guidelines for effective sample size determination. *American Statistician, 55*(3), 187–193.

Levin, M. E., Pistorello, J., Seeley, J. R., & Hayes, S. C. (2014). Feasibility of a prototype web-based acceptance and commitment therapy prevention program for college students. *Journal of American College Health, 62*(1), 20–30.

Locey, M. L. (2020). The evolution of behavior analysis: Toward a replication crisis? *Perspectives on Behavior Science, 43*(4), 655–675.

Matthews, B. A., Shimoff, E., Catania, A. C., & Sagvolden, T. (1977). Uninstructed human responding: Sensitivity to ratio and interval contingencies. *Journal of the Experimental Analysis of Behavior, 27*(3), 453–467.

McBride, D. M. (2018). *The process of statistical analysis in psychology*. SAGE.

Mukerjee, R., & Wu, C. F. J. (2006). *A modern theory of factorial designs*. Springer Science+Business Media.

National Research Council. (2011). *Guide for the care and use of laboratory animals: Edition 8*. National Academies Press.

Oehlert, G. W. (2010). A first course in design and analysis of experiments. Retrieved from *https://hdl.handle.net/11299/168002*.

Open Science Collaboration. (2015). Estimating the reproducibility of psychological science. *Science, 349*(6251), aac4716.

Perone, M. (1999). Statistical inference in behavior analysis: Experimental control is better. *Behavior Analyst, 22*(2), 109–116.

Peterson, K. M., Piazza, C. C., & Volkert, V. M. (2016). A comparison of a modified sequential oral sensory approach to an applied behavior-analytic approach in the treatment of food selectivity in children with autism spectrum disorder. *Journal of Applied Behavior Analysis, 49*(3), 485–511.

Pickard, K. E., & Ingersoll, B. R. (2016). Quality versus quantity: The role of socioeconomic status on parent-reported service knowledge, service use, unmet service needs, and barriers to service use. *Autism, 20*(1), 106–115.

R Core Team. (2021). R: A language and environment for statistical computing. Retrieved from *www.r-project.org*.

Richards, J. B., Sabol, K. E., & de Wit, H. (1999). Effects of methamphetamine on the adjusting amount procedure, a model of impulsive behavior in rats. *Psychopharmacology, 146*(4), 432–439.

Richardson, J. T. E. (2018). The use of Latin-square designs in educational and psychological research. *Educational Research Review, 24*, 84–97.

Rosales-Ruiz, J., & Baer, D. M. (1997). Behavioral cusps: A developmental and pragmatic concept for behavior analysis. *Journal of Applied Behavior Analysis, 30*(3), 533–544.

Russell, W. M. S., & Burch, R. L. (1959). *The principles of humane experimental technique.* Methuen.

Shahan, T. A., Browning, K. O., Nist, A. N., & Sutton, G. M. (2020). Resurgence and downshifts in alternative reinforcement rate. *Journal of the Experimental Analysis of Behavior, 114*(2), 163–178.

Sidman, M. (1960). *Tactics of scientific research.* Authors Cooperative.

Sloman, K. N., Vollmer, T. R., Cotnoir, N. M., Borrero, C. S., Borrero, J. C., Samaha, A. L., & St Peter, C. C. (2005). Descriptive analyses of caregiver reprimands. *Journal of Applied Behavior Analysis, 38*(3), 373–383.

Smith, G. C. S., & Pell, J. P. (2003). Parachute use to prevent death and major trauma related to gravitational challenge: Systematic review of randomised controlled trials. *British Medical Journal, 327*(7429), 1459–1461.

Thye, S. R. (2007). Logical and philosophical foundations of experimental research in the social sciences. In M. Webster, Jr., & J. Sell (Eds.), *Laboratory experiments in the social sciences* (pp. 53–82). Academic Press.

Tincani, M., & Travers, J. (2019). Replication research, publication bias, and applied behavior analysis. *Perspectives on Behavior Science, 42*(1), 59–75.

Toth, L. A., & Gardiner, T. W. (2000). Food and water restriction protocols: Physiological and behavioral considerations. *Contemporary Topics in Laboratory Animal Science, 39*(6), 9–17.

Tufte, E. R. (1983). *The visual display of quantitative information.* Graphics Press.

Wasserstein, R. L., & Lazar, N. A. (2016). The ASA's statement on *p*-values: Context, process, and purpose. *American Statistician, 70*(2), 129–131.

Wasserstein, R. L., Schirm, A. L., & Lazar, N. A. (2019). Moving to a world beyond "p < 0.05." *American Statistician, 73*(Suppl. 1), 1–19.

Webster, M., Jr., & Sell, J. (Eds.). (2007). *Laboratory experiments in the social sciences.* Academic Press.

CHAPTER 5

Some Frequently Asked Questions about Measuring Behavior

Elizabeth G. E. Kyonka
Shrinidhi Subramaniam

Science cannot progress without reliable and accurate
measurement of what it is you are trying to study.
The key is measurement, simple as that.
—ROBERT HARE (in Spiegel & Hare, 2011)

Reliable, accurate measures of behavior must be the foundation for any scientific analysis of behavior. In psychology and other behavioral sciences, reliable and accurate measurement of dependent variables and representative, statistically robust datasets are achieved through a combination of experimental and statistical control procedures (e.g., Shadish et al., 2002). The basic principles of data collection and measurement are not discipline-specific, but the specific means of achieving experimental and statistical control necessarily depend on the research design, analytic approach, and philosophy of science. Even though we may study the same phenomena, "behavior analysts do things differently than members of other sciences" (Petursdottir & Carr, 2018, p. 228). Our collective interest in behavior for its own sake rather than as an operationalization of underlying hypothetical constructs, our emphasis on analyzing large samples of behavior from the same subject, and the relatively high priority we place on experimental control all provide a unique context for interpretations of accuracy, reliability, and validity that may differ from traditional psychometric interpretations.

Within behavior analysis, differences in experimental and analytic design can require different approaches to data collection and measurement. Single-subject experiments that use laboratory animals in operant chambers to study learning, human-operant experiments that use group designs to elucidate behavioral mechanisms, and applied research evaluating the efficacy of a new intervention for eliminating problem behavior for a specific client all require behavioral observations that are reliable, accurate, representative of the behavior, and sufficiently numerous, but the methods used to obtain such samples necessarily differ.

This chapter considers some issues that are peculiar to behavior analysis, some of which may be particularly relevant to behavior analysts operating across a translational spectrum. The chapter is structured as a series of questions and answers, in which the answers consider research that may examine phenomena at different levels of social significance, along a translational spectrum with five tiers (Kyonka & Subramaniam, 2018). This spectrum does not divide behavior analysis into basic, translational, and applied subdisciplines. Instead, tiers are based on whether the subjects, target behaviors, relevant stimuli and setting were selected for experimental control or social importance. According to this taxonomy, the more applied elements a study has, the higher the tier. Blue-sky basic research (Tier 0) privileges experimental control, often using convenient subjects such as laboratory animals, arbitrary stimuli, and laboratory settings to answer fundamental questions about behavior. Use-inspired (Tier 1) and solution-oriented (Tier 2) research rely on elements of convenience or artificiality to generate new knowledge about behavior or new behavioral technology. Applied research (Tier 3) and impact assessment (Tier 4) provide solutions to specific problems faced in naturalistic scenarios (i.e., without researcher intervention).

The five tiers of our translational spectrum are designed to be applied to datasets, not to individual behavior analysts (Kyonka & Subramaniam, 2018). Like others (e.g., Critchfield, 2011; Lerman, 2003; Mace & Critchfield, 2010), we hope that individual behavior analysts will continue to equip themselves to conduct research across tiers as their interests and needs dictate, and we hope that this chapter will help them to do so.

How Do Behavior Analysts Ensure Behavioral Observations Are Valid?

In psychometrics, *validity* is the degree to which a recorded outcome or event measures what it is supposed to measure. A valid measure is internally consistent (comprising multiple data points that assess the same thing) with high test–retest reliability (response patterns are consistent over time), a consistent factor structure (the same structure is found in multiple/all datasets), and measurement invariance (scale details are consistent across populations, time, and context[1]; Hussey & Hughes, 2020). Conclusions drawn from measures that are not valid are not useful, even if the measurements are reliable.

In behavior analysis, valid behavioral measures are generally achieved by developing clear, effective operational definitions and ensuring they are recorded without systematic biases (to the extent that it is possible to do so). There are behavior-analytic analogues to most of the features of psychometrically valid measures. Whether automated or human-transduced, observations are calibrated to ensure that responses are recorded consistently. Behavior analysts apply stability criteria in steady-state procedures to ensure that differences in results are attributable to experimental manipulations rather than other adaptive processes (Killeen, 1978), similar to test–retest reliability in questionnaires. Discovering invariant environment–behavior relations is arguably the objective of experimental analyses of behavior (Nevin, 1984) and is important in determining the effectiveness of intervention in more applied research.

---

[1] For example, if a self-report questionnaire is designed to measure severity of depressive symptoms on a scale of 1–10, a numeric score of 7 should mean the same thing regardless of the demographic characteristics of the client, method of administration, or point in treatment. If a score of 7 is interpreted as indicating moderate to severe symptoms before treatment begins for one client, it should be interpreted the same way when produced at follow-up, with different clients, and in other situations.

What Makes an Operational Definition Effective?

An *operational definition* is a concrete, specific description of a behavior in strictly behavioral terms (Kazdin, 2016). Operational definitions of behavior can be topographical or functional. *Topographical operational definitions* specify the form of the response. By contrast, *functional operational definitions* specify the response's effect on the environment and include "all relevant forms of the response class" (Cooper et al., 2020, p. 67). For example, the National Football League (2021, p. 7) defines a *drop kick* as "a kick by a player who drops the ball and kicks it as, or immediately after, it touches the ground" and a safety kick as "a kick that puts the ball in play after a safety."

The topographical definition of drop kick specifies a necessary posture or physical orientation of the kicker relative to the ball, but the functional definition of safety kick does not. The definition for drop kick enables referees to distinguish drop kicks from place kicks and punts. The definition for safety kick helps determine when and how game play proceeds after a safety. Each definition is effective in the context in which it is used. In blue-sky basic behavior analysis, researchers can typically contrive or control key environment–behavior relations. Topographical definitions of behavior can enable researchers to engineer those relations with precision, making it possible to discover the fundamental behavioral processes involved. In some applied contexts, functional definitions that specify consequences are needed to differentiate between potentially dangerous behavior and less dangerous and borderline appropriate behavior. Whether topographical or functional, and regardless of where data collection falls along the spectrum of translation, effective operational definitions are designed for a specific context. They are objective, clear, and complete (Cooper et al., 2020) within the confines of the context in which they are used.

Clear and objective operational definitions can be recorded accurately in the observation context; that is, there is no ambiguity about how to classify behavioral events, or which responses count, as instances of the behavior. For example, "hitting with an open hand or fist, kicking, pinching, biting, or pulling hair" (e.g., Johnson et al., 2004) is a clearer operational definition for *aggression* than "hostile or violent behavior or attitudes toward another." The first (topographical) definition includes observable behaviors exclusively. The second definition specifies adjectives that describe aggressive behavior but are subject to individual interpretation. Recording the occurrence of aggressive behavior by human observers is likely to be easier (and to produce greater agreement) with the first definition than with the second.

Complete operational definitions specify all relevant aspects of the behavior being measured, so that there are no misclassifications; that is, a complete operational definition for aggression enables the observer to record all instances of aggression as aggression, and no non-instances of aggression as aggression. For example, a definition of aggression that specifies hitting, pinching, and pulling hair would be incomplete if the subject also kicks and bites people. Conversely, a too-broad definition (e.g., "any forceful motor movement") is also incomplete, even though it captures all relevant aggressive behaviors, because many nonaggressive behaviors (e.g., running and jumping) would also be classified as aggression incorrectly.

Effective operational definitions include details about the context in which they apply. There is a necessary tradeoff between brevity (which is important for clarity) and completeness. An exhaustive topographical operational definition for aggression would require a long and detailed list of movements, and an exhaustive functional definition would need to specify many outcomes and exceptions. Either would necessarily include elements that would be irrelevant or inappropriate in some contexts. Johnson et al.'s (2004) definition for aggression would be inadequate as a general operational definition of aggression, but was suited to the context in which it was used.

In laboratory research, factors that place physiological or electronic limits on what "counts" as a response shape the operational definition of target responses. For example, when a target response involves pressing a lever or plastic response disc, the manipulandum must move a minimum amount for the response to be detected. These detection thresholds can be adapted in different ways. Adjusting the size, protrusion, and tension of a response lever affects the amount of force required to produce a detectable response (MedAssociates, 2021). In some cases, very forceful pressing or pecking can cause a lever or response key to bounce, such that the input system records multiple responses. One way to address this "jitter" is to place restrictions on the minimum interresponse time (e.g., Blough, 1966). If a lever is retractable, the time it takes the lever to extend and retract can impact maximum response rates on some schedules (e.g., continuous reinforcement). The temporal resolution of the operating system that records responses also limits the maximum response rate that can be detected, although contemporary systems are generally able to record events with millisecond accuracy or better, and biological organisms making voluntary motor movements are unlikely to exceed those limits. Operational definitions do not necessarily receive as much attention in laboratory experimental research as they do in applied research and practice, but equipment settings and other practical considerations impact operational definitions of responses and determine (in part) the generality of results.

Constructing operational definitions that are clear, complete, and context-specific is a necessary foundation for valid and reliable experimental research and empirically informed practice. It is a concern that is as relevant in laboratory experiments involving responses detected exclusively by mechanical or electronic means as in applied research and practice.

Now That I Have an Effective Operational Definition, How Should I Measure the Target Behavior?

Behavior-analytic measurement can be direct or indirect. *Direct measurement* involves using humans or machines to observe the behavior as it occurs by counting its frequency, timing its duration, and/or calculating its magnitude, among other strategies. *Indirect measurement* involves measuring a behavior through its impact on the environment, archival records of the behavior, or self-reports such as rating scales and interviews. When overt behavior is targeted for assessment and intervention, the preferred option is to directly observe the behavior.

I Can Directly Observe the Behavior; What Should I Measure, and Which Measurement Strategy Should I Use?

First, define the *observation period,* the window in which you observe one or more dimensions of the behavior as it occurs, and decide whether to collect an event record or estimate of the behavior. Depending on the goals of the research and the resources at their disposal, behavior analysts can use continuous or discontinuous recording procedures. Both approaches should be designed to obtain a representative sample of behavior. *Continuous recording* involves observing one or more dimensions of behavior and/or other events during a defined observation period. *Discontinuous recording* involves estimating behavior and/or events using interval recording procedures (partial- and whole-interval recording) and time sampling (momentary time sampling). Much has been written about the process and relative merit of each procedure (Cooper et al., 2020; Miltenberger, 2016), and guides are available to help clinicians decide which procedure to use for a specific target behavior (LeBlanc et al., 2016).

To obtain a representative sample of behavior, define your observation period based on the behavior of interest. For example, behavior that occurs at a high frequency and steady rate can be observed during shorter observation periods than behavior that occurs at a high frequency, but in bouts. Furthermore, design of the interval size of a discontinuous procedure should also be based on dimensions of the target behavior at baseline. For example, behavior that occurs at a high frequency and steady rate might be overestimated using partial-interval recording unless the intervals are limited to a few seconds. One guide suggests arranging for shorter intervals with shorter observation periods and longer intervals with longer observation periods (Devine et al., 2011).

Once you define the observation period, select the most appropriate strategy to measure the behavior directly. Below, we draw from and expand on the measurement strategies listed in the fifth edition of the *Behavior Analyst Certification Board (BACB) Task List* (2017).

Measure Occurrence

Occurrence is defined as the count, frequency, rate, or percentage of a target behavior. Table 5.1 illustrates how the same occurrence measure, the number of clicks on a computer mouse, can be used across the translational spectrum. A researcher conducting a blue-sky basic experiment might measure the number of mouse clicks per minute emitted by a human subject to describe relative rate of responding under different concurrent variable-interval schedules of reinforcement. In use-inspired and solution-oriented research, a researcher might use the same procedure to compare choice making in typically developing participants versus a clinical population (e.g., people with addiction). In applied research and impact assessment, a researcher could offer participants choices in treatment and use computer key presses to determine and deliver preferred treatments.

Research on human learning processes has often used computer key presses as target behaviors. Analyses of the count, frequency, rate, or percentage of computer key presses have yielded important insights into environment–behavior relations that generalize in many ways. For example, Allan and Gibbon (1991) developed a temporal bisection task to measure human temporal discrimination. On each trial, a computer played an auditory tone (the sample stimulus). Once the tone was complete, the participant's task was to categorize its duration as short by typing "S," or long by typing "L." They found that the proportion of long responses as a function of time conformed to an S-shaped psychophysical function much like those produced by nonhumans in similar tasks. The top panel of Figure 5.1 lists stimuli and feedback presented in each block of one condition of Allan and Gibbon's Experiment 1. In other conditions, short and long tone durations were 0.75 second and 1 second, 1 second and 1.5 seconds, 1.4 seconds and 2.1 seconds. The bottom

TABLE 5.1. Examples of Different Ways to Measure Behavior

Measure	Blue-sky basic	Use-inspired/solution-oriented	Applied research and impact assessment
Occurrence • Count • Frequency • Rate • Percentage	Computer key presses to describe relative response rate under different VI schedules (choice, matching)	Computer key presses in an intertemporal choice procedure for people with and without addiction	Computer key presses to choose an intervention
Temporal dimensions of behavior • Duration • Latency • Interresponse time	Examining frequencies of IRT distributions in a DRL schedule to determine what operant is reinforced	Comparing IRT distributions in humans and other animals in DRL schedules	IRT in a spaced-responding DRL to reduce requests for attention in a classroom
Form and strength of behavior • Topography • Magnitude	Setting response force requirements for a lever press to earn a reinforcer to model the relation between effort and response rate	Measuring the effectiveness of a canvas arm splint to keep hands in pockets in a convenience sample of adults	Calibrating minimum force requirements in canvas arm splint to decrease self-injurious behavior
Trials to criterion • Count of responses required to meet a goal or standard	Measuring the number of trials for acquisition of preference in a concurrent schedule with different reinforcer ratios	Measuring the number of discrete trials it takes to discriminate arbitrary stimuli with high and low preferred consequences	Measuring the number of discrete trials to master academically relevant targets with high and low frequency of preferred consequences
Variability • Bounce in a single variable across observations • The extent to which multiple topographies/forms/patterns of behavior are present	Modeling response patterns in lag schedules with pigeons	Comparing response pattern distributions in pigeons under varying lag schedules with and without D-amphetamine.	Reducing stereotypy using lag schedules of reinforcement in a client with autism
Product measures Observable impact of behavior on environment	Counting the number of food pellets left in a hopper to describe motivating operations in pigeons	Measuring antecedents to food consumption in healthy participants by measuring the weight of ad libitum food	Body weight as a measure of food acceptance during an antecedent intervention in a client with food refusal
Standardized questionnaires Quantifiable self-reports	Scale validation to establish reliability and validity of a scale measuring intertemporal choice	Comparing real and hypothetical intertemporal choice-delay discounting (with and without actual contact with the outcomes)	Reducing delay discounting using acceptance and commitment therapy
Interviews	Open ended questions about choice in human operant concurrent schedule arrangement to add context to preference	Varying question wording in an interview-based preference assessment with clients to understand the influence of the experimenter	Interview based preference assessment with teachers to identify potential reinforcers to use in interventions

Note. DRL = differential reinforcement of low rates of behavior; IRT = interresponse time; and VI = variable interval.

Trial Type	Stimulus Duration (s)	Feedback provided?	Trials per Block
Short	1	"Short" on 50% of trials	14
Intermediate	1.1	none	7
	1.2	none	7
	1.3	none	7
	1.4	none	7
	1.5	none	7
	1.6	none	7
	1.7	none	7
	1.8	none	7
	1.9	none	7
Long	2	"Long" on 50% of trials	14

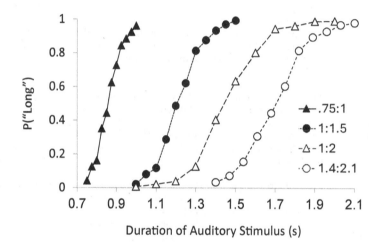

FIGURE 5.1. Procedure and results of a temporal bisection experiment. Procedure and results of Allan and Gibbon's (1991) Experiment 1. P("L") is the probability that a participant typed "L" to indicate that the duration of the auditory stimulus was long. Graph reprinted with permission of Elsevier.

panel shows the probability of choosing "L," averaged over subjects. Allan and Gibbon showed that regardless of the duration of short and long tones, the point of subjective equality (when a participant was equally likely to choose "S" or "L") was always close to the geometric mean of short and long durations. They explained this result in terms of the scalar expectancy model of interval timing.

Allan and Gibbon's (1991) experiments typified blue-sky basic research with respect to aims, procedural details, and analytic approach. Based on citations of the work in other peer-reviewed publications, the impact of the temporal bisection task was broad. It is most frequently cited by other empirical reports of temporal learning and time perception in experimental psychology journals such as the *Quarterly Journal of Psychology* and *Behavioural Processes*, but it has been cited by articles published in over 70 different journals, including in work about veterinary sciences (Cliff et al., 2019), people with type 2 diabetes and people who smoke tobacco (Vázquez & Torres, 2017), and people with schizophrenia (Reed & Randell, 2014), Alzheimer's disease (Caselli et al., 2009), autism (Gil et al., 2012), and Parkinson's disease (Shea-Brown et al., 2006). In research investigating timing in children (Droit-Volet et al., 2004; Droit-Volet & Rattat, 2007; Droit-Volet, 2013) older children integrated temporal and numeric properties of stimuli, but younger children did not, and children overestimated durations when the presented stimuli were aversive or threatening. Results like these have implications for teaching children music and safety skills. The experimental method was developed to test predictions of a theoretical model of interval timing. It was successfully adapted with few changes to inform a range of use-inspired, solution-oriented, and applied research, providing an example of successful translation.

In the area of education, behavior analysts have recognized that learning objectives should not always be based on counts of correct responses (i.e., accuracy) alone, but also on rate (count/time). For example, a student could add two numbers together accurately, but they may take a very long time to arrive at the correct answer. To achieve computational fluency, the student must be able to add numbers together accurately and quickly. According to an Association for Behavior Analysis International policy statement on students' right to effective education (Barrett et al., 1991, p. 81), "Curriculum and instructional objectives should . . . specify mastery criteria that include both the accuracy and the speed dimensions of fluent performance." Fluency is thus a measure of behavior that combines occurrence, time, and accuracy to characterize performance. From bench to bedside, research on fluency has led to instructional techniques such as precision teaching and direct instruction that can improve reading and math performance in students with a wide range of skills (Johnson & Street, 2014) and highlights the importance of measuring occurrence.

Measure Temporal Dimensions of Behavior

All behavior occurs in time. It follows that an important category of direct measurement involves measuring the temporal dimensions of behavior such as duration, how long a continuous behavior is observed; latency, how long it takes for a behavior to occur after some other event; and interresponse time (IRT), the time between two instances of the behavior. Table 5.1 illustrates measures of IRT across the translational spectrum. A basic researcher might examine a frequency distribution of IRTs to describe response spacing in a differential reinforcement of low rates (DRL) schedule. In use-inspired research, college students might respond in the same DRL schedule to compare temporal discrimination and differentiation across species. In more applied research, a teacher might implement a spaced-responding DRL, in which they measure the IRT of a students' requests for attention, and honor the requests if the IRT is greater than 15 minutes.

Duration, latency, and IRT are important dimensions of behavior in research on human learning across the translational spectrum. Baum and Rachlin (1969) characterized choice as allocation of time across two or more alternatives. They found that the time pigeons spent on different sides of a long experimental chamber matched the relative rate of food they received from each side. Similarly, use-inspired research by Conger and Killeen (1974) reported that the time participants spent talking in a discussion group matched the relative rate of verbal approval from confederate members of the group. In a more solution-oriented study, Neef et al. (1992) measured the time that special education students spent on math problems and found that time allocation matched relative reinforcement rate for correct responses.

Measure Form and Strength of Behavior

Sometimes, the form and strength of behavior is of interest. The *form* of a behavior can be described as the topography or structure of the behavior. The *strength* of a behavior can be described as the magnitude, force, or intensity of the behavior. Table 5.1 illustrates how response force can be measured across the translational spectrum. A researcher conducting a blue-sky basic experiment might change the force requirements on a response option to develop a model of response effort. In solution-oriented research, the experimenter might invent a canvas arm splint restraint using typically developing or adult participants to observe and calibrate the settings on the restraint. In applications of this research, the tightness of the canvas arm splint restraint might be manipulated as a treatment to decrease a client's self-injurious behavior (e.g., Fisher et al., 1997).

Defining the strength or magnitude of a response may involve the force of a response, units of energy burned, the displacement of objects, the distance traveled, sensory outcomes, or even counts of the behavior. In organizational behavior management, response effort has been manipulated by moving objects necessary to complete a task at a distance from the employee (e.g., Casella et al., 2010). Occurrence of the task is the direct measure of behavior, but effort is also measured as the movement of the employee to complete the task.

The magnitude of sound emitted by subjects can be measured in behavioral research. Here, the magnitude of behavior is measured as the decibel level of noise at a specified location. Research on active learning in a college classroom has used decibel analysis to quantify the magnitude of discussion during classroom activities (Owens et al., 2017). In the workplace, loud discussions between employees may be discouraged, so a decibel analysis can be used to intervene on unprofessional behavior (Sigurdsson et al., 2011).

The form of behavior is often important in applied research and impact assessment involving training subjects to master motor skills. Research on the acquisition of motor skills may include topographical and functional operational definitions (see section "What Makes an Operational Definition Effective?") and multiple measurement strategies to ensure that the correct form meets the desired function. For example, in training typing, a teacher might be interested in not only in the number of correct characters (count) but also the placement of the fingers on the keyboard (form) (Dillon et al., 2004).

Measure Trials to Criterion

In learning and skill-acquisition research, the *direct measure of a target behavior* can be defined as the number of trials to criterion. *Trials to criterion* is defined as "the number of responses it takes for someone to meet the standard set for success" (Cooper et al., 2020, p. 131). Table 5.1 illustrates the measurement of trials to criterion across the translational spectrum. A researcher conducting blue-sky basic research might measure the number of interreinforcer intervals it takes for a subject to develop a stable preference for one schedule of reinforcement over another. In solution-oriented research, the standard for success might be the number of trials to a correct discrimination of arbitrary targets, while applied research may involve the same procedure with academically relevant targets.

Research that uses trials to criterion can use one or more of the measurement strategies described in this section along with a definition for mastery. For example, in the study by Dillon et al. (2004), the researchers evaluated trials to criterion by measuring the *rate of acquisition*—the number of training hours it took to reach a critical step in the typing and keypad training programs. Training on life skills can also be evaluated using trials to criterion measures. Sprague and Horner (1984) taught individuals with disabilities to purchase items from vending machines and measured the generalization of that skill to untrained machines. During training, trials to criterion represented the number of purchases the learner made until they mastered the skill. *Mastery* was defined as the individual purchasing an item independently and without errors on three consecutive attempts.

Measure Variability

A behavior might be measured using one of the aforementioned direct measures, but the target is really the variability of the behavior. *Variability* can be defined as the bounce in a single variable across observations or the extent to which multiple topographies, forms, or sequences of behavior are present. In one line of research that spans the translational spectrum, experimenters attempted to promote novel response patterns using lag schedules of reinforcement (Lee et al., 2002; Page & Neuringer, 1985). Table 5.2 illustrates this measurement of variability. A basic researcher might set up several keys in a pigeon operant chamber and program reinforcers for novel key peck sequences. Use-inspired research

TABLE 5.2. Methods of Assessing Reliability for Target Responses That Can Be Automated

Target response	Observer/recorder	Reliability assessment
Singular nonverbal response: Lever press, key peck, nose poke, mouse click, or swipe to a touchscreen	Automated (e.g., computer or electrical relay)	Regular calibration by the researcher to ensure equipment is functioning
Singular verbal response: Likert scale rating, binary choice (e.g., yes–no questions, responses in most discounting tasks), typed numeric estimates, computerized visual analogue scales	Automated	Repeated administration, manipulation checks
	Human (e.g., measuring visual analogue scale ratings with a ruler)	Calculate IOA
Verbal description: Written or otherwise recorded description of behavior (e.g., by the subject or a teacher or caregiver)	Fully automated (e.g., using data analytics/natural language processing type analysis)	Occasional recalibration of the classification system may be valuable
	Recorded by computer but counted, classified, or otherwise interpreted by human observer	Calculate IOA on the classification but not on topographical details (e.g., number of words or word length)
Response class with multiple response topographies (e.g., aggression)	Human	Calculate IOA

might involve evaluating effects of D-amphetamine on these novel key peck sequences. In applied research, the same lag schedule could be used to reduce stereotypy in a client with autism.

How Do I Measure Behavior If I Can't Observe the Target in Real Time?

Behavior analysts can measure a target behavior of interest indirectly by identifying a proxy for the behavior and observing it. Indirect measurement strategies include obtaining permanent products, having participants complete standardized questionnaires or rating scales, and conducting interviews with participants. In behavior analysis, direct measurement of the target behavior is generally preferred over indirect measurement. Indirect measures of behavior such as verbal reports could have dubious correspondence with the behavior of interest. For example, a participant may report that they engaged in a target behavior even when they did not for social approval or some other desirable outcome. Furthermore, verbal reports of behavior may be subject to biases in remembering and could be influenced by other events. Observing the behavior as it occurs is not always a feasible method, and there are preferred ways to measure behavior indirectly and to convince others of the correspondence between indirect measures and the behavior of interest.

What Is the Preferred Way to Measure Behavior Indirectly?

Indirect measurement generally occurs at a delay following the target behavior. If the target behavior changes the environment in a measurable way, recording the behavior indirectly using a product measure is preferred over self-reports (LeBlanc et al., 2016).

When the target behavior has an impact on the environment, this impact is the "product" of behavior. For example, a client with self-injurious behavior (SIB) might have observable tissue damage on their body from repeated instances of the behavior. For a permanent product measure to be used appropriately, the behavior analyst should be confident in the validity and reliability of the behavior that generated the product (LeBlanc et al., 2016); that is, the SIB must lead to the tissue damage, and the tissue damage must reliably follow the SIB and not follow other events.

Product measures can be obtained from archival records or by measuring physical traces of the target behavior (Kazdin, 1979). Kazdin described archival records as reports of behavior that have been collected and stored by institutions or governments. For example, a behavior-analytic researcher interested in a subject's employment history might review Social Security earnings reports that have been collected and stored by the U.S. government. Kazdin described physical traces as displacements in the environment due to a behavior. Table 5.1 illustrates examples of physical traces across the translational spectrum. A basic researcher measures the number of food pellets remaining in a hopper after an experimental session with different levels of food deprivation as a measure of motivating operations in pigeons. For a use-inspired or solution-oriented project, a researcher might conduct a similar study with healthy adults where they instruct the individual to fast for some amount of time, then present freely available snacks. They then measure the weight of the remaining snacks to determine the conditions under which people eat different snack foods. In more applied research, a client's weight might be monitored as a permanent product measure of food acceptance.

Behavioral researchers evaluating interventions to curb addiction often use permanent product recording to measure drug use. Drug use is typically a target behavior that often occurs privately, but there is a well-developed technology to measure its occurrence after the fact. In abstinence-based contingency management interventions, the absence of drug use is often reinforced with financial incentives (Silverman et al., 2021). Rather than continuously observing subjects or asking them whether they used substances, biological samples are obtained under direct observation and tested for the presence of drug metabolites. Testing for recent cocaine use, for example, can occur by measuring the concentration of benzoylecgonine in the urine (Holtyn et al., 2017).

Permanent products have historically been used in applied behavior analysis research as a measure of academic performance in school settings (see Kelly, 1976, 1977). These measures can include written responses on a worksheet (Deshais et al., 2019), number of assignments completed (Cushing & Kennedy, 1997), and questions answered correctly (Knapczyk, 1989), among others (see Cooper et al., 2020, p. 93).

How Do I Measure the Target Behavior Indirectly When I Am Not Confident of the Validity and Reliability of Its Impact on the Environment?

In verbal human subjects, other- and self-reports of behavior can be obtained through standardized questionnaires, rating scales, and interviews. This form of indirect measurement may involve the subject remembering and describing past behavior, reporting tendencies, or engaging with hypothetical scenarios and reporting hypothetical behavior.

What Is the Function of Measuring a Target Behavior Using Self-Report?

Although the spectrum of behavior analytic research tends to focus on direct measures of observable behavior or permanent product recording, self-reports can serve several functions (for reviews, see Critchfield et al., 1998; Perone, 1988). First, when behavior is covert or private, self-report is the most feasible method to observe the target behavior. Questionnaires, scales, and interviews help pinpoint what a person is thinking and feeling or doing inside and outside the experiential environment. Second, self-reports can help the researcher understand a person's tendencies by measuring average responses to questionnaire items. A rating scale may be able to identify preferences for a variety of outcomes quickly, while a direct measure of the behavior could take a long time.[2] Third, perhaps because they are practical and convenient, self-reports are sometimes obtained to explain human behavior as a "short-cut around the difficulties of a true experimental analysis" (Perone, 1988, p. 74). In these cases, if obtained in valid and reliable ways, self-

---

[2] For example, a client with specific phobia of dentistry might visit the dentist rarely, if at all, and a therapist may have limited opportunity to observe the client in situations when symptoms manifest. Standardized self-report assessments can direct the therapist's attention to situations that may require more detailed assessment and evaluation, provide additional information about dimensions of the phobia, and may be useful as indices of change throughout treatment (Hood & Antony, 2012).

reports can help a researcher generate hypotheses about behavior. Finally, behavior analysts might be interested in the content of what people say in its own right. For example, there is a large body of translational research on say–do correspondence wherein what people say is the operationally defined target behavior.

What Are Some Ways Behavior Analysts Have Used Self-Report Measures in Quantitative Research?

In behavior-analytic research, standardized questionnaires have been used to gain information about choice and preferences, and in more applied research, to relate them to problems of social significance and target behavioral processes for intervention. Table 5.1 illustrates research using standardized questionnaires and rating scales measuring intertemporal choice along a translational spectrum. Basic research may involve developing a scale on intertemporal choice and establishing its validity and reliability in a convenience sample. Use-inspired and solution-oriented research might take that scale and relate choices in situations under which the outcomes are hypothetical or when participants experience the outcomes. Applied and impact assessment research may attempt to reduce impulsive choices on these questionnaires using a treatment such as acceptance and commitment therapy.

This kind of translational research program has resulted in several standardized questionnaires measuring intertemporal choice, risky choice, and impulsivity. These questionnaires include the Monetary Choice Questionnaire (Kirby et al., 1999) and the Probability Discounting Questionnaire (Madden et al., 2009). Applied behavior-analytic studies have related choices on these standardized questionnaires to health behaviors such as drug use (Bickel & Marsch, 2001), pathological gambling (Andrade & Petry, 2012), texting while driving (Hayashi et al., 2018), and binge eating (Stojek & MacKillop, 2017), among others.

In addition to measuring intertemporal and risky choices, behavior analysts have used standardized questionnaires and rating scales to help identify preferred outcomes that can serve as potentially reinforcing consequences for clients or research subjects. These preference assessments have taken the form of rating scales (Green et al., 1991; Parsons & Reid, 1990) and standardized checklists (Matson et al., 1999), responses on which have been validated using reinforcer assessments.

Standardized questionnaires and rating scales are sometimes used to gain more information or generate more hypotheses about learning processes under study. For example, Baumann and Odum (2012) related delay discounting with other processes such as impulsivity, temporal discrimination, and time perspective. They studied these different phenomena with direct and indirect measures of behavior. A temporal bisection task measured temporal discrimination directly. A delay and probability discounting task with hypothetical outcomes indirectly, but behaviorally measured impulsive and risky choices, respectively. They measured other related constructs using validated rating scales—the Barratt Impulsiveness Scale measured motor, attentional, and nonplanning impulsivity, and the Zimbardo Time Perspective Inventory measured past negative, present hedonistic, future, past positive, and present fatalistic perspectives of time.

Researchers conducting applied behavior analysis experiments often use standardized rating scales and questionnaires to measure social validity of assessment and treatment (see Common & Lane, 2017, for a review). These include Kazdin's (1980) Treatment

Acceptability Inventory, which evaluates judgments of treatments by recipients or stakeholders; the Treatment Acceptability Rating Form—Revised (TARF-R; Reimers & Wacker, 1988); and the Intervention Rating Profile (Witt et al., 1984).

What Are Some Ways Behavior Analysts Have Used Interviews?

Self- and other-reports of behavior or contextual variables can be measured using interviews, which typically involve the researcher presenting the subject with questions about their behavior and/or environment.

Table 5.1 illustrates research using interviews along a translational spectrum. In the human-operant laboratory, a researcher conducting a blue-sky basic experiment might use an interview following a session of exposure to a concurrent-schedule choice arrangement. The interviewer could ask participants about their choices and their understanding of the contingencies in the experiment to determine whether participants generated self-statements and rules that predicted their response/time allocation. Use-inspired and solution-oriented research may involve studying question variations in an interview-based preference assessment to understand response biases driven by question wording. A more applied approach might use the Preference Assessment Interview to identify potential reinforcers a teacher can use for students in a classroom.

Several basic, use-inspired, and solution-oriented behavior-analytic studies with human subjects have used interviews with open-ended questions to help identify and describe functional relations between behavior and environment. For example, Horne and Lowe (1993) evaluated human responding in a concurrent schedule. At the end of the experiment, they asked participants the following interview questions: "What did you think the experiment was about?"; "How did you set about winning points?" Similarly, Wearden and Shimp (1985) studied spaced responding in a paced random-interval schedule in which an appropriately timed interresponse interval led to "GOOD" and points (vs. "POOR" and no points). At the end of the experiment, they asked participants, "What did you have to do to get a 'GOOD'?" and "What did you have to do to get a 'POOR'?" Fox and Kyonka (2017) administered poststudy questionnaires in which participants reported their response strategies in a diminishing-returns procedure in which a rule given to the participants was or was not the optimal way to earn points (see Hackenberg & Joker, 1994). The researchers coded whether the self-reported response strategy was consistent or inconsistent with the rule and compared response strategies of rule followers versus rule breakers.

For the most part, interviews in the spectrum of behavior-analytic research are designed to solve problems. For example, assessment of problem behavior in organizational behavior management involves identifying the causes of performance problems in employees. These problems may be difficult to detect with field observations. If field observations are possible, preliminary interviews can inform logistics of the observations. The Performance Diagnostic Checklist (PDC; Austin, 2000) and PDC–Human Services (Carr et al., 2013) are interviews conducted by behavior analysts with supervisors and managers to gain information about the function of employee problem behavior.

Structured interviews have been developed for functional behavior assessment in a variety of other settings. For example, the Functional Analysis Screening Tool (FAST; Iwata et al., 2013) asks parents, instructors, therapists, staff or other informants about problem behavior, medical and physical problems, what happens before the problem behavior, and what happens after the problem behavior. Similarly, the Functional Assessment Informant Record for Teachers (FAIR-T; Dufrene et al., 2007) is a structured interview given by a behavior analyst to a teacher or classroom aide about a student's problem behavior. This interviewer also asks about a student's academic skills and deficits. The Reinforcer Assessment for Individuals with Severe Disability (RAISD; Fisher et al., 1996) is an interview-based preference assessment. Like the preference assessment surveys and rating scales, the RAISD attempts to identify preferred stimuli that may function as reinforcers in treatment. Because it is in an interview, the behavior analyst asks follow-up questions to add detail to the self-report.

What Are Sources of Bias in Behavioral Measurements and How Can I Address Them?

Measurement error is any deviation of a recorded measurement from the so-called true value being measured. Eliminating all measurement error is not possible when the true values are unknown or unknowable, as is typically the case in behavior analysis. Although it is impossible to eliminate all measurement error, minimizing potential sources of *bias*, defined as nonrandom errors in measurement, is an essential part of ensuring the validity of behavioral observations.

Measurement is fully automated if a computer or other device detects and classifies responses directly without human transduction or interpretation. Typical examples include pigeons or other animal subjects pecking plastic discs, rats pressing levers, humans or other animal subjects swiping at touchscreens, and humans rating their agreement with statements using Likert scales. Bias can occur in automated recording of behavior due to equipment fatigue or malfunction. For example, a touchscreen might have reduced sensitivity in high-traffic locations on the screen, making it less likely that taps or swipes in those positions are recorded. Regular recalibration (e.g., a researcher responds at each position on a touchscreen in a systematic manner, ideally with response topography that is consistent with participants' or subjects' typical response topography, then confirms that each response was recorded) can detect this kind of error, and counterbalancing the locations where response options appear throughout a session can minimize or eliminate any systematic impact of such errors on dependent variables.

Some form of regular calibration to detect equipment issues is likely needed in most behavioral measurement that relies on automated recording. In laboratory operant conditioning research with pigeons, calibration might involve a daily equipment check protocol run by a researcher before the first session of the day. We recommend that equipment check protocols evaluate all automated inputs and outputs. In a pigeon operant conditioning chamber, a researcher might "peck" each response key a specified number of times to confirm that each "peck" is recorded as a separate response (and only one response). The computer might be programmed to change the key color or stimulus presented with each response, so the researcher can determine visually whether any bulbs are burnt out. In addition to checking manipulanda, the protocol should include activation and deactivation of the hopper or dipper to ensure that food or liquid is available when it is programmed to be available (and not otherwise). The researcher might also visually inspect the hopper to ensure that there is enough food available to last until it can be refilled.

Regular calibration can detect equipment malfunctions and ensure that they are addressed relatively quickly. When issues are not detected or are not quickly fixed, counterbalancing can ensure that errors associated with equipment problems are distributed evenly throughout the experiment rather than concentrated in a particular condition or response class. In repeated-measures group experimental designs, counterbalancing is a technique used to deal with serial order effects in which all subjects experience the same experimental conditions, but different subgroups experience the conditions in different orders (see DePuy & Berger, 2014, for a description of different types of complete and partial counterbalancing). In behavior-analytic research, counterbalancing is extended to include varied or randomized presentation of events in time or space to minimize order and position effects within data collected from an individual subject. For example, in concurrent chain schedules in which red and green initial-link keys signal different terminal-link outcomes, counterbalancing the location of red and green initial links (i.e., as left or right) would involve changing the location where the red initial link is programmed to appear randomly or pseudo-randomly from trial to trial or from one interreinforcer interval to the next. In addition to addressing potential equipment failures, this kind of counterbalancing can also be a way to address certain subject biases (e.g., side key or color biases). It is important to note that counterbalancing does not reduce measurement error; it minimizes bias by equalizing the distribution of errors throughout experiments.

Reactivity, which is the change in subject's behavior as a result of observation, is another source of bias. In some cases (e.g., self-management interventions), reactivity is desirable; however, in others, reactivity may lead to errors in judgment of treatment effects. Reactivity can be minimized by using minimally obtrusive measures such as one-way mirrors or cameras present at all times. Reactivity tends to be a transient phenomenon, so giving subjects a chance to habituate to the presence of observers or recording equipment such as cameras should minimize its impact. A heuristic might be to record the behavior across at least three observation periods that occur on different days. Measuring behavior through archival records and permanent products can reduce the chances that reactivity will impact the target behavior.

Self-report report instruments and other indirect measures of behavior are associated with different types of response bias and require different approaches to minimizing bias than direct observations. The demands associated with answering questionnaires can produce reactivity. Responses can be affected by the amount of attention the respondent devotes to the task. Reactive inhibition or fatigue related to the demands of answering questions can be expected to increase as sessions continue, making responses to items that appear later in a questionnaire potentially less reliable than responses to earlier items. Self-reports can be biased due to the respondent's desire to agree with the questioner (acquiescence bias) to provide the answers they believe the questioner wants to receive (courtesy bias), or to underestimate supposedly undesirable behaviors (social desirability bias).

Strategies for minimizing response bias in self-report (and caregiver- or other-report) instruments can involve adapting the wording of individual items and considering the structure of the questionnaire as a whole. For example, reverse-worded items measure the "opposite" of the construct or variable being measured. If a higher rating indicates the respondent experiences more reinforcement related to a particular consequence on a behavior rating scale, items for which a lower rating indicates more reinforcement are reverse-worded. Although they do not necessarily reduce careless responding and thus have implications for factor analysis (Woods, 2006), including reverse-worded items can minimize acquiescence and attention biases. To minimize courtesy and social desirability biases, avoid administering instruments with items that are worded in a way that implies there is a particular correct or virtuous answer. As with counterbalancing, randomizing the order of presentation of items should distribute errors related to response fatigue throughout all items (at least across subjects).

Some biases are present when a human observer records the target behavior and other events. *Observer bias* is the impact that the observer's expectations and skills have on their data collection practices. For example, an observer who has knowledge of study hypotheses may produce systematic recording errors in favor of the hypotheses. Having observers who are blind to study hypotheses is one way to prevent this expectancy error; however, this practice might not be possible in behavior-analytic research in which the environment changes in obvious ways. Another source of bias is *observer drift*, which is the change in control by operational definitions over recording with time. Observer bias and drift can be assessed with reliability checks. Having a second observer present at all times permits calibration and recalibration of measurement, which can minimize these sources of bias (Mudford et al., 2011). Furthermore, newly trained observers can conduct intermittent checks to ensure appropriate control of measurement by the operational definitions of the target behavior and events. Behavior analysts should consider observer bias and drift when defining the target behavior and developing a measurement system. Restricting duration and difficulty of observations can limit the opportunity for observer drift, while automating data collection can avoid observer bias.

Ambiguity in operational definitions of target responses can be another source of bias. If different observers interpret the operational definition for a target behavior in different ways, there may be systematic differences in measurement depending on who is recording the behavior. Having multiple observers record the same sample of behavior and comparing records to assess interobserver agreement (IOA) is an empirical means of evaluating whether operational definitions are interpreted consistently. Calibrating IOA on a regular basis can assist with mitigating this source of bias.

How Do Behavior Analysts Assess Agreement?

Although it has been discussed as a measure of believability rather than reliability (Johnston et al., 2020), interrater reliability in behavior analysis is often assessed in the form of IOA, "the degree to which two or more independent observers report the same observed values after measuring the same events" (Cooper et al., 2020, p. 111). Behavior analysts can calculate IOA by dividing agreements by the sum of agreements and disagreements—or taking the ratio of obtained frequencies or durations of behavior—and multiplying by 100 to obtain a percentage.

Behavior analysts have written extensively about IOA. The comprehensive body of literature on IOA in applied behavior analysis includes detailed descriptions of appropriate ways to calculate IOA depending on the target behavior and temporal window (e.g., Cooper et al., 2020; House et al., 1981; Johnston et al., 2020; Miltenberger, 2016), which include total agreement, exact agreement, interval agreement, and agreement on the occurrence or nonoccurrence of behavior. Behavior-analysis researchers have conducted evaluations of the relative utility of IOA calculations in different circumstances (e.g., Mudford et al., 2009), created tools to facilitate the calculation of IOA (e.g., Reed & Azulay, 2010), and listed recommendations for best practice (e.g., Vollmer et al., 2008).

Should I Calculate Interobserver Agreement?

An extensive body of literature in applied behavior analysis outlines the benefits of calculating IOA and specifies different methods of calculation (e.g., Cooper et al., 2020), but few, if any, of these resources address the issue of whether calculating IOA for a particular target behavior is necessary or valuable. The absence of clear guidelines about when to calculate IOA may lead some behavior analysts to assume it is necessary to report IOA on all behavior in all circumstances. Calculating and reporting IOA when it is not useful to do so (e.g., providing independent human confirmation of computer readouts of counts of automatically recorded responses) is not a good use of a behavior analyst's time or effort.

As Figure 5.2 illustrates, the answer to this question is deceptively simple: IOA is useful when there is potential for disagreement regarding the record of behavioral events among researchers or practitioners, as is the case when human observers record the duration or frequency of responses defined by function-based operational definitions. Other circumstances require different methods of assessing reliability, such as equipment calibration.

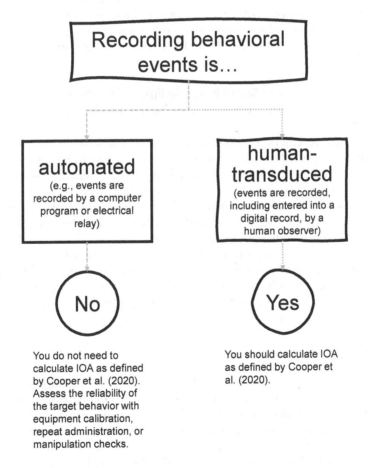

FIGURE 5.2. Should I calculate interobserver agreement (IOA)?

Fully automated observation does not require IOA as traditionally calculated and reported by behavior analysts. *Fully automated* means that a computer or other electronic device detects and classifies responses directly, without human transduction or interpretation. Typical examples include pigeons or other animal subjects pecking plastic discs, rats pressing levers, humans or other animal subjects swiping at touchscreens, and humans rating their agreement with statements using Likert scales. When an electronic input device registers responses and a computer program records them, it is important to ensure that the equipment and program are functioning properly throughout data collection, but little is gained by having multiple human observers independently examine readouts of event records then compare their observations of what they have read. If the automated behavioral recording had been unreliable in some way (e.g., a key was sticking or a written item was worded in a way that participants did not interpret it consistently), calculating IOA as defined by Cooper et al. (2020) would not reveal the irregularity. Conversely, if IOA on a fully automated recording is less than 100%, the discrepancy reflects an issue with the legibility of the readout or the skill of the readers rather than with the reliability of the record.

Calculating and reporting IOA on automatically recorded events is not necessary, but this does not mean that automated behavioral records are automatically reliable. Behavior analysts using automated recording must evaluate the reliability of observations in other ways (e.g., with regular equipment recalibration or manipulation checks). Table 5.2 suggests methods of assessing reliability for some commonly automated responses.

What Are Some Possible Future Directions for Measurement in Behavior Analysis?

It is difficult to make predictions, the saying goes, especially about the future. Research methods might be expected to change more slowly than research topics do. In a hypothetical second edition of this textbook published 10 years hence, topical chapters will have 10 years of new research and (we hope) unanticipated insights to incorporate, but the ways behavior analysts conceptualize reliable, valid measures of behavior might not change much. Nevertheless, as behavior analysis adapts and changes, our methods must as well. We venture two predictions about the future of data collection and measurement in behavior analysis: Technological advancements will transform the way we observe behavior and the types of dependent variables we choose to analyze, and behavior analysts will become increasingly aware and considerate of justice, equity, diversity, and inclusion (JEDI) issues as they relate to the generality, external validity, and social significance of behavioral observations.

Continued Integration of New Technology

Behavior analysis has witnessed increased integration of technology in research and practice. For many years, behavior analysts have used data collection and measurement procedures that involve video recording the behavior or observing the behavior in real time via streaming services. These technologies make direct observation possible in real time or decrease the delay between target behavior and recording. Despite this common practice, a general set of best practices (logistical, ethical, etc.) for using video recording and videoconferencing in research and clinical settings has yet to be explicitly outlined in the field.

Technological advancements may change which behaviors we measure. Reports of biometric recordings of different aspects of behavior, such as actigraphy (Lesser et al., 2019; van Camp & Hayes, 2012), eye tracking (Dube et al., 2010; Paeye & Madelain, 2013), and the volume of vocalizations (Jackson & Wallace, 1974), may become more prevalent in behavior-analytic journals. Touchscreen swipes and taps are becoming more common in laboratory research with human (e.g., Ritchey et al., 2021) and nonhuman (e.g., Tan & Hackenberg, 2015; Toegel et al., 2021) subjects. Increased utilization of behavioral measures that can be recorded automatically may lead to less dependence on human-transduced data collection and less need to report IOA, but more emphasis on equipment calibration and manipulation checks. The increased availability of more continuous measures (rather than simple counts and response rates) and more nuanced information about each event will impact experimental design, for example, by increasing parametric analyses.

JEDI in Measurement

In many ways, behavior analysis has only recently awakened to many of the injustices, inequities, and the lack of diversity and inclusion in our field. Fortunately, awareness of these issues is increasing, leading to calls for behavior analysts to incorporate restorative justice into behavior analysis (Pavlacic et al., 2021); adopt meaningful antiracist perspectives and practices (Gingles, 2021; Levy et al., 2021); engage in professional development to improve cultural responsiveness and diversity in themselves, supervisees, and trainees (BACB, 2020; Beaulieu & Jimenez-Gomez, 2022; Jimenez-Gomez & Baulieu, 2022); and otherwise do the work to ensure that behavior analysis is open to anyone as a researcher, practitioner, or client. Selecting and defining target behaviors can be influenced by principles of JEDI in a variety of ways. In clinical practice, behavior analysts have an ethical obligation to involve clients and stakeholders throughout assessment and treatment (BACB, 2020). In applied research, participants and other stakeholders can be involved in operationally defining the target behavior and creating the measurement system, thus enhancing the social significance of the research. Focus groups comprising ultimate stakeholders can be used to inform data collection and measurement in use-inspired and solution-oriented research as well. Compassionate, antiracist, culturally relevant practice involves strengths-based assessment rather than a focus on the subject's deficits (Gingles, 2021). Thus, behavior analysts are encouraged to select and measure target behaviors that acknowledge and promote strengths rather than highlight and reduce deficits.

To enable the analysis of generality, method sections should include reports of participants' sociodemographic characteristics. It remains unclear to many researchers which variables to include and how to create appropriate groupings. General guidance for what to report in manuscripts is provided in *Journal Article Reporting Standards* by the American Psychological Association. Other guides include *Consolidated Standards of Reporting Trials* (CONSORT) for clinical trials and *Single-Case Reporting Guideline in Behavioral Interventions* (SCRIBE) for single-case research. For example, Tate et al. (2016) developed SCRIBE and recommended that researchers "describe the demographic characteristics [of each participant] and clinical (or other) features relevant to the research question, such that anonymity is ensured" (p. 18). They listed, "age, sex, ethnicity, socioeconomic status, geographic location, as well as diagnoses where indicated, and functional or developmental abilities" (p. 19) as relevant demographic characteristics in single-case research. Many of these variables (i.e., race, ethnicity, culture, language, and socioeconomic status) are underreported in behavior-analysis research published in journals such as the *Journal of Applied Behavior Analysis* (Brodhead et al., 2014; Jones et al., 2020; Li et al., 2017) and *The Analysis of Verbal Behavior* (Brodhead et al., 2014), signaling an important future direction in data collection and measurement.

We hope behavior analysts will continue to build cultural competence through self-assessment, professional development, and training in culturally responsive practices (Beaulieu & Jimenez-Gomez, 2022; Jimenez-Gomez & Beaulieu, 2022). To develop and inform these practices in a data-driven manner, behavior analysts might collaborate with experts in the incorporation of culturally responsive practices into reporting and analyzing demographic data. Developing systems to measure structural variables (institutional characteristics, policies, etc.) in addition to the target behavior and demographic variables is an important aspect of contextualizing analysis (Pearson et al., 2022). Standardizing these systems will facilitate comparison and longitudinal analysis, which will enable behavior analysts to refine and improve reporting standards.

Recognizing that so-called "objective" measures of behavior are never truly objective is an important and necessary step toward a just and equitable analysis of behavior. All systems of measurement, even those using programmed or automated data collection systems, are products of the behavior of scientists. All operational definitions of behaviors, including those applied to key pecks, lever presses, licks, and nose pokes are similarly determined by human scientists in particular sociocultural contexts. Presumptions of scientific objectivity can function to obscure the influence of cultural, demographic, economic, linguistic, and other contextual biases over who gets to determine the status quo in behavior analysis and other sciences (Levitt et al., 2022). For example, Pearson et al. (2022) questioned whether using high school grade point average (GPA) and college coursework rather than ostensibly objective American College Testing/Scholastic Aptitude Test (ACT/SAT) scores as a measure of preparation for higher education would alter the population of science, technology, engineering, and math (STEM) undergraduates from which professional scientists are ultimately drawn. Behavior analysts could begin to pursue an explicitly humanized and humanizing science of behavior by acknowledging that behavioral observations and behavioral data are socially constructed (Castillo & Gillborn, 2022; Gillborn et al., 2018; Kyonka & Subramaniam, 2023) and through critical examination of functional relations among social categories and methods of data collection and measurement.

Conclusion

Most principles of good data collection and measurement apply to multiple scientific disciplines and across the spectrum of translation. This chapter is not an exhaustive review of behavior-analytic systems of measurement, nor is it necessarily designed to enable researchers to select a system of measurement. Instead, it highlights select issues where interpreting and applying the general principles may be challenging for behavior analysts attempting translational work.

Pioneering computer scientist Grace Murray Hopper is supposed to have said that "one accurate measurement is worth a thousand expert opinions." Her statement seems to imply that accurate, useful measurements are, if not easy to obtain, at least readily recognized and universally valued. Whether the target behavior is a broad and varied response class or a precise, discrete response, the potential exists for nuances in the definition to alter what "counts" as a response (and consequently affect results) in meaningful ways. Whether topographical or functional, operational definitions that specify observable behaviors are considered effective when they are clear and complete within the specified context in which they are used. With direct observation, before data collection can begin, behavior analysts specify the observation period and whether recording is continuous or discontinuous. Direct observation can involve measuring the occurrence, latency, form, strength, or other dimensions of behavior. Indirect measures such as permanent product recording, self- or other-reports of behavior through rating scales, and interviews can serve various functions in behavior analysis research, including generation of new hypotheses about functional relations.

Accurate measurement that is free from any error is not achievable in natural science when true values are unknown. In developing any data collection and measurement system, behavior analysts cannot expect to record behavior without error. Instead, we should aim to address sources of systematic bias (e.g., reactivity, response bias, and observer bias) with regular calibration of human or machine observers. Similarly, using IOA to assess the believability of human-transduced data enables behavior analysts to evaluate whether there are systematic biases in the interpretation of operational definitions, but it does not ensure or even estimate the accuracy of the measurements. As modern life becomes increasingly intertwined with and dependent on digital technologies, fully human-transduced measurement may become a rarity. Nevertheless, all measurement is specified, if not conducted, by human scientists. As such, considering the social contexts in which data collection and measurement occur, critically questioning the methodological status quo, and developing frameworks for building the cultural competence of observers can be expected to help behavior analysts achieve a just and equitable science of behavior that is open to all.

REFERENCES

Allan, L. G., & Gibbon, J. (1991). Human bisection at the geometric mean. *Learning and Motivation, 22*(1–2), 39–58.

Andrade, L. F., & Petry, N. M. (2012). Delay and probability discounting in pathological gamblers with and without a history of substance use problems. *Psychopharmacology, 219*(2), 491–499.

Austin, J. (2000). Performance analysis and performance diagnostics. In J. Austin & J. Carr (Eds.), *Handbook of applied behavior analysis* (pp. 321–349). Context Press.

Barrett, B. H., Beck, R., Binder, C., Cook, D. A., Engelmann, S., Greer, R. D., . . . Watkins, C. L. (1991). The right to effective education. *The Behavior Analyst, 14*(1), 79–82.

Baum, W. M., & Rachlin, H. C. (1969). Choice as time allocation. *Journal of the Experimental Analysis of Behavior, 12*(6), 861–874.

Baumann, A. A., & Odum, A. L. (2012). Impulsivity, risk taking, and timing. *Behavioural Processes, 90*(3), 408–414.

Beaulieu, L., & Jimenez-Gomez, C. (2022). Cultural responsiveness in applied behavior analysis: Self-assessment. *Journal of Applied Behavior Analysis, 55*(2), 337–356.

Behavior Analyst Certification Board. (2017). *BCBA/BCaBA task list* (5th ed.). Author.

Behavior Analyst Certification Board. (2020). Ethics code for behavior analysts. Retrieved from *https://bacb.com/wp-content/ethics-code-for-behavior-analysts*.

Bickel, W. K., & Marsch, L. A. (2001). Toward a behavioral economic understanding of drug dependence: Delay discounting processes. *Addiction, 96*(1), 73–86.

Blough, D. S. (1966). The reinforcement of least-frequent interresponse times. *Journal of the*

Experimental Analysis of Behavior, 9(5), 581–591.

Brodhead, M. T., Durán, L., & Bloom, S. E. (2014). Cultural and linguistic diversity in recent verbal behavior research on individuals with disabilities: A review and implications for research and practice. *Analysis of Verbal Behavior, 30*(1), 75–86.

Carr, J. E., Wilder, D. A., Majdalany, L., Mathisen, D., & Strain, L. A. (2013). An assessment-based solution to a human-service employee performance problem. *Behavior Analysis in Practice, 6*(1), 16–32.

Casella, S. E., Wilder, D. A., Neidert, P., Rey, C., Compton, M., & Chong, I. (2010). The effects of response effort on safe performance by therapists at an autism treatment facility. *Journal of Applied Behavior Analysis, 43*(4), 729–734.

Caselli, L., Iaboli, L., & Nichelli, P. (2009). Time estimation in mild Alzheimer's disease patients. *Behavioral and Brain Functions, 5*(1), 1–10.

Castillo, W., & Gillborn, D. (2022). How to "QuantCrit:" Practices and questions for education data researchers and users. *EdWorkingPapers.com.*

Cliff, J. H., Jackson, S. M., McEwan, J. S., & Bizo, L. A. (2019). Weber's Law and the Scalar Property of Timing: A test of canine timing. *Animals, 9*(10), 801.

Common, E. A., & Lane, K. L. (2017). Social validity assessment. In J. K. Luiselli (Ed.), *Applied behavior analysis advanced guidebook* (pp. 73–92). Academic Press.

Conger, R., & Killeen, P. (1974). Use of concurrent operants in small group research: A demonstration. *Pacific Sociological Review, 17*(4), 399–416.

Cooper, J. O., Heron, T. E., & Heward, W. L. (2020). *Applied behavior analysis.* Pearson UK.

Critchfield, T. S. (2011). To a young basic scientist, about to embark on a program of translational research. *The Behavior Analyst, 34*(2), 137–148.

Critchfield, T. S., Tucker, J. A., & Vuchinich, R. E. (1998). Self-report methods. In K. L. Lattal & M. Perone (Eds.), *Handbook of research methods in human operant behavior* (pp. 435–470). Springer.

Cushing, L. S., & Kennedy, C. H. (1997). Academic effects of providing peer support in general education classrooms on students without disabilities. *Journal of Applied Behavior Analysis, 30*(1), 139–151.

DePuy, V., & Berger, V. W. (2014). Counterbalancing. Retrieved from *www.wiley.com/learn/wileystatsref.*

Deshais, M. A., Fisher, A. B., & Kahng, S. (2019). A comparison of group contingencies on academic compliance. *Journal of Applied Behavior Analysis, 52*(1), 116–131.

Devine, S. L., Rapp, J. T., Testa, J. R., Henrickson, M. L., & Schnerch, G. (2011). Detecting changes in simulated events using partial-interval recording and momentary time sampling: III. Evaluating sensitivity as a function of session length. *Behavioral Interventions, 26*(2), 103–124.

Dillon, E. M., Wong, C. J., Sylvest, C. E., Crone-Todd, D. E., & Silverman, K. (2004). Computer-based typing and keypad skills training outcomes of unemployed injection drug users in a therapeutic workplace. *Substance Use and Misuse, 39*(13–14), 2325–2353.

Droit-Volet, S. (2013). Time perception in children: A neurodevelopmental approach. *Neuropsychologia, 51*(2), 220–234.

Droit-Volet, S., & Rattat, A. C. (2007). A further analysis of time bisection behavior in children with and without reference memory: The similarity and the partition task. *Acta Psychologica, 125*(2), 240–256.

Droit-Volet, S., Tourret, S., & Wearden, J. (2004). Perception of the duration of auditory and visual stimuli in children and adults. *Quarterly Journal of Experimental Psychology Section A, 57*(5), 797–818.

Dube, W. V., Dickson, C. A., Balsamo, L. M., O'Donnell, K. L., Tomanari, G. Y., Farren, K. M., . . . McIlvane, W. J. (2010). Observing behavior and atypically restricted stimulus control. *Journal of the Experimental Analysis of Behavior, 94*(3), 297–313.

Dufrene, B. A., Doggett, R. A., Henington, C., & Watson, T. S. (2007). Functional assessment and intervention for disruptive classroom behaviors in preschool and head start classrooms. *Journal of Behavioral Education, 16*(4), 368–388.

Fisher, W. W., Piazza, C. C., Bowman, L. G., & Amari, A. (1996). Integrating caregiver report with a systematic choice assessment to enhance reinforcer identification. *American Journal on Mental Retardation, 101*, 15–25.

Fisher, W. W., Piazza, C. C., Bowman, L. G., Hanley, G. P., & Adelinis, J. D. (1997). Direct and collateral effects of restraints and restraint fading. *Journal of Applied Behavior Analysis, 30*(1), 105–120.

Fox, A. E., & Kyonka, E. G. (2017). Searching for the variables that control human rule-governed "insensitivity." *Journal of the Experimental Analysis of Behavior, 108*(2), 236–254.

Gil, S., Chambres, P., Hyvert, C., Fanget, M., & Droit-Volet, S. (2012). Children with autism spectrum disorders have "the working raw material" for time perception. *PLOS One, 7*(11), Article e49116.

Gillborn, D., Warmington, P., & Demack, S. (2018). QuantCrit: Education, policy, "Big Data" and principles for a critical race theory of statistics. *Race Ethnicity and Education, 21*(2), 158–179.

Gingles, D. (2021). Igniting collective freedom: An integrative behavioral model of acceptance and commitment toward Black liberation. *Behavior Analysis in Practice, 15*(4), 1050–1065.

Green, C. W., Reid, D. H., Canipe, V. S., & Gardner, S. M. (1991). A comprehensive evaluation of reinforcer identification processes for persons with profound multiple handicaps. *Journal of Applied Behavior Analysis, 24*(3), 537–552.

Hackenberg, T. D., & Joker, V. R. (1994). Instructional versus schedule control of humans' choices in situations of diminishing returns. *Journal of the Experimental Analysis of Behavior, 62*(3), 367–383.

Hayashi, Y., Fessler, H. J., Friedel, J. E., Foreman, A. M., & Wirth, O. (2018). The roles of delay and probability discounting in texting while driving: Toward the development of a translational scientific program. *Journal of the Experimental Analysis of Behavior, 110*(2), 229–242.

Holtyn, A. F., Knealing, T. W., Jarvis, B. P., Subramaniam, S., & Silverman, K. (2017). Monitoring cocaine use and abstinence among cocaine users for contingency management interventions. *Psychological Record, 67*(2), 253–259.

Hood, H. K., & Antony, M. M. (2012). Evidence-based assessment and treatment of specific phobias in adults. In T. E. Davis III, T. H. Ollendick, & L.-G. Öst (Eds.), *Intensive one-session treatment of specific phobias* (pp. 19–42). Springer.

Horne, P. J., & Lowe, C. F. (1993). Determinants of human performance on concurrent schedules. *Journal of the Experimental Analysis of Behavior, 59*(1), 29–60.

House, A. E., House, B. J., & Campbell, M. B. (1981). Measures of interobserver agreement: Calculation formulas and distribution effects. *Journal of Behavioral Assessment, 3*(1), 37–57.

Hussey, I., & Hughes, S. (2020). Hidden invalidity among 15 commonly used measures in social and personality psychology. *Advances in Methods and Practices in Psychological Science, 3*(2), 166–184.

Iwata, B. A., DeLeon, I. G., & Roscoe, E. M. (2013). Reliability and validity of the Functional Analysis Screening Tool. *Journal of Applied Behavior Analysis, 46*(1), 271–284.

Jackson, D. A., & Wallace, R. F. (1974). The modification and generalization of voice loudness in a fifteen-year-old retarded girl. *Journal of Applied Behavior Analysis, 7*(3), 461–471.

Jimenez-Gomez, C., & Beaulieu, L. (2022). Cultural responsiveness in applied behavior analysis: Research and practice. *Journal of Applied Behavior Analysis, 55*(3), 650–673.

Johnson, K., & Street, E. M. (2014). Precision teaching: The legacy of Ogden Lindsley. In F. K. McSweeney & E. S. Murphy (Eds.), *The Wiley Blackwell handbook of operant and classical conditioning* (pp. 581–609). Wiley Blackwell.

Johnson, L., McComas, J., Thompson, A., & Symons, F. J. (2004). Obtained versus programmed reinforcement: Practical considerations in the treatment of escape-reinforced aggression. *Journal of Applied Behavior Analysis, 37*(2), 239–242.

Johnston, J. M., Pennypacker, H. S., & Green, G. (2020). *Strategies and tactics of behavioral research and practice*. Routledge.

Jones, S. H., St. Peter, C. C., & Ruckle, M. M. (2020). Reporting of demographic variables in the *Journal of Applied Behavior Analysis. Journal of Applied Behavior Analysis, 53*(3), 1304–1315.

Kazdin, A. E. (1979). Unobtrusive measures in behavioral assessment. *Journal of Applied Behavior Analysis, 12*(4), 713–724.

Kazdin, A. E. (1980). Acceptability of alternative treatments for deviant child behavior. *Journal of Applied Behavior Analysis, 13*(2), 259–273.

Kazdin, A. E. (2016). Single-case experimental research designs. In A. E. Kazdin (Ed.), *Methodological issues and strategies in clinical research* (pp. 459–483). American Psychological Association.

Kelly, M. B. (1976). A review of academic permanent-product data collection and reliability procedures in applied behavior analysis research. *Journal of Applied Behavior Analysis, 9*(2), 211–211.

Kelly, M. B. (1977). A review of the observational data-collection and reliability procedures reported in the *Journal of Applied Behavior Analysis*. *Journal of Applied Behavior Analysis, 10*(1), 97–101.

Killeen, P. R. (1978). Stability criteria. *Journal of the Experimental Analysis of Behavior, 29*(1), 17–25.

Kirby, K. N., Petry, N. M., & Bickel, W. K. (1999). Heroin addicts have higher discount rates for delayed rewards than non-drug-using controls. *Journal of Experimental Psychology: General, 128*(1), 78–87.

Knapczyk, D. R. (1989). Generalization of student question asking from special class to regular class settings. *Journal of Applied Behavior Analysis, 22*(1), 77–83.

Kyonka, E. G., & Subramaniam, S. (2018). Translating behavior analysis: A spectrum rather than a road map. *Perspectives on Behavior Science, 41*(2), 591–613.

Kyonka, E. G. E., & Subramaniam, S. (2023). *Justice, equity, diversity, and inclusion in behavior analysis research.* Manuscript in preparation.

LeBlanc, L. A., Raetz, P. B., Sellers, T. P., & Carr, J. E. (2016). A proposed model for selecting measurement procedures for the assessment and treatment of problem behavior. *Behavior Analysis in Practice, 9*(1), 77–83.

Lee, R., McComas, J. J., & Jawor, J. (2002). The effects of differential and lag reinforcement schedules on varied verbal responding by individuals with autism. *Journal of Applied Behavior Analysis, 35*(4), 391–402.

Lerman, D. C. (2003). From the laboratory to community application: Translational research in behavior analysis. *Journal of Applied Behavior Analysis, 36*(4), 415.

Lesser, A. D., Luczynski, K. C., & Hood, S. A. (2019). Evaluating motion detection to score sleep disturbance for children: A translational approach to developing a measurement system. *Journal of Applied Behavior Analysis, 52*(2), 580–599.

Levitt, H. M., Surace, F. I., Wu, M. B., Chapin, B., Hargrove, J. G., Herbitter, C., . . . Hochman, A. L. (2022). The meaning of scientific objectivity and subjectivity: From the perspective of methodologists. *Psychological Methods, 27*(4), 589–605.

Levy, S., Siebold, A., Vaidya, J., Truchon, M. M., Dettmering, J., & Mittelman, C. A. (2021).

A look in the mirror: How the field of behavior analysis can become anti-racist. *Behavior Analysis in Practice, 15*(4), 1112–1125.

Li, A., Wallace, L., Ehrhardt, K. E., & Poling, A. (2017). Reporting participant characteristics in intervention articles published in five behavior-analytic journals, 2013–2015. *Behavior Analysis: Research and Practice, 17*(1), 84–91.

Mace, F. C., & Critchfield, T. S. (2010). Translational research in behavior analysis: Historical traditions and imperative for the future. *Journal of the Experimental Analysis of Behavior, 93*(3), 293–312.

Madden, G. J., Petry, N. M., & Johnson, P. S. (2009). Pathological gamblers discount probabilistic rewards less steeply than matched controls. *Experimental and Clinical Psychopharmacology, 17*(5), 283–290.

Matson, J. L., Bielecki, J., Mayville, E. A., Smalls, Y., Bamburg, J. W., & Baglio, C. S. (1999). The development of a reinforcer choice assessment scale for persons with severe and profound mental retardation. *Research in Developmental Disabilities, 20*(5), 379–384.

MedAssociates. (2021). Illuminated retractable lever for rat. Retrieved from *www.med-associates.com/product/illuminated-retractable-lever-for-rat.*

Miltenberger, R. G. (2016). *Behavior modification: Principles and procedures.* Cengage Learning.

Mudford, O. C., Taylor, S. A., & Martin, N. T. (2009). Continuous recording and interobserver agreement algorithms reported in the *Journal of Applied Behavior Analysis* (1995–2005). *Journal of Applied Behavior Analysis, 42*(1), 165–169.

Mudford, O. C., Zeleny, J. R., Fisher, W. W., Klum, M. E., & Owen, T. M. (2011). Calibration of observational measurement of rate of responding. *Journal of Applied Behavior Analysis, 44*(3), 571–586.

National Football League. (2021). 2021 Official Playing Rules of the National Football League. Retrieved July 28, 2022, from *https://operations.nfl.com/media/5427/2021-nfl-rulebook.pdf.*

Neef, N. A., Mace, F. C., Shea, M. C., & Shade, D. (1992). Effects of reinforcer rate and reinforcer quality on time allocation: Extensions of matching theory to educational settings. *Journal of Applied Behavior Analysis, 25*(3), 691–699.

Nevin, J. A. (1984). Quantitative analysis. *Jour-*

nal of the Experimental Analysis of Behavior, 42(3), 421–434.

Owens, M. T., Seidel, S. B., Wong, M., Bejines, T. E., Lietz, S., Perez, J. R., . . . Tanner, K. D. (2017). Classroom sound can be used to classify teaching practices in college science courses. *Proceedings of the National Academy of Sciences of the USA, 114*(12), 3085–3090.

Paeye, C., & Madelain, L. (2013). Reinforcing saccadic amplitude variability. *Journal of the Experimental Analysis of Behavior, 95*(2), 149–162.

Page, S., & Neuringer, A. (1985). Variability is an operant. *Journal of Experimental Psychology: Animal Behavior Processes, 11*(3), 429–452.

Parsons, M. B., & Reid, D. H. (1990). Assessing food preferences among persons with profound mental retardation: Providing opportunities to make choices. *Journal of Applied Behavior Analysis, 23*(2), 183–195.

Pavlacic, J. M., Kellum, K. K., & Schulenberg, S. E. (2021). Advocating for the use of restorative justice practices: Examining the overlap between restorative justice and behavior analysis. *Behavior Analysis in Practice, 15*(4), 1237–1246.

Pearson, M. I., Castle, S. D., Matz, R. L., Koester, B. P., & Byrd, W. C. (2022). Integrating critical approaches into quantitative STEM equity work. *CBE—Life Sciences Education, 21*(1), es1.

Perone, M. (1988). Laboratory lore and research practices in the experimental analysis of human behavior: Use and abuse of subjects' verbal reports. *Behavior Analyst, 11*(1), 71–75.

Petursdottir, A. I., & Carr, J. E. (2018). Applying the taxonomy of validity threats from mainstream research design to single-case experiments in applied behavior analysis. *Behavior Analysis in Practice, 11*(3), 228–240.

Reed, D. D., & Azulay, R. L. (2011). A Microsoft Excel® 2010 based tool for calculating interobserver agreement. *Behavior Analysis in Practice, 4*(2), 45–52.

Reed, P., & Randell, J. (2014). Altered time-perception performance in individuals with high schizotypy levels. *Psychiatry Research, 220*(1–2), 211–216.

Reimers, T. M., & Wacker, D. P. (1988). Parents' ratings of the acceptability of behavioral treatment recommendations made in an outpatient clinic: A preliminary analysis of the influence of treatment effectiveness. *Behavioral Disorders, 14*(1), 7–15.

Ritchey, C. M., Mizutani, Y., Kuroda, T., Gil-

roy, S., & Podlesnik, C. A. (2021). Examining effects of training duration on humans' resurgence and variability using a novel touchscreen procedure. *Journal of the Experimental Analysis of Behavior, 116*(3), 344–358.

Shadish, W. R., Cook, T. D., & Campbell, D. T. (2002). *Experimental and quasi-experimental designs for generalized causal inference.* Houghton Mifflin.

Shea-Brown, E., Rinzel, J., Rakitin, B. C., & Malapani, C. (2006). A firing rate model of Parkinsonian deficits in interval timing. *Brain Research, 1070*(1), 189–201.

Sigurdsson, S. O., Aklin, W., Ring, B. M., Needham, M., Boscoe, J., & Silverman, K. (2011). Automated measurement of noise violations in the therapeutic workplace. *Behavior Analysis in Practice, 4*(1), 47–52.

Silverman, K., Holtyn, A. F., Jarvis, B. P., & Subramaniam, S. (2021). Behavior analysis and treatment of drug addiction: Recent advances in research on abstinence reinforcement. In W. W. Fisher, C. C. Piazza, & H. S. Roane (Eds.), *Handbook of applied behavior analysis* (2nd ed., pp. 490–511). Guilford Press.

Spiegel, A. (Interviewer), & Hare, R. (Interviewee). (2011). Creator of psychopathy test worries about its use [Interview transcript]. Retrieved from *www.npr.org/2011/05/27/136723357/creator-of-psychopathy-test-worries-about-its-use.*

Sprague, J. R., & Horner, R. H. (1984). The effects of single instance, multiple instance, and general case training on generalized vending machine use by moderately and severely handicapped students. *Journal of Applied Behavior Analysis, 17*(2), 273–278.

Stojek, M. M., & MacKillop, J. (2017). Relative reinforcing value of food and delayed reward discounting in obesity and disordered eating: A systematic review. *Clinical Psychology Review, 55*, 1–11.

Tan, L., & Hackenberg, T. D. (2015). Pigeons' demand and preference for specific and generalized conditioned reinforcers in a token economy. *Journal of the Experimental Analysis of Behavior, 104*(3), 296–314.

Tate, R. L., Perdices, M., Rosenkoetter, U., McDonald, S., Togher, L., Shadish, W., . . . Vohra, S. (2016). The Single-Case Reporting Guideline in Behavioral Interventions (SCRIBE) 2016: Explanation and elaboration. *Archives of Scientific Psychology, 4*(1), 10–31.

Toegel, F., Toegel, C., & Perone, M. (2021). Design and evaluation of a touchscreen apparatus for operant research with pigeons. *Journal of the Experimental Analysis of Behavior, 116*(2), 249–264.

Van Camp, C. M., & Hayes, L. B. (2012). Assessing and increasing physical activity. *Journal of Applied Behavior Analysis, 45*(4), 871–875.

Vázquez Lira, R., & Torres, A. (2017). Assessment of intertemporal preferences in type-2 diabetes patients and smokers. *International Journal of Psychological Research, 10*(1), 35–44.

Vollmer, T. R., Sloman, K. N., & Pipkin, C. S. P. (2008). Practical implications of data reliability and treatment integrity monitoring. *Behavior Analysis in Practice, 1*(2), 4–11.

Wearden, J. H., & Shimp, C. P. (1985). Local temporal patterning of operant behavior in humans. *Journal of the Experimental Analysis of Behavior, 44*(3), 315–324.

Witt, J. C., Elliott, S. N., & Martens, B. K. (1984). Acceptability of behavioral interventions used in classrooms: The influence of amount of teacher time, severity of behavior problem, and type of intervention. *Behavioral Disorders, 9*(2), 95–104.

Woods, C. M. (2006). Careless responding to reverse-worded items: Implications for confirmatory factor analysis. *Journal of Psychopathology and Behavioral Assessment, 28*(3), 186–191.

PART III

PAVLOVIAN CONDITIONING

CHAPTER 6

Pavlovian Conditioning
PRINCIPLES TO GUIDE APPLICATION

Eric A. Thrailkill
Catalina N. Rey

Classical conditioning, sometimes referred to as Pavlovian or respondent conditioning, was first studied systematically in the laboratory of Ivan Pavlov (1927) in St. Petersburg, Russia. In his best-known experiment, Pavlov rang a bell, then gave a dog some food. After a few pairings of the bell and food, the dog began to salivate to the bell, and thus anticipated the presentation of food. The events in Pavlov's experiment can be described in broadly applicable terms. The food is the *unconditioned stimulus* (US), because it unconditionally elicits salivation before the experiment begins. The natural response to the food itself, salivation, is the *unconditioned response* (UR). The bell is known as the *conditioned stimulus* (CS), because it only elicits the salivary response conditional on the bell–food pairings. The new salivation response to the bell is correspondingly called the *conditioned response* (CR).

This chapter provides a contemporary understanding of Pavlovian conditioning as a fundamental psychological process. The standard behavior-analytic approach should be to incorporate and consider Pavlovian conditioning processes when developing treatment, instruction, and intervention protocols. We assume that readers are familiar with basic concepts and principles of operant conditioning. Pavlovian conditioning and operant conditioning differ in several ways. One of the most fundamental differences is that the responses observed in Pavlov's experiment are *elicited* and thus controlled by presentation of an antecedent stimulus. In contrast, the response observed in operant conditioning is (partially) controlled by its consequences. In this chapter, we discuss Pavlovian influences on operant behavior and provide a wide range of examples throughout to emphasize the applied and translational relevance of these processes.

The Various Impacts of Pavlovian Conditioning

To begin, we acknowledge a persistent cultural impression that Pavlovian conditioning is a rigid and simplistic reflex process in which a fixed event comes to elicit a fixed response. Our goal is to convey that, in fact, conditioning is a nuanced and dynamic process, and that Pavlovian and instrumental (operant) behaviors are not mutually exclusive in their occurrence. For example, as a result of Pavlovian conditioning, signals for food may evoke a large set of responses that prepare the organism to digest food: They can elicit secretion of gastric acid, pancreatic enzymes, and insulin, in addition to salivation. The stimulus that predicts food can also elicit approach behavior, an increase in body temperature, and a state of arousal or excitement. An animal may get up and eat more food even when sated and quiescent when presented with a signal for food. In another realm, food cues that trigger food consumption and craving have potential to influence overeating and obesity. Someone who routinely eats dinner while watching TV at home may find themself craving food shortly after returning home and turning on the TV after dining out. Signals for food evoke a diverse array of food-related behaviors or a "behavior system" that is functionally organized to facilitate eating (Timberlake, 1994). In other words, Pavlovian conditioned stimuli (CSs) impact not only reflex responses but also operant behavior.

Pavlovian conditioning is involved in other important aspects of eating, such as how one learns to like or dislike different foods. In nonhuman animals, such as rats, flavors associated with nutrients (sugars, starches, calories, proteins, or fats) come to be preferred, while bitter flavors that may be associated with noxious chemicals or poisons, are avoided (Holman, 1975; Sclafani, 1997). The fact that flavor CSs can be associated with a range of positive and negative biological consequences (USs) is important for omnivorous animals that need to learn about which new foods to approach and which to avoid. Flavors associated with illness become disliked, as illustrated by the college student who gets sick drinking tequila and consequently learns to hate the flavor. Likewise, a child might learn to dislike carrots if they were the last thing he ate before getting nauseous and vomiting.

It is easy to see how conditioning of likes and dislikes can be useful to clinicians. A famous example is the pairing of novel flavors with chemotherapy (Bernstein, 1978). Chemotherapy can make cancer patients sick, which may then result in the conditioning of an aversion to a food that was eaten recently (or to the clinic itself). One successful approach to avoid establishing the clinic or familiar foods as aversive is to pair the distinct flavor of a candy or ice cream with chemotherapy with the intent to develop a nausea CR to the distinct flavor and not the clinic itself or other familiar foods. Bernstein et al. (1982) applied this method to reduce food aversions in children undergoing chemotherapy for cancer. They found that exposing children to a distinct flavored ice cream before chemotherapy treatments reduced aversion to foods in their normal diets.

Pavlovian conditioning is also important for understanding how drugs influence behavior. Whenever a drug is taken, it constitutes a US and may be associated with potential CSs that are present at the time. The analysis of Pavlovian conditioning with drugs as the US illustrates an important phenomenon: The conditioned response elicited by a drug can be "opposite" to the unconditional effect of the drug (Siegel, 1999). For example, although morphine reduces sensitivity to pain, a CS associated with morphine elicits an opposite increase in sensitivity to pain, not a reduction (Siegel, 1975). As a result, some patients who receive opioids for the treatment of chronic pain sometimes become more sensitive to certain painful stimuli following prolonged use (i.e., opioid-induced hyperalgesia). Similarly, although alcohol causes body temperature to decrease, an alcohol CS elicits an increase in body temperature (Mansfield & Cunningham, 1980). In each case, the CR is referred to as *compensatory* because it counteracts the drug effect.

Compensatory CRs are an example of how Pavlovian conditioning plays an important role in preparing organisms for biologically significant events.

Compensatory responses have implications for drug addiction. First, repeated administrations of the drug consist of repeated drug and CS (e.g., people, settings, odors, rituals) pairings. These exposures cause the compensatory response to the CS to become stronger and more effective at counteracting the effect of the drug. The result is drug tolerance; that is, more and more of the drug must be taken to experience the same drug effect. One disastrous implication of drug tolerance is that tolerance will be lost if the drug is taken without being signaled by the usual CS; that is, taking a drug around new people, in a new setting, around unfamiliar sights/sound/scents, or without engaging in the usual preparatory routine can result in a loss of tolerance and increase the likelihood of drug overdose. Second, the fact that conditioned compensatory responses oppose the drug effect and may be uncomfortable or unpleasant suggests that drug CSs play a crucial role in understanding drug addiction and relapse. For example, a CS associated with effects of an opioid may elicit compensatory responses, such as increased sensitivity to pain, changes in body temperature, and hyperactivity (the opposite of the unconditional morphine effect). These withdrawal symptoms then motivate the user to take the drug in order to get rid of (or escape) these unpleasant responses (Siegel, 1999). Compensatory responses contribute to the strong urge to take drugs in the presence of drug-associated CSs. The hypothesis is also consistent with self-reports of individuals who are tempted to resume taking the drug when they are exposed to drug-associated cues after a period of abstinence (Heilig, 2015).

It is also important to note that individuals do not always develop conditioned compensatory responses to USs. Even with drugs, sometimes compensatory responses do not develop. One example is the phenomenon of sensitization with cocaine or amphetamine. When one of these drugs is associated with an environment, the environment evokes an increase in activity that is consistent with the drug effect, not opposite to it. For example, after repeated exposure to cocaine in a specific chamber, rats exhibit an enhanced locomotor response when subsequently challenged with the drug in that specific chamber, but not in a different environment (Post et al., 1981). Similarly, studies have shown that once a person has experienced amphetamine-induced psychosis, continued substance use often induces further episodes with smaller doses and more rapid onsets (Bartlett et al., 1997; Satel et al., 1991; Ujike & Sato, 2004). Some have also reported stress alone to induce psychosis in people who abuse amphetamines (Sato et al., 1992). Furthermore, drug-associated CSs may develop salient properties that capture a person's attention and enhance drug craving (Berridge & Robinson, 2016; Watson et al., 2019). For instance, several studies revealed that smoking-related cues selectively attract the eye gaze of individuals who smoke cigarettes (e.g., Bradley et al., 2003; for an extension to food-related cues, see Brand et al., 2020; van Ens et al., 2019).

In addition to their role in drug effects, CSs are relevant for understanding how Pavlovian conditioning influences immune system and neuroendocrine responses (see Hadamitzky et al., 2020, for a review). An early example is a report of a learned allergic response in a patient allergic to roses when that patient was exposed to an artificial rose (Mackenzie, 1886). Another area with considerable applied significance is conditioned fertility (Domjan & Gutiérrez, 2019; Hoffmann, 2017). As a result of being associated with access to a sexual partner, the presentation of a Pavlovian CS can significantly increase rates of fertilization and the number of offspring that result from a sexual encounter (Adkins-Regan & MacKillop, 2003, Domjan et al., 2012; Hollis et al., 1997).

A CS associated with a frightening US can elicit a whole system of conditioned fear responses that are broadly designed to help the organism cope with the fearful situation and find safety (Bolles, 1970; Hoffman et al., 2022). A fear CS elicits changes in respiration, heart rate, blood pressure, and even a (compensatory) decrease in sensitivity to pain. A brief CS that occurs close in time to an aversive US can also elicit adaptively timed protective reflexes. For example, the rabbit blinks to a brief CS that predicts a mild electric shock US near the eye. If one increases the duration of the same CS paired with the same US, then it will elicit mainly fear responses (e.g., change in heart rate). The fear elicited by a CS may potentiate the response elicited by another CS or a startle response to a sudden noise (e.g., Davis, 1986). A common example is when someone is watching a scary movie and it elicits various fear responses. A sudden noise such as a ringing phone might elicit a startle response, although it would not usually do so otherwise.

Fear conditioning has broad clinical relevance, as it can contribute to anxiety disorders, including phobias, panic disorder, and posttraumatic stress disorder (PTSD). For example, in panic disorder, people who experience unexpected panic attacks can become anxious about having another one. In this case, the panic attack (the US or UR) may condition anxiety to the external situation in which it occurs (e.g., crowded bus, elevator, airplane) and also internal (interoceptive) CSs created by early symptoms of the attack (e.g., sweaty palms, dizziness, a sudden pounding of the heart). These CSs may then come to evoke anxiety or panic responses (Bouton et al., 2001). It is interesting to note here that CSs may elicit emotional reactions without conscious awareness (e.g., LeDoux, 1996). A good example comes from an experiment that used a masking protocol that prevents awareness of a stimulus by following it with a second, brief stimulus. People selected to be highly afraid of snakes (but not of spiders) or of spiders (but not of snakes) show elevated skin-conductance (autonomic) responses to masked presentations of their feared (but not of their not feared) animal (Öhman & Soares, 1994). In addition to eliciting conditioned responses, CSs motivate ongoing behavior. For example, presenting a CS that elicits anxiety can increase the vigor of operant behaviors that avoid or escape the frightening US (Davis, 2006; Lissek et al., 2008). Similarly, a CS associated with a drug or a sugary food may motivate the individual to seek the drug or sugary food (e.g., Watson et al., 2014).

The Learning Process in Pavlovian Conditioning

Research since the late 1900s has revealed several important details about the learning process that underlies Pavlovian conditioning (Rescorla, 1988). Several findings are especially important. First, pairing a CS with a US does not always result in conditioning. This finding is best illustrated by Leon Kamin's (1969) experiment sketched in Figure 6.1a. In a conditioning phase, Phase 2, two groups of rats received fear conditioning in which presentations of a CS were followed by a mild foot shock US. This procedure resulted in the suppression of ongoing activity during the presentation of the CS. For each group, the CS consisted of a light (A) and noise (X) presented simultaneously (AX) prior to the shock. Of interest was the amount of conditioning gained by the noise, X, when tested by itself in a subsequent test phase. It is important to note here that the test consisted of CS presentations without the US. This method separates the measure of learning (the ability of the CS to evoke the CR) from performance with the US present (see Rescorla & Holland, 1982, for further discussion). The groups differed in their history prior to the conditioning of the compound. In Phase 1, one group (the "blocking" group) received pairings of the light, A, by itself with the shock, and the other (the "control" group) did

a.

Group	Phase 1	Phase 2	Test	Result
"Blocking"	A - US	AX - US	X?	cr
Control	—	AX - US	X?	CR

b.

Group	Conditioning	Test	Result
"Correlated"	AX - US	X?	cr
	AX - US		
	BX - no US		
	BX - no US		
"Uncorrelated"	AX - US	X?	CR
	AX - no US		
	BX - US		
	BX - no US		

FIGURE 6.1. Experimental designs that result in blocking and relative validity effects. A, B, and X refer to CSs that differ in sensory characteristics; US refers to the unconditioned stimulus; CR and cr refer to a large/strong and small/weak conditioned response, respectively. See text for details.

not. In the test, Kamin (1969) found substantial fear in response to the noise, X, in the control group. The blocking group, however, showed little to no fear in response to X. Training with A blocked conditioning of X that would have otherwise occurred when AX was followed by shock. Importantly, both groups received the same number of X–shock pairings, yet the levels of conditioning differed substantially. For the pretrained animals, A already signaled the shock. The pairing of X and shock was negated by the absence of an informational relation: A already signaled the shock, and X was redundant. The blocking effect suggests that a CS must provide new information about the US if learning is to occur.

The blocking effect has clear clinical implications. One example is slower word recognition after pairing pictures with words (Dittlinger & Lerman, 2011; Singh & Solman, 1990). Children are often taught to read by pairing new written words with pictures. This procedure may actually slow word recognition because the pictures can block learning of the written word. The blocking effect also has implications for the selection of therapist/caregiver prompts and the transfer of stimulus control. That is, prompts with established strong discriminative properties might be more difficult to fade because they block the transfer of stimulus control to the intended discriminative stimulus, creating prompt dependency (see Cengher et al., 2018, for a discussion regarding stimulus and response prompts).

An experiment by Rescorla (1968) further illustrates the importance of informational relation between CS and US, also referred to as their *contingency,* as distinct from CS–US contiguity in producing conditioning. The typical Pavlovian conditioning experiment arranges for the CS and US to occur close together in time, such as having the US delivered at the offset or during the CS. Moreover, it arranges the CS to be informative about the US. The likelihood of the US is much greater given the presentation of the CS than it is when the CS is absent. In a fear conditioning experiment with rats, Rescorla separated CS–US contiguity from informativeness by systematically varying the probability of the US in the presence and the absence of the CS. In this experiment, groups of rats received the same number of CS and US presentations but differed in the probability of having the US delivered during the CS versus some point during the time that separated CS presentations (the *intertrial interval*). Rescorla found that conditioning to the CS systematically increased as the probability of the US during the CS increased. Put another way, the greater the likelihood of the US in the absence of the CS, the weaker the conditioning to the CS (and presumably stronger conditioning to the background cues). If the probability of the US was the same during the CS and the absence of the CS, there was little or no evidence of conditioning. This provided the insight that in order to predict the success of conditioning, one needs to know two probabilities: the probability of the US given the CS, and the probability of the US given no CS. Conditioning will not occur unless the CS signals a change in the ongoing likelihood of the US.

Such an informational relation between CS and US is important to consider when using pairing procedures to condition reinforcers or punishers (see da Silva & Williams, 2020, for more discussion). If a therapist, for example, aims to condition a specific praise statement as a reinforcer by pairing it with candy delivered to a child, she must consider how often the child receives the praise statement absent the candy and vice versa. Note that the child will treat the CS as a signal for "no US" if the probability of the US is less in the presence of the CS than in its absence. In this case, the signal is called a *conditioned inhibitor,* because it will inhibit performance elicited by other CSs (Pavlov, 1927; Rescorla, 1969). Informativeness is also relevant to teaching compliance with small children. If a teacher consistently follows through with prompting a child after providing an instruction, the child will quickly learn to comply with the instruction. Alternatively, if instructions result in follow through only half the time, a teacher is more likely to have students who "don't listen."

Consistent with the role of information, conditioning mainly accrues to the most valid predictors of the US. An experiment by Wagner et al. (1968) provides the classic example. In the experimental design (illustrated in Figure 6.1b), two groups of rats received subtly different treatments that had markedly different consequences on learning and behavior. For some of the trials in the "correlated" group, CSs A and X (high-frequency tone and light) were presented together and always paired with a foot shock US. On other trials, B and X (low-frequency tone and light) occurred together, and the US was never presented. After a number of such AX and BX trials, conditioning, indexed as suppression of ongoing lever pressing for food, was strongest to A (A blocked learning to X) and weakest to B. X supported a weak CR despite the fact that X was paired with the US on half the occasions on which it was presented. In contrast, in the "uncorrelated" group, which received the same number of AX and BX trials, X was also paired with the US half the time, but the results were very different. For this group, A and B were no more predictive of the US than X (the US was presented on half the trials with either A or B). Here, X was as valid a predictor as A or B, and there was substantial learning to X. (In fact, X was the best predictor of the US, as it was actually paired with the US twice as often as A or B.) The "relative validity" effect has been observed over a very wide range of conditioning methods, from fear conditioning in rats to category learning in humans (Soto & Wasserman, 2010) to sucrose conditioning in honeybees (Couvillon et al., 1983).

The fact that the validity of the CS as a predictor of the US has such a strong influence on conditioning suggests that subtle differences in conditioning history can have a profound influence on an individual's learning and behavior. Returning to the drug conditioning example, if two people were to take a drug in a manner analogous to that of the correlated and uncorrelated groups, one person would have tolerance and craving elicited almost exclusively by CS A, whereas the other would have tolerance and craving elicited strongly by A, B, and especially X.

By now it should be clear that conditioning is not determined by CS–US pairings. Instead, theorists have proposed that Pavlovian conditioning can be better accounted for by the discrepancy between (1) the US predicted by all CSs present on a trial and (2) the US that actually happens on the trial (Rescorla & Wagner, 1972; Wagner & Rescorla, 1972). This discrepancy is often referred to as *prediction error*. The size and direction of the discrepancy or error will determine whether the pairing of a CS and US causes an increase in conditioning, no change in conditioning, or even a decrease in conditioning. To expand on the latter idea, a new CS can acquire a negative value, and inhibit behavior, if the US is smaller than that which other CSs present predict; that is, a conditioned inhibitor is a CS that predicts "less US than expected," and a conditioned excitor is a CS that predicts "more US than expected." The Rescorla–Wagner model (Rescorla & Wagner, 1972) formalizes these principles and asserts that on any conditioning trial, the change in associative strength to a CS will be a function of the difference between the strength of the US that occurs on that trial and the extent to which the US is predicted by other CSs that are also present: $\Delta V_{CS} = \alpha\beta\,(\lambda - \Sigma V)$. Where, for each CS–US pairing, ΔV_{CS} is the change in associative strength (V), or conditioning, to the CS. This is determined by the difference between, λ, the strength (i.e., magnitude, intensity, salience) of the US, and ΣV, the summed associative strengths of all other CSs that are present on the trial (the extent to which the US is already predicted). The α and β terms are fractions based on the salience of the CS and US, respectively. These influence the rate of learning by influencing the amount of associative change that will occur on the trial. This theory allows CSs to acquire either positive or negative values that correspond to excitation and inhibition, respectively. The Rescorla–Wagner model set the stage for several later theories that have emphasized a number of psychological processes, such as surprisingness of the US and the CS (Pearce & Hall, 1980), short-term memory (Wagner, 1976), memory priming (Wagner, 1981), and also attention to the CS (Mackintosh, 1975; Pearce & Mackintosh, 2010) in accounting for Pavlovian conditioning.

Pavlovian conditioning is most robust if the CS and US are intense or salient (Annau & Kamin, 1961; Fanselow, 1980; Holland, 1977). It is also best if the CS and US are novel (Lubow, 1973; Randich & LoLordo, 1979). For example, in latent inhibition, repeated exposure to the CS alone before conditioning can diminish its ability to elicit responding when it is paired with the US (Lubow & Moore, 1959). In the US preexposure effect, repeated exposure to the US before conditioning can likewise decrease the conditioning that later occurs when a CS and the US are paired (Taylor, 1956). One idea captured in each of the theories just described is that the CS and the US must be "surprising" at the time of their pairing for learning to occur. Thus, the effects of pairing a CS with positive reinforcers, trauma, or drug USs may depend in subtle ways on the individual's prior experience with the CS and the US. One clear suggestion for clinicians is to consider the history and surprisingness of the CS and US when conditioning reinforcers or other important stimuli.

There are important variants of Pavlovian conditioning. In sensory preconditioning, two CSs (A and B) are first paired, and then one of them (A) is later paired with the US (Brogden, 1939). Stimulus A evokes conditioned responding, of course, but so does stimulus B—indirectly, through its association with A. For example, Jose, Roy, and Ben are all in the same class at school. Roy and Ben are best friends and always hang out together. One day, Jose is walking home from school and Ben beats him up and takes his lunch money. The next day, Jose sees Roy at school and becomes anxious, even though Roy was not present when Ben beat up Jose. A related finding is second-order conditioning (Rizley & Rescorla, 1972). Here, stimulus A is paired with a US first and then subsequently with stimulus B. Once again, both A and B will evoke responding. This process might be useful for conditioning reinforcers to deliver contingent on desired behavior in applied settings. If a clinician first pairs their praise (A) with edible reinforcers (US) and later pairs their praise with tokens (B), both praise and tokens may function as conditioned reinforcers. Sensory preconditioning and second-order conditioning increase the range of stimuli that can control the conditioned response.

Procedures That Result in Pavlovian Conditioning

So far, we have considered the results of pairing a CS and US; however, it is also useful to further describe how the arrangement of CS and US influences conditioning. Sketches of four pairing arrangements are shown in Figure 6.2. "Delay" conditioning refers to the presentation of the CS prior to the delivery of the US, such that the CS predicts that US. The presentation of the US typically coincides with the offset of the CS. Delay conditioning is the most common and effective pairing procedure. "Trace" conditioning introduces a gap, or trace interval, separating the end of the CS and the delivery of the US. Trace conditioning results in a weaker conditioned response than delay conditioning and is thought to reflect conditioning to a memory trace of the CS that is present when the US occurs. Consistent with this idea, neuroscience research has implicated brain areas involved in working memory (e.g., the hippocampus) as particularly important for trace conditioning but not delay conditioning (e.g., Solomon et al., 1986). The CS and US can also be arranged in "backward" order; that is, the beginning of the CS occurs after or during the US presentation. This arrangement can result in either excitatory or inhibitory conditioning to the CS (Cole & Miller, 1999; Tait & Saladin, 1986). Backward pairings can result in excitatory conditioning if the US is unpredicted or "surprising" (Wagner & Terry, 1975). However, it is more common for organisms to treat a backward-paired CS

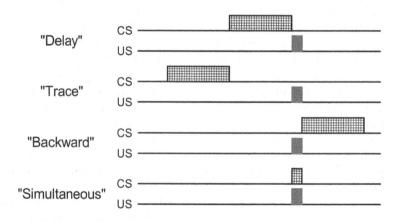

FIGURE 6.2. Arrangements of CS and US presentation during Pavlovian conditioning. CS and US refer to conditioned and unconditioned stimulus, respectively.

as a signal for "no US" and inhibit their response accordingly (e.g., Ewing et al., 1985; see also Delamater et al., 2003). Finally, in "simultaneous" CS–US pairings, the onset and offset of the CS and US both coincide. Simultaneous pairings can also result in excitatory or inhibitory conditioning under certain circumstances (Heth, 1976). Simultaneous conditioning arrangements are less common but may be particularly important for conditioning of flavor preferences (e.g., Holman, 1980) and perceptual learning (Gibson & Walk, 1956; McLaren & Mackintosh, 2000). Factors such as the CS duration and the intertrial interval separating CS–US pairings influence the strength of conditioning in each arrangement of CS and US (e.g., Thrailkill et al., 2020; for review, see Gottlieb & Begej, 2014). Moreover, each procedure interacts with the previously described characteristic properties of the CSs and USs in interesting and important ways to influence Pavlovian conditioning.

How to Change Behavior

For close to a century, researchers have asked the natural question of how to eliminate Pavlovian conditioned responses. Pavlov (1927) studied *extinction,* which refers to the decrease in the conditioned response when the CS is presented repeatedly without the US after conditioning. Note that extinction has since been studied in many areas as a method for reducing Pavlovian and operant conditioned behavior, and much has been discovered about the behavioral and brain processes involved in extinction (Bouton et al., 2021). The overall message is that extinction is fundamental to most response elimination processes. For example, extinction is the basis of many behavioral or cognitive-behavioral therapies designed to reduce pathological conditioned responding through repeated exposure to the CS (e.g., exposure therapy; Foa, 2011; Vervliet et al., 2013). Another response elimination procedure is *counterconditioning,* in which the CS is paired with a very different US–UR (Keller et al., 2020; Scavio, 1974). For instance, counterconditioning was the inspiration for systematic desensitization, a behavior therapy technique in which frightening CSs are deliberately associated with relaxation during therapy (Wolpe, 1954).

Pavlovian extinction and counterconditioning likely play an important role in clinical interventions, even when the treatments focus on operant behavior. For example, many children with feeding disorders have a history of medical problems (e.g., gastroesophageal reflux disease) that have made eating painful (Di Lorenzo et al., 2005), resulting in taste aversions (Garb & Stunkard, 1974). One critical component of behavioral treatments for pediatric feeding disorders involves repeated presentations of the target food without allowing food refusal behaviors to terminate the trial (Piazza et al., 2003). This approach, known as escape extinction, targets operant inappropriate mealtime behavior; however, this procedure likely often involves Pavlovian extinction as well because foods (CSs) are being presented repeatedly without the US (pain). Note that this treatment also involves counterconditioning by presenting reinforcers contingent on food acceptance. Extinction and counterconditioning are also important aspects of medical desensitization procedures used to teach individuals to tolerate necessary medical treatments. For example, Shabani and Fisher (2006) successfully implemented these procedures to teach an autistic adolescent with type 2 diabetes to tolerate blood drawings necessary to monitor his blood glucose levels. The procedures involved gradual increases in needle exposure and reinforcement for tolerating the procedure without moving his arm away. Though the authors focused on operant behavior (pulling arm away), research shows that medical desensitization procedures also reduce emotions of fear (McMurtry et al., 2015).

Although extinction and counterconditioning reduce unwanted conditioned responses, they do not destroy the original learning, which remains in the brain, ready to return to behavior under the right circumstances (Bouton & Balleine, 2019). Again, we note that each of the following response recovery phenomena have been shown to apply to Pavlovian and operant conditioned responses. Conditioned responses that have been eliminated by extinction or counterconditioning can recover if time passes before the CS is presented again (spontaneous recovery; Rescorla, 2004). Medical desensitization, for instance, is an effective treatment for needle phobias; however, treatment effects are often not detected at 1-year follow-up assessments (McMurtry et al., 2015). Conditioned responses can also return if the patient returns to the context of conditioning after extinction in another context; that is, if fear conditioning to needles occurred in a hospital setting (Context A), and the successful treatment occurred in a clinic setting (Context B), fear responses can return when needles are presented at the next medical appointment in the hospital setting (Context A). Conditioned responses can also return if the extinguished CS is in a different context. For example, if food aversion was conditioned in the home setting (Context A) and treatment was conducted in a clinic (Context B), the food aversion can return when food is presented at school or restaurants (Context C). Likewise, a similar recovery could also occur if food-aversion conditioning and treatment both occurred in the home (Context A) and the CS is encountered in a new context (Context B). The ABC and AAB examples illustrate the context-specific property of extinction learning, which is well-established with Pavlovian and operant responses in animals (see Bouton, 2019). Such so-called "renewal" effects emphasize that extinction, as well as other retroactive interference treatments (e.g., counterconditioning, omission training, differential reinforcement of alternative behavior) do not erase the original learning but instead produce new learning that is particularly context specific. This new learning may consist of CS–no US learning in Pavlovian conditioning, and response inhibition learning in operant conditioning (Bouton, 2019). As with an ambiguous word, which likewise has more than one meaning, the new learning about the response that has occurred during extinction or counterconditioning depends fundamentally on the current context (Bouton, 1993, 2002).

Research on context effects in both animal and human learning and memory suggests that a wide variety of stimuli can play the role of context. Drugs, for example, can be very salient in this regard. When rats are given fear extinction while under the influence of a benzodiazepine tranquilizer or alcohol, fear is renewed when the CS is tested in the absence of the context provided by the drug (Bouton et al., 1990). This is an example of state-dependent learning (Overton, 1966, 1991), in which retention of information is best when tested in the same state in which it was originally learned (see also Schepers & Bouton, 2017, 2019). State-dependent learning has many implications for practitioners, because many of the clients they serve are often taking prescription medication. For example, if a child learns to tolerate medical procedures through medical desensitization treatment while taking psychotropic medications, problem behavior and noncompliance could reemerge if there are medication changes. State-dependent learning also has implications for the administration of drugs more generally. For example, if a person were to take a drug to reduce anxiety, the anxiety reduction would reinforce drug taking. State-dependent extinction might further preserve any anxiety that might otherwise extinguish during natural exposure to the anxiety-eliciting cues. Thus, drug use could, paradoxically, preserve the original anxiety, creating a self-perpetuating cycle that could provide a possible explanation of the link between anxiety disorders and substance abuse (see, e.g., Koob et al., 2020).

One point of this discussion is that drugs can play multiple roles in learning: They can be USs or reinforcers on the one hand, and CSs or contexts on the other. The possible complex behavioral effects of drugs are worth bearing in mind. Another general message is that contemporary theory emphasizes the fact that extinction (and other processes like counterconditioning) entails new learning rather than a destruction of older learning. Instead of trying to destroy the original memory (or behavior) with treatment, another therapeutic strategy might be to build therapies that allow the organism to prevent or cope with the original memory (or behavior; Bouton, 2014). One possibility is to conduct extinction exposure in many contexts, including those where relapse might be most problematic to the patient (e.g., Bustamante et al., 2016; Gunther et al., 1998). Another approach would be to encourage retrieval strategies (e.g., retrieval cues such as reminder cards or text messages) that increase the similarity of the current context and the treatment context, and help remind the patient of the therapy experience (e.g., Collins & Brandon, 2002; Craske et al., 2018; Thrailkill et al., 2019; Trask, 2019).

As noted earlier, operant learning has many parallels with Pavlovian learning. Thorndike (1911) emphasized the role of the reinforcer as "stamping in" the response. More recent approaches to operant learning tend to view the reinforcer as a sort of guide or motivator of behavior (e.g., Bolles, 1975). A modern, "synthetic" view of operant conditioning (see later discussion) holds that responses and outcomes are associated in the same way that stimulus–outcome learning is thought to be involved in Pavlovian learning (Bouton, 2016). Historically, operant behavior has been studied as its own topic. This distinction reflects the idea that much of human behavior appears to be voluntary, or goal-directed, and not directly attributable to antecedent cues. Human behavior is influenced by a wide variety of primary, conditioned, generalized, derived, and social reinforcers. For example, simple attention from teachers or hospital staff members has been shown to reinforce disruptive or problematic behavior exhibited by students or patients. In either case, when the attention is withheld and redirected toward other activities, the problematic behaviors can decrease (i.e., undergo extinction). Human behavior is influenced by verbal reinforcers, such as praise, and more generally, by conditioned reinforcers, such as money, which have no intrinsic value except for the value derived through (Pavlovian) association with more basic, biologically relevant, and/or "primary" rewards. Conditioned reinforcers have been used to modify behavior in schools and other congregate settings. For instance, in a token economy, appropriate behaviors are reinforced with tokens that can be used to purchase other valued items (Hackenberg, 2009). In more natural settings, reinforcers are always delivered in social relationships, where their effects are dynamic and reciprocal (e.g., Conger & Killeen, 1974; FeldmanHall & Dunsmoor, 2019). Like Pavlovian learning, operant learning is always operating and always influencing behavior.

Pavlovian and Operant Learning Together

From the previous discussion, it should be fairly clear that there is more going on in operant learning than merely associating antecedent, behavior, and consequence (see, e.g., Domjan, 2016, for more discussion). Theories of the motivating effects of reinforcers usually emphasize the fact that Pavlovian CSs in the background are also associated with the reinforcer, and that the expectancy of the reinforcer (or conditioned motivational state) they arouse increases the vigor of the operant response (de Wit & Dickinson, 2009; Rescorla & Solomon, 1967). These theories emphasize the influence of Pavlovian and operant factors: Pavlovian learning occurs simultaneously and motivates behavior during operant learning.

Avoidance Learning

The interaction of Pavlovian and operant learning is especially important in understanding avoidance learning. The avoidance learning situation requires organisms to learn a response that prevents the presentation of an aversive event. Note that avoidance requires a subtle explanation, because there is no obvious reinforcer; that is, preventing the aversive event is obviously important, but how can the nonoccurrence of an event function as a reinforcer? Though other explanations have been proposed, a large empirical literature suggests the answer is that Pavlovian CSs present in the environment come to predict the occurrence of the aversive event, and consequently arouse anxiety or fear (Cain, 2019; Mineka, 1979; Mineka & Zinbarg, 2006). The avoidance response can therefore be reinforced if it results in escape from or reduces that fear. For example, the sight of a needle at a medical appointment could evoke an avoidance response in the form of a tantrum that prevents the delivery of the vaccination. Pavlovian and operant factors are thus both important: Pavlovian conditioning of fear motivates and allows reinforcement of an operant response through its reduction. Escape from fear or anxiety is thought to play a significant role in many human behavior disorders, including anxiety disorders. Other examples include the individual with obsessive–compulsive disorder who counts, checks, or washes his hands repeatedly to reduce anxiety, the individual with fear of certain places and situations (agoraphobia) stays at home to avoid fear of places associated with panic attacks, and the individual with an eating disorder learns to vomit after a meal in order to reduce the learned anxiety evoked by eating the meal.

Excellent avoidance can be obtained in the laboratory without the repeated presentation of the aversive stimulus (and corresponding negative reinforcement in the form of escape). If an animal is required to perform a response that resembles one of its natural and prepared fear responses, it will quickly learn to avoid successfully. These responses are referred to as species-specific defensive reactions (SSDRs; Bolles, 1970; Fanselow, 1997). For example, rats will readily learn to freeze (remain motionless) or flee (run to another environment) to avoid shock, two behaviors that have evolved to escape or avoid predation. Freezing and fleeing are also respondents rather than operants; they are controlled by antecedent Pavlovian CSs that predict shock rather than the consequences of escape from fear (Fanselow, 1980). Thus, the rat learns about environmental cues associated with danger, and these arouse fear and evoke natural defensive behaviors including withdrawal and escape. When the rat can use an SSDR to avoid, the only necessary learning is Pavlovian. Note that learning to perform a response that differs from a natural SSDR requires more feedback or reinforcement through fear reduction. Lever pressing, for example, is easy for the rat to learn when the reinforcer is a food pellet but difficult to learn when the same behavior avoids shock (Bolles, 1972). Work with avoidance in humans suggests an important role for expectancies; that is, the CS predicts an aversive event and the response predicts no aversive event (Lovibond, 2006). Altogether, many years of research support the importance of Pavlovian learning in avoidance learning.

When an SSDR is available, it is the only learning necessary; when the required response is not an SSDR, Pavlovian learning allows the organism to expect something bad. Likewise, clinicians should be mindful of CSs that might be conditioned when paired with aversive events. For example, a therapist may allow a client access to videos on an iPad as a reinforcer for completing school work tasks. If the therapist only approaches the client while she is watching a video to remove the iPad and prompt her to get back to work, the approaching therapist could easily become a CS that predicts iPad loss and evoke avoidance problem behavior.

This perspective is also encouraged by studies of learned helplessness (Seligman & Maier, 1967). In this phenomenon, exposure to either controllable or uncontrollable aversive events results in different levels of reactivity to later aversive events. In a typical experiment, subjects exposed to inescapable shock in one phase are less successful at learning a new behavior that escapes shock in a second phase in comparison to subjects exposed to escapable shock. Subjects in each treatment are exposed to the same shock, but its controllability (a psychological dimension) creates a difference. Some have suggested that exposure to inescapable shock results in learning that shock and behavior are independent (Seligman & Maier, 1967). Although learned helplessness (and this interpretation) was once thought to model features of depression, the current view is that controllability modulates the stressfulness and negative impact of aversive events (Maier & Seligman, 2016).

At a theoretical level, learned helplessness also implies that learning operant contingencies in which behaviors lead to reinforcers might involve learning something about the controllability of those reinforcers. This appears to be the case in clinical settings. For example, escape extinction is a common behavioral intervention for problem behavior maintained by escape or avoidance. In the prior examples of medical desensitization and treatments for feeding disorders/food refusal, escape extinction is often a component of the treatment. Here, problem behavior that used to be successful in terminating or avoiding the medical procedure or food presentation no longer produces escape. Escape extinction is also a common intervention component for problem behavior maintained by escape from demands such as educational activities. In this case, if instructional demands evoke problem behavior, the child would be prompted to follow through with the instruction and not allowed escape (oftentimes they are also taught how to appropriately request a break when needed as an alternative response). One of the main conclusions of work on aversive learning is thus that there are both biological (i.e., evolutionary, SSDR) and cognitive dimensions (i.e., controllability, predictability) to operant learning.

Approach Learning

The possibility that much of operant behavior can be influenced by Pavlovian contingencies is also consistent with research with positive reinforcers. For example, in the typical experiment with pigeons (e.g., Skinner, 1938), the bird learns to peck at a plastic disk on a wall of the chamber (a response "key") to earn food. Although pecking seems to be an operant response, it turns out that the pigeon can be trained to peck by merely illuminating the key for a few seconds before presenting the reinforcer (Brown & Jenkins, 1968). Although there is no requirement for the bird to peck the key, the bird will begin to peck at the illuminated key anyway. The illuminated key is a Pavlovian predictor of food. This phenomenon is sometimes referred to as "sign tracking," or "autoshaping" in reference to result of seemingly automatic shaping of key pecking (Boakes, 1977; Brown & Jenkins, 1968). The pigeon does this even if the experimenter arranges things so that pecks actually prevent delivery of food (which is otherwise delivered on trials without pecks); here, the birds will continue to peck over many trials. Although the peck has a negative correlation with food, key illumination remains a weakly positive predictor of food (Williams & Williams, 1969; see also Robinson & Berridge, 2013). Pavlovian contingencies cannot be ignored. When rats' lever pressing for food is punished with mild foot shock, the rats stop lever pressing at least partly (and perhaps predominantly) because they learn that the lever now predicts shock and withdraw from it (Rescorla & Solomon, 1967). A child might likewise learn to stay away from the parent or caregiver who delivers punishment rather than refrain from performing the punished behavior. A great deal of operant behavior may actually be controlled by Pavlovian learning.

A Synthetic View of Operant Behavior

The idea, then, is that operant behavior is controlled by several hypothetical associations. As just discussed, much of operant behavior can be controlled by a Pavlovian factor, in which background cues (CSs) are associated with the reinforcing outcome (O). As discussed earlier, this can allow the CS (S) to evoke a variety of behaviors, as well as emotional reactions (and motivational states) that can additionally motivate operant behavior. In modern terms, the operant behavior is represented by the organism learning a direct (and similar) association between the operant response (R) and the reinforcing outcome (O). Evidence for this sort of learning comes from experiments on reinforcer devaluation (Adams & Dickinson, 1981; Dickinson, 1985; Thrailkill & Bouton, 2015). In a classic experiment, Colwill and Rescorla (1985) trained rats to perform two operant responses (e.g., pressing a lever and pulling a chain), each paired with a different reinforcer (e.g., food pellet vs. a liquid sucrose solution). After conditioning, rats received a separate second phase in which one of the reinforcers (e.g., pellet) was paired with illness. This created a powerful taste aversion to the reinforcer. Importantly, the rats learned the aversion separate from the response; the response operandum (e.g., lever/chain) was not available. In a final test, the organism was presented with the response operanda and allowed to perform either response. No reinforcers were presented during the test. The result was that the rats no longer emitted the response that produced the now-aversive reinforcer. In order to perform this way, an organism must have (1) learned which response produced which reinforcer (R–O) and (2) combined this knowledge with the knowledge that it no longer likes or values that reinforcer (O–illness). The result cannot be explained by the simpler, more traditional view that reinforcers merely stamp in or strengthen operant behavior (S–R; Dickinson, 1994; see also Bouton, 2021). Another crucial point is that organisms need to learn how reinforcers influence a particular motivational state—this process is referred to as "incentive learning" (Balleine, 1992, 2001), which is a process through which the organism learns the value of the reinforcer. Thus, in a reinforcer devaluation experiment, the organism must actually contact the reinforcer in the changed motivational state in order to learn that it does not like it. Incentive learning is probably always involved in making reinforcers more or less desirable.

To further integrate the discussion, recall that earning reinforcers involves learning to associate cues in the environment with them. Such stimulus–outcome, or S–O (Pavlovian), learning can have many effects on behavior: As we have seen, S may evoke approach behaviors and may elicit many other responses that generally get the organism ready for the reinforcer. Consider the example of learning to respond to one's name: In learning to associate hearing their name with a reinforcer delivery from the person who says the name, a child learns to attend to or approach a person when they call their name. On the other hand, if a child learns to associate the word, "no" with an aversive event, they may learn to pause or stop what they are doing when they hear the word "no." As also mentioned earlier, the presentation of S may excite or inhibit the operant response. This feature of operant behavior is illustrated by Pavlovian-instrumental transfer: When a CS (S) that is associated with a US (O) is presented while an organism performs an operant response that earns O, the rate of responding increases. CSs that predict the O (excitors) increase the rate of the operant response (Lovibond, 1983; Lovibond & Colagiuri, 2013), whereas CSs that predict the nonoccurrence of O (inhibitors) decrease it (Laurent & Balleine, 2015; Quail et al., 2017). A CS that predicts O can also excite operant behaviors that lead to other Os that are motivationally similar, such as two different types of food. However, CSs are especially likely to increase responses that are associated with the same O. Thus, in addition to influencing general motivation of operant behavior, Pavlovian cues can influence choice of a specific response over others (Corbit & Balleine, 2005; Ostlund & Marshall, 2021). This capacity is presumably exploited by advertisers who create Ss in the form of television commercials or targeted advertisements on social media, for example, whose presentation can motivate the consumer to buy a particular brand of pizza or beer.

Finally, cues in the environment can also enter into modulating relationships with S-O (Pavlovian) or R-O (operant) associations. Such cues are often referred to as *occasion setters* in Pavlovian conditioning and *discriminative stimuli* in operant conditioning. In the earlier examples of Pavlovian influences on operant behavior, the CS has general and specific influences on the rate and selection of operant responding. Each example shows the direct influence of a Pavlovian cue on the operant response via its association with O. In contrast, a modulating stimulus is not directly associated with the outcome; instead, it provides information about the S-O or R-O association, and therefore has an indirect influence on the response.

A Pavlovian occasion setter is a stimulus that does not elicit a response when presented alone but instead influences, or modulates, responding to a CS that has its own relationship with the US. Whereas the CS signals when the US is going to occur, the modulating stimulus (occasion setter) indicates whether the CS will be followed by the US (Holland, 1992; Trask et al., 2017). There are two main types of arrangements that result in occasion setting. The occasion setting stimulus may predict that a US will not occur when it otherwise would. For example, a rat receives intermixed presentations of a tone (T) paired with a foot shock US and a tone–light compound (TL) that is not followed by the US. Eventually, the rat will learn to freeze in response to T and not TL. This is referred to as a "feature-negative" discrimination, because L is a feature that indicates the US will *not* be presented. An analogous example would be a small child who first yells (CS) and then hits (US) his sister when they fight—unless a parent is present in which case, he will still yell but not hit his sibling in their presence. The yelling could function as a CS that elicits the activation syndrome or a fear response except for when a parent (occasion setter) is present. The opposite, "feature-positive" discrimination, can be arranged in which L indicates the US will be presented. Here, the rat eventually freezes to TL but not T after TL–US pairings intermixed with T without the US (Rescorla, 1986, 1987; see also Hearst, 1978; Ross & Holland, 1981). Again, L modulates the T–US association but now indicates the presence of US. For instance, say a person usually drinks decaffeinated coffee except when they visit their in-laws, who offer only regular (caffeinated) coffee (US). This person might come to find that they feel more alert when they simply smell the scent of coffee (CS), but only when they are at their in-laws' home (occasion setter), despite the identical aroma of decaf and caffeinated coffee.

One important and unique property of occasion setters is their ability to modulate other CS–US associations if these had been subject to modulation by an occasion setter in a similar discrimination (Holland, 1986, 1989); that is, if the rat in the earlier feature-negative example had also learned a second feature-negative discrimination, such that a click (C) was followed by a foot shock US and flashing light-click (FC) was not. The light (L) trained as a negative feature would also reduce responding when presented in compound with the click (LC). Note, however, that for transfer to occur, the occasion setter must have been trained in the same (positive–negative feature) relation previously; the L from the feature-negative example would not function to modulate a US trained in a feature-positive discrimination. A large and careful empirical literature has identified several important characteristics of Pavlovian occasion setters that are outside the scope of this chapter, and we refer interested readers to reviews dedicated to the subject (Holland, 1992; Trask et al., 2017).

In a typical operant learning situation, a response (R) is followed by a reinforcing outcome (O) in the presence of some discriminative stimulus. Like a Pavlovian CS, a discriminative stimulus can signal the presentation and identity of the O (Colwill & Rescorla, 1988). Discriminative stimuli can also function to modulate operant behavior in a manner analogous to Pavlovian occasion setting; that is, a discriminative stimulus can enter into a hierarchical relation with the R-O association and signal whether an R will be followed by an O, as well as which R will be followed by which O (Colwill & Rescorla, 1990). Whether a discriminative stimulus functions to signal the O, a Pavlovian association, or plays a hierarchical role, modulation or occasion setting, will depend on its learning history. Clearly, discriminated operants are relevant to human behavior as most of our everyday behavior, such as checking email, refueling our vehicles, and cooking meals, is under the control of distinct and identifiable antecedent stimuli (Thrailkill et al., 2018, 2021; Thrailkill, 2023). A synthetic approach emphasizes the importance of understanding the relationships and interactions between events that comprise stimuli, responses, and outcomes.

Conclusion

This chapter provides an up-to-date survey of Pavlovian conditioning from a translational perspective. Pavlovian conditioning as a subject is not distinct, simple, esoteric, outdated, or irrelevant to behavior analysis. Rather, it should be clear that the principles of Pavlovian learning have a rich tradition of translation and application, and therefore offer useful tools for addressing behavior in translational, applied, and clinical settings. From a synthetic perspective, Pavlovian and operant conditioning result from common learning processes. Such an approach can generate hypotheses for how to understand and change behavior by targeting underlying learning mechanisms (Bouton, 2014; Bouton & Balleine, 2019). The study of Pavlovian conditioning has led to a wealth of systematic data and theories that are enduring, interesting, and fundamental to anyone interested in understanding behavior.

ACKNOWLEDGMENTS

Preparation of this chapter was supported by Grant Nos. K01 DA044456 and P20 GM103644 (EAT) from the National Institutes of Health. We thank Mark Bouton for helpful discussions on this chapter.

REFERENCES

Adams, C. D., & Dickinson, A. (1981). Instrumental responding following reinforcer devaluation. *Quarterly Journal of Experimental Psychology Section B, 33*, 109–121.

Adkins-Regan, E., & MacKillop, E. A. (2003). Japanese quail (*Coturnix japonica*) inseminations are more likely to fertilize eggs in a context predicting mating opportunities. *Proceedings of the Royal Society of London B: Biological Sciences, 270*(1525), 1685–1689.

Annau, Z., & Kamin, L. J. (1961). The conditioned emotional response as a function of intensity of the US. *Journal of Comparative and Physiological Psychology, 54*(4), 428–432.

Balleine, B. (1992). Instrumental performance following a shift in primary motivation depends on incentive learning. *Journal of Experimental Psychology: Animal Behavior Processes, 18*, 236–250.

Balleine, B. W. (2001). Incentive processes in instrumental conditioning. In R. R. Mowrer & S. B. Klein (Eds.), *Handbook of contemporary learning theories* (pp. 307–366). Erlbaum.

Bartlett, E., Hallin, A., Chapman, B., & Angrist, B. (1997). Selective sensitization to the psychosis-inducing effects of cocaine: A possible marker for addiction relapse vulnerability? *Neuropsychopharmacology, 16*(1), 77–82.

Bernstein, I. L. (1978). Learned taste aversions in children receiving chemotherapy. *Science, 200*, 1302–1303.

Bernstein, I. L., Webster, M. M., & Bernstein, I. D. (1982). Food aversions in children receiving chemotherapy for cancer. *Cancer, 50*(12), 2961–2963.

Berridge, K. C., & Robinson, T. E. (2016). Liking, wanting, and the incentive-sensitization theory of addiction. *American Psychologist, 71*, 670–679.

Boakes, R. A. (1977). Performance on learning to associate a stimulus with positive reinforcement. In H. Davis & H. M. B. Hurwitz (Eds.), *Operant–Pavlovian interactions* (pp. 67–97). Erlbaum.

Bolles, R. C. (1970). Species-specific defense reactions and avoidance learning. *Psychological Review, 77*, 32–48.

Bolles, R. C. (1972). The avoidance learning problem. In G. H. Bower (Ed.), *The psychology of learning and motivation* (Vol. 6, pp. 97–145). Academic Press.

Bolles, R. C. (1975). *Theory of motivation* (2nd ed.). Harper & Row.

Bouton, M. E. (1993). Context, time, and memory retrieval in the interference paradigms of Pavlovian learning. *Psychological Bulletin, 114*, 80–99.

Bouton, M. E. (2002). Context, ambiguity, and unlearning: Sources of relapse after behavioral extinction. *Biological Psychiatry, 52*, 976–986.

Bouton, M. E. (2014). Why behavior change is difficult to sustain. *Preventive Medicine, 68*, 29–36.

Bouton, M. E. (2016). *Learning and behavior: A contemporary synthesis* (2nd ed.). Sinauer.

Bouton, M. E. (2019). Extinction of instrumental (operant) learning: Interference, varieties of context, and mechanisms of contextual control. *Psychopharmacology, 236*(1), 7–19.

Bouton, M. E. (2021). Context, attention, and the switch between habit and goal-direction in behavior. *Learning and Behavior, 49*, 349–362.

Bouton, M. E., & Balleine, B. W. (2019). Prediction and control of operant behavior: What you see is not all there is. *Behavior Analysis: Research and Practice, 19*, 202–212.

Bouton, M. E., Kenney, F. A., & Rosengard, C. (1990). State-dependent fear extinction with two benzodiazepine tranquilizers. *Behavioral Neuroscience, 104*(1), 44–55.

Bouton, M. E., Maren, S., & McNally, G. P. (2021). Behavioral and neurobiological mechanisms of Pavlovian and instrumental extinction learning. *Physiological Reviews, 101*, 611–681.

Bouton, M. E., Mineka, S., & Barlow, D. H. (2001). A modern learning theory perspective on the etiology of panic disorder. *Psychological Review, 108*, 4–32.

Bradley, B. P., Mogg, K., Wright, T., & Field, M. (2003). Attentional bias in drug dependence: Vigilance for cigarette-related cues in smokers. *Psychology of Addictive Behaviors, 17*, 66–72.

Brand, J., Masterson, T. D., Emond, J. A., Lansigan, R., & Gilbert-Diamond, D. (2020). Measuring attentional bias to food cues in young children using a visual search task: An eye-tracking study. *Appetite, 148*, Article 104610.

Brogden, W. J. (1939). Sensory pre-conditioning. *Journal of Experimental Psychology, 25*(4), 323–332.

Brown, P. L., & Jenkins, H. M. (1968). Auto-shaping of the pigeon's key-peck. *Journal of the Experimental Analysis of Behavior, 11*, 1–8.

Bustamante, J., Uengoer, M., Thorwart, A., & Lachnit, H. (2016). Extinction in multiple contexts: Effects on the rate of extinction and the strength of response recovery. *Learning and Behavior, 44*(3), 283–294.

Cain, C. K. (2019). Avoidance problems reconsidered. *Current Opinion in Behavioral Sciences, 26*, 9–17.

Cengher, M., Budd, A., Farrell, N., & Fienup, D. M. (2018). A review of prompt-fading procedures: Implications for effective and efficient skill acquisition. *Journal of Developmental and Physical Disabilities, 30*, 155–173.

Cole, R. P., & Miller, R. R. (1999). Conditioned excitation and conditioned inhibition acquired through backward conditioning. *Learning and Motivation, 30*, 129–156.

Collins, B. N., & Brandon, T. H. (2002). Effects of extinction context and retrieval cues on alcohol cue reactivity among nonalcoholic drinkers. *Journal of Consulting and Clinical Psychology, 70*(2), 390–397.

Colwill, R. M., & Rescorla, R. A. (1985). Post-conditioning devaluation of a reinforcer affects instrumental responding. *Journal of Experimental Psychology: Animal Behavior Processes, 11*, 120–132.

Colwill, R. M., & Rescorla, R. A. (1988). Associations between the discriminative stimulus and the reinforcer in instrumental learning. *Journal of Experimental Psychology: Animal Behavior Processes, 14*(2), 155–164.

Colwill, R. M., & Rescorla, R. A. (1990). Evidence for the hierarchical structure of instrumental learning. *Animal Learning and Behavior, 18*(1), 71–82.

Conger, R., & Killeen, P. (1974). Use of concurrent operants in small group research: A demonstration. *Pacific Sociological Review, 17*, 399–416.

Corbit, L. H., & Balleine, B. W. (2005). Double dissociation of basolateral and central amygdala lesions on the general and outcome-specific forms of Pavlovian-instrumental transfer. *Journal of Neuroscience, 25*, 962–970.

Couvillon, P. A., Klosterhalfen, S., & Bitterman, M. E. (1983). Analysis of overshadowing in honeybees. *Journal of Comparative Psychology, 97*(2), 154–166.

Craske, M. G., Hermans, D., & Vervliet, B. (2018). State-of-the-art and future directions for extinction as a translational model for fear and anxiety. *Philosophical Transactions of the Royal Society B: Biological Sciences, 373*(1742), Article 20170025.

da Silva, S. P., & Williams, A. M. (2020). Translations in stimulus–stimulus pairing: Autoshaping of learner vocalizations. *Perspectives on Behavior Science, 43*(1), 57–103.

Davis, M. (1986). Pharmacological and anatomical analysis of fear conditioning using the fear-potentiated startle paradigm. *Behavioral Neuroscience, 100*, 814–824.

Davis, M. (2006). Neural systems involved in fear and anxiety measured with fear-potentiated startle. *American Psychologist, 61*(8), 741–756.

Delamater, A. R., Sosa, W., & LoLordo, V. M. (2003). Outcome-specific conditioned inhibition in Pavlovian backward conditioning. *Animal Learning and Behavior, 31*(4), 393–402.

de Wit, S., & Dickinson, A. (2009). Associative theories of goal-directed behaviour: A case for animal–human translational models. *Psychological Research, 73*, 463–476.

Dickinson, A. (1985). Actions and habits: The development of behavioural autonomy. *Philosophical Transactions of the Royal Society of London B: Biological Sciences, 308*, 67–78.

Dickinson, A. (1994). Instrumental conditioning. In N. J. Mackintosh (Ed.), *Handbook of perception and cognition series: Animal learning and cognition* (2nd ed., pp. 45–79). Academic Press.

Di Lorenzo, C., Colletti, R. B., Lehmann, H. P., Boyle, J. T., Gerson, W. T., Hyams, J. S., . . . NASPGHAN Committee on Chronic Abdominal Pain. (2005). Chronic abdominal pain in children: A technical report of the American Academy of Pediatrics and the North American Society for Pediatric Gastroenterology, Hepatology and Nutrition. *Journal of Pediatric Gastroenterology and Nutrition, 40*(3), 249–261.

Dittlinger, L. H., & Lerman, D. C. (2011). Further analysis of picture interference when teaching word recognition to children with autism. *Journal of Applied Behavior Analysis, 44,* 341–349.

Domjan, M. (2016). Elicited versus emitted behavior: Time to abandon the distinction. *Journal of the Experimental Analysis of Behavior, 105*(2), 231–245.

Domjan, M., & Gutiérrez, G. (2019). The behavior system for sexual learning. *Behavioural Processes, 162,* 184–196.

Domjan, M., Mahometa, M., & Matthews, R. N. (2012). Learning in intimate connections: Conditioned fertility and its role in sexual competition. *Socioaffective Neuroscience and Psychology, 2*(1), Article 17333.

Ewing, M. F., Larew, M. B., & Wagner, A. R. (1985). Distribution-of-trials effects in Pavlovian conditioning: An apparent involvement of inhibitory backward conditioning with short intertrial intervals. *Journal of Experimental Psychology: Animal Behavior Processes, 11,* 537–547.

Fanselow, M. S. (1980). Conditional and unconditional components of post-shock freezing. *Pavlovian Journal of Biological Science, 15,* 177–182.

Fanselow, M. (1997). Species-specific defense reactions: Retrospect and prospect. In M. E. Bouton (Ed.), *Learning, motivation, and cognition* (pp. 321–341). American Psychological Association.

FeldmanHall, O., & Dunsmoor, J. E. (2019). Viewing adaptive social choice through the lens of associative learning. *Perspectives on Psychological Science, 14*(2), 175–196.

Foa, E. B. (2011). Prolonged exposure therapy: Past, present, and future. *Depression and Anxiety, 28*(12), 1043–1047.

Garb, J. L., & Stunkard, A. J. (1974). Taste aversions in man. *American Journal of Psychiatry, 131*(11), 1204–1207.

Gibson, E. J., & Walk, R. D. (1956). The effect of prolonged exposure to visually presented patterns on learning to discriminate them. *Journal of Comparative and Physiological Psychology, 49*(3), 239–242.

Gottlieb, D., & Begej, E. (2014). Principles of Pavlovian conditioning. In F. McSweeney & E.

Murphy (Eds.), *The Wiley–Blackwell handbook of operant and classical conditioning* (pp. 3–26). Wiley-Blackwell.

Gunther, L. M., Denniston, J. C., & Miller, R. R. (1998). Conducting exposure treatment in multiple contexts can prevent relapse. *Behaviour Research and Therapy, 36*(1), 75–91.

Hackenberg, T. D. (2009). Token reinforcement: A review and analysis. *Journal of the Experimental Analysis of Behavior, 91,* 257–286.

Hadamitzky, M., Lückemann, L., Pacheco-López, G., & Schedlowski, M. (2020). Pavlovian conditioning of immunological and neuroendocrine functions. *Physiological Reviews, 100,* 357–405.

Hearst, E. (1978). Stimulus relationships and feature selection in learning and behavior. In S. H. Hulse, H. Fowler, & W. K. Honig (Eds.), *Cognitive processes in animal behavior* (pp. 51–88). Erlbaum.

Heilig, M. (2015). *The thirteenth step: Addiction in the age of brain science.* Columbia University Press.

Heth, C. D. (1976). Simultaneous and backward fear conditioning as a function of number of CS-UCS pairings. *Journal of Experimental Psychology: Animal Behavior Processes, 2,* 117–129.

Hoffman, A. N., Trott, J. M., Makridis, A., & Fanselow, M. S. (2022). Anxiety, fear, panic: An approach to assessing the defensive behavior system across the predatory imminence continuum. *Learning and Behavior, 50,* 339–348.

Hoffmann, H. (2017). Situating human sexual conditioning. *Archives of Sexual Behavior, 46*(8), 2213–2229.

Holland, P. C. (1977). Conditioned stimulus as a determinant of the form of the Pavlovian conditioned response. *Journal of Experimental Psychology: Animal Behavior Processes, 3*(1), 77–104.

Holland, P. C. (1986). Transfer after serial feature positive discrimination training. *Learning and Motivation, 17*(3), 243–268.

Holland, P. C. (1989). Transfer of negative occasion setting and conditioned inhibition across conditioned and unconditioned stimuli. *Journal of Experimental Psychology: Animal Behavior Processes, 15*(4), 311–328.

Holland, P. C. (1992). Occasion setting in Pavlovian conditioning. In D. Medin (Ed.), *The psychology of learning and motivation* (Vol. 28, pp. 69–125). Academic Press.

Hollis, K. L., Pharr, V. L., Dumas, M. J., Britton, G. B., & Field, J. (1997). Classical conditioning provides paternity advantage for territorial male blue gouramis (*Trichogaster trichopterus*). *Journal of Comparative Psychology, 111*(3), 219–225.

Holman, E. W. (1975). Immediate and delayed reinforcers for flavor preferences in rats. *Learning and Motivation, 6*(1), 91–100.

Holman, E. W. (1980). Irrelevant-incentive learning with flavors in rats. *Journal of Experimental Psychology: Animal Behavior Processes, 6*, 126–136.

Kamin, L. J. (1969). Selective association and conditioning. In N. J. Mackintosh & W. K. Honig (Eds.), *Fundamental issues in associative learning* (pp. 42–64). Dalhousie University Press.

Keller, N. E., Hennings, A. C., & Dunsmoor, J. E. (2020). Behavioral and neural processes in counterconditioning: Past and future directions. *Behaviour Research and Therapy, 125*, Article 103532.

Koob, G. F., Powell, P., & White, A. (2020). Addiction as a coping response: Hyperkatifeia, deaths of despair, and COVID-19. *American Journal of Psychiatry, 177*(11), 1031–1037.

Laurent, V., & Balleine, B. W. (2015). Factual and counterfactual action-outcome mappings control choice between goal-directed actions in rats. *Current Biology, 25*(8), 1074–1079.

LeDoux, J. E. (1996). *The emotional brain: The mysterious underpinnings of emotional life.* Simon & Schuster.

Lissek, S., Biggs, A. L., Rabin, S. J., Cornwell, B. R., Alvarez, R. P., Pine, D. S., & Grillon, C. (2008). Generalization of conditioned fear-potentiated startle in humans: Experimental validation and clinical relevance. *Behaviour Research and Therapy, 46*(5), 678–687.

Lovibond, P. F. (1983). Facilitation of instrumental behavior by a Pavlovian appetitive conditioned stimulus. *Journal of Experimental Psychology: Animal Behavior Processes, 9*, 225–247.

Lovibond, P. F. (2006). Fear and avoidance: An integrated expectancy model. In M. G. Craske, D. Hermans, & D. Vansteenwegen (Eds.), *Fear and learning: From basic processes to clinical implications* (pp. 117–132). American Psychological Association.

Lovibond, P. F., & Colagiuri, B. (2013). Facilitation of voluntary goal-directed action by reward cues. *Psychological Science, 24*, 2030–2037.

Lubow, R. E. (1973). Latent inhibition. *Psychological Bulletin, 79*(6), 398–407.

Lubow, R. E., & Moore, A. U. (1959). Latent inhibition: The effect of nonreinforced preexposure to the conditional stimulus. *Journal of Comparative and Physiological Psychology, 52*(4), 415–419.

Mackenzie, J. N. (1886). The production of the so-called "rose cold" by means of an artificial rose, with remarks and historical notes. *American Journal of the Medical Sciences, 91*(181), 45–57.

Mackintosh, N. J. (1975). A theory of attention: Variations in the associability of stimuli with reinforcement. *Psychological Review, 82*, 276–298.

Maier, S. F., & Seligman, M. E. P. (2016). Learned helplessness at fifty: Insights from neuroscience. *Psychological Review, 123*, 349–367.

Mansfield, J. G., & Cunningham, C. L. (1980). Conditioning and extinction of tolerance to the hypothermic effect of ethanol in rats. *Journal of Comparative and Physiological Psychology, 94*, 962–969.

McLaren, I. P. L., & Mackintosh, N. J. (2000). An elemental model of associative learning: I. Latent inhibition and perceptual learning. *Animal Learning and Behavior, 28*, 211–246.

McMurtry, C. M., Noel, M., Taddio, A., Antony, M. M., Asmundson, G. J., Riddell, R. P., . . . HELPinKids & Adults Team. (2015). Interventions for individuals with high levels of needle fear: Systematic review of randomized controlled trials and quasi-randomized controlled trials. *Clinical Journal of Pain, 31*(10, Suppl.), S109–S123.

Mineka, S. (1979). The role of fear in theories of avoidance learning, flooding, and extinction. *Psychological Bulletin, 86*, 985–1010.

Mineka, S., & Zinbarg, R. (2006). A contemporary learning theory perspective on the etiology of anxiety disorders: It's not what you thought it was. *American Psychologist, 61*(1), 10–26.

Öhman, A., & Soares, J. J. (1994). "Unconscious anxiety": Phobic responses to masked stimuli. *Journal of Abnormal Psychology, 103*(2), 231–240.

Ostlund, S. B., & Marshall, A. T. (2021). Probing the role of reward expectancy in Pavlovian-instrumental transfer. *Current Opinion in Behavioral Sciences, 41*, 106–113.

Overton, D. A. (1966). State-dependent learning produced by depressant and atropine-like drugs. *Psychopharmacologia, 10*(1), 6–31.

Overton, D. A. (1991). Historical context of state dependent learning and discriminative drug effects. *Behavioural Pharmacology, 2*(4), 253–264.

Pavlov, I. P. (1927). *Conditioned reflexes: An investigation of the physiological activity of the cerebral cortex* (G. V. Anrep, Trans.). Oxford University Press.

Pearce, J. M., & Hall, G. (1980). A model for Pavlovian learning: Variations in the effectiveness of conditioned but not of unconditioned stimuli. *Psychological Review, 87*, 532–552.

Pearce, J. M., & Mackintosh, N. J. (2010). Two theories of attention: A review and a possible integration. In C. J. Mitchell & M. E. Le Pelley (Eds.), *Attention and associative learning: From brain to behaviour* (pp. 11–40). Oxford University Press.

Piazza, C. C., Patel, M. R., Gulotta, C. S., Sevin, B. M., & Layer, S. A. (2003). On the relative contributions of positive reinforcement and escape extinction in the treatment of food refusal. *Journal of Applied Behavior Analysis, 36*(3), 309–324.

Post, R. M., Lockfeld, A., Squillace, K. M., & Contel, N. R. (1981). Drug–environment interaction: Context dependency of cocaine-induced behavioral sensitization. *Life Sciences, 28*(7), 755–760.

Quail, S. L., Laurent, V., & Balleine, B. W. (2017). Inhibitory Pavlovian–instrumental transfer in humans. *Journal of Experimental Psychology: Animal Learning and Cognition, 43*, 315–324.

Randich, A., & LoLordo, V. M. (1979). Associative and nonassociative theories of the UCS preexposure phenomenon: Implications for Pavlovian conditioning. *Psychological Bulletin, 86*(3), 523–548.

Rescorla, R. A. (1968). Probability of shock in the presence and absence of CS in fear conditioning. *Journal of Comparative and Physiological Psychology, 66*, 1–5.

Rescorla, R. A. (1969). Pavlovian conditioned inhibition. *Psychological Bulletin, 72*(2), 77–94.

Rescorla, R. A. (1986). Facilitation and excitation. *Journal of Experimental Psychology: Animal Behavior Processes, 12*(4), 325–332.

Rescorla, R. A. (1987). Facilitation and inhibition. *Journal of Experimental Psychology: Animal Behavior Processes, 13*(3), 250–259.

Rescorla, R. A. (1988). Pavlovian conditioning: It's not what you think it is. *American Psychologist, 43*, 151–160.

Rescorla, R. A. (2004). Spontaneous recovery. *Learning and Memory, 11*, 501–509.

Rescorla, R. A., & Holland, P. C. (1982). Behavioral studies of associative learning in animals. *Annual Review of Psychology, 33*, 265–308.

Rescorla, R. A., & Solomon, R. L. (1967). Two-process learning theory: Relationships between Pavlovian conditioning and instrumental learning. *Psychological Review, 74*, 151–182.

Rescorla, R. A., & Wagner, A. R. (1972). A theory of Pavlovian conditioning: Variations in the effectiveness of reinforcement and nonreinforcement. In A. H. Black & W. F. Prokasy (Eds.), *Classical conditioning: II. Current theory and research* (pp. 64–99). Appleton-Century-Crofts.

Rizley, R. C., & Rescorla, R. A. (1972). Associations in second-order conditioning and sensory preconditioning. *Journal of Comparative and Physiological Psychology, 81*(1), 1–11.

Robinson, M. J. F., & Berridge, K. C. (2013). Instant transformation of learned repulsion into motivational "wanting." *Current Biology, 23*, 282–289.

Ross, R. T., & Holland, P. C. (1981). Conditioning of simultaneous and serial feature-positive discriminations. *Animal Learning and Behavior, 9*(3), 293–303.

Satel, S. L., Southwick, S. M., & Gawin, F. H. (1991). Clinical features of cocaine-induced paranoia. *American Journal of Psychiatry, 148*(4), 495–498.

Sato, M., Numachi, Y., & Hamamura, T. (1992). Relapse of paranoid psychotic state in methamphetamine model of schizophrenia. *Schizophrenia Bulletin, 18*(1), 115–122.

Scavio, M. J. (1974). Classical–classical transfer: Effects of prior aversive conditions upon appetitive conditioning in rabbits (*Oryctolagus cuniculus*). *Journal of Comparative and Physiological Psychology, 86*(1), 107–115.

Schepers, S. T., & Bouton, M. E. (2017). Hunger as a context: Food seeking that is inhibited during hunger can renew in the context of satiety. *Psychological Science, 28*(11), 1640–1648.

Schepers, S. T., & Bouton, M. E. (2019). Stress as a context: Stress causes relapse of inhibited food seeking if it has been associated with prior food seeking. *Appetite, 132*, 131–138.

Sclafani, A. (1997). Learned controls of ingestive behaviour. *Appetite, 29*, 153–158.

Seligman, M. E., & Maier, S. F. (1967). Failure to escape traumatic shock. *Journal of Experimental Psychology, 74*, 1–9.

Shabani, D. B., & Fisher, W. W. (2006). Stimulus fading and differential reinforcement for the treatment of needle phobia in a youth with autism. *Journal of Applied Behavior Analysis, 39*(4), 449–452.

Siegel, S. (1975). Evidence from rats that morphine tolerance is a learned response. *Journal of Comparative and Physiological Psychology, 89,* 498–506.

Siegel, S. (1999). Drug anticipation and drug addiction. The 1998 H. David Archibald lecture. *Addiction, 94,* 1113–1124.

Singh, N. N., & Solman, R. T. (1990). A stimulus control analysis of the picture-word problem in children who are mentally retarded: The blocking effect. *Journal of Applied Behavior Analysis, 23,* 525–532.

Skinner, B. F. (1938). *The behavior of organisms: An experimental analysis.* Appleton-Century.

Solomon, P. R, Vander Schaaf, E. R., Thompson, R. F., & Weisz, D. J. (1986). Hippocampus and trace conditioning of the rabbit's classically conditioned nictitating membrane response. *Behavioral Neuroscience, 100,* 729–744.

Soto, F. A., & Wasserman, E. A. (2010). Error-driven learning in visual categorization and object recognition: A common-elements model. *Psychological Review, 117*(2), 349–381.

Tait, R. W., & Saladin, M. E. (1986). Concurrent development of excitatory and inhibitory associations during backward conditioning. *Animal Learning and Behavior, 14,* 133–137.

Taylor, J. A. (1956). Level of conditioning and intensity of the adaptation stimulus. *Journal of Experimental Psychology, 51*(2), 127–130.

Thorndike, E. L. (1911). *Animal intelligence.* Macmillan.

Thrailkill, E. A. (2023). Partial reinforcement extinction and omission effects in the elimination and recovery of discriminated operant behavior. *Journal of Experimental Psychology: Animal Learning and Cognition.* [Epub ahead of print]

Thrailkill, E. A., Ameden, W. C., & Bouton, M. E. (2019). Resurgence in humans: Reducing relapse by increasing generalization between treatment and testing. *Journal of Experimental Psychology: Animal Learning and Cognition, 45*(3), 338–349.

Thrailkill, E. A., & Bouton, M. E. (2015). Contextual control of instrumental actions and habits. *Journal of Experimental Psychology: Animal Learning and Cognition, 41*(1), 69–80.

Thrailkill, E. A., Michaud, N. L., & Bouton, M. E. (2021). Reinforcer predictability and stimulus salience promote discriminated habit learning. *Journal of Experimental Psychology: Animal Learning and Cognition, 47*(2), 183–199.

Thrailkill, E. A., Todd, T. P., & Bouton, M. E. (2020). Effects of conditioned stimulus (CS) duration, intertrial interval, and I/T ratio on appetitive Pavlovian conditioning. *Journal of Experimental Psychology: Animal Learning and Cognition, 46*(3), 243–255.

Thrailkill, E. A., Trask, S., Vidal, P., Alcalá, J. A., & Bouton, M. E. (2018). Stimulus control of actions and habits: A role for reinforcer predictability and attention in the development of habitual behavior. *Journal of Experimental Psychology: Animal Learning and Cognition, 44*(4), 370–384.

Timberlake, W. (1994). Behavior systems, associationism, and Pavlovian conditioning. *Psychonomic Bulletin and Review, 1,* 405–420.

Trask, S. (2019). Cues associated with alternative reinforcement during extinction can attenuate resurgence of an extinguished instrumental response. *Learning and Behavior, 47*(1), 66–79.

Trask, S., Thrailkill, E. A., & Bouton, M. E. (2017). Occasion setting, inhibition, and the contextual control of extinction in Pavlovian and instrumental (operant) learning. *Behavioural Processes, 137,* 64–72.

Ujike, H., & Sato, M. (2004). Clinical features of sensitization to methamphetamine observed in patients with methamphetamine dependence and psychosis. *Annals of the New York Academy of Sciences, 1025,* 279–287.

van Ens, W., Schmidt, U., Campbell, I. C., Roefs, A., & Werthmann, J. (2019). Test–retest reliability of attention bias for food: Robust eye-tracking and reaction time indices. *Appetite, 136,* 86–92.

Vervliet, B., Craske, M. G., & Hermans, D. (2013). Fear extinction and relapse: State of the art. *Annual Review of Clinical Psychology, 9,* 215–248.

Wagner, A. R. (1976). Priming in STM: An information-processing mechanism for self-generated or retrieval-generated depression in performance. In T. J. Tighe & R. N. Leaton (Eds.), *Habituation: Perspectives from child development, animal behavior, and neuropsychology* (pp. 95–128). Erlbaum.

Wagner, A. R. (1981). SOP: A model of automatic memory processing in animal behavior. In N. E. Spear & R. R. Miller (Eds.), *Information processing in animals: Memory mechanisms* (pp. 5–47). Erlbaum.

Wagner, A. R., Logan, F. A., Haberlandt, K., & Price, T. (1968). Stimulus selection in animal discrimination learning. *Journal of Experimental Psychology, 76*, 171–180.

Wagner, A. R., & Rescorla, R. A. (1972). Inhibition in Pavlovian conditioning: Application of a theory. In R. A. Boakes & S. Halliday (Eds.), *Inhibition in learning* (pp. 301–336). Academic Press.

Wagner, A. R., & Terry, W. S. (1975). Backward conditioning to a CS following an expected vs. a surprising UCS. *Animal Learning and Behavior, 3*, 370–374.

Watson, P., Pearson, D., Most, S. B., Theeuwes, J., Wiers, R. W., & Le Pelley, M. E. (2019). Attentional capture by Pavlovian reward-signaling distractors in visual search persists when rewards are removed. *PLOS One, 14*(12), Article e0226284.

Watson, P., Wiers, R. W., Hommel, B., & de Wit, S. (2014). Working for food you don't desire: Cues interfere with goal-directed food-seeking. *Appetite, 79*, 139–148.

Williams, D. R., & Williams, H. (1969). Automaintenance in the pigeon: Sustained pecking despite contingent non-reinforcement. *Journal of the Experimental Analysis of Behavior, 12*, 511–520.

Wolpe, J. (1954). Reciprocal inhibition as the main basis of psychotherapeutic effects. *Archives of Neurology and Psychiatry, 72*(2), 205–226.

CHAPTER 7

Stimulus Selection and Stimulus Competition

Martha Escobar
Zebulon K. Bell
Francisco Arcediano

A few years ago, the neighbors of one of us (M. E.) decided to foster two dogs: A large, short-coated dog, and a small, curly-haired dog. Their daughter, who was not very familiar with dogs, entered the house loudly, startling the dogs, which snapped at her in what could have been a terrible outcome had the parents not intervened on time. Although the girl sustained no injuries, she became terrified of the foster dogs, who had to be removed from the home. In this situation, the dogs became a stimulus that controlled a fear response. Many emotional responses are acquired in this manner: A previously neutral stimulus (in this case, the dogs) comes to be associated with an emotion-inducing stimulus (in this case, the dog's aggressive behavior), and the stimulus comes to elicit the emotional response (fear). Typically, we state that the neutral stimulus has become *conditioned* and, thus, the fear it produces is a *conditioned fear response* (cf. Pavlov, 1927). We refer to the stimulus that comes to trigger the conditioned response (the dogs) as the *conditioned stimulus* (CS), the stimulus that naturally elicits a response (the dog's aggressive behavior) as the *unconditioned stimulus*, and the emotional response that comes to be elicited by the CS (fear) as the *conditioned response*.

The conditioned fear response that the girl in this example developed was actually more complex than her being afraid of her foster dogs. The girl was afraid of not only the dogs that attacked her but also other, large, short-coated dogs, regardless of breed or color; that is, the fear response was not *specific* to the stimuli that were part of the learning episode, but *generalized* to other, similar stimuli. The girl also displayed significantly less fear of small, curly-coated dogs than she did of large short-coated dogs. This reflected not only a *discrimination* among the two dog stimuli based on their physical features but also a *stimulus competition* effect: The more salient stimulus (the larger dog) was more effective in controlling behavior than the less salient stimulus (the smaller dog), despite both dogs having been involved in the learning episode.

This situation exemplifies the complexities we encounter when determining which stimulus or stimuli control behavior, and the somewhat paradoxical observations that, in some instances, behavioral control by a given stimulus seems to fail. We begin by discussing how conditioned responses are determined by the similarity between the stimuli encountered in a given situation and the stimuli that were present during training (i.e., generalization vs. discrimination), how stimuli are selected from the environment and interact to determine behavioral control (i.e., *stimulus competition effects*), and the extent to which these effects are conditional on the acquisition and retrieval conditions (*specificity effects*). We use classical conditioning as a framework, and provide links and extensions between this basic research and applied situations.[1]

What Comes to Control Behavior?: Stimulus Generalization and Discrimination

The situation described at the beginning of this chapter presents examples of both *stimulus generalization*, the observation that the response elicited by a given stimulus is directly proportional to its similarity to the training stimulus, and *stimulus discrimination*, the observation that the response elicited by a given stimulus is inversely proportional to its dissimilarity to the training stimulus. Simply put, stimuli that are similar to the training stimulus will also elicit the response, whereas stimuli that are very different from the training stimulus will not. Generalization and discrimination are usually related to the physical properties of the stimulus in a single dimension (e.g., frequencies or wavelengths can be close to each other or far away from each other in the spectrum). However, generalization and discrimination can be changed through training.

Stimulus discrimination training (e.g., Ginat-Frolich et al., 2017; Shechner et al., 2015) can be used to get an organism to respond to a target stimulus but not to similar stimuli. A standard stimulus discrimination training preparation involves the reinforcement of behavior in the presence of one stimulus (the discriminative stimulus, S^D), but not in the presence of another stimulus (S^Δ). Stimulus discrimination training seems also to lead to learning of the relative, as opposed to the absolute, value of stimuli. Kohler (1918/1938) reinforced chickens for pecking a light gray stimulus (S^D), but not a dark gray stimulus (S^Δ). After the discrimination was acquired, chickens were offered a choice between the original light gray stimulus and a new, even lighter gray stimulus. The chickens (as well as apes in a later study) responded to the new, lighter gray stimulus in over 70% of trials, suggesting that subjects preferred to select the "relationally correct" stimulus. Kohler called this concept in relational learning "transposition," suggesting that the relation between stimuli holds regardless of where the stimulus is moved along a gradient (e.g., wavelength of visible light; Lazareva, 2012). The counterpart of stimulus discrimination training, *stimulus equivalence training*, is used to increase stimulus generalization across a broad array of similar stimuli. To accomplish this goal, two different stimuli receive equivalent training, either by pairing them with a common outcome or by requiring a common response (Delius et al., 2000; Honey & Hall, 1989; Rehfeldt, 2011).

Sidman (1994) suggested that stimulus equivalence training can lead to the development of *equivalence classes*, which may in turn lead to the occurrence of *emergent*

---

[1] Although we use classical conditioning principles when referring to associative learning, the principles we describe can easily be applied to operant conditioning situations.

relations (behavior control by relations that have not been explicitly trained). For example, if training occurs with three stimuli, A, B, and C, these three stimuli would be considered to be within an equivalence class if they exhibit the logical relationships of *reflexivity* (also known as *sameness*, A = A, B = B, and C = C), *symmetry* (if A leads to B, then B leads to A), and *transitivity* (if A leads to B and A leads to C, then B should lead to C). Equivalence classes can lead to emergent relations, in which relationships that have not been explicitly trained (e.g., B leads to C in the previous example) can develop and control behavior.

Elemental and Configural Perception

The example at the beginning of the chapter suggests that the girl became afraid of one of the dogs that attacked her, but not both. Thus, one may wonder what exactly elicited her fear response. Was it the size, coat, or color of the dog? Maybe it was the way the dog moved, or the shape of its snout? Or maybe it was the smell of the dog? Although we usually talk about complex stimuli (like a dog) as a unitary entity, the reality is that behavior can come under the control of any feature (or many features) of a stimulus. In the laboratory, this question can be studied by creating complex stimuli and analyzing the specific features of that complex stimulus that come to control behavior. In a classic study, Reynolds (1961) tried to determine which aspects of a complex visual stimulus would control the pecking response of pigeons. Pigeons tend to "peck" (hit with their beak) stimuli that have become associated with food outcomes. Reynolds trained pigeons to peck an illuminated key that featured a white triangle superimposed onto a red background. Pigeons were rewarded when pecking at this particular compound visual stimulus, but they received no reward for pecking a key showing a white circle on a green background. At test, each feature of the training stimulus was presented separately; specifically, the pigeons were presented with an illuminated key showing either a white triangle or the key itself was illuminated red. Reynolds observed that each pigeon produced the response when presented with different features of the training stimulus: One pigeon responded more vigorously to the presence of the triangle (even without the red background), whereas the other pigeon responded more vigorously to a red illuminated key (even without the triangle).

Most learning theories (e.g., Miller & Matzel, 1988; Rescorla & Wagner, 1972) assume that subjects perceive stimuli elementally but, as mentioned earlier, the concept of "element" usually refers to a set of features. For example, we usually consider a sound to be an element, even though the sound itself is a compound of features (e.g., frequency, amplitude, timbre, location). Configural theories assume that all events that impinge on the senses at any given time are part of a configuration, and subjects come to discriminate among different configurations (e.g., Pearce, 1987, 1994). In this situation, behavioral control would be determined by the extent to which the stimulus presented is similar to the stimulus that was previously paired with the outcome (i.e., *generalization decrement*). Configural theories assume that each configuration comprises a large number of elements, a portion of which become activated with the stimulus presentation. The more times a stimulus is presented, the more likely it is that the same elements become activated and create strong associations between them and the outcome (e.g., Estes, 1950). Generalization, then, would be a direct function of the number of common elements that get activated when similar stimuli are presented, and discrimination would be an inverse function of this common activation (see Figure 7.1).

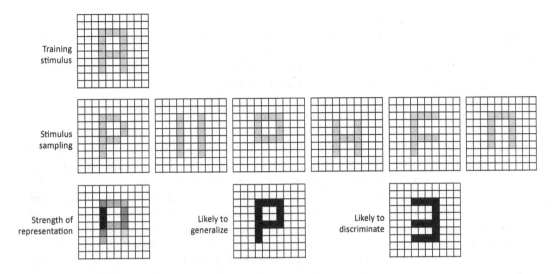

FIGURE 7.1. Representation of a stimulus sampling theory. When a stimulus is presented during training (*top panel*), a sample of its elements is activated each time the stimulus is presented. The *middle panel* presents the hypothetical stimulus sampling that may occur over six presentations of the stimulus (assuming that 75% of the stimulus elements are sampled in each presentation). Each element has a certain probability of being sampled in each presentation, and the strength of its association with the outcome is a direct function of the number of times it has been sampled across trials (*bottom panel*; darker shades represent stronger activation). Generalization is more likely to occur to stimuli that share elements with the elements that have been strongly associated with the outcome, and less likely to stimuli that share few of these elements (*bottom panel*).

Stimulus Generalization and Discrimination: Summary and Applications

After acquisition of an association, conditioned responding may generalize to other, similar stimuli, but not to other, dissimilar stimuli (discrimination). Generalization and discrimination can be enhanced via training, either by pairing different stimuli with different outcomes or responses (*discrimination training*) or with the same outcome or response (*equivalence training*). Equivalence training is essential to develop equivalence classes, in which a collection of stimuli can elicit the same behavior. Stimuli within an equivalence class exhibit the logical relationships of reflexivity (A = A), symmetry (if A → B, then B → A), and transitivity (if A → B and A → C, then B → C). Equivalence classes can lead to *emergent relations*, in which relationships that have not been explicitly trained (e.g., B → C in the previous example) can develop and control behavior. The development of equivalence classes is essential for language training. For example, a child learning to tact can be presented with a picture of a red apple and a cartoon drawing of a red apple, both associated with the word *apple*. The child should be able to pick the picture of a red apple from a field of choices if presented with the picture of a red apple (apple = apple), thus exhibiting *reflexivity*. If presented with the word *apple*, the child should be able to pick a picture of the red apple from a field of choices (*symmetry*; picture → word and word → picture). If the child is now presented with the picture of an apple associated with the word *fruit*, the child should pick the cartoon drawing of the red apple when presented with the word *fruit* (picture → cartoon, picture → word, word → cartoon; *transitivity*).

Note that the association between the word *fruit* and the cartoon was not trained, but emerged as a consequence of the development of an equivalence class (Sidman, 2009). Despite the essential role of equivalence classes for language acquisition, language abilities are not required to develop equivalence classes. Nonetheless, the capacity to add verbal labels to a class greatly facilitate the process of acquiring such equivalence classes (e.g., Miguel, 2018).

A common idiom is that a person "cannot see the forest for the trees," suggesting that someone focuses on the details rather than the big picture. We can use this saying as an analogy to the problem of what comes to control behavior: Stimuli may be perceived as a combination of details or features, such as shape, color, and size (in an *elemental* manner), or as a unitary event composed of a large number of features (in a *configural* manner). Determining whether subjects perceive the stimulus elementally or configurally may assist in determining whether behavior is controlled by an individual feature of the stimulus or the stimulus as a whole. For example, face processing (which includes the capacity to recognize and discriminate among faces) requires configural processing of the face; elemental processing, which focuses on individual features of the face, leads to difficulties with recognition and discrimination. Seemingly, neurotypical individuals use configural processing of face stimuli, whereas neuroatypical individuals use more local features to process faces, resulting in slower processing and difficulties with discrimination of face stimuli (e.g., Behrmann et al., 2006).

Stimuli Interact to Determine Behavioral Control: Stimulus Competition

At the beginning of the chapter, we described a situation in which a girl had been attacked by two dogs (a large, short-coated dog, and a small, curly-coated dog). Objectively, if both dogs came toward her, both dogs were part of the episode that resulted in her being afraid of dogs. However, she displayed significantly more fear toward large and short-coated dogs than toward small and curly-coated dogs. This outcome is surprising, because the two stimuli (the two dogs) share many elements in common and generalization should be expected. We should also expect some equivalence between the two stimuli, because they have been paired with various common outcomes (the category of "dog," the experience with the aggression, etc.). Thus, despite an experience that should lead to both stimuli having equivalent behavioral control, one of them fails to exert behavioral control. One possible explanation for this observation is that the larger dog is a more salient stimulus than the smaller dog, and this difference in salience resulted in the less salient stimulus failing to elicit a response; that is, the stimuli *competed* with each other for behavioral control.

Overshadowing

Most examples of conditioning involve a single stimulus paired with an outcome, but, in reality, multiple stimuli can precede the occurrence of an outcome. Consider the study by Reynolds (1961) described earlier, in which pigeons were trained to peck an illuminated key featuring a white triangle on a red background. At test, some pigeons pecked when presented with the white triangle, whereas others pecked when presented with a red key. Thus, the stimulus that was most salient for each subject (either the white triangle or the red key) came to control behavior despite both features having the same contingency with the outcome. In other words, the more salient feature *overshadowed* the less salient feature. The typical overshadowing preparation is presented in Figure 7.2A. In the overshadowing paradigm, two stimuli are presented simultaneously and paired with an outcome, resulting in less responding to the less salient stimulus than to the more salient stimulus (i.e., the less salient stimulus is overshadowed by the more salient, overshadowing, stimulus). Importantly, the overshadowed stimulus is salient enough to support behavioral control if paired with the outcome by itself; that is, overshadowing is not simply due to the subject failing to perceive the overshadowed stimulus (comparison condition, Figure 7.2A).

What makes a stimulus more salient than other stimuli? In most cases, the intensity of the stimulus is equated to saliency, such that a brighter light is more salient than a

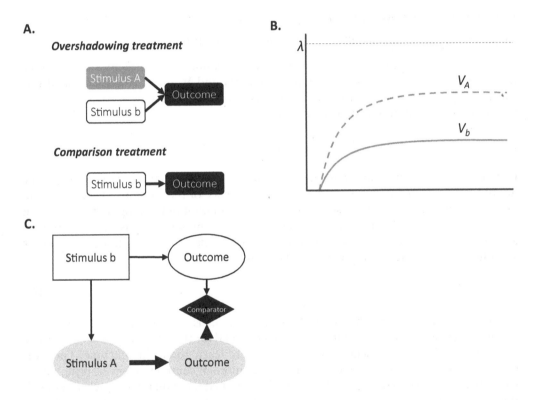

FIGURE 7.2. (A) Schematic representation of the overshadowing treatment and a typical comparison treatment. The overshadowing stimulus, b, is of lower salience than the overshadowing stimulus, A. As a consequence of the compound training, Stimulus b exhibits less behavioral control in the overshadowing than the comparison group. (B) Representation of overshadowing using Rescorla and Wagner's (1972) model. For this simulation, α_A was set to a value double that of α_b. Due to its larger salience (α), Stimulus A acquires most of the available associative strength (V). (C) Representation of overshadowing using the comparator model of Miller and Mazel (1988). Presentation of Stimulus b activates memories of its associates, the outcome and Stimulus A. In turn, Stimulus A activates a memory of the outcome. The strength of the memory of the outcome activated through A (which has a strength equal to the product of the strength with which Stimulus b activates Stimulus A and the strength with which Stimulus A activates the outcome) is larger than that activated directly by Stimulus b, reducing behavioral control by Stimulus b.

dimmer light, and a louder sound is more salient than a softer sound. Stimulus intensity is known to favor behavioral control by the more salient stimulus to the detriment of behavioral control by less salient stimuli (e.g., Mackintosh, 1976). Salience can also be related to the discrete properties of the stimulus, such that stimuli that are constantly present over time tend to be of lower salience than stimuli that have a discrete onset and offset (Odling-Smee, 1978). Stimuli that extend over time are known as *contextual stimuli*, and they may lose salience or relevance as predictors of changes in the environment (e.g., delivery of outcomes). Stimuli of equivalent salience can also exert *reciprocal overshadowing*, a situation in which responding to both members of the compound is decreased relative to control groups in which the stimuli are trained separately (Arcediano et al., 2004; March et al., 1992).

Why Does Overshadowing Occur?

OVERSHADOWING AS A FAILURE TO ACQUIRE AN ASSOCIATION

Some theorists suggest that overshadowing reflects a failure to acquire information about the overshadowed stimulus. For example, Rescorla and Wagner (1972) suggested that learning is a function of salience and the extent to which the outcome is already predicted by the stimuli that antecede it, as predicted by

$$\Delta V^n = \alpha \cdot \beta \cdot (\lambda - \Sigma V^{n-1}) \tag{7.1}$$

in which ΔV^n represents the change in the strength of the association between the stimulus and the outcome in trial n, α represents the salience of the stimulus, β represents the salience of the outcome, λ represents the maximum amount of learning that the outcome can support (i.e., the learning asymptote), and ΣV^{n-1} represents the associative strength at trial $n - 1$ of all stimuli presented in trial n. The strength of association between each stimulus and outcome would then be updated using

$$V^n = V^{n-1} + \Delta V^n \tag{7.2}$$

In very simple terms, the more times the stimulus is paired with the outcome, the larger the strength of the association between them (V for that stimulus). The parenthetical term, $(\lambda - \Sigma V^{n-1})$ represents how much is left to learn about the outcome: The more times the stimulus and outcome are paired, the more V subtracts from λ, bringing the parenthetical term closer to zero. The formula is applied individually for each stimulus in the compound. For example, a child goes into the pediatric clinic and a nurse in a white coat and wearing vinyl gloves gives the child a shot. The observation is that, in future visits, the child begins to cry when nurses wearing a white coat enter the examination room, but not when the pediatrician wearing street clothes and vinyl gloves enters the examination room. This outcome suggests that the stimulus "gloves" acquired less behavioral control than the stimulus "white coat." The Rescorla–Wagner model would assume that the less salient stimulus (the gloves) would have a lower salience than the white coat.[2]

---

[2]Note that in complex situations, it is possible for the salience of a given feature be different for different subjects, or for features reciprocally to overshadow each other.

That is, α_{gloves} would be lower than α_{coat}. Because the values for β and λ remain the same, ΔV^n_{gloves} would be lower than ΔV^n_{coat}. Furthermore, because the term ΣV^{n-1} reflects the sum of V^n_{gloves} and V^n_{coat}, the learning asymptote would be acquired soon and there would be little opportunity for the subject to acquire much information about the gloves stimulus. This type of approach is simple: The lack of behavioral control by the overshadowed stimulus reflects a failure to acquire information about it (see Figure 7.2B).

Despite the great success of models such as that of Rescorla and Wagner (1972) in explaining overshadowing, there are situations that suggest overshadowing reflects processes other than the failure to learn the relationship between the overshadowed stimulus and the outcome. For example, overshadowing can occur in as little as one trial (Haesen et al., 2017; James & Wagner, 1980; Mackintosh & Reese, 1979). In order for an explanation such as that of Rescorla and Wagner (1972) to be applicable, the compound must be presented at least twice: In in the first trial, ΣV^{n-1} is zero, because both the overshadowing and overshadowed stimuli are neutral; thus, the overshadowed stimulus should acquire the same association to the outcome whether it is presented in compound or by itself. Overshadowing would develop after the two (overshadowing and overshadowed) stimuli have acquired associative strength (i.e., in the second trial), because ΣV^{n-1} would be much larger in the group in which the overshadowed stimulus is trained in compound than in the group in which it is trained alone. This failure of the model can be overcome if instead of focusing solely on salience and predictability of the outcome, we focus on the allocation of attentional resources to the stimulus. If the more salient stimulus commands most of the subject's attention, little attention can be devoted to the less salient stimulus, and if learning is a function of attention to the stimulus, overshadowing should be observed, even with a single trial (e.g., Kruschke, 2005; Mackintosh, 1975). Some other authors have suggested that attenuated behavior control by the overshadowed stimulus may reflect a failure to generalize from the compound to the test stimulus; that is, subjects may view the compound as a single, complex stimulus (a so-called "configuration"), and respond in proportion to how similar the test stimulus is to the configural stimulus (e.g., Pearce, 1987, 1994). Salience should increase the generalization between the compound and the stimulus, resulting in the more salient stimulus commanding more behavioral control than the less salient stimulus.

OVERSHADOWING AS A FAILURE TO RETRIEVE AN ASSOCIATION

If overshadowing reflects the failure to acquire an association between the overshadowed stimulus and the outcome, the overshadowed stimulus should not acquire behavioral control if it is trained in compound with the overshadowing stimulus. However, there is evidence that the association between the overshadowed stimulus and the outcome is acquired, albeit at a slower rate than the association between the overshadowing stimulus and the outcome. For example, if the number of training trials is extended well beyond the point at which behavioral control by the overshadowing stimulus is observed, the overshadowed stimulus exhibits unimpaired behavioral control. Stout et al. (2003; also see Azorlosa & Cicala, 1988) reported overshadowing of a mild auditory stimulus by a more salient auditory stimulus if the compound was paired with a mild electrical stimulus four times, but this overshadowing dissipated if the compound was paired with the outcome 36 times. Behavioral control by the overshadowed stimulus can also be "uncovered" through manipulations that do not involve further training with the overshadowed stimulus. If time lapses between overshadowing training and assessment of behavioral control, the common observation is that responding to the overshadowed stimulus "spontaneously recovers" (Kraemer et al., 1988). Manipulations of the association between the overshadowing stimulus and the outcome can also change behavioral control by the overshadowed stimulus. Kaufman and Bolles (1981) trained rats with a compound of a mild noise and a bright light, and observed attenuated behavioral control by the noise (as compared to a group in which the noise had been presented alone). Subsequently, they presented the light repeatedly, until behavioral control by the light ceased (i.e., extinction; cf. Pavlov, 1927). When the noise was retested, it was observed to control behavior just as well as in the group in which the tone had been trained alone (also see De Houwer & Beckers, 2002; Matzel et al., 1985; Wasserman & Berglan, 1998).

If behavioral control by the overshadowed stimulus can be reestablished without providing further pairings with the outcome, learning about its predictive value must have occurred during the compound training trials; that is, the failure to observe behavioral control by the overshadowed stimulus must reflect not a failure to *acquire* the association, but a failure to *retrieve* the association. Models based on memory competition are well suited to explain why responding to the overshadowed stimulus can reoccur. Miller and Matzel (1988; also see Denniston et al., 2001; Stout & Miller, 2007) proposed a retrieval model in which all stimuli acquire associations to each other and the outcome with which they were paired but compete for behavioral control at the time of memory retrieval. Figure 7.2C presents a schematic representation of this *comparator hypothesis*. Consider again the example in which a child receives a painful shot from a nurse wearing a white coat and vinyl gloves, with the coat coming to control the fear response more effectively than the vinyl gloves. In this case, the model assumes that both the overshadowing (coat) and overshadowed (gloves) stimuli become associated with the outcome of pain and have the *potential* of eliciting the fear response. However, because the salience of the coat is greater than the salience of the gloves, the strength of association between the coat and the outcome is also greater than the strength of association between the gloves and the outcome. At the moment of retrieval (i.e., when the child is presented with gloves), the strength with which the gloves activate a memory of the outcome is compared to the strength with which stimuli that also have an association to the gloves (in this case, the coat) also activate a memory of the outcome. If the gloves more effectively activate a memory of the outcome than its comparator stimuli, then a response will be observed. If, in contrast, the comparator stimuli more effectively activate a memory of the outcome, then a response will not be observed (Figure 7.2C). In this model, manipulating the strength of association between the target stimulus (the gloves) and its comparator stimuli (the coat) or the strength of association between the comparator stimuli and the outcome can change the extent to which the gloves can elicit a response. This is because these associations can change how effectively the comparator stimulus activates the memory of the outcome, Thus, extinction of the overshadowing stimulus (i.e., presenting the overshadowing stimulus alone and without the outcome), which results in a decrease in the strength of both the overshadowed–overshadowing stimuli and overshadowing stimulus–outcome associations, should increase responding to the overshadowed stimulus.[3]

---

[3] Modifications to the Rescorla and Wagner (1972) model have been proposed to account for recovery from overshadowing (e.g., Van Hamme & Wasserman, 1994; for discussion, see Witnauer et al., 2018).

Blocking

Imagine a situation in which the caretaker of a preverbal child points to two signs, each containing a picture, one of an open left hand with the palm facing up and the fingers of a right hand approaching the palm (let's call this sign "plate"), and another picture of a face and the right hand bringing the fingers close to the mouth (let's call this sign "eat"). Pointing at the pictures is followed by the child getting a snack, to which the child responds with obvious excitement. On a subsequent day, the signs are separated, the child is presented only with the "eat" sign, and responds very excitedly. Now, imagine that a different caretaker presents a different child with the "plate" sign prior to providing the snack. At some point, the caretaker begins presenting both the "plate" and the "eat" signs prior to providing the snack. Then, she is asked to use only the "eat" sign but, when she presents it to the child, the child shows no excitement and acts as if no snack was anticipated. Note that, in both situations, the "eat" sign has the same relationship to the snack outcome. However, in the second case, the child had prior experience with the "plate" sign, and this prior experience seems to have *blocked* behavioral control by the "eat" sign.

First described by Kamin (1969), blocking occurs when a novel stimulus (in the previous example, the "eat" sign) is paired with the outcome in the presence of reliable predictor of the outcome (in the previous example, the "plate" sign). The consequence is reduced behavioral control by the *blocked* stimulus due to it having been trained in the presence of the *blocking* stimulus (Figure 7.3A). The phenomenon of blocking suggests that learning is a function of the extent to which a stimulus can predict the outcome: There should be no learning to a stimulus that does not predict a change in the subsequent event; that is, learning depends on the extent to which an outcome is *surprising* and, if the extent to which the outcome is not yet predicted is considered to be "error," then each learning trial represents an error correction (e.g., Rescorla & Wagner, 1972). Blocking has been reported in many species and with a variety of preparations (Prados et al., 2013). In humans, blocking has usually been reported in causal-inference tasks, in which participants are asked to rate the likelihood of occurrence of an outcome given a particular cause or predictor (Dickinson & Burke, 1996; Jones et al., 2019; Le Pelley et al., 2005; Wasserman & Berglan, 1998). There are also analogues to animal procedures that record behavioral responses to assess the development of blocking (e.g., Arcediano et al., 2001), as well as examples of blocking among social stimuli (e.g., Sanbonmatsu et al., 1994) suggesting that the blocking effect is somewhat general across different learning domains (but see further discussion below).

Why Does Blocking Occur?

BLOCKING AS A FAILURE TO ACQUIRE AN ASSOCIATION

Consider the Rescorla–Wagner equation (7.1). The parenthetical term, $(\lambda - \Sigma V^{n-1})$ represents the discrepancy between what can be learned about the outcome (λ) and what is known about the outcome given the stimuli that are present on a given trial (ΣV^{n-1}). Thus, the parenthetical term represents the extent to which the outcome is "surprising" and, as learning progresses and ΣV^{n-1} becomes larger, there is less of the outcome left to predict (the outcome is no longer surprising). In the case of blocking, the initial learning about the blocking stimulus as a predictor of the outcome leads to its associative strength

A.

Blocking treatment

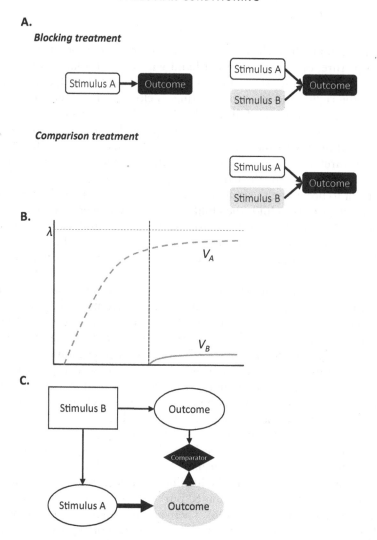

Comparison treatment

B.

C.

FIGURE 7.3. (A) Schematic representation of the blocking treatment and a possible comparison treatment (other comparison treatments include presentations of Stimulus A alone, unpaired presentations of Stimulus A and the outcome, or pairings of an irrelevant stimulus, C, and the outcome). The blocking stimulus, A, is becomes a reliable predictor of the outcome in the first stage of training. When Stimulus B is introduced, it does not provide new information about the outcome and subsequently exhibits less behavioral control than in the comparison group. (B) Representation of blocking using Rescorla and Wagner's (1972) model. For this simulation, $\alpha_A = \alpha_B$. The vertical, dotted, line divides the treatment phases. During Phase 1, Stimulus A acquires most of the available associative strength and, in Phase 2, there is little associative strength for Stimulus B to acquire. (C) Representation of blocking using the comparator model of Miller and Mazel (1988). Presentation of Stimulus B activates memories of its associates, the outcome and Stimulus A. In turn, Stimulus A activates a memory of the outcome. The strength of the memory of the outcome activated through A (which has a strength equal to the product of the strength with which Stimulus B activates Stimulus A and the strength with which Stimulus A activates the outcome) is larger than that activated directly by Stimulus B, reducing behavioral control by Stimulus B.

($V_{blocking}$) growing large. When the blocked stimulus is introduced, the value of ΣV^{n-1} reflects the current value of $V_{blocking}$; because this value is large, the "surprise" value of the outcome is very low, and little can be learned about the blocked stimulus (Figure 7.3B). There is experimental support for the idea that blocking is related to a lack of a surprising outcome, as changes in the outcome (e.g., adding a second outcome or changing the intensity of the outcome) can increase behavioral control by the blocked stimulus (e.g., Mackintosh et al., 1980).

As is the case with overshadowing, blocking has also been explained in terms of attentional mechanisms: If the blocking stimulus, which has been previously paired with the outcome, commands most of the available attentional resources, a failure to shift attention to the (redundant) blocked stimulus can result in the blocking effect (Kruschke, 2005).

BLOCKING AS A FAILURE TO RETRIEVE AN ASSOCIATION

Despite the success of acquisition models such as that of Rescorla and Wagner (1972) in explaining blocking, they can do so only if there is more than one pairing of the blocking–blocked stimulus compound and the outcome, and blocking has been observed after a single compound trial (e.g., Balaz et al., 1982; Mackintosh et al., 1980). Blocking can also dissipate under certain circumstances. Behavioral control by the blocked stimulus can "spontaneously recover" if time is allowed to elapse between blocking training and testing (e.g., Pineño et al., 2005), or dissipate if reminder cues that were present during blocking training (the blocked stimulus, the blocking stimulus, or the outcome) are presented prior to testing (e.g., Balaz et al., 1982). As is the case with overshadowing, manipulating the association between the blocking stimulus and the outcome can reestablish behavioral control by the blocked stimulus. In a video-game-like preparation, Arcediano et al. (2001) asked participants to move a figure around a jail-like room that they could escape by pressing on a lever. Pressing on the lever lifted the bars that were blocking the escape route. Colored panels on the walls (the conditioned stimuli) signaled an imminent "shock" that lowered the bars to the escape route (the unconditioned stimulus) unless they moved the figure to a safe place. Thus, participants could be pressing the lever or running away to safety, which resulted in suppression of the lever-pressing response. With this task, Arcediano et al. observed not only blocking but also recovery from blocking if the blocking stimulus underwent extinction. Thus, as is the case with overshadowing, blocking does not seem to reflect a lack of learning about the relationship between the blocked stimulus and the outcome.

Memory retrieval models are well-suited to explain these recovery effects. Consider again the comparator model. Presentation of the blocked stimulus activates memories of stimuli that are associated with it, including the blocking stimulus and the outcome. Because the blocking stimulus already has a history of pairings with the outcome, it can more strongly activate the memory of the outcome than the blocked stimulus, and responding to the blocked stimulus is attenuated (Figure 7.3C). If the blocking stimulus undergoes extinction, it will activate the memory of the outcome less strongly than the blocked stimulus, and responding will be restored. Further support for memory retrieval models comes from the observation that behavioral control by the blocking stimulus is also attenuated due to its being paired with the blocked stimulus (Arcediano et al., 2004).

Other Forms of Stimulus Competition

Relative Stimulus Validity

Relative stimulus validity (Matute et al., 1996; Wagner et al., 1968) is a form of stimulus competition in which behavioral control by a stimulus is decreased due to it being paired with another stimulus that is more reliably paired with the same outcome. Imagine a situation in which two groups of participants are asked to rate the extent to which certain behaviors are predictive of contracting a virus. Group A learns that 100% of individuals who visited a grocery store and attended a concert contracted the virus, and 0% of individuals who visited a grocery store and a swimming pool contracted the virus. Group B learns that 50% of individuals who visited a grocery store and attended a concert contracted the virus, and 50% of individuals who visited a grocery store and a swimming pool contracted the virus. The usual observation would be that individuals in Group A would rate the relative risk of going to the grocery store as much lower than would individuals in Group B, despite the fact that the relationship between going to the grocery store and contracting the virus is the same in Groups A and B (50% of those visiting a grocery store contracted the virus); that is, the extent to which visiting a grocery store is rated as predictive of the outcome (contracting the virus) is relative to the validity of the stimuli that accompany it. In Group A, there is a stimulus that predicts the outcome 100% of the time (attending a concert) and a stimulus that predicts the outcome will occur 0% of the time (visiting a swimming pool), whereas both stimuli are equally predictive of the outcome and the absence of the outcome in Group B.

Overexpectation

What would happen if an outcome was independently predicted by two stimuli, A and B, and those two stimuli were presented together, followed by the outcome? Intuitively, we can assume the subject would expect double the outcome. But what if the outcome that follows the compound is the same that followed elements A and B? The usual observation is that behavioral control by stimuli A and B decreases, so that they control behavior fully when presented together, but only partially when presented apart (Rescorla, 1970). This is a surprising prediction of the Rescorla–Wagner (1972) model, which assumes that all outcomes have an asymptote for the associative value they can support (λ). If stimuli A and B have both been trained to asymptote (i.e., to a value close to λ), the parenthetical term in the equation, $(\lambda - \Sigma V^{n-1})$, is a negative value ($\Sigma V^{n-1} = V_A{}^{n-1} + V_B{}^{n-1} \approx 2\lambda$). Thus, pairings of the AB compound and the outcome will result in a loss, rather than a gain, of associative value to stimuli A and B (for more surprising predictions of the Rescorla–Wagner model, as well as an analysis of its failures, see R. R. Miller et al., 1995).

Does Stimulus Competition Always Occur?

Stimulus competition is at the core of the development of learning theory, and it is assumed that stimuli compete for behavioral control under most circumstances. However, one must note that stimulus competition effects can be difficult to obtain in the laboratory, and may be highly dependent on parameters. Maes et al. (2016) presented various failures to obtain the blocking effect, and questioned whether the effect was robust enough to be central to our understanding of stimulus interaction and the development of learning theories. Soto (2018; also see Urcelay, 2017) suggested that based on existing theories of learning, these failures can be expected, because all theories are parameter-dependent, and using theory to make predictions should lead to expectations of failure to obtain blocking under some circumstances (but see Maes et al., 2018).

The training procedures used to obtain overshadowing and blocking can also lead to enhanced, rather than impaired, responding to the potentially overshadowed and blocked stimuli. When the overshadowing procedure leads to enhanced responding to the to-be-overshadowed stimulus, we talk about *potentiation* (Clarke et al., 1979), and when the blocking procedure leads to enhanced responding to the to-be-blocked stimulus, we talk about *augmentation* (Batson & Batsell, 2000). Typically, these response-enhancement effects are observed among stimuli that have a close physiological connection, namely, taste stimuli and internal malaise outcomes, but sometimes they can be observed with nongustatory stimuli such as odors and environmental stimuli (J. S. Miller et al., 1995).

Competition Can Occur in the Absence of Compound Training

Typically, we think about stimulus competition occurring when two stimuli are trained together and predict a common outcome. However, stimuli can be trained apart to predict a common outcome, or the same stimulus can be trained to predict different outcomes. Consider, for example, the case of extinction (cf. Pavlov, 1927). In extinction, a stimulus that predicted an outcome is now trained to predict the absence of the outcome, and behavioral control by the stimulus decreases. In this situation, a common stimulus predicts two subsequent events (delivery and omission of the outcome). The situation can be reversed, and the stimulus could initially predict no outcome and then be trained to predict an outcome. In this situation, behavioral control by the stimulus slows in development, and *latent inhibition* (cf. Lubow & Moore, 1959) is said to occur (latent inhibition is also known as the *CS-preexposure effect,* because there is exposure to the stimulus prior to conditioning). Stimuli trained apart to predict a common outcome can also affect responding to each other (e.g., Amundson et al., 2003; Escobar et al., 2001b; González-Martín et al., 2012). Typically, these phenomena are explained in terms of memory interference, with the association most active at the moment of retrieval coming to control behavior at the expense of other associations that share a common term (Escobar et al., 2001a). Miller and Escobar (2002) suggested that all instances of competition, whether stimuli are or are not presented in compound, can be explained in terms of this type of interference. However, interference models may not be suitable to explain all instances of stimulus competition.

Context Dependence and Specificity

Escobar et al. (2003) presented human participants with a computer task in which the screen was divided into four quarters, each with a different background. Participants were asked to look at the screen, and block letters were presented in one or more of the quarters. In one condition, participants saw multiple presentations of one letter (Stimulus A) in one of the quarters and, suddenly, Stimulus A was followed by the outcome (a white cross). Participants were then asked to rate the likelihood with which the white cross would follow the presentation of Stimulus A, in comparison to a second stimulus (Stimulus B), which did not receive multiple exposures prior to the pairing with the white cross outcome. Participants rated Stimulus A to be a less reliable predictor of the outcome than Stimulus B; that is, they exhibited *latent inhibition*. In a second condition, Stimulus

A was repeatedly presented in one of the quarters, and then it was paired with the white cross outcome in a different quarter. Despite the total number of preexposures being the same, participants in the second condition exhibited less latent inhibition (i.e., they rated Stimulus A as a better predictor of the white cross outcome) than participants in the first condition. This exemplifies a key feature of interference effects: They are highly context-specific (Bouton, 1994, 2002, 2004).

Contexts can act as powerful retrieval cues, and they can serve as strong modulators of responding in situations in which there is ambiguity as to the predictive value of a stimulus (Bouton, 1994, 2002, 2004; Escobar et al., 2001b). In the case of latent inhibition and extinction, there are two conflicting associations: between the stimulus and the outcome and between the stimulus and the absence of the outcome. The context can help disambiguate which association should come to control behavior. If the subject is in the environment in which the stimulus–outcome association was acquired, behavioral control will be observed, whereas if the subject is in the environment in which the stimulus–no outcome association was acquired, little behavioral control will be observed.

What about situations in which competition occurs between stimuli that were trained in compound? In these situations, there is much less context specificity. The target stimulus (e.g., the overshadowed or blocked stimulus) is not ambiguous, but rather has less relative value as a predictor of the outcome. Thus, it is the value of its associated stimulus (e.g., the overshadowing or blocking stimulus) that determines whether the target stimulus will elicit a response and control behavior.

Stimulus Competition: Summary and Applications

Stimulus competition is observed in situations in which more than one stimulus can potentially come to control behavior. Whether it reflects failure to acquire all possible associations, or failure to retrieve a particular association, the common observation is that one stimulus tends to acquire behavioral control, whereas other stimuli do not. In some cases, stimulus competition is a matter of saliency. *Overshadowing* occurs when a more salient stimulus controls behavior, while other less salient (but also predictive) stimuli do not. In other cases, stimulus competition is a matter of predictability. *Blocking* occurs when there is a reliable predictor of the outcome; in this case, other, redundant, stimuli acquire little behavioral control. Other instances of stimulus competition may be related to the extent to which a stimulus predicts the outcome reliably (*relative validity*) or whether the outcome that occurs matches what is expected based on the stimulus training history (*overexpectation*).

Stimulus competition is a valuable behavioral adaptation: The strongest or more reliable predictor of an outcome comes to control behavior. However, sometimes its occurrence may hinder training of desired associations. For example, in some situations, instructional prompts (e.g., pictures) may delay acquisition of some responses (e.g., word reading). Dittlinger and Lerman (2011) presented children with cards that contained either a word alone, a picture alone, or both the word and a picture. The children were presented with the target stimulus and five distractor stimuli, and were tasked with touching the stimulus that corresponded to a spoken word. Acquisition of a response to the word was delayed whenever a picture was also presented, a result that the authors explained in terms of overshadowing of the word stimulus by the picture stimulus. Didden et al. (2000) used a similar procedure and observed that acquisition of a response to the word was more delayed when the word was presented with a "known" picture (a picture that was already associated to the spoken word) than an "unknown" picture, an observation that they attributed to blocking. Understanding that stimulus competition may be a factor in delayed acquisition of a response allows for correction strategies. For example, Singh and Solman (1990) observed that increasing the salience of the words by changing their position and size relative to the pictures decreased the potential negative impact of the pictures on acquisition of the response to the words. Figure 7.4 presents a schematic representation of the blocking and overshadowing procedures. Note that the two stimulus competition effects can co-occur; the blocking procedure involves compound training, and some overshadowing can co-occur (see Didden et al., 2000, for discussion).

Stimulus Selection and Competition in Autism Spectrum Disorders

Thus far in this chapter, we have focused on how the *experimental analysis of behavior* investigates and explains stimulus competition and selection effects. Although much has been said of the relationship between applied behavior analysis and the experimental analysis of behavior, we should also be concerned about the extent to which the divergence of the two fields can prevent extensions of laboratory research to applied practice (Marr, 2017; Rider, 1991). Laboratory and applied research have been fruitful and the divergence between the two has been regarded as an inevitable development of the disciplines; however, there are also many supporters of a unified study of behavior (Marr & Zilio, 2013). For the purposes of this chapter, we focus on stimulus competition effects

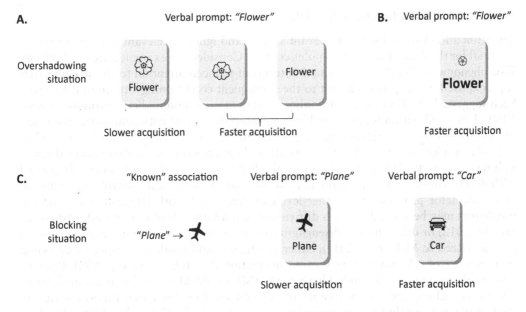

FIGURE 7.4. (A) Schematic representation of the overshadowing procedure. A response to the word stimulus is acquired slower when presented in compound with the picture stimulus than when it is presented on its own. (B) Increasing the salience of the word stimulus can decrease overshadowing. (C) Schematic representation of the blocking procedure. A response to the word stimulus is acquired slower when presented in compound with a picture that has already been associated to the verbal prompt than when the picture is not "known" prior to the compound training.

in individuals diagnosed with autism spectrum disorders (ASDs). Rather than a comprehensive review, we wish to highlight the connections between our current understanding of stimulus competition theory and observations in the ASD literature.

Generalization and Discrimination in ASD

Humans tend to resort to configural perception; this is what allows us to view objects holistically rather than as the sum of their parts. However, it has been proposed that individuals with ASD differ from neurotypical individuals on the central coherence of their cognitive system (Frith, 1989). Rather than a deficit in using the global aspects of a stimulus, it seems that this deficit stems from a bias to process information more locally, but this bias can be overcome under some conditions if attention is directed to the global features of the stimulus (Happé & Frith, 2006; Plaisted et al., 2003). A focus on local aspects of stimuli is more closely related to enhanced discrimination in individuals with ASD than in typically developing controls in both the visual (Litrownik et al., 1978) and auditory (O'Riordan & Passetti, 2006), but not the tactile (O'Riordan & Passetti, 2006) domains. Enhanced discrimination is accompanied by reduced generalization in ASD. This may make it difficult to generalize skills to similar situations, as the focus will be on small details of the antecedent stimuli. This difficulty with generalization may lead to issues with transferability of identical tasks to different materials, or in social situations in which complex stimuli have multiple elements that vary from situation to situation (e.g., determining a person's gender or emotions; Deruelle et al., 2008).

Attention and Stimulus Overselectivity

Attention allows us to focus on relevant stimuli and ignore irrelevant stimuli, a process essential for the development of stimulus control. Consider, for example, latent inhibition. This phenomenon has been explained in terms of reduced attention to the stimulus that is preexposed, making it irrelevant to the subsequent conditioning situation; it has even been suggested to reflect the conditioning of inattention to nonpredictive stimuli (Lubow, 1989). Latent inhibition is attenuated in individuals diagnosed with conditions that result in hyperattention (e.g., schizophrenia and attention deficit disorders) and enhanced in individuals with conditions known to result in hypoattention (e.g., Parkinson's disease; Lubow & Gewirtz, 1995). Remington et al. (2009) observed that individuals diagnosed with ASD exhibit greater perceptual capacity than neurotypical controls, engaging in more distractor processing at higher levels of perceptual load. Difficulties in ignoring distractors may be associated with difficulties in inhibiting distractor stimuli (Adams & Jarrold, 2012) or difficulties in disengaging attention from one stimulus and focusing on another (Reed & McCarthy, 2011), either of which would result in nonspecific encoding into memory of relevant and irrelevant information (Courchesne et al., 1994). It seems reasonable to assume that individuals with ASD would also exhibit attenuated latent inhibition, although we are not aware of any empirical evidence that this is the case in clinical populations (but for an animal model, see Kosaki & Watanabe, 2016). Toddlers with ASD show deficits in habituation to faces (Webb et al., 2010), suggesting that hyperattention may indeed reduce the inhibitory processes that aid stimulus selection.

Lovaas et al. (1966, 1971) first coined the term *stimulus overselectivity* to describe an individual's overselective attention to a restricted element or set of elements of an overall complex stimulus. Stimulus overselectivity can be conceptualized as too narrow a focus, a partial neglect of sensory inputs (in which detail-oriented focus detracts from perceiving the bigger picture), or a genuine issue with attention (Ploog, 2010). At the time, stimulus overselectivity was regarded as an attentional deficit, with a notable prevalence in individuals with ASD. In an adaptation of Reynolds's (1961) work on attention in the pigeon, Lovaas et al. (1971) presented participants with a compound stimulus comprising three elements (auditory, visual, and tactile elements), and later tested each of these elements in isolation to examine which element, if any, came to control behavior. Although all participants learned to respond to the compound, individuals with ASD tended to respond to only one element of the compound, children with developmental delay responded to two components, and neurotypical controls responded equally to all three components. Later studies have shown that stimulus overselectivity is not an exclusive cognitive trait of individuals with ASD; stimulus overselectivity has been observed across a variety of age ranges (Ploog, 2010). More recent studies suggest that stimulus overselectivity is equally likely to occur among individuals diagnosed with ASD and individuals diagnosed with other intellectual disabilities (Dube et al., 2016), and the prevalence of stimulus overselectivity in ASD is decreasing over time, potentially due to improvements in intervention techniques (Rieth et al., 2015).

Stimulus Competition in ASD

Individuals with ASD tend to show dysfunctions in associative memory (Southwick et al., 2011). Deficits in associative learning (e.g., fear conditioning) appear to be related to difficulties in gaining awareness of the stimulus–outcome contingency (Powell et al., 2016) and lower responsiveness to expectancy violations (the extent to which the outcome is surprising; Lawson et al., 2017).

Stimulus competition effects have been observed in individuals with ASD. Dittlinger and Lerman (2011) examined the observation that pictures may delay acquisition when teaching word recognition to children diagnosed with ASD. Participants learned target words more quickly when those words were presented alone than when they were paired with pictures, which is consistent with stimulus overshadowing. Their participants were also given trials in which words were presented alongside pictures that they could or could not identify prior to training (i.e., pictures that were relevant or irrelevant to the word item, respectively). Words presented together with irrelevant pictures were learned more quickly than words presented together with relevant pictures, which is consistent with a blocking effect.

Overshadowing and blocking have also been proposed as relevant mechanisms underlying prompt-fading procedures, which are used to encourage skill acquisition in individuals with developmental disabilities (Cengher et al., 2018). Prompts are supplemental stimuli that can evoke correct responding either by prompting the stimulus (emphasizing a feature of a stimulus; e.g., exaggerating the arm-up vs. arm-down features when discriminating between the letters *b* and *p*) or by prompting the response (evoking the correct response; e.g., pointing; Deitz & Malone, 1985). Either type of prompt is then faded as the contingency is acquired. Stimulus-prompting procedures appear to be more effective than response-prompting procedures, despite response-prompting actually emphasizing the correct response. Cengher et al. (2018) suggested that this difference in effectiveness of prompting procedures could be due to stimulus competition between the prompt and the training contingency. Stimulus prompts are novel, whereas response prompts are typically familiar stimuli that have a conditioning history and already possess discriminative properties. Thus, when the contingency is introduced, response prompts have the potential to block behavioral control by the discriminative stimulus that is intended to trigger the response, whereas stimulus prompts do not. Even if the response prompt was novel, overshadowing could also determine the greater effectiveness of stimulus over response prompting. In stimulus prompting, only one stimulus is presented during conditioning, whereas in response prompting, the prompt and the discriminative stimulus are presented together, so overshadowing is more likely to occur in response than in stimulus prompting. The advantage of using a stimulus competition analysis for prompting procedures is that understanding the stimulus competition effect can lead to a more successful prompting implementation. For example, blocking in response prompting could be reduced by using prompts that have no previous conditioning history, and overshadowing could be fully avoided in stimulus prompting by ensuring that the prompt's salience is lower than that of the discriminative stimulus (see Cengher et al., 2018, for further discussion).

A Departure from Attentional Models

Although attentional processes have been emphasized in many developmental and psychopathological conditions (e.g., autism, attention deficit disorder, schizophrenia), associative models designed to account for stimulus competition effects have suggested an emphasis on processes other than attention to explain and understand cognitive dysfunctions in these conditions. For example, Escobar et al. (2002) suggested that some of the so-called "attentional deficits" in schizophrenia could be better modeled using a retrieval-deficit approach, such as Miller and Matzel's (1988) comparator theory. Escobar et al. (2002) proposed that failures to observe stimulus competition phenomena in schizophrenia resulted from a deficit in the comparison of associations' relative strength (i.e., an *underactive* comparator mechanism) rather than attentional dysfunctions. Reed (2007) proposed a similar analysis to explain stimulus overselectivity effects in ASD. In Reed's view, ASD may lead to an *overactive* comparator mechanism, such that small differences among stimuli can activate the comparator mechanism and lead to behavioral control by minor stimulus features (i.e., overselectivity). The use of a learning model to explain overselectivity has advantages that go beyond explanation, as they can lead to prediction. For example, if overselectivity were the result of a comparison between relative association strengths, extinguishing the overselected features of the stimulus could restore behavioral control to the underselected features of the stimulus (just as extinguishing the overshadowing stimulus can restore behavioral control by the overshadowed stimulus), an assumption that has some empirical support (Broomfield et al., 2009). This approach could explain many features of cognition in autism, such as reactivity to salience, novelty, and isolated areas of expertise (see Reed, 2007, for discussion).

Conclusion

Conditioning procedures can lead to robust behavioral control by stimuli that are paired with an outcome. However, under some circumstances, closely related stimuli can also elicit a response (*generalization*), while mildly different stimuli may fail to elicit the response (*discrimination*). Stimuli that are paired with an outcome may also fail to elicit a response based not only on their physical properties but also the circumstances under which they were trained or the associative status of other, associated stimuli (*stimulus competition*). Stimulus competition can account for situations in which behavioral control by a trained stimulus fail (e.g., overshadowing), as well as situations in which behavior appears to suddenly "develop" to a stimulus that did not previously elicit a response (e.g., recovery from overshadowing). An understanding of the possible underlying principles of stimulus competition can also suggest different ways to understand and address behavioral concerns. For example, using a framework such as that provided by error-correction theories (e.g., Rescorla & Wagner, 1972) can explain why two trained signals may become less effective when used together than in isolation (e.g., overexpectation) and comparator theories (e.g., Miller & Matzel, 1988; Reed, 2007) can suggest strategies to address issues such as stimulus overselectivity (e.g., extinguish the overselected features of the stimulus).

REFERENCES

Adams, N. C., & Jarrold, C. (2012). Inhibition in autism: Children with autism have difficulty inhibiting irrelevant distractors but not prepotent responses. *Journal of Autism and Developmental Disorders, 42,* 1052–1063.

Amundson, J. C., Escobar, M., & Miller, R. R. (2003). Proactive interference between cues trained with a common outcome in first-order Pavlovian conditioning. *Journal of Experimental Psychology: Animal Behavior Processes, 29,* 311–322.

Arcediano, F., Escobar, M., & Matute, H. (2001). Reversal from blocking in humans as a result of posttraining extinction of the blocking stimulus. *Animal Learning & Behavior, 29,* 354–366.

Arcediano, F., Escobar, M., & Miller, R. R. (2004). Is stimulus competition an acquisition deficit or a performance deficit? *Psychonomic Bulletin & Review, 11,* 1105–1110.

Arcediano, F., Matute, H., Escobar, M., & Miller, R. R. (2005). Competition between antecedent and between subsequent stimuli in causal judgments. *Journal of Experimental Psychology: Learning, Memory, and Cognition, 31,* 228–237.

Azorlosa, J. L., & Cicala, G. A. (1988). Increased conditioning in rats to a blocked CS after the first compound trial. *Bulletin of the Psychonomic Society, 26,* 254–257.

Balaz, M. A., Kasprow, W. J., & Miller, R. R. (1982). Blocking with a single compound trial. *Animal Learning and Behavior, 10,* 271–276.

Batson, J. D., & Batsell, W. R., Jr. (2000). Augmentation, not blocking, in an A+/AX+ flavor-conditioning procedure. *Psychonomic Bulletin and Review, 7,* 466–471.

Behrmann, M., Avidan, G., Leonard, G. K.,

Kimchi, R., Luna, B., Humphreys, K., & Minshew, N. (2006). Configural processing in autism and its relationship to face processing. *Neuropsychologia, 44,* 110–129.

Bouton, M. E. (1994). Context, ambiguity, and classical conditioning. *Current Directions in Psychological Science, 3,* 49–53.

Bouton, M. E. (2002). Context, ambiguity, and unlearning: Sources of relapse after behavioral extinction. *Biological Psychiatry, 52,* 976–986.

Bouton, M. E. (2004). Context and behavioral processes in extinction. *Learning and Memory, 11,* 485–494.

Broomfield, L., McHugh, L., & Reed, P. (2009). Extinction of over-selected stimuli causes re-emergence of previously under-selected cues in children with autistic spectrum disorders. *Journal of Autism and Developmental Disabilities, 39,* 290–298.

Cengher, M., Budd, A., Farrell, N., & Fienup, D. M. (2018). A review of prompt-fading procedures: Implications for effective and efficient skill acquisition. *Journal of Developmental and Physical Disabilities, 30,* 155–173.

Clarke, J. C., Westbrook, R. F., & Irwin, J. (1979). Potentiation instead of overshadowing in the pigeon. *Behavioral and Neural Biology, 25,* 18–29.

Courchesne, E., Townsend, J., Akshoomoff, N. A., Saitoh, O., Yeung-Courchesne, R., Lincoln, A. J., . . . Lau, L. (1994). Impairment in shifting attention in autistic and cerebellar patients. *Behavioral Neuroscience, 108,* 848–865.

De Houwer, J., & Beckers, T. (2002). Higher-order retrospective revaluation in human causal learning. *Quarterly Journal of Experimental Psychology, 55B,* 137–151.

Deitz, S. M., & Malone, L. W. (1985). On terms: Stimulus control terminology. *Behavior Analyst, 8*, 259–264.

Delius, J. D., Jitsumori, M., & Siemann, M. (2000). Stimulus equivalencies through discrimination reversals. In C. Heyes & L. Huber (Eds.), *The evolution of cognition* (pp. 103–122). Bradford/MIT Press.

Denniston, J. C., Savastano, H. I., & Miller, R. R. (2001). The extended comparator hypothesis: Learning by contiguity, responding by relative strength. In R. R. Mowrer & S. B. Klein (Eds.), *Handbook of contemporary learning theories* (pp. 65–117). Erlbaum.

Deruelle, C., Rondan, C., Salle-Collemiche, X., Bastard-Rosset, D., & Da Fonséca, D. (2008). Attention to low- and high-spatial frequencies in categorizing facial identities, emotions and gender in children with autism. *Brain and Cognition, 66*, 115–212.

Dickinson, A., & Burke, J. (1996). Within-compound associations mediate the retrospective revaluation of causality judgements. *Quarterly Journal of Experimental Psychology, 49B*, 60–80.

Didden, R., Prinsen, H., & Sigafoos, J. (2000). The blocking effect of pictorial prompts on sight-word reading. *Journal of Applied Behavior Analysis, 33*, 317–320.

Dittlinger, L. H., & Lerman, D. C. (2011). Further analysis of picture interference when teaching word recognition to children with autism. *Journal of Applied Behavior Analysis, 44*(2), 341–349.

Dube, W. V., Farber, R. S., Mueller, M. R., Grant, E., Lorin, L., & Deutsch, C. K. (2016). Stimulus overselectivity in autism, Down syndrome, and typical development. *American Journal on Intellectual and Developmental Disabilities, 121*(3), 219–235.

Escobar, M., Arcediano, F., & Miller, R. R. (2001a). Conditions favoring retroactive interference between antecedent events and between subsequent events. *Psychonomic Bulletin and Review, 8*, 691–697.

Escobar, M., Arcediano, F., & Miller, R. R. (2003). Latent inhibition in human adults without masking. *Journal of Experimental Psychology: Learning, Memory, and Cognition, 29*, 1028–1040.

Escobar, M., Matute, H., & Miller, R. R. (2001b). Cues trained apart compete for behavioral control in rats: Convergence with the associative interference literature. *Journal of Experimental Psychology: General, 130*, 97–115.

Escobar, M., Miller, R. R., & Oberling, P. (2002). Associative deficit accounts of disrupted latent inhibition and blocking in schizophrenia. *Neuroscience and Biobehavioral Reviews, 26*, 203–216.

Estes, W. K. (1950). Toward a statistical theory of learning. *Psychological Review, 57*, 94–107.

Frith, U. (1989). *Autism: Explaining the enigma.* Blackwell.

Ginat-Frolich, R., Klein, Z., Katz, O., & Shechner, T. (2017). A novel perceptual discrimination training task: Reducing fear overgeneralization in the context of fear learning. *Behavior Research and Therapy, 93*, 29–37.

González-Martín, E., Cobos, P. L., Morís, J., & López, F. J. (2012). Interference between outcomes, spontaneous recovery, and context effects as measured by a cued response reaction time task: Evidence for associative retrieval models. *Journal of Experimental Psychology: Animal Behavior Processes, 38*, 419–432.

Haesen, K., Beckers, T., Baeyens, F., & Vervliet, B. (2017). One-trial overshadowing: Evidence for fast specific fear learning in humans. *Behaviour Research and Therapy, 90*, 16–24.

Happé, F., & Frith, U. (2006). The weak coherence account: Detail-focused cognitive style in autism spectrum disorders. *Journal of Autism and Developmental Disorders, 36*(1), 5–25.

Honey, R. C., & Hall, G. (1989). Enhanced discriminability and reduced associability following flavor preexposure. *Learning and Motivation, 20*, 262–277.

James, J. H., & Wagner, A. R. (1980). One-trial overshadowing: Evidence of distributive processing. *Journal of Experimental Psychology: Animal Behavior Processes, 6*, 188–205.

Jones, P., Zaksaite, T., & Mitchell, C. (2019). Uncertainty and blocking in human causal learning. *Journal of Experimental Psychology: Animal Learning and Cognition, 45*, 111–124.

Kamin, L. J. (1969). Predictability, surprise, attention, and conditioning. In B. Campbell & R. Church (Eds.), *Punishment and aversive behavior* (pp. 279–276). Appleton-Century-Crofts.

Kaufman, M. A., & Bolles, R. C. (1981). A non-associative aspect of overshadowing. *Bulletin of the Psychonomic Society, 18*, 318–320.

Kohler, W. (1938). Simple structural functions in the chimpanzee and in the chicken. In W. D. Ellis (Ed.), *A source book of Gestalt psychol-*

ogy (pp. 217–227). Routledge & Kegan Paul. (Original work published 1918)

Kosaki, Y., & Watanabe, S. (2016). Impaired Pavlovian predictive learning between temporally phasic but not static events in autism-model strain mice. *Neurobiology of Learning and Memory, 134*, 304–316.

Kraemer, P. J., Lariviere, N. A., & Spear, N. E. (1988). Expression of a taste aversion conditioned with an odor-taste compound: Overshadowing is relatively weak in weanlings and decreases over a retention interval in adults. *Animal Learning and Behavior, 16*, 164–168.

Kruschke, J. K. (2005). Learning involves attention. In G. Houghton (Ed.), *Connectionist models in cognitive psychology* (pp. 113–140). Psychology Press.

Lawson, R. P., Mathys, C., & Rees, G. (2017). Adults with autism overestimate the volatility of the sensory environment. *Nature Neuroscience, 20*, 1293–1299.

Lazareva, O. F. (2012). Relational learning in a context of transposition: A review. *Journal of the Experimental Analysis of Behavior, 97*(2), 231–248.

Le Pelley, M. E., Oakeshott, S. M., & McLaren, I. P. L. (2005). Blocking and unblocking in human causal learning. *Journal of Experimental Psychology: Animal Behavior Processes, 31*, 56–70.

Litrownik, A. J., McInnis, E. T., Wetzel-Pritchard, A. M., & Filipelli, D. L. (1978). Restricted stimulus control and inferred attentional deficits in autistic and retarded children. *Journal of Abnormal Psychology, 87*, 554–562.

Lovaas, O. I., Berberich, J. P., Perloff, B. F., & Schaeffer, B. (1966). Acquisition of imitative speech in schizophrenic children. *Science, 151*, 705–707.

Lovaas, O. I., Schreibman, L., Koegel, R. L., & Rehm, R. (1971). Selective responding by autistic children to multiple sensory input. *Journal of Abnormal Psychology, 77*, 211–222.

Lubow, R. E. (1989). *Latent inhibition and conditioned attention theory.* Cambridge University Press.

Lubow, R. E., & Gewirtz, J. C. (1995). Latent inhibition in humans: Data, theory, and implications for schizophrenia. *Psychological Bulletin, 117*, 87–103.

Lubow, R. E., & Moore, A. U. (1959). Latent inhibition: The effect of nonreinforced preexposure to the conditioned stimulus. *Journal of*

Comparative and Physiological Psychology, 52, 415–419.

Mackintosh, N. J. (1975). A theory of attention: Variations in the associability of stimuli with reinforcement. *Psychological Review, 82*, 276–298.

Mackintosh, N. J. (1976). Overshadowing and stimulus intensity. *Animal Learning and Behavior, 4*, 186–192.

Mackintosh, N. J., & Reese, B. (1979). One-trial overshadowing. *Quarterly Journal of Experimental Psychology, 31*, 519–526.

Mackintosh, N. J., Dickinson, A., & Cotton, M. M. (1980). Surprise and blocking: Effects of the number of compound trials. *Animal Learning and Behavior, 8*, 387–391.

Maes, E., Boddez, Y., Alfei, J. M., Krypotos, A.-M., D'Hooge, R., De Houwer, J., & Beckers, T. (2016). The elusive nature of the blocking effect: 15 failures to replicate. *Journal of Experimental Psychology: General, 145*, e49–e71.

Maes, E., Krypotos, A. M., Boddez, Y., Alfei Palloni, J. M., D'Hooge, R., De Houwer, J., & Beckers, T. (2018). Failures to replicate blocking are surprising and informative—Reply to Soto (2018). *Journal of Experimental Psychology: General, 147*, 603–610.

March, J., Chamizo, V. D., & Mackintosh, N. J. (1992). Reciprocal overshadowing between intra-maze and extra-maze cues. *Quarterly Journal of Experimental Psychology, 45B*, 49–63.

Marr, M. J. (2017). The future of behavior analysis: Foxes and hedgehogs revisited. *Behavior Analyst, 40*, 197–207.

Marr, M. J., & Zilio, D. (2013). No island entire of itself: Reductionism and behavior analysis. *European Journal of Behavior Analysis, 14*(2), 241–257.

Matute, H., Arcediano, F., & Miller, R. R. (1996). Test question modulates cue competition between causes and between effects. *Journal of Experimental Psychology: Learning, Memory, and Cognition, 22*, 182–196.

Matzel, L. D., Schachtman, T. R., & Miller, R. R. (1985). Recovery of an overshadowed association achieved by extinction of the overshadowed stimulus. *Learning and Motivation, 16*, 398–412.

Miguel, C. F. (2018). Problem-solving, bidirectional naming, and the development of verbal repertoires. *Behavior Analysis: Research and Practice, 18*, 340–353.

Miller, J. S., Scherer, S. L., & Jagielo, J. A. (1995). Enhancement of conditioning by a nongustatory CS: Ontogenetic differences in the mechanisms underlying potentiation. *Learning and Motivation, 26*, 43–62.

Miller, R. R., Barnet, R. C., & Grahame, N. J. (1995). Assessment of the Rescorla–Wagner model. *Psychological Bulletin, 117*, 363–386.

Miller, R. R., & Escobar, M. (2002). Associative interference between cues and between outcomes presented together and presented apart: An integration. *Behavioural Processes, 57*, 163–185.

Miller, R. R., & Matzel, L. D. (1988). The comparator hypothesis: A response rule for the expression of associations. In G. H. Bower (Ed.), *The psychology of learning and motivation* (Vol. 22, pp. 51–92). Academic Press.

O'Riordan, M. A., & Passetti, F. (2006). Discrimination in autism within different sensory modalities. *Journal of Autism and Developmental Disorders, 36*, 665–675.

Odling-Smee, F. J. (1978). The overshadowing of background stimuli by an informative CS in aversive Pavlovian conditioning with rats. *Animal Learning and Behavior, 6*, 43–51.

Pavlov, I. P. (1927). *Conditioned reflexes*. Oxford University Press.

Pearce, J. M. (1987). A model for stimulus generalization in Pavlovian conditioning. *Psychological Review, 94*, 61–73.

Pearce, J. M. (1994). Similarity and discrimination: A selective review and a connectionist model. *Psychological Review, 101*, 587–607.

Pineño, O., Urushihara, K., & Miller, R. R. (2005). Spontaneous recovery from forward and backward blocking. *Journal of Experimental Psychology: Animal Behavior Processes, 31*, 172–183.

Plaisted, K. C., Saksida, L., Alcantara, J., & Weisblatt, E. (2003). Towards an understanding of the mechanisms of weak ventral coherence effects: Experiments in visual configural learning and auditory perception. *Philosophical Transactions, 358*, 375–386.

Ploog, B. O. (2010). Stimulus overselectivity four decades later: A review of the literature and its implications for current research in autism spectrum disorder. *Journal of Autism and Developmental Disorders, 40*, 1332–1349.

Powell, P. S., Travers, B. G., Klinger, L. G., & Klinger, M. R. (2016). Difficulties with multisensory fear conditioning in individuals with autism spectrum disorder. *Research in Autism Spectrum Disorder, 25*, 137–146.

Prados, J., Alvarez, B., Acebes, F., Loy, I., Sansa, J., & Moreno-Fernández, M. M. (2013). Blocking in rats, humans and snails using a within-subjects design. *Behavioural Processes, 100*, 23–31.

Reed, P. (2007). Comparator deficits in autism during discrimination learning: Theory to treatment. In P. C. Carlisle (Ed.), *Progress in autism research* (pp. 187–219). Nova Science.

Reed, P., & McCarthy, J. (2011). Cross-modal attention switching is impaired in autism spectrum disorder. *Journal of Autism and Developmental Disorders, 42*, 947–953.

Rehfeldt, R. A. (2011). Toward a technology of derived stimulus relations: An analysis of articles published in the *Journal of Applied Behavior Analysis*, 1992–2009. *Journal of Applied Behavior Analysis, 44*, 109–119.

Remington, A., Swettenham, J., Campbell, R., & Coleman, M. (2009). Selective attention and perceptual load in autism spectrum disorder. *Psychological Science, 20*(11), 1388–1393.

Rescorla, R. A. (1970). Reduction in the effectiveness of reinforcement after prior excitatory conditioning. *Learning and Motivation, 1*, 372–381.

Rescorla, R. A., & Wagner, A. R. (1972). A theory of Pavlovian conditioning: Variations in the effectiveness of reinforcement and nonreinforcement. In A. Black & W. R. Prokasy (Eds.), *Classical conditioning II* (pp. 64–99). Academic Press.

Reynolds, G. S. (1961). Attention in the pigeon. *Journal of the Experimental Analysis of Behavior, 4*, 203–208.

Rider, D. P. (1991). The speciation of behavior analysis. *The Behavior Analyst, 14*(2), 171–181.

Rieth, S. R., Stahmer, A. C., Suhrenreich, J., & Schreibman, L. (2015). Examination of the prevalence of stimulus overselectivity in children with ASD. *Journal of Applied Behavior Analysis, 48*(1), 71–84.

Sanbonmatsu, D. M., Akimoto, S. A., & Gibson, B. D. (1994). Stereotype-based blocking in social explanation. *Personality and Social Psychology Bulletin, 20*, 71–81.

Shechner, T., Britton, J. C., Ronkin, E. G., Jarcho, J. M., Mash, J. A., Michalska, K. J., . . . Pine, D. S. (2015). Fear conditioning and extinction in anxious and nonanxious youth and adults: Examining a novel developmentally-appropriate fear-conditioning task. *Depression and Anxiety, 32*(4), 277–288.

Sidman, M. (1994). *Equivalence relations and*

behavior: A research story. Authors Cooperative.

Sidman, M. (2009). Equivalence relations and behavior: An introductory tutorial. *Analysis of Verbal Behavior, 25*, 1–13.

Singh, N. N., & Solman, R. T. (1990). A stimulus control analysis of the picture-word problem in children who are mentally retarded: The blocking effect. *Journal of Applied Behavior Analysis, 23*, 525–532.

Soto, F. A. (2018). Contemporary associative learning theory predicts failures to obtain blocking: Comment on Maes et al. (2016). *Journal of Experimental Psychology: General, 147*, 597–602.

Southwick, J. S., Bigler, E. D., Froehlich, A., Dubray, M. B., Alexander, A. K., Lange, N., & Lainhart, J. E. (2011). Memory functioning in children and adults with autism. *Neuropsychology, 25*, 702–710.

Stout, S. C., Arcediano, F., Escobar, M., & Miller, R. R. (2003). Overshadowing as a function of trial number: Dynamics of first- and second-order comparator effects. *Learning and Behavior, 31*, 85–97.

Stout, S. C., & Miller, R. R. (2007). Sometimes-competing retrieval: A formalization of the comparator hypothesis. *Psychological Review, 114*(3), 759–783.

Urcelay, G. (2017). Competition and facilitation in compound conditioning. *Journal of Experimental Psychology: Animal Learning and Cognition, 43*, 303–314.

Van Hamme, L. J., & Wasserman, E. A. (1994). Cue competition in causality judgments: The role of nonpresentation of compound stimulus elements. *Learning and Motivation, 25*, 127–151.

Wagner, A. R., Logan, F. A., Haberlandt, K., & Price, T. (1968). Stimulus selection in animal discrimination learning. *Journal of Experimental Psychology, 76*, 171–180.

Wasserman, E., & Berglan, L. (1998). Backward blocking and recovery from overshadowing in human causal judgement: The role of within-compound associations. *Quarterly Journal of Experimental Psychology, 51B*, 121–138.

Webb, S. J., Jones, E. J. H., Merkle, K., Namkung, J., Toth, K., Greenson, J., . . . Dawson, G. (2010). Toddlers with elevated autism symptoms show slowed habituation to faces. *Child Neuropsychology, 16*, 255–278.

Witnauer, J., Rhodes, J., Kysor, S., & Narasiwodeyar, S. (2018). The sometimes competing retrieval model and Van Hamme & Wasserman models predict the selective role of within-compound associations in retrospective revaluation. *Behavioural Processes, 154*, 27–35.

CHAPTER 8

Fear Conditioning, Anxiety, and Phobias
CONSIDERATIONS FOR
OPERANT–RESPONDENT INTERACTIONS

Adam Brewer
Yanerys Leon
Stephanie C. Kuhn
David Kuhn
Michael W. Schlund

Among the general population, approximately 31.9% of adolescents (ages 13–17) are diagnosed with an anxiety disorder (Kessler et al., 2005). Applied behavior analysts may be interested in reports of fear that are positively correlated with maladaptive behaviors (Evans et al., 2005). Applied behavior analysts working in clinical contexts have historically taken a primarily operant approach to assessment and treatment of maladaptive behavior. Operant approaches to treatment evaluate environmental determinants of behavior through the lens of the three-term contingency (i.e., antecedents, behavior, consequences) under the influence of motivating operations. For instance, after identifying the function of maladaptive behavior, a therapist may aim to reinforce a communicative response that serves the same function of the maladaptive behavior with or without removing the consequence maintaining problem behavior (Kurtz et al., 2011). Although this approach has been successful in producing effective, empirically validated treatments, sometimes progress is poor or treatment fails (Briggs et al., 2018). In some instances, functional analyses and treatment development could be informed by investigation of Pavlovian associative learning processes in the acquisition, maintenance, and reduction of dysfunctional emotional and behavioral responses.

We propose that behavior-analytic researchers and practitioners would find the experimental and clinical psychopathology literature a valuable source of inspiration and knowledge for informing treatment development. A large basic and clinical research literature exists that has highlighted the role of Pavlovian learning processes in the acquisition, maintenance, and reduction of anxiety, fear, and phobic responses and other dysfunctional behavior (for reviews, see De Houwer, 2020; Vervliet et al., 2013; Davidson et al., 1994; Lissek et al., 2005). In this chapter, we discuss findings from basic and clinical mainstream research that highlight the role of Pavlovian learning processes in learning fear, extinction of fear, fear generalization, relapse of fear, and relations between fear and avoidance. This chapter is designed to provide another perspective or lens from which to view common emotional and behavioral problems. Our discussion is not intended as a guide for treating individuals who exhibit long-lasting anxiety or phobias that meet clinically significant levels as outlined by the criteria established by the *Diagnostic and Statistical Manual of Mental Disorders* (American Psychiatric Association, 2022). We focus on treating maladaptive behaviors that are elicited by common encounters and routines that are developmentally or age appropriate. Finally, we discuss ethical considerations related to risk assessment associated with treatment and scope of practice and competency for behavior analysis practitioners.

Fear

Acquisition

Environmental stimuli can become threatening when they are associated with and predictive of aversive stimuli (e.g., loud sounds, physical pain; for a review, see Delgado et al., 2006). To study how one acquires learned fear or threat in the laboratory, researchers employ various Pavlovian fear conditioning paradigms (Figure 8.1, left column, row A). In the typical fear conditioning paradigm with nonhuman animals and humans, an aversive unconditioned stimulus (US) such as electric shock is paired with a neutral stimulus (NS), such as yellow light (which does not elicit fear), and a distinctly different color (e.g., a red light) is paired with the absence of the US. It is important to note that the US (i.e., the electric shock) requires no ontogenetic history such as fear conditioning or operant consequences to elicit a response that is automatic (or reflexive). Prior to stimulus–stimulus pairing of CS+ (i.e., the yellow light) and US (yellow light-to-shock), the unconditioned elicited response (UCR) to the shock can include defecation/urination, sweating, startle, aggressive behavior, and physical immobility ("freezing"). Moreover, prior to fear conditioning, the presentation of neither the CS+ nor the CS– elicit reflexive behavior similar to the UCR; they are neutral stimuli. During fear conditioning trials, the presentation of electric shock (US) is reliably paired and predicted by the yellow light (CS+); the red light (control CS–) is never paired with the US. To test for acquisition of fear, each cue is presented without electric shock to assess whether CS+ or CS– elicits fear (UCR) associated with the presentation of the electric shock (US). Only the CS+ elicits behavior associated with presentation of the US. Thus, the yellow light becomes the CS+ (i.e., the yellow light directly paired with shock). The yellow light (CS+) has acquired a similar stimulus function as the electric shock and now is said to be associated with the US (i.e., Pavlovian or respondent acquisition). In other words, the subject engages in a conditioned response (CR) to the CS+ as if they were being threatened that a shock is coming. Note that the colors in Figures 8.1 and 8.2 are depicted by shades of gray where lighter shades represent yellow and darker shades represent red.

Human laboratory studies of fear conditioning often involve (1) typically developing adults and children or (2) clinical populations diagnosed with an anxiety disorder or autism spectrum disorder (ASD) (for reviews, see Fullana et al., 2020; Lissek et al., 2005; South et al., 2011; Top et al., 2016; Vervliet et al., 2013). In these studies, fear CRs are measured in the form of physiological arousal (for a review, see Lonsdorf et al., 2017).

Additionally, researchers typically gather self-report data from participants to include subjective ratings of feelings of fear and anxiety (affective) and thoughts/beliefs regarding the expected CS–US probabilities, or how the likely threat cue will be followed by the aversive event (cognitive; Lovibond et al., 2009).

We can apply knowledge of fear processes to clinically relevant populations that are frequent recipients of behavior-analytic intervention. For example, anxiety disorders are more prevalent for individuals with ASD compared to others (Evans et al., 2005). It is well established that individuals with ASD exhibit a wide range of fears and phobias (American Psychiatric Association, 2022; Leyfer et al., 2006; Muris et al., 1998; Simonoff et al., 2008; Sukhodolsky et al., 2008) to seemingly benign events or routines (e.g., Kanner, 1943; Evans et al., 2005; Gillis et al., 2009; Richman et al., 2012; Turner & Romanczyk, 2012). An example of a common learned fear of children with ASD (for a review, see Lydon et al., 2015; Turner & Romanczyk, 2012) and many other populations is the receipt of a medical injection (i.e., Shabani & Fisher, 2006; Meindl et al., 2019; Wolff & Symons, 2013). Despite the benefits to the individual (and others) of receiving shots, the pain associated with this procedure often leads to fears. In Figure 8.1 (right column, row A), the pain from the shot (US) may be paired with the sight of the needle, medical personnel (i.e., doctor with lab coat), and other contextual stimuli (e.g., room, medical equipment) that may all come to function as CS+ (threat stimuli) and elicit fear responses (CR). Such maladaptive CRs are likely to make subsequent medical procedures stressful for the client, caregivers, and medical personnel.

Generalization

Laboratory models have been developed to understand how fear may transfer to stimuli that have never been paired with the US (for reviews, see Dymond et al., 2015; Honig & Urcuioli, 1981). Let us return to the earlier example of pairing a yellow light with an electric shock. Consider a yellow cue of moderate intensity that is used for fear acquisition. To assess whether fear generalizes or spreads to other stimuli (Figure 8.1: left column, row B) that have no direct fear conditioning history (CS–), the subject is exposed to different light intensities (e.g., from left to right: least bright, less bright, the intensity of the CS+, more bright, most bright). Subjects typically exhibit a stronger CR to intensities that are more similar to the CS+ (relatively more or less bright) than other wavelengths (most and least bright). This outcome is illustrated in Figure 8.1 as a fear generalization gradient depicted by the size of the cartoon's emotional response. Because generalization was programmed and tested using topographically similar stimuli with different dimensional properties (i.e., intensity), this is known as *perceptual* generalization.

Another type of generalization is related to the context associated with fear conditioning (e.g., Pryce et al., 1999). For instance, fear conditioning trials might occur in the context of an experimental chamber. During additional tests for fear generalization, subjects might be exposed to a different context (e.g., a different experimental chamber without a history of the presentation of the light or the shock; CS–). The result is that a conditioned fear response occurs in the novel experimental chamber, which is evidence for *contextual* generalization. In both generalization paradigms (perceptual and contextual), conditioned fear may indirectly transfer to stimuli not associated with the US.

Recall the situation in which the child experienced the injection that caused pain (US) associated with a syringe and the doctor (CS+). Fear generalization may occur with similar lab coats (Figure 8.1, right column, row B). Conditioned fear may also generalize

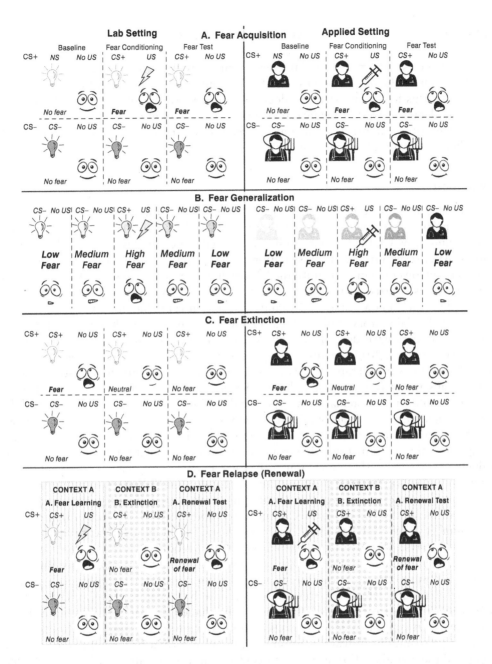

FIGURE 8.1. The left column depicts a laboratory example using a yellow light (depicted as gray outline and white fill) as a CS+ (red light depicted with black outline and dark gray fill as a CS–) and an electric shock as the US; the right column illustrates a parallel, applied example using a doctor as the CS+ (janitor as a CS–) and injections as the US. More specifically, Row A shows the process of fear conditioning in which a neutral stimulus (NS) is paired with an aversive unconditioned stimulus (US); the CS– is paired with the absence of the US. Thereafter, the NS acquires properties of the US and becomes a CS+; like the US, the CS+ elicits fear. Fear generalization (Row B) is shown using different intensities of a CS+ (yellow light or lab coat); these different intensities have never been directly paired with the US (CS–). More fear is elicited by a CS– that resembles the intensity of the CS–. Row C highlights how fears are eliminated using fear extinction in which the CS+ systematically is paired with the absence of the US (a doctor visit without an injection); across trials, fear gradually decreases. Last, Row D illustrates how a previously extinguished fear response can return if fear is learned in one context (A), such as a medical office associated with a doctor administering an injection and treated in separate context (B) such as behavior analytic clinic's simulation. Thereafter, relapse of fear can occur upon returning to the original context (the medical office) in which fear was acquired (context A).

to other doctors, others wearing lab coats, syringes without needles (e.g., oral syringes to administer medicine), or other contextual stimuli; that is, by way of contextual generalization, this fear may extend to doctor's offices more broadly, other medical buildings (e.g., dental offices) or medical personnel (e.g., school nurses), and equipment (e.g., disposable saliva ejector). Fear may also spread to a parent or caregiver who has been reliably paired with taking the child to get a shot.

Extinction

Conditioned fears have been systematically eliminated in the laboratory by disrupting CS–US pairings (i.e., repeated presentation of the CS without the US). In Figure 8.1 (left column, row C), the CS+ (cue light) is repeatedly presented without the US (electric shock). After several trials, the presentation of the CS+ elicits a conditioned fear response of lower and lower magnitude, until the CR reaches near-zero or zero levels. This respondent process is referred to as *respondent extinction* (or *fear extinction*) and was initially designed to teach a new stimulus–stimulus association via habituation to the CS+.

Rooted in laboratory studies of fear extinction, clinicians working with adults with anxiety disorders have developed a number of treatments involving exposure therapy (e.g., Vervliet et al., 2013). Figure 8.1 (right column, row C) shows that one mechanism underlying exposure therapy involves systematically pairing threatening stimuli (CS+) with the absence of aversive events (thus rendering them into a CS–). In our applied example, that would entail systematically exposing the child to the doctor without a scheduled shot for multiple visits. To accomplish this, exposure-based therapy relies on the creation of a fear hierarchy of the stimuli that range from lesser to more fearful stimuli and vary along some stimulus dimension. For example, when working with someone with a fear of a doctor associated with an injection, a therapist may begin by asking a (verbally proficient) client to imagine interacting with the doctor (less fearful). This would be followed by a range of intermediate steps on the fear hierarchy and end with receiving an injection from the doctor (more fearful). Progression along the fear hierarchy often depends on a number of overt operant responses (e.g., the client exhibiting appropriate approach responses), physiological respondent behaviors (e.g., blood pressure), as well as verbal report of their fear at each level, before moving onto the next step. An important limitation of exposure therapy in its aforementioned form is that it often contains aspects of imaginal exposure, which requires an advanced verbal repertoire (e.g., imagining and labeling private physiological events). This may be challenging for children with ASD and others without sophisticated verbal repertoires. More recently, clinicians have utilized digital representations of feared stimuli (e.g., in video format or virtual reality environments; Maskey et al., 2014) as a way to control and present different levels of the fear hierarchy. Advances that utilize digital stimuli are promising for use in exposure-based therapy with populations with limited verbal skills.

Hereafter, we highlight the literature on evidence-based approaches that have modified traditional exposure-based therapies (inspired by fear extinction) to meet the individual needs of children with ASD exhibiting challenging behavior (for a review, see Hagopian & Jennett, 2008). For example, Ricciardi et al. (2006) created a fear hierarchy for a child with ASD who was afraid of animatronic toys. The fear hierarchy varied along the single dimension of distance from the toy; the progression was 5 meters, 4 meters, 3 meters, 2 meters, and 1 meter. Initially, if the child remained at a 5-meter distance for 90% of the observation period for two consecutive sessions, then the child was exposed to the next closest distance of 4 meters, until the child was finally within 1 meter of the toy. In this study, operant procedures were not explicitly arranged (i.e., differential reinforcement was not programmed) and traditional escape–extinction procedures were unnecessary (i.e., the child did not attempt to escape the treatment context).

Despite the effects reported by Ricciardi et al. (2006), other researchers have suggested that graduated exposure without operant positive reinforcement may not be sufficient to reduce fears. For example, Jones and Friman (1999) used graduated exposure, using duration as a dimension, to treat the challenging and emotional behavior of a child with ASD associated with a fear of bugs. Such fear responses interfered with academic responding (i.e., conducting math calculations), which prevented the child from contacting available positive reinforcement (e.g., praise, good grades) for correct responding. During the graduated exposure sessions, the participant was exposed to a fear hierarchy that started with holding a jar of crickets and progressed through touching and eventually holding a cricket in each hand for 20 seconds. Although graduated exposure produced some initial treatment gains, contingent positive reinforcement (delivery of an appetitive stimulus contingent upon a target response; see Bernstein et al., Chapter 11, this volume) for approach (differential reinforcement of alternative behavior [DRA]) and absence of problem behavior (differential reinforcement of other behavior [DRO]) was necessary to maintain an increase the rate of math calculations in the presence of bugs.

Additional studies have demonstrated that graduated exposure (sometimes referred to as *contact desensitization* or *stimulus fading*) plus contingent positive reinforcement were effective for increasing approach toward a fearful stimulus (e.g., getting insulin shots) for a child with comorbid ASD and diabetes (Shabani & Fisher, 2006; see also dog phobias, Tyner et al., 2016). A common feature of these studies is that they relied on observable behavior (e.g., approach response and absence of problem behavior) to assess progress on a fear hierarchy. In a notable exception, Chok et al. (2010) assessed both observable behavior and a physiological response (e.g., heart rate) to help guide treatment decisions regarding progression on the fear hierarchy for a child with ASD who was fearful of dogs. It is worth noting that heart rate may increase for a variety of reasons (e.g., arousal, physical activity) other than exposure to a CS+ elicited conditioned fear response. Taken together, exposure-based therapies, in isolation or in combination with operant positive reinforcement, can be effective in the treatment of challenging behaviors associated with fearful stimuli and essential routines.

Renewal of Fear

A major challenge to exposure-based treatment of fears is relapse (for a review, see Vervliet et al., 2013). A well-established finding in both the laboratory and the clinic is that a CR that has previously undergone fear extinction in which respondent behaviors are reduced to zero or near-zero levels may return or relapse, such that treatment effects fail to generalize to targeted contexts (Craske et al., 2018). At least three types of procedures have been used to study relapse of extinguished fear: contextual renewal (e.g., Bouton, 1994; Bouton & King, 1983), spontaneous recovery (e.g., Pavlov, 1927; Huff et al., 2009), and reinstatement (e.g., LaBar & Phelps, 2005; Rescorla & Heth, 1975).

In contextual renewal (e.g., Abramowitz, 2013; Bouton, 2002; Tiwari et al., 2013), fear acquisition occurs in Context A (yellow light paired with shock), in which the light is paired with shock (Figure 8.1, left column, row D). Next, fear extinction occurs in a different context, B (i.e., yellow light presented without shock in a different chamber), and the cue no longer elicits fear. Last, the subject transitions back to Context A (the same chamber in which fear was acquired); however, the cue light is no longer followed by shock. The typical finding is that the original context once again elicits fear (e.g., increased skin conductance), that was previously extinguished in different context B, before dissipating after several trials (e.g., Thomas et al., 2003). Contextual renewal of fear is a robust finding across procedural variants such as ABC, in which the subject transitions to an entirely novel context in the last phase (instead of the initial fear acquisition Context A). In addition, AAB renewal in which fears are extinguished in the same context in which fears are acquired (compared to different contexts such as ABA and ABC) is followed by testing to a new context (similar to ABC).

These findings are particularly relevant for clinicians working with individuals to treat preclinical problem behavior (Figure 8.1, right column, row D). Returning to the example of the injection fear acquired in the doctor's office (Context A), a clinician may expose an individual to an increasing fear hierarchy (sight of lab coats, medical personnel, sight of needle, needle touches arms but does not penetrate, etc.) in a controlled simulation in a clinical setting (Context B) and successfully extinguish the elicited fear response in that context. However, upon return to the doctor's office (Context A) the stimuli that were present during the initial fear acquisition context and were not present in the structured clinical setting (e.g., unique artwork) may now elicit a fear response and ultimately result in relapse (ABA renewal). Intervention may be successful in that environment; however, the client may still experience fear of those stimuli at school or in the community (Context B) or other nontreatment settings (AAB renewal). Considering the likelihood of fear relapse based on the aforementioned processes, the general notion that extinction eliminates or removes a response entirely from an organism's repertoire is a common misconception. Practitioners must be equipped with more robust and effective treatment approaches to treating this class of persistent, and often pervasive, avoidant behavior.

Basic and applied researchers have examined factors that can be protective against relapse and renewal of fears and phobias. One such strategy that has been implemented involves exposure to multiple stimuli that resemble the feared stimulus (i.e., CS+ and stimuli that share formal similarity to the CS+ along one dimension). For example, basic researchers have shown that subjects exposed to fear extinction trials in multiple contexts have a lower probability of CR in a new context in relapse trials relative to subjects who were exposed to all respondent extinction trials in one context alone (Chelonis et al., 1999). Applied researchers treating spider phobias using exposure therapy have shown that exposure to images of multiple spiders in different contexts was protective against relapse (Rowe & Craske, 1998), providing evidence for perceptual generalization of extinction effects. More recently, applied researchers have examined the effects of extinction trials in the context of exposure therapy across multiple contexts (i.e., programming for contextual generalization of extinction effects) conducted in a virtual reality context, and showed similar results (i.e., multiple context exposure was protective against relapse in a renewal test; Shiban et al., 2013).

Results of these studies have important implications for treatment of fear and phobias in practice. There has been an increase in the use of virtual reality within the context of exposure therapy for typically developing adults with anxiety disorders and specific phobias. Given the basic literature on contextual renewal, one can anticipate a greater likelihood of relapse and renewal if exposure therapy occurs in a strictly virtual environment, particularly when such treatment is applied to individuals with ASD. Although the use of virtual reality is promising for exposure-based therapy (i.e., stimuli can be precisely arranged, presented, and scaled), there are limitations inherent to generalization using such procedures; this can be particularly problematic for individuals with ASD for whom generalization of skills often must be specifically programmed.

Collectively, the studies of relapse of fear have highlighted that CS–US is not directly weakened by exposure-based treatment; exposure-based therapy is believed to rely on a habituation model of respondent extinction (e.g., Benito & Walther, 2015); that is, these treatment mechanisms were designed to weaken the conditioned fear response by targeting the CS–US association and repeatedly presenting the CS in the absence of the aversive event (Wolpe, 1958). For instance, behavioral evidence from studies of fear renewal illustrates that respondent extinction may not generalize beyond contextual stimuli (i.e., original setting in which therapy was conducted). Exposure-based therapy may not directly alter the original CS–US association; rather, these therapies might create a new association, such that the CS does not predict the US (Craske et al., 2014). Thus, the CS+ has acquired two Pavlovian associations. One is the original fear-eliciting CS–US relation combined with the new, second association from exposure-based therapy, the CS–no US relation. These two associations interact to determine the response strength of the conditioned fear response (for a theoretical alternative, see Shahan & Craig, 2017).

This inhibitory learning approach to exposure-based therapy has inspired translational researchers in anxiety disorders to engineer novel prevention and mitigation strategies to maximize treatment gains and maintenance in exposure-based therapy (Craske et al., 2014; Lipp et al., 2020). For example, rather than instructing a client to tolerate or wait until their fear subsides before progressing to the next step of the fear hierarchy, clinicians may attempt to teach what needs to be learned or create an expectancy violation (i.e., a mismatch between an expected outcome and the actual outcome). For example, if a client states they expect that the dog will bite them, the clinician could ask them "to test this out" by petting a therapy dog (associated with a very low probability of biting). Before prompting this response, the clinician can ask the client how fearful they are on a scale of 0–100. Following the client successfully petting the dog, the clinician may ask them if petting the dog resulted in a bite. If the answer is no (a mismatch of the expected outcome), the clinician may follow by asking them (1) how they know and (2) what they learned as a result of exposure to the US (or consequence). It is worth noting that expectancy violation may not be appropriate for fears that require tolerating a painful stimulus such as receiving an injection. Another inhibitory learning strategy may entail programming for variability in the time between exposure sessions or varying the order of the fear hierarchy (e.g., starting with an intermediate step before the initial step), which may initially produce higher levels of fear but has benefits in long-term maintenance. Removing distracting stimuli from the treatment environment may also be beneficial. For example, if the client has access to another activity (e.g., iPad) during the exposure-based therapy, that stimulus should be faded or removed such that the client is only attending to the treatment procedures and not simply being distracted. More applied research is needed to determine if these prevention and mitigation strategies generalize to individuals with autism.

Avoidance

Acquisition and Maintenance

In laboratory studies of operant avoidance, a conditioned threat (CS+) is used to signal an aversive event such as electric shock (US). If the subject actively responds on the operandum (e.g., pressing a lever, pecking a key, clicking a mouse button) in the presence of a discriminable threat stimulus, then, as a consequence, the aversive event is postponed or terminated. Thus, a negative reinforcement contingency is arranged that maintains avoidance. Due to the presentation of a discriminable threat, this procedure is usually referred to as *signaled avoidance* (e.g., Cándido et al., 1988; Weisman & Litner, 1969). Although there is some debate regarding the specific processes involved in avoidance (see one- versus two-factor theory: Baron & Perone, 2001), studies of signaled avoidance have provided important insights in clinical behavior analysis broadly (Hayes et al., 2011) and fear, phobias, and anxiety, specifically (Craske & Mystkowski, 2006; Dymond et al., 2018).

Pavlovian fear conditioning can produce an elicited response that contacts and is ultimately maintained via consequences (i.e., negative reinforcement). Row A of Figure 8.2 (left column) shows how the threat stimulus (CS+), which also signals an aversive consequence, acquired its aversive properties due to Pavlovian fear conditioning via pairing with the shock (US). Next, in Row B of Figure 8.2, if the conditioned fear response (e.g., button pressing, running away, aggression) terminates or postpones shock, then fear may have contacted secondary gain in the form of negative reinforcement. If the elicited fear

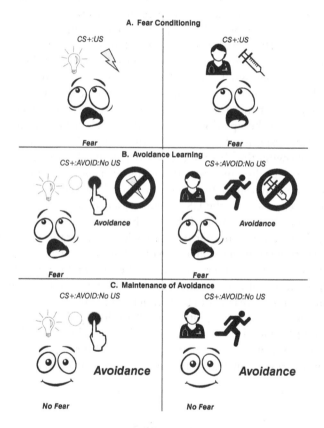

FIGURE 8.2. The left column depicts a laboratory example using a yellow light as a CS+ (depicted as gray outline with white fill) and an electric shock as the US; the right column illustrates a parallel, applied example using a doctor as the CS+ and injections as the US. Row A illustrates the Pavlovian learning processes in which fear is acquired. Row B depicts how the Pavlovian CS–US relations can motivate a response (button pressing in the lab or running away from the doctor), which can postpone or prevent the presentation of the US. Row C highlights that once this response contacts operant consequences, avoidance as a "coping strategy" can eliminate fear and be maintained via negative reinforcement.

topography (e.g., freezing) is incompatible with the avoidance response (e.g., pecking a key), then active avoidance may not be successful (Estes & Skinner, 1941). From an operant perspective, fear conditioning renders the removal of the threat stimulus negatively reinforcing (an establishing operation). Thus, the threat stimulus may have both respondent and operant functions, such that the conditioned threat can elicit both conditioned fear (respondent) and evoke avoidant (operant) behavior. Thereafter, the threat stimulus may acquire an operant, discriminative function by virtue of signaling an opportunity to avoid harm. Thus, during maintenance of avoidance (a coping strategy), fear may no longer be elicited (Figure 8.2, left column; Row C). Consequently, the respondent–operant interaction may reflect a transition from a respondent fear conditioned cue (CS+) to an operant discriminative stimulus that signals the opportunity to prevent harm and motivates and maintains avoidance. Although avoidance is highly resistant to change because of its successful consequence of preventing or terminating an aversive consequence, it may also create a new Pavlovian association such that the CS+ is no longer followed by a US. Due to weakening of the CS–US relation, the subject may occasionally fail to avoid and receive a shock. As a result, the cycle of avoidance will continue, presumably due to a recent, intermittent repairing of the CS+ and US association and exposure to aversive consequences.

Let's revisit the applied example described previously in this chapter to illustrate how respondent and operant processes can interact to result in maintenance of fear responses. Consider the example of the child who is avoidant of a doctor due to an injection phobia. This child may emit extreme overt operant behavior that makes visits to the doctor's office extremely difficult (e.g., crying, screaming, aggression,). Initially (Figure 8.2, right column, Row A), emotional responding may be primarily reflexive in nature (i.e., crying from the injection that causes pain). At subsequent visits (Figure 8.2, right column, Row B), contextual stimuli, such as the doctor (CS+), may elicit similar emotional, fear responses that produce escape (i.e., parent or medical personnel terminate medical procedure due to escalating problem behavior), avoidance (i.e., parent attempts to bring child into medical office but leaves before initiating medical procedure because of escalating problem behavior), and other appetitive consequences (i.e., comfort, tangible items, treats; often referred to as *secondary gain*; Friman & Dymond, 2020). Once avoidance is a successful coping strategy for threats, emotional responding may be replaced by chronic avoidance without a fear response (Figure 8.2, right column; Row C).

Clinical treatments for avoidance in the context of fears and phobias typically involve asking the client to approach the feared stimulus. The process typically begins with a clinician working with the individual to create a fear hierarchy ranging from least to most fearful stimuli. For individuals with intact verbal repertoires, the hierarchy is typically developed based on self-report. However, when working with individuals with limited verbal skills, clinicians may create the fear hierarchy based on direct observation (Jennett & Hagopian, 2008) or by modifying the feared stimulus on some relevant dimension (e.g., size, distance, salience in the environment; Erfanian & Miltenberger, 1990). Differential reinforcement is often programmed for approaching or tolerating the feared stimulus. For example, Shabani and Fisher (2006) treated problem behavior related to a needle phobia exhibited by an adolescent diagnosed with ASD and diabetes. Using graduated exposure and DRO, they successfully taught the participant to tolerate a blood draw via finger prick without escape extinction. Moreover, they demonstrated that (1) procedures that have been used to treat fears and phobias emitted by typically developing persons can be successful for individuals with developmental disabilities with limited language and (2) a fear hierarchy can be developed by practitioners based on participant overt behavior.

There are several implications and considerations for practitioners working with vulnerable populations in the context of assessment and treatment of fears and phobias that are worth noting as they relate to the use of operant reinforcement and extinction. First, previous researchers have shown that operant escape extinction may not always be a necessary component in the treatment of fears and phobias (Jennett & Hagopian, 2008; Rosen et al., 2016; Shabani & Fisher, 2006); that is, in some cases, allowing the individual to escape or avoid the aversive stimulus/event may still be allowed without compromising the integrity or effects of the treatment. Moreover, Jennet and Hagopian (2008) cautioned against the use of escape extinction in this context, particularly for individuals with ASD. They suggest that in order for fear extinction to take place, the feared stimulus should not be paired with any aversive event. Thus, operant escape extinction may induce more emotional responding (Rasmussen et al., 2022) and other extinction-induced side effects (e.g., extinction bursts, aggression) relative to positively reinforced behavior (Lerman et al., 1999). As such, implementing escape extinction in this context may be countertherapeutic if it results in extinction-induced emotional responding whereby the physiological response mimics an extreme anxiety response (i.e., increased heart rate, rapid breathing; see Friman & Dymond, 2020, for a discussion of induced anxiety via disrupted breathing patterns). Second, differential reinforcement contingencies can be arranged in a number of ways depending on the context and specific behavioral (avoidant) presentation. Clinicians can opt to arrange a DRA contingency, such that the reinforced operant would likely be an overt, approach response (e.g., Tyner et al., 2016). Alternatively, clinicians may opt to arrange a DRO contingency whereby the reinforced operant is the absence of the escape response (e.g., Shabani & Fisher, 2006).

Indirect Pathways to Fear and Avoidance

Beyond the direct pathway to learn to avoid via "trial and error," fear conditioning may also spread through instructions and social observation, thereby motivating avoidance (e.g., Rachman, 1977; Bandura, 2021; Gerull & Rapee, 2002; Egliston & Rapee, 2007; Dubi et al., 2008; Askew & Field, 2007). For example, Cameron et al. (2015) used a between-groups design to demonstrate the role of direct, instructed, and observational learning pathways for fear and avoidance. For the direct conditioning group, participants learned through differential consequences to press an avoidance key in the presence of a threat cue (CS+) to prevent electric shock (US). For the verbal instructions group, participants were given written rules on how to avoid an upcoming shock. For example, when the yellow circle was presented (instructed CS+) they were told to press an avoidance key; shock never followed the CS–. For the social observation group, participants watched a video of a demonstrator participating in the same exact study as the participant. Participants watched the trials in which avoidance occurred in the presence of CS+ but not in the presence of the CS–. During the test condition, novel CSs were presented, and no shocks were arranged. Results showed that all three groups learned to avoid a novel CS+ (but not CS–) and that self-reported CS–US expectancies were higher for the CS+ than CS–. Thus, despite differences in fear acquisition pathway (etiology), avoidance was motivated by fear in a similar fashion. Other indirect pathways include symbolic generalization, stimulus equivalence, and other derived relations (see Belisle & Tarbox, Chapter 24, this volume).

In practice, children may learn to fear and avoid previously neutral/benign stimuli based on observations of another's (e.g., caregiver) behavior or explicit caregiver instruction. For example, a child may see a dog while on a walk with a caregiver. For the child, the dog may function as a neutral stimulus and may even occasion an approach response.

However, for the caregiver, the dog may elicit fear and fearful behavior (i.e., screaming, walking away, holding the child). Additionally, the caregiver may instruct the child to avoid the dog and include verbal descriptions of fearful situations (e.g., "Don't touch, he can bite"). In both of these contexts, the dog may now acquire eliciting functions (i.e., respondent, fear responses) and evoke avoidant behavior (i.e., keep away from dogs) for the child. The pattern of avoidance (i.e., no contact with dogs outside of the observational and/or instructed fear context) may continue to strengthen via negative reinforcement, as the child does not encounter the dog in the absence of those eliciting stimuli.

Relapse of Avoidance

In practice, fears and avoidance are reduced via a variety of approaches, such as exposure-based therapy and medication (Hagopian & Jennett, 2008). While these approaches are often initially effective, individuals with anxiety are at increased risk for treatment relapse (i.e., the return of symptoms after a period of improvement with treatment; Lissek et al., 2005). A significant threat to long-term gains is that relapse occurs in 19–62% of cases after completing therapy when returning to the setting that initially triggered fear (Craske & Mystkowski, 2006). A prominent way to teach individuals to cope with phobias is to simply choose to avoid threats (American Psychiatric Association, 2022). Despite many important discoveries afforded by using physiological measures in laboratory models of respondent fear and relapse, an important aspect that is missing and crucial for understanding fears, phobias, and anxiety is the behavioral measure of choosing to avoid or approach threats associated with phobias.

To study relapse of fear and avoidance (and generalization), Cameron et al. (2015) exposed groups of participants to respondent fear conditioning in which a circle (CS+), was paired with electric shock, along with different-size circles (indirect CS–), and a triangle (CS–) that was paired the absence of shock. The dependent measures used were skin conductance and ratings of CS–US expectancies. Next, groups were taught how to avoid the shock in the presence of the CS+ through instructions or observational learning (watching a movie demonstrating the avoidance of shock). Generalization of fear and avoidance were observed. After fear and avoidance were eliminated using fear extinction, reinstatement was tested for by exposing both groups to three unpredictable electric shock presentations. Relapse of fear and avoidance occurred for both groups due to reinstatement of the US via unsignaled presentations. Similar processes can result in reinstatement of fear in applied contexts. For example, the child with an injection phobia who had undergone treatment and for whom the phobia has been extinguished may experience a reinstatement of fear and avoidance following another, physically similar experience in a different context (e.g., a nose swab or a bee sting).

To study renewal of fear and avoidance, Schlund et al. (2020) arranged a computerized approach–avoidance decision-making task that examined the effects of escalating threat on choice for a positive reinforcer or negative reinforcer. Pavlovian fear conditioning established that different vertical positions (CS+) on a threat meter were associated with an increased probability of money loss (US) fear conditioning. During the conflict test (Context A), participants were provided a decision to either (1) approach a reward (positive reinforcement) with the added risk of money loss or (2) avoid, which prevented money loss (negative reinforcement). Across trials, reward amounts remained fixed, while the level of threat varied unpredictably. Results showed significantly elevated indices of fear (i.e., increased galvanic skin response, and self-reports of threat expectancies and anxiety) and avoidance at higher threat levels. Using a different-color background to simulate a treatment setting, participants were exposed to Pavlovian threat extinction in which threats (CS+) signaled no money loss (US; Context B). As a result, both CS–US expectancies, avoidance, and skin conductance decreased. Returning to Context A in which fear and avoidance were acquired, renewal occurred in the form of increased avoidance and ratings (no increase in skin conductance).

Taken together, these results demonstrate major challenges to long-term maintenance of treatment gains related to reductions in conditioned fear and avoidance. Understanding how respondent fear conditioning interacts with avoidance and other forms of relapse (e.g., resurgence, spontaneous recovery) await further investigation. A better understanding of these basic processes may yield effective mitigation and prevention strategies that have been largely successful for challenging behavior maintained by appetitive stimuli (Wathen & Podlesnik, 2018; see Saini et al., Chapter 19, this volume). An area that is ripe for further research on operant–respondent interactions in the development and maintenance of phobias is in the context of exposure therapy delivered via virtual and augmented reality environments. This technology may also be able to more closely simulate the stimuli used in the target setting to prevent relapse, such as context renewal. Virtual reality environments are promising in that fear hierarchies can be carefully and systematically arranged and presented in a therapeutic session. Given the controlled nature of the sessions, physiological measures can more easily be obtained during exposures and used to inform progression within individual treatment sessions (e.g., biofeedback; Tolin et al., 2020). One noteworthy limitation of treatment in a fully virtual environment is that it is likely that some relevant, fear-inducing stimuli may not be experienced (i.e., may not contact respondent extinction); thus, relapse may be more likely. A promising alternative may be the use of augmented reality (rather than a fully immersive, virtual environment). In augmented reality, the individual wears a headset that produces digital stimuli that are superimposed on the individual's environment. For example, a client that has a fear of needles may wear the device in their home environment and digital stimuli (i.e., digital representations of doctor's office, medical personnel, medical equipment) may be present in that environment and progress according to a prespecified fear hierarchy. Given that this individual is in their home environment, any additional stimuli that have come to acquire eliciting properties by way of higher-order conditioning (e.g., presence of the parent) may now come under the appropriate control during therapeutic sessions and may make relapse less likely. Additionally, idiosyncratic features of the doctor's office (e.g., unique artwork) can be replicated in a digital format and presented during extinction trials to induce respondent extinction of any contextual stimuli that may have acquired fear-eliciting properties during acquisition.

Ethics

There are several ethical issues related to behavioral assessment and treatment of fear and phobias, most of which are related to the discomfort of the individual participating in treatment. Interventions for fears and phobias all involve some type of exposure to the feared stimulus, whether that exposure is abrupt, gradual, conducted in conjunction with a positive reinforcement procedure, implemented with or without escape extinction, accompanied by "distracting" stimuli, or involves preexposure. Although risks exist with exposure therapy, it is a generally safe and effective intervention that is rated as acceptably safe and tolerable by clients (Deacon, 2012).

The *Ethics Code for Behavior Analysts* (the Code; Behavior Analyst Certification Board® [BACB], 2020) guides the professional activities of behavior analysts and provides a framework for behavior analysts and others to evaluate their own behavior and to assess whether a behavior analyst has violated their ethical obligations. Similar to codes of ethics and responsible conduct in other human service fields, the Code states that behavior analysts work to "maximize benefits and do no harm" and that analysts do this by understanding and working within the boundaries of their competence. Additionally, the Code provides some guidance around ethical decision making. The code recommends a structured decision-making process to address ethical dilemmas that considers the full context and the function of the applicable ethics standards. The structured decision-making process recommended is a multi-step process. Several of these steps are especially relevant to the assessment and treatment of fears and phobias, including (1) considering the potential risk of harm to relevant individuals, (2) identifying the relevant core principles (e.g., do no harm) and Code standards (see below for discussion), (3) consulting available resources, (4) developing several possible actions to reduce or remove risk of harm, and (5) prioritizing the best interests of clients.

There are several specific standards that stand out as related to the assessment and treatment of fears and phobias. Code 2.01, *Providing Effective Treatment*, states that analysts prioritize clients' rights and needs in service delivery, and that services are designed to maximize desired outcomes for and protect all clients. Relatedly, Code 2.15, *Minimizing Risk of Behavior-Change Interventions*, states that behavior analysts select, design, and implement behavior-change interventions with a focus on minimizing risk of harm to the client and stakeholders, and provides some guidance about only implementing restrictive and punishment-based procedures such that the risk of harm to the client without intervention outweighs the risk associated with the behavior-change intervention. These codes are related to some of the broad ethical concerns that may be involved during treatments that incorporate exposure to aversive stimuli. Although exposure-based interventions are not restrictive or punishment-based, they do involve the presentation of aversive stimuli. Specifically, it's important to plan the intervention so that exposures are arranged in such a manner as to protect clients by minimizing discomfort and distress while obtaining optimal treatment results (i.e., risk of harm with failure to intervene is greater than the risk associated with intervention). Moreover, although the interventions for fears and phobias involve some level of exposure to the aversive stimulus, individuals seek treatment for these conditions due to the negative impact that the avoidant and related behaviors have on their lives. Discomfort can be minimized by evaluating the effects of exposure-based interventions with escape first, before using escape prevention (i.e., escape extinction; Ricciardi et al., 2006). Implementing procedures that involve graduated exposure can reduce the exposure to the most aversive "dose" of the feared stimuli and therefore lessen discomfort. However, although this may often be the appropriate course of treatment, it is also important to consider the risk of the delay of a meaningful treatment effect. For example, a graduated exposure intervention may take more sessions than a more direct exposure procedure. This may or may not be acceptable in a given situation depending on the level of impact the fear-related behavior has on the individual's daily life; that is, there may be ethical concerns with failing to consider exposure therapy in favor of less effective interventions (Deacon, 2012).

The position that exposure therapy poses an unacceptably high level of risk is associated with inaccurate information about exposure therapy (e.g., beliefs that exposure therapy leads to high attrition rates and generalization failures; Olatunji et al., 2009). Bailey and Burch (2016) developed a four-step procedure for determining risks and benefits of behavioral interventions: (1) assess the general risk factors for behavioral treatment, (2) assess the benefits of behavioral treatment, (3) assess the risk factors for each procedure, and (4) reconcile the risks and benefits with key parties involved. They go on to discuss how general risk factors can affect the outcome of a treatment plan and provide considerations that are applicable to behavioral intervention of fears and phobias. These risk factors include the nature of the behavior to be treated, sufficient personnel, the skill and training of the mediator, appropriateness of the setting, experience of behavior analyst, risk to others in the setting, buy-in from the key people associated with the case, and the liability to the behavior analyst.

With fear and phobias, the more severe the behavior related to the phobia, the greater the risk of failure to effectively intervene. The behavior analyst may implement the plan themselves or in conjunction with a caregiver, such as an educator or parent. If a parent is involved as a mediator (i.e., individual implementing the intervention) the extent to which they have been properly trained to implement the intervention and the extent to which they do so is a consideration as is the buy-in from this mediator. Consider a parent whose child becomes very distressed when participating in an intervention for an injection phobia that has spread to the doctor and medical offices. The child's emotional response may be so aversive to the parent that the parent is motivated to escape that situation and abandon the intervention (this also relates to the buy-in risk factor). The risk factors associated with the setting include the hygiene of the instruments, as well as risk to the client and others in the case of avoidant behavior that involves a struggle when the materials are within reach or when an injection is being administered. The behavior analyst's experience in this type of intervention is also a potential risk factor. While assessment and treatment of fear and phobias are within the scope of *practice* for behavior analysts, they are not necessarily in the scope of *competence* for any given behavior analyst. An analyst who implements this type of assessment and treatment must have proper education and practical training with appropriate supervision prior to implementing these procedures. This scope of competence may exist on a continuum where the higher the risk of failure, the higher the level of competence required. Bailey and Burch (2016) recommend evaluating the benefits of behavioral treatments by examining the following factors: client direct benefit, indirect benefit to setting, benefits to mediators and caregivers, benefits to peers in the setting, and general liability to the setting is decreased. Exposure-based interventions may temporarily increase discomfort, however. By assessing and managing the risk that exists, analysts can reduce the risk of harm to clients, while providing a powerful and effective intervention procedure (Deacon, 2012).

Conclusion

In summary, in this chapter we have discussed how respondent fear conditioning can elicit emotional behavior related to fears, phobias, and anxiety. We have illustrated how knowledge of respondent learning processes (respondent extinction) has inspired treatment (contact desensitization) and identified challenges to treatment success in the form of relapse (e.g., renewal, reinstatement). We have examined the dynamics of how fear-elicited behavior can be maintained through operant learning processes in the form of negative reinforcement. Beyond direct conditioning of fear and avoidance, we have provided an overview of indirect pathways for fear and avoidance (instructions, observational learning). We have also highlighted how conditioned fear can spread through generalization, and the impact this could have on the individual's quality of life. Last, we have provided ethical considerations related to treatment of these complex contingencies (assessment, risk factors, scope of practice, and competency).

ACKNOWLEDGMENTS

Special thanks to Drs. Laura Turner, Corina Jimenez-Gomez, and Christopher Podlesnik for their feedback on this topic. This chapter was written with the support of a Western Connecticut State University/American Association of University Professors research grant.

REFERENCES

Abramowitz, J. S. (2013). The practice of exposure therapy: Relevance of cognitive-behavioral theory and extinction theory. *Behavior Therapy, 44,* 548–558.

American Psychiatric Association. (2022). *Diagnostic and statistical manual of mental disorders* (5th ed., text rev.). Author.

Askew, C., & Field, A. P. (2007). Vicarious learning and the development of fears in childhood. *Behaviour Research and Therapy, 45,* 2616–2627.

Bailey, J., & Burch, M. (2016). *Ethics for behavior analysts* (3rd ed.). Routledge.

Bandura, A. (2021). Analysis of modeling processes. In A. Bandura (Ed.), *Psychological modeling* (pp. 1–62). Routledge.

Baron, A., & Perone, M. (2001). Explaining avoidance: Two factors are still better than one. *Journal of the Experimental Analysis of Behavior, 75*(3), 357–361.

Behavior Analyst Certification Board. (2020). *Ethics code for behavior analysts.* Author.

Benito, K. G., & Walther, M. (2015). Therapeutic process during exposure: Habituation model. *Journal of Obsessive–Compulsive and Related Disorders, 6,* 147–157.

Bouton, M. E. (1994). Conditioning, remembering, and forgetting. *Journal of Experimental Psychology: Animal Behavior Processes, 20,* 219–231.

Bouton, M. E. (2002). Context, ambiguity, and unlearning: Sources of relapse after behavioral extinction. *Biological Psychiatry, 52,* 976–986.

Bouton, M. E., & King, D. A. (1983). Contextual control of the extinction of conditioned fear: Tests for the associative value of the context. *Journal of Experimental Psychology: Animal Behavior Processes, 9,* 248–265.

Briggs, A. M., Fisher, W. W., Greer, B. D., & Kimball, R. T. (2018). Prevalence of resurgence of destructive behavior when thinning reinforcement schedules during functional communication training. *Journal of Applied Behavior Analysis, 51,* 620–633.

Cameron, G., Schlund, M. W., & Dymond, S. (2015). Generalization of socially transmitted and instructed avoidance. *Frontiers in Behavioral Neuroscience, 9,* Article 159.

Cándido, A., Maldonado, A., & Vila, J. (1988). Vertical jumping and signaled avoidance. *Journal of the Experimental Analysis of Behavior, 50,* 273–276.

Chelonis, J. J., Calton, J. L., Hart, J. A., & Schachtman, T. R. (1999). Attenuation of the renewal effect by extinction in multiple contexts. *Learning and Motivation, 30,* 1–14.

Chok, J. T., Demanche, J., Kennedy, A., & Studer, L. (2010). Utilizing physiological measures to facilitate phobia treatment with individuals with autism and intellectual disability: A case study. *Behavioral Interventions, 25,* 325–337.

Craske, M. G., Hermans, D., & Vervliet, B. (2018). State-of-the-art and future directions for extinction as a translational model for fear and anxiety. *Philosophical Transactions of the Royal Society B: Biological Sciences, 373,* Article 20170025.

Craske, M. G., & Mystkowski, J. L. (2006). Exposure therapy and extinction: Clinical studies. In M. G. Craske, D. Hermans, & D. Vansteenwegen (Eds.), *Fear and learning: From basic processes to clinical implications* (pp. 217–233). American Psychological Association.

Craske, M. G., Treanor, M., Conway, C. C., Zbozinek, T., & Vervliet, B. (2014). Maximizing exposure therapy: An inhibitory learning approach. *Behaviour Research and Therapy,* *58,* 10–23.

Davidson, J. R., Tupler, L. A., & Potts, N. L. (1994). Treatment of social phobia with benzodiazepines. *Journal of Clinical Psychiatry,* *55,* 28–32.

Deacon B. (2012) The ethics of exposure therapy for anxiety disorders. In P. Neudeck & H. U. Wittchen (Eds.), *Exposure therapy* (pp. 9–22). Springer.

De Houwer, J. (2020). Revisiting classical conditioning as a model for anxiety disorders: A conceptual analysis and brief review. *Behaviour Research and Therapy, 127,* Article 103558.

Delgado, M. R., Olsson, A., & Phelps, E. A. (2006). Extending animal models of fear conditioning to humans. *Biological Psychology,* *73,* 39–48.

Dubi, K., Rapee, R. M., Emerton, J. L., & Schniering, C. A. (2008). Maternal modeling and the acquisition of fear and avoidance in toddlers: Influence of stimulus preparedness and child temperament. *Journal of Abnormal Child Psychology, 36,* 499–512.

Dymond, S., Bennett, M., Boyle, S., Roche, B., & Schlund, M. (2018). Related to anxiety: Arbitrarily applicable relational responding and experimental psychopathology research on fear and avoidance. *Perspectives on Behavior Science, 41,* 189–213.

Dymond, S., Dunsmoor, J. E., Vervliet, B., Roche, B., & Hermans, D. (2015). Fear generalization in humans: Systematic review and implications for anxiety disorder research. *Behavior Therapy, 46,* 561–582.

Egliston, K. A., & Rapee, R. (2007). Inhibition of fear acquisition in toddlers following positive modelling by their mothers. *Behaviour Research and Therapy, 45,* 1871–1882.

Erfanian, N., & Miltenberger, R. G. (1990). Brief report: Contact desensitization in the treatment of dog phobias in persons who have mental retardation. *Behavioral Interventions, 5,* 55–60.

Estes, W. K., & Skinner, B. F. (1941). Some quantitative properties of anxiety. *Journal of Experimental Psychology, 29,* 390–400.

Evans, D. W., Canavera, K., Kleinpeter, F. L., Maccubbin, E., & Taga, K. (2005). The fears, phobias and anxieties of children with autism spectrum disorders and down syndrome: Comparisons with developmentally and chronologically age matched children. *Child Psychiatry and Human Development, 36,* 3–26.

Friman, P. C., & Dymond, S. (2020). The fear factor: A functional perspective on anxiety. In P. Sturmey (Ed.), *Functional analysis in clinical treatment* (pp. 375–397). Academic Press.

Fullana, M. A., Dunsmoor, J. E., Schruers, K. R. J., Savage, H. S., Bach, D. R., & Harrison, B. J. (2020). Human fear conditioning: From neuroscience to the clinic. *Behaviour Research and Therapy, 124,* Article 103528.

Gerull, F., & Rapee, R. (2002). Mother knows best: Effects of maternal modelling on the acquisition of fear and avoidance behaviour in toddlers. *Behaviour Research and Therapy, 40,* 279–287.

Gillis, J. M., Hammond Natof, T., Lockshin, S. B., & Romanczyk, R. G. (2009). Fear of routine physical exams in children with autism spectrum disorders: Prevalence and intervention effectiveness. *Focus on Autism and Other Developmental Disabilities, 24,* 156–168.

Hagopian, L. P., & Jennett, H. K. (2008). Behavioral assessment and treatment of anxiety in individuals with intellectual disabilities and autism. *Journal of Developmental and Physical Disabilities, 20,* 467–483.

Hayes, S. C., Strosahl, K. D., & Wilson, K. G. (2011). *Acceptance and commitment therapy: The process and practice of mindful change.* Guilford Press.

Honig, W. K., & Urcuioli, P. J. (1981). The legacy of Guttman and Kalish (1956): 25 years of research on stimulus generalization. *Journal of the Experimental Analysis of Behavior, 36,* 405–445.

Huff, N. C., Hernandez, J. A., Blanding, N. Q., & LaBar, K. S. (2009). Delayed extinction attenuates conditioned fear renewal and spontaneous recovery in humans. *Behavioral Neuroscience, 123,* 834–843.

Jennett, H. K., & Hagopian, L. P. (2008). Identifying empirically supported treatments for phobic avoidance in individuals with intellectual disabilities. *Behavior Therapy, 39,* 151–161.

Jones, K. M., & Friman, P. C. (1999). A case study of behavioral assessment and treatment of insect phobia. *Journal of Applied Behavior Analysis, 32,* 95–98.

Kanner, L. (1943). Autistic disturbances of affective contact. *Nervous Child, 2,* 217–250.

Kessler, R. C., Chiu, W. T., Demler, O., & Walters, E. E. (2005). Prevalence, severity, and comorbidity of 12-month DSM-IV disorders in the National Comorbidity Survey Replication. *Archives of General Psychiatry, 62,* 617–627.

Kurtz, P. F., Boelter, E. W., Jarmolowicz, D. P., Chin, M. D., & Hagopian, L. P. (2011). An analysis of functional communication training as an empirically supported treatment for problem behavior displayed by individuals with intellectual disabilities. *Research in Developmental Disabilities, 32,* 2935–2942.

LaBar, K. S., & Phelps, E. A. (2005). Reinstatement of conditioned fear in humans is context dependent and impaired in amnesia. *Behavioral Neuroscience, 119,* 677–686.

Lerman, D. C., Iwata, B. A., & Wallace, M. D. (1999). Side effects of extinction: Prevalence of bursting and aggression during the treatment of self-injurious behavior. *Journal of Applied Behavior Analysis, 32,* 1–8.

Leyfer, O. T., Folstein, S. E., Bacalman, S., Davis, N. O., Dinh, E., Morgan, J., . . . Lainhart, J. E. (2006). Comorbid psychiatric disorders in children with autism: Interview development and rates of disorders. *Journal of Autism and Developmental Disorders, 36,* 849–861.

Lipp, O. V., Waters, A. M., Luck, C. C., Ryan, K. M., & Craske, M. G. (2020). Novel approaches for strengthening human fear extinction: The roles of novelty, additional USs, and additional GSs. *Behaviour Research and Therapy, 124,* Article 103529.

Lissek, S., Powers, A. S., McClure, E. B., Phelps, E. A., Woldehawariat, G., Grillon, C., & Pine, D. S. (2005). Classical fear conditioning in the anxiety disorders: A meta-analysis. *Behaviour Research and Therapy, 43,* 1391–1424.

Lonsdorf, T. B., Menz, M. M., Andreatta, M., Fullana, M. A., Golkar, A., Haaker, J., . . . Merz, C. J. (2017). Don't fear "fear conditioning": Methodological considerations for the design and analysis of studies on human fear acquisition, extinction, and return of fear. *Neuroscience and Biobehavioral Reviews, 77,* 247–285.

Lovibond, P. F., Mitchell, C. J., Minard, E., Brady, A., & Menzies, R. G. (2009). Safety behaviours preserve threat beliefs: Protection from extinction of human fear conditioning by an avoidance response. *Behaviour Research and Therapy, 47,* 716–720.

Lydon, S., Healy, O., O'Callaghan, O., Mulhern, T., & Holloway, J. (2015). A systematic review of the treatment of fears and phobias among children with autism spectrum disorders. *Review Journal of Autism and Developmental Disorders, 2,* 141–154.

Maskey, M., Lowry, J., Rodgers, J., McConachie, H., & Parr, J. R. (2014). Reducing specific phobia/fear in young people with autism spectrum disorders (ASDs) through a virtual reality environment intervention. *PLOS One, 9,* Article e100374.

Meindl, J. N., Saba, S., Gray, M., Stuebing, L., & Jarvis, A. (2019). Reducing blood draw phobia in an adult with autism spectrum disorder using low-cost virtual reality exposure therapy. *Journal of Applied Research in Intellectual Disabilities, 32,* 1446–1452.

Muris, P., Steerneman, P., Merckelbach, H., Holdrinet, I., & Meesters, C. (1998). Comorbid anxiety symptoms in children with pervasive developmental disorders. *Journal of Anxiety Disorders, 12,* 387–393.

Olatunji, B. O., Deacon, B. J., & Abramowitz, J. S. (2009). The cruelest cure?: Ethical issues in the implementation of exposure-based treatments. *Cognitive and Behavioral Practice, 16*(2), 172–180.

Pavlov, I. P. (1927). *Conditioned reflexes.* Oxford University Press.

Pryce, C. R., Lehmann, J., & Feldon, J. (1999). Effect of sex on fear conditioning is similar for context and discrete CS in Wistar, Lewis and Fischer rat strains. *Pharmacology Biochemistry and Behavior, 64,* 753–759.

Rachman, S. J. (1977). The conditioning theory of fear acquisition: A critical examination. *Behaviour Research and Therapy, 15,* 375–387.

Rasmussen, E. B., Clay, C. J., Pierce, W. D., & Cheney, C. D. (2022). *Behavior analysis and learning: A biobehavioral approach.* Taylor & Francis.

Rescorla, R. A., & Heth, C. D. (1975). Reinstatement of fear to an extinguished conditioned stimulus. *Journal of Experimental Psychology: Animal Behavior Processes, 1,* 88–96.

Ricciardi, J. N., Luiselli, J. K., & Camare, M. (2006). Shaping approach responses as intervention for specific phobia in a child with autism. *Journal of Applied Behavior Analysis, 39,* 445–448.

Richman, D. M., Dotson, W. H., Rose, C. A., Thompson, S., & Abby, L. (2012). Effects of age on the types and severity of excessive fear or the absence of fear in children and young adults with autism. *Journal of Mental Health Research in Intellectual Disabilities, 5,* 215–235.

Rosen, T. E., Connell, J. E., & Kerns, C. M. (2016). A review of behavioral interventions for anxiety-related behaviors in lower-functioning individuals with autism. *Behavioral Interventions, 31,* 120–143.

Rowe, M. K., & Craske, M. G. (1998). Effects of varied-stimulus exposure training on fear reduction and return of fear. *Behaviour Research and Therapy, 36*(7–8), 719–734.

Schlund, M. W., Ludlum, M., Magee, S. K.,

Tone, E. B., Brewer, A., Richman, D. M., & Dymond, S. (2020). Renewal of fear and avoidance in humans to escalating threat: Implications for translational research on anxiety disorders. *Journal of the Experimental Analysis of Behavior, 113*, 153–171.

Shabani, D. B., & Fisher, W. W. (2006). Stimulus fading and differential reinforcement for the treatment of needle phobia in a youth with autism. *Journal of Applied Behavior Analysis, 39*, 449–452.

Shahan, T. A., & Craig, A. R. (2017). Resurgence as choice. *Behavioural Processes, 141*, 100–127.

Shiban, Y., Pauli, P., & Mühlberger, A. (2013). Effect of multiple context exposure on renewal in spider phobia. *Behaviour Research and Therapy, 51*, 68–74.

Simonoff, E., Pickles, A., Charman, T., Chandler, S., Loucas, T., & Baird, G. (2008). Psychiatric disorders in children with autism spectrum disorders: Prevalence, comorbidity, and associated factors in a population-derived sample. *Journal of the American Academy of Child and Adolescent Psychiatry, 47*, 921–929.

South, M., Larson, M. J., White, S. E., Dana, J., & Crowley, M. J. (2011). Better fear conditioning is associated with reduced symptom severity in autism spectrum disorders. *Autism Research, 4*, 412–421.

Sukhodolsky, D. G., Scahill, L., Gadow, K. D., Arnold, L. E., Aman, M. G., McDougle, C. J., . . . Vitiello, B. (2008). Parent-rated anxiety symptoms in children with pervasive developmental disorders: Frequency and association with core autism symptoms and cognitive functioning. *Journal of Abnormal Child Psychology, 36*, 117–128.

Thomas, B. L., Larsen, N., & Ayres, J. J. (2003). Role of context similarity in ABA, ABC, and AAB renewal paradigms: Implications for theories of renewal and for treating human phobias. *Learning and Motivation, 34*, 410–436.

Tiwari, S., Kendall, P. C., Hoff, A. L., Harrison, J. P., & Fizur, P. (2013). Characteristics of exposure sessions as predictors of treatment response in anxious youth. *Journal of Clinical Child and Adolescent Psychology, 42*, 34–43.

Tolin, D. F., Davies, C. D., Moskow, D. M., & Hofmann, S. G. (2020). Biofeedback and neurofeedback for anxiety disorders: A quantitative and qualitative systematic review. *Anxiety Disorders, 1191*, 265–289.

Top, D. N., Jr., Stephenson, K. G., Doxey, C. R., Crowley, M. J., Kirwan, C. B., & South, M. (2016). Atypical amygdala response to fear conditioning in autism spectrum disorder. *Biological Psychiatry: Cognitive Neuroscience and Neuroimaging, 1*, 308–315.

Turner, L. B., & Romanczyk, R. G. (2012). Assessment of fear in children with an autism spectrum disorder. *Research in Autism Spectrum Disorders, 6*, 1203–1210.

Tyner, S., Brewer, A., Helman, M., Leon, Y., Pritchard, J., & Schlund, M. (2016). Nice doggie!: Contact desensitization plus reinforcement decreases dog phobias for children with autism. *Behavior Analysis in Practice, 9*, 54–57.

Vervliet, B., Craske, M. G., & Hermans, D. (2013). Fear extinction and relapse: State of the art. *Annual Review of Clinical Psychology, 9*, 215–248.

Wathen, S. N., & Podlesnik, C. A. (2018). Laboratory models of treatment relapse and mitigation techniques. *Behavior Analysis: Research and Practice, 18*, 362–387.

Weisman, R. G., & Litner, J. S. (1969). Positive conditioned reinforcement of Sidman avoidance behavior in rats. *Journal of Comparative and Physiological Psychology, 68*, 597–603.

Wolff, J. J., & Symons, F. J. (2013). An evaluation of multi-component exposure treatment of needle phobia in an adult with autism and intellectual disability. *Journal of Applied Research in Intellectual Disabilities, 26*, 344–348.

Wolpe, J. (1958). *Psychotherapy by reciprocal inhibition.* Stanford University Press.

OPERANT CONDITIONING

CHAPTER 9

Reinforcement

FOUNDATIONAL PRINCIPLES AND THEIR APPLICATIONS

Charlene N. Agnew
Rafaela M. Fontes
Nicole M. DeRosa
Andrew R. Craig

Reinforcement is among the most fundamental principles of learning. It is a topic that is covered in every textbook on behavior, and nearly every introductory textbook on psychology. Authors have described reinforcement in different ways. For example, Keller and Schoenfeld (1950) described "positive reinforcers as those stimuli which strengthen responses when presented (e.g., food strengthens bar-pressing or loop-pulling behavior), and negative reinforcers as those which strengthen when they are removed" (p. 61). Alternatively, Powell et al. (2017) suggested that "an event is a reinforcer if it (1) follows a behavior, and (2) the future probability of that behavior increases" (p. 218). Domjam (2015) defined reinforcement through a focus on the procedural aspects of reinforcement, stating that "positive reinforcement is a procedure in which the instrumental response produces an appetitive stimulus" (p. 131), as did Chance (2014), who stated that "in positive reinforcement, the consequence of a behavior is the appearance of, or an increase in the intensity of, a stimulus" (p. 133). Regardless of how one defines *reinforcement,* the principle underscores many of the other concepts presented in this text, including stimulus control, extinction, differential reinforcement, motivation, choice, and verbal behavior. Reinforcement plays an important role in our everyday behavior, whether those behaviors are desirable or undesirable.

The principle of reinforcement also carries substantial theoretical baggage. The way behavior analysts have conceptualized reinforcement has evolved over the years (for discussion, see Shahan, 2017), leaving practitioners and researchers in what may feel like an uncomfortable position; that is, behavior analysts *use* reinforcement daily to promote socially significant behavior change or to uncover the complexities of behavior in laboratory situations, but the concept itself has been and continues to be a dynamic one and one that is the center of debate in the science of behavior analysis.

In this chapter, we provide a historical overview of the concept of reinforcement and, in doing so, shed light on the way behavior analysts have discussed and thought about reinforcement throughout the development of the field of behavior analysis. Next, we describe theories of reinforcement that are meant to help behavior analysts understand why and how reinforcement affects behavior. We do not aim to settle any debates that center on the concept of reinforcement, but we do wish to provide information to readers, so that they can appreciate how the concept has evolved over time. We also provide information about how reinforcement is used in clinical applications of behavior-analytic principles.

History of the Concept of Reinforcement

The idea that behavior is affected by its consequences was first proposed as the *law of effect* by Thorndike (1898, 1911, 1932; Thorndike & Columbia University, 1932) in his studies with nonhuman animals such as cats in puzzle boxes. In those studies, Thorndike observed that responses that were followed by *satisfactory* or *pleasant* consequences were more likely to reoccur, while responses followed by *uncomfortable* or *unpleasant* consequences were less likely to reoccur. Thorndike's notion that behavior is impacted by its consequences set the foundation for the scientific approach to explaining behavior later proposed by Skinner (1938). However, contrary to Thorndike (1898, 1911), Skinner (1938) focused on observable events and rejected explanations that referred to unobservable mental states and feelings. Skinner (1938) abandoned the use of Thorndike's subjective terms such as *satisfying, pleasant,* or *unpleasant* and instead referred to the consequences that increase/strengthen behavior as *reinforcers*.[1] This term allowed Skinner to do two things. First, it allowed him to establish a technical term that was not associated with other meanings in popular speech, such as "reward" (Michael, 1975; Skinner, 1938). His goal was to use a scientific vocabulary and avoid resorting to unobservable constructs, thereby setting the stage for increased parsimony and a focus on observable behavior. Second, it allowed Skinner to map onto the terms already in use within classical conditioning, where *reinforcer* referred to the unconditioned stimuli that were assumed to strengthen the relationship between the conditioned stimulus and the unconditioned stimulus (Michael, 1975). In his description of operant behavior, however, Skinner (1938, 1953a, 1953b) defined *reinforcer* as any stimulus that follows a behavior and increases the frequency (or probability) of that behavior in the future.

Skinner's definition of *reinforcer* contains two essential features (Sidman, 1989). First, a reinforcer must be contingent on a response, in that it is a consequence for a given behavior. Second, a reinforcer must increase the frequency and/or the probability of that behavior. Therefore, the definition of *reinforcer* is conditional upon its effects on behavior. One of the advantages of this conditional definition is a shift in focus to the function of the stimulus (i.e., how the stimulus impacts behavior) rather than its topography, thus excluding from the definition any reference to mental states or feelings caused by the presentation of the reinforcing stimulus (i.e., pleasure, satisfaction). This functional definition is the crucial difference between Skinner's and Thorndike's approaches to explain behavior.

---

[1] The term *reinforcer* refers to the stimulus presented or removed following an operant response that increases the frequency of that response. The term *reinforcement* refers to both (1) the procedure of using reinforcers to increase the frequency of a given response and (2) the behavioral process that results in increases in response rates during reinforcement procedures.

Reinforcers are further categorized as either positive reinforcers and negative reinforcers. Skinner (1938) initially used the terms *positive* and *negative* to distinguish between stimuli that increase or decrease, respectively, the frequency of behavior; that is, where positive reinforcers referred to consequences that increase (i.e., strengthen) the behavior they follow, and negative reinforcers referred to consequences that decrease (i.e., weaken) the behavior they follow. Since that time, the concept of reinforcement and the distinction between positive and negative reinforcers has been refined to a more technical definition throughout several iterations. For example, in 1950, Keller and Schoenfeld proposed that the term *reinforcer* should only refer to consequences that increase the frequency of behavior and that *punisher* should be used to refer to consequences that decrease the frequency of behavior. Furthermore, they suggested the distinction between positive and negative should indicate the addition or subtraction of the stimulus from the situation, instead of the effects of those operations on behavior. Therefore, according to Keller and Schoenfeld's definition, an increase in the frequency of a response following the addition of a stimulus that was previously absent should be classified as positive reinforcement. For example, if presenting food contingent on a response increases the frequency of that response, food is then considered a positive reinforcer because it was "added" (+) to the situation following the response. Conversely, negative reinforcement is the increase in the frequency of a response following the removal of a stimulus that was present. For example, if removing a loud sound contingent on a response increases the future probability of that response occurring, removal of the sound is then considered a negative reinforcer, because the sound was "subtracted" (–) from the situation. These definitions of positive and negative reinforcers/reinforcement became standard and were adopted by Skinner (1953a) himself.

The effects of reinforcers on behavior have been extensively demonstrated empirically with nonhuman animals since the term was proposed in the 1930s (e.g., Ferster & Skinner, 1957; Guercio, 2018; Lattal, 1998, 2013; Skinner, 1953b; we return to these topics below). However, it was only in the late 1950s and early 1960s that the concept of reinforcement was extended to the study of human behavior. Initial studies focused on replicating the findings from nonhuman animals in the laboratory with both clinical and nonclinical populations (Morris et al., 2013). For example, in one of the first applied studies using operant procedures, Fuller (1949) demonstrated that contingent reinforcer delivery resulted in an increase in the arm movement of a comatose patient.

Conditioning principles then began to be applied by researchers and clinicians to the treatment of behavioral disorders in humans (e.g., Azrin & Lindsley, 1956; Barrett, 1962; Bijou, 1955, 1957; Ferster & DeMyer, 1962; Wolf et al., 1964) and to be used in psychiatric facilities to shape and maintain certain behaviors and decrease other behaviors among patients (e.g., Ayllon & Azrin, 1964, 1965; Ayllon & Haughton, 1964; Bensberg et al., 1965). For example, Ayllon and Azrin (1965) conducted a series of experiments in a mental hospital using reinforcers to increase responses among patients such as serving meals, sorting laundry, and cleaning dishes. The results demonstrated that selected behaviors could be maintained while interventions were in place, but the same behaviors decreased once reinforcement was no longer delivered (a process known as *extinction*; see Schieltz et al., Chapter 12, this volume).

The successful application of reinforcement procedures to diverse settings and populations speaks to the generality of reinforcement principles. Indeed, subsequent decades of research with both human participants and nonhuman subjects provided substantial empirical evidence that behavior is established and maintained by both positive and negative reinforcement contingencies (e.g., Beavers et al., 2013; Hanley et al., 2003; Guercio, 2018; Lattal, 1998; Morris et al., 2013). We next describe some of the conceptual nuances associated with, and empirical work dedicated to, positive and negative reinforcement to provide readers with a better understanding of the role these processes play within behavior analysis.

Positive and Negative Reinforcement

Although positive and negative reinforcers have similar effects on behavior (i.e., increase its frequency), they have been described and studied as separate behavioral processes. The distinction between positive and negative reinforcers is mainly based on the procedures used in each case and the transitions between stimulus situations they entail (Baron & Galizio, 2005; Michael, 1975; Nevin & Mandell, 2017). With positive reinforcement, the response results in the presentation of a stimulus that was previously absent. Thus, responding results in a transition from a condition where the reinforcing stimulus (e.g., food) is absent (i.e., before the response) to a condition where the reinforcing stimulus is present (i.e., after the response).

Conversely, negative reinforcement encompasses two types of responses, *escape* and *avoidance*, and thus two types of transitions. During escape, the response results in the removal of a (typically aversive) stimulus that was previously present. For example, escape is studied in the laboratory by presenting an aversive stimulus (e.g., shock) that is only removed after the animal emits a response (e.g., pressing a lever). Thus, during escape, responding results in a transition from a condition where the aversive stimulus is present (i.e., shock presented before a lever press) to a condition where the aversive stimulus is absent (i.e., removal of shock after a lever press; e.g., Boren et al., 1959; Dinsmoor et al., 1958; Kelsey, 1977).

During avoidance, a response results in the cancellation of the future presentation of an aversive stimulus. In the laboratory, avoidance is studied by presenting the aversive stimulus (e.g., shock) according to programmed intervals (e.g., shocks are delivered every 30 seconds). In such procedures, responding (e.g., pressing the lever) during the interval between shocks delays the next shock presentation (e.g., Boren et al., 1959; Hineline & Rachlin, 1969; Sidman, 1953a, 1953b). Thus, the transition produced by responding during avoidance is less clear, because responding occurs before the aversive stimulus is presented. If the avoidance response is successful, the aversive stimulus is absent both before and after the response. This peculiarity of the avoidance procedure has generated much debate as to what maintains responding in such conditions (see the section "Theories of Negative Reinforcement" for more detail).

These differences in procedure and the type of stimulus involved in each case (i.e., appetitive vs. aversive) are the main aspects maintaining the conceptual distinction between positive and negative reinforcement (Michael, 1975; Sidman, 1989). However, the validity and utility of such distinction have been challenged by many. Michael (1975, 2006) and Baron and Galizio (2005, 2006) have argued that in many situations, the distinction between positive and negative reinforcement is ambiguous, making it hard to identify which consequence is controlling a behavior. These authors have suggested that every situation can be interpreted as a positive or negative reinforcement contingency, depending on the aspect of the situation to which one is attending. For example, is "turning on the light" maintained by the addition of the light to the room (i.e., positive reinforcement) or the removal of the darkness (i.e., negative reinforcement)? Are responses followed by food maintained by the presentation of food (i.e., positive reinforcement) or by the reduction in hunger (i.e., negative reinforcement)? Besides the difficulty in distinguishing whether the presentation or removal of a stimulus is the variable maintaining a behavior, in many situations, behavior may be maintained by both types of reinforcers concomitantly. For example, an employee may dedicate themself to work because doing so results in a bonus at the end of the month and also avoids reprimands from a boss. For these reasons, Michael (1975) suggested that the positive–negative distinction is unnecessary and it would be more parsimonious to abandon it and refer to all contingencies that increase the frequency of behavior as reinforcement, and all contingencies that decrease the frequency of behavior as punishment.

Although Michael's (1975) position has been accepted as logical and coherent (e.g., Baron & Galizio, 2005, 2006; Lattal & Lattal, 2006; Jackson Marr, 2006), the positive-negative distinction has persisted in the field and continues to be used and taught to new generations of behavior analysts. One possible reason for the preservation of this distinction is that identifying the consequences maintaining behavior based on aspects of the procedure (i.e., addition or removal of a stimulus) serves a function within the verbal community (Chase, 2006; Iwata, 2006). For example, this distinction can be especially practical for treatment of certain types of behavior disorders in applied settings, as it allows clinicians to describe the stimuli to be added or removed throughout various treatment procedures. Importantly, regardless of the positive or negative label and the arbitrariness of this distinction, data from basic, translational, and applied research have provided strong empirical evidence for the relevance and impact of reinforcement on our daily lives.

Theories of Reinforcement

Despite a large amount of empirical evidence showing that reinforcers increase the frequency of the behavior they follow, there has been much debate over how reinforcement works as a process. Several theories have been proposed in an attempt to provide an accurate description of the mechanisms underlying reinforcement; that is, practice shows us *that* reinforcement works to increase the future probability of behavior. Theories of reinforcement attempt to tell us *why* it does so. In this section, we describe several of these positions. Our goal is not to resolve any disagreements between theories or to point to one theory over others as the best approximation of process. Instead, we hope only to provide readers with a survey of different ways of conceptualizing reinforcement.

The Reflex Reserve

The main theoretical assumption underlying the model Skinner (1938, 1948) proposed is that a reinforcer functions by *strengthening* the response it follows. According to Skinner (1938), of all possible responses to be emitted by the organism, "stronger" responses have a higher probability of occurring than weak responses, and the strength of a given response is a function of its past consequences. Because reinforcers work by strengthening the response they follow, responses that are reinforced become stronger and thus more likely to occur.

To explain the strengthening process, Skinner (1938) initially used the concept of the *reflex reserve*. Although the mechanisms operating the reflex reserve were never described in detail, the basic premise was that reinforcers work by filling a reservoir that controls the rate of responding (Killeen, 1988; Shahan, 2017). The level of the reservoir was hypothesized to be a direct function of the rate of reinforcers, and the fuller the reservoir is, the stronger the response becomes. Because stronger responses were assumed to be emitted at higher rates, absolute response rate was used as an index of response strength. Therefore, higher reinforcer rates should result in stronger responses that would be emitted at high rates (for a more detailed discussion on the functioning of the reflex reserve, see Catania, 2005; Killeen, 1988).

However, studies showing higher response rates with partial (i.e., intermittent) schedules of reinforcement than with continuous schedules of reinforcement challenged the assumption that higher reinforcer rates result in stronger responses. If response strength, and consequently response rate, are a direct function of reinforcer rates, continuous schedules should result in stronger responses and higher response rates than partial schedules. Partial reinforcement effects also posed problems for the use of response rate as a measure of response strength by showing that response rates do not always increase with increases in reinforcer rate. For example, ratio schedules produce higher response rates than interval schedules, even when the same reinforcer rate is programmed by both schedules (e.g., Baum, 1993; Ferster & Skinner, 1957; Zuriff, 1970).

These and other findings brought to light some fundamental problems with the concept of response strength as a complete explanation for reinforcement (Hursh, 1980, 1984; Hursh & Silberberg, 2008) and challenged the reflex reserve as a theory of behavior. Perhaps this explains why Skinner abandoned the notion of reflex reserve and never fully described the mechanisms underlying the effects of reinforcers on response strength (Killeen, 1988; Hursh & Silberberg, 2008). Regardless, the strengthening assumption implicit in Skinner's writings has guided how behavior analysts explain and understand the relation between response and reinforcer (e.g., Shahan, 2010, 2017; Simon et al., 2020).

The Matching Law

A special challenge for response rate as an index of strength was posed by Herrnstein in his experiments with concurrent schedules of reinforcement (1961, 1970, 1974). Herrnstein's findings revealed a new type of orderliness between response and reinforcer rates. More specifically, when different response options are available and those options are associated with different conditions of reinforcement, the proportion of responses allocated to one of the options matches the proportion of reinforcers obtained from that option. To describe this relationship between the distribution of responses and reinforcers in concurrent-schedule situations, Herrnstein proposed a quantitative model known as the *matching law* (see McComas et al., Chapter 16, this volume).

Besides providing an accurate description of response allocation in choice situations, the matching law also pointed to a new response-strength index that could overcome the limitations noted earlier with absolute response rates. From a matching law approach, response strength should be measured through relative instead of absolute response rates; that is, the strength of a given response should be measured by the proportion of responses allocated to one option relative to another, because response allocation is more sensitive to changes in parameters of reinforcement than absolute response rates (Killeen & Hall, 2001).

This change in measurement also resulted in an extension of the concept of strength, with studies showing that response allocation matches not only relative reinforcer rates but also relative reinforcer magnitude (e.g., Catania, 1963) and relative reinforcer immediacy (e.g., Chung & Herrnstein, 1967). As a result, strength was no longer described as a function of reinforcer rate, but of reinforcer value, where value resulted from the combination of reinforcer parameters such as rate, magnitude, and delay (Baum & Rachlin, 1969). Importantly, more valuable reinforcers were assumed to have a greater strengthening power than less valuable ones, and the value of a given reinforcer (i.e., its strengthening power) was not to be measured in absolute terms, but in relation to another reinforcer through changes in response allocation.

The use of relative measures as an index of response strength was superior to the absolute rates used by Skinner, because this measure was more sensitive to changes in reinforcer parameters and did not assume a linear relationship between rate of responding and absolute rate (or amount) of reinforcers. However, Herrnstein's approach did assume a linear relation between response allocation and reinforcer *value* (Rachlin, 1971). This assumption has been challenged by empirical evidence showing that changes in allocation can be impacted by variables other than reinforcer parameters, such as the availability of other sources of reinforcement (i.e., open vs. closed economies of reinforcement—see more below; Hursh, 1980, 1984; Rachlin et al., 1980; Schwartz et al., 2016). Another limitation of Herrnstein's approach is that response allocation does not provide any way to measure the absolute value of a reinforcer in isolation, only the value of a reinforcer relative to another (Hursh, 1980). Last, matching-based models are only suitable to compare the value of reinforcers that are substitutable with one another (i.e., one reinforcer can replace another; food vs. food) as opposed to reinforcers that are complementary with (i.e., consumption of one reinforcer directly varies with consumption of another; chips and salsa) or independent of (i.e., reinforcers that share no relation; milk and gasoline) one another (Hursh & Roma, 2016; Hursh & Silberberg, 2008; see also Madden et al., Chapter 21, this volume).

Although these limitations have raised questions about the adequacy of response allocation as a scale for reinforcement value, the matching law still is one of the most popular and influential quantitative theories in behavior analysis and its principles underlie many other behavioral theories (e.g., Deluty, 1976; de Villiers, 1980; Fantino, 1969; Mazur, 1987; Shahan & Craig, 2017). The matching law also has important implications for behavioral treatments in applied settings and has informed how reinforcers should be programmed during interventions (Fisher & Mazur, 1997). As one example, differential reinforcement of alternative behavior (DRA), a procedure commonly used during behavioral interventions, is based on the idea that responding to one option (i.e., problem behavior) can be decreased by increasing response allocation toward a competing option (i.e., alternative behavior) that is associated with a more valuable reinforcer (McDowell, 1988, 1989). Choice-based preference assessments are also inspired by the matching law assumption that the value of a reinforcer can be measured through response allocation in concurrent-schedule situations. Thus, more valuable reinforcers should be chosen more often than less valuable ones (Fisher et al., 1992; Piazza et al., 1996; Roscoe et al., 1999).

Behavioral Momentum Theory

Nevin's studies of behavior under multiple schedules of reinforcement further extended our understanding of response strength. In his seminal study, Nevin (1974) trained pigeons to peck keys on two separate components, each associated with different reinforcer rates and signaled by distinct discriminative stimuli. Nevin then observed that when responding was disrupted by the delivery of response-independent food or extinction, responding in the presence of the stimulus associated with the richer schedule of reinforcement was more resistant to change (i.e., responding decreased slower) than responding in the presence of the stimulus associated with the leaner schedule of reinforcement.

The variables thought to give rise to these findings were formalized by *behavioral momentum theory* (BMT; Nevin et al., 1983), which was built as a metaphor relating persistence of behavior to Newton's second law of motion, which states that the changes in velocity of a moving object are a direct function of the magnitude of force applied to the object and an inverse function of the object's mass. In behavioral terms, BMT proposes that when a disruptor is applied to an ongoing behavior, the decrease in response rate is a direct function of the magnitude of the disruptor and an inverse function of response strength (Nevin & Grace, 2000; Nevin & Shahan, 2011).

Importantly, according to BMT, response strength (i.e., "behavioral mass") is a function of the reinforcement rate delivered in a stimulus situation. Additionally, BMT proposes that response rate and resistance to change are two different aspects of operant behavior and result from distinct relations within the three-term contingency.[2] While response rate is governed by the relation between the reinforcers and the responses that produce them, resistance to change is governed by the relation between the reinforcer and the discriminative stimulus present when the reinforcer is delivered. Therefore, resistance to change is controlled by the rate (or magnitude) of reinforcers delivered in the presence of a specific stimulus, regardless of the response rate in the presence of that stimulus.

Indeed, several studies in both basic and applied settings have demonstrated that responding in multiple-schedule components associated with richer schedules of reinforcement is more resistant to change than responding in components associated with leaner schedules of reinforcement (e.g., Mace & Belfiore, 1990; Mace et al., 1988; Nevin et al., 1990). Furthermore, many of these studies provide evidence that reinforcers increase response strength (i.e., increase resistance to change) independently of changes in response rates (for review, see Craig et al., Chapter 18, this volume).

The BMT approach to response strength is similar to Skinner's approach in that both are based on the assumption that reinforcers increase response strength and that responses associated with higher reinforcer rates are stronger than responses associated with lower reinforcer rates. However, contrary to Skinner, BMT proposes that the strength of a response should be measured through its resistance to change in the face of a disruptor instead of response rate, because stronger responses are more resistant to disruption than weaker responses. The BMT approach also differs from the matching law approach in how it suggests one ought to measure response strength. While the matching law measures strength through relative response rates in concurrent schedules (i.e., response allocation between different options), BMT measures strength through response rates in the components of a multiple schedule as proportion of their preceding baselines. However, it is important to note that, similar to relative response rates, resistance to change is also a function of *relative* reinforcer rates delivered in the presence of a given discriminative stimulus; that is, a component is considered rich or lean in relation to the reinforcer rate delivered in the other component of the multiple schedule.

Although BMT has accounted for data from multiple schedules, the theory has been challenged as an adequate theory for understanding response strength by several empirical findings that run counter to the theory's assertions. For example, BMT has failed

---

[2] The three-term contingency (S^D: B → C) describes the relation between an antecedent stimulus (S^D), the behavior (B), and the consequence (C).

to predict data generated from single schedules (e.g., Cohen, 1998; Cohen et al., 1993), which suggests that resistance to change may not be a measure of the true strength of a response but only a measure of strength under specific conditions. Furthermore, the assumption of independence between response rate and resistance to change has also been challenged. For example, studies manipulating response rates across the components of a multiple schedule while equating reinforcer rate across components have demonstrated that, under some conditions, low rates of responding are more resistant to change than higher rates (e.g., Blackman, 1968; Lattal, 1989; Nevin et al., 2012). Last, evidence showing no differential resistance to change with extreme (i.e., 1:100 reinforcer-rate differential) differences in reinforcer rates between multiple-schedule components has also posed a challenge to BMT (McLean et al., 2012). If response strength is a direct function of reinforcer rates, as assumed by the theory, increasing reinforcer rate in a discriminative context should increase resistance to change, and decreasing reinforcer rate in a discriminative context should decrease resistance to change.

Nonetheless, BMT is still an influential behavioral theory, and extensions of BMT have been proposed to account for more complex phenomena, such as relapse (e.g., Shahan & Sweeney, 2011; but for a discussion on the limitations of the BMT model of relapse, see Craig & Shahan, 2016; Nevin et al., 2017). Furthermore, BMT has important implications for the treatment of problem behavior (Plaud & Gaither, 1996; Pritchard et al., 2014). For example, studies based on BMT demonstrated that the use of DRA during treatment can increase the strength of problem behavior by increasing the reinforcer rate in the stimulus condition wherein the problem behavior was reinforced. As a result, DRA may increase the resistance to change of problem behavior (e.g., Mace et al., 2010; Wacker et al., 2011). Such findings have provided important information to practitioners and offer insights about some of the undesirable side effects of procedures typically used during behavioral interventions.

Behavior-Economics Framework

Another approach to understanding reinforcer value was proposed by Hursh (1980, 1984), who drew from the field of microeconomics to explain differences in responding to similar schedules of reinforcement across studies. In this analysis, discrepancies in performance when parameters of reinforcement are held constant can indicate other variables that affect responding. For example, in studies wherein all the food available to the animal is earned during the experimental session (i.e., closed economy), animals respond at higher and more consistent rates than in studies wherein supplemental feeding is received after the sessions (i.e., open economy). Roane et al. (2005) demonstrated this difference in responding in an applied setting as well when they compared rates of adaptive behavior emitted by participants with intellectual and developmental disabilities when they received reinforcers after completion of a session (open economy) and when reinforcers were only available during sessions (closed economy). These authors found more responding within the closed-economy than in the open-economy arrangement.

The findings just described could not be accommodated by any approach that regarded *value* solely as a function of reinforcer dimensions such as rate or amount. Instead, Hursh proposed that value is not an intrinsic property of the reinforcing stimulus but instead the result of the relation between consumption (i.e., obtained reinforcers) and cost (i.e., the number of responses required per reinforcer; Hursh & Roma, 2016; Hursh & Silberberg, 2008; Madden, 2000). Thus, from a behavioral-economic perspective, reinforcer value is better measured by demand curves that describe changes in consumption as a function of changes in the cost to obtain each reinforcer (Hursh, 1980, 1984; Hursh & Silberberg, 2008). Because consumption decreases with increases in cost, the rate of decrease provides a measure of elasticity of demand. If demand is elastic, consumption is highly impacted by increases in price. If demand is inelastic, changes in price will result in minimal, if any, changes in consumption. Thus, elasticity of demand indicates the sensitivity of consumption to increases in cost and is assumed to be inversely related to reinforcer value, because organisms work harder across a range of prices for more valuable reinforcers than for less valuable reinforcers (e.g., Christensen et al., 2008; Hursh et al., 1988; Madden et al., 2007a, 2007b).

Drawing from the idea that reinforcer value is an inverse function of elasticity of demand, and using the model put forth by Hursh et al. (1988) as a foundation, Hursh and Silberberg (2008) proposed an augmented quantitative model (i.e., exponential model of demand [EMD]) that provides a metric to compare the value of qualitatively different reinforcing stimuli that may compete with the those behavioral measures described so far (i.e., response rate, relative response rate, and resistance to change). The EMD has been useful for evaluating variables that affect reinforcer value (e.g., the reinforcing stimulus and the economic context into which that stimulus is delivered) separately from variables that affect responding (e.g., changes in reinforcer magnitude or response effort). Therefore, the model may provide a more sensitive measure of changes in value than response allocation or resistance to change (Hursh & Silberberg, 2008; Johnson & Bickel, 2006; Schwartz et al., 2016). Furthermore, because reinforcer value is measured by the rate of decrease in consumption when cost increases, EMD provides a way to measure the value of single reinforcers and also serves as an adequate metric for directly comparing the value of qualitatively and functionally different reinforcers, overcoming some of the main limitations of the matching law and BMT.

The behavior-economic framework also has important implications for application and has been used to study factors that impact problem behavior in several contexts (e.g., Avcu et al., 2019; Bickel et al., 1993; Borrero et al., 2007; Cassidy & Kurti, 2018). Analysis of demand has also been shown to be a useful tool for identifying reinforcers to be used during treatment (Delmendo et al., 2009; Reed et al., 2013). For example, Roane et al. (2001) used a progressive-ratio assessment informed by behavioral economics and demand analyses to examine the correspondence between the reinforcer efficacy of specific toys and outcomes from interventions for problem behavior that incorporated those specific toys as reinforcers within intervention. In this study, the "cost" of each reinforcer was progressively increased until the break point, or the point at which responding stopped. The authors found that toys that were associated with higher break points also were more effective when used to treat problem behavior than toys associated with lower break points. Behavior economics principles and procedures also have been used to inform public policy related to treatment for myriad health-related behaviors such as substance use (see Hursh, 1991; Hursh & Roma, 2013). This work demonstrates the importance of the concept of reinforcement for human health and safety.

Theories of Negative Reinforcement

The theories mentioned earlier have mainly focused on positive reinforcers, and limited attempts to extend the theories to negative reinforcers have been made. Extensions are often based on the assumption that positive and negative reinforcers have similar effects on response strength. For example, studies using concurrent schedules of negative reinforcement have suggested that when shock reduction is considered the reinforcer, response allocation is a function of relative reinforcer rates (Baum, 1973; de Villiers, 1974). These findings suggest that responses maintained by negative reinforcers can also be described by the matching law. Furthermore, studies investigating the effects of negative reinforcer rate on resistance to change have suggested that higher rates of negative reinforcers result in greater resistance to change compared to lower rates (Romani et al., 2016; Zuj et al., 2020), which suggests that BMT can account for the effects of negative reinforcers on response strength. The behavior-economics framework and EMD also have been used to investigate the value of negative reinforcers and to compare the value of negative and positive reinforcers (e.g., Avcu et al., 2019; Fragale et al., 2017; Spiegler et al., 2018). Furthermore, research in this area has demonstrated that elasticity of demand is a reliable measure for the value of both positive and negative reinforcers. There is also evidence that the value of a negative reinforcer is a function of the aversive nature of the stimulus to be escaped from or avoided, because increases in the intensity of the aversive stimulus increase consumption and decrease elasticity of demand (Fragale et al., 2017).

As previously mentioned, the avoidance procedure is peculiar in that it lacks a clear and immediate consequence following the response. This peculiarity has generated discussion about the consequences that maintain avoidance responses. Two main theories have been proposed to account for the variables maintaining avoidance: the two-factor theory and the shock-reduction theory (Hineline & Rosales-Ruiz, 2013). The two-factor theory of avoidance is based on the idea that avoidance functionally serves as escape from stimuli associated with the unconditioned aversive stimulus. The two-factor theory was based on the findings from studies arranging a warning signal (e.g., light or tone) indicating that a shock was imminent. Responding during the warning signal removed the warning stimulus and canceled the next presentation of shock. The results from such studies showed that organisms quickly learned to respond while the warning signal was on to avoid the shock (e.g., Dinsmoor & Sears, 1973; Kamin, 1957; Rescorla, 1969). Thus, the first factor in two-factor theory is the development of an aversive Pavlovian association between a warning signal and the aversive outcome delivered at the end of the signal. The second factor involves operant escape, wherein engaging in some operant response is reinforced by termination of the aversive conditioned stimulus (i.e., the warning signal).

However, studies using the Sidman avoidance procedure, wherein avoidance is maintained in the absence of a warning signal (e.g., Sidman, 1953a, 1962a), have challenged the two-factor theory, and have given rise to the one-factor shock-reduction theory. The shock-reduction theory is based on a molar approach (e.g., Baum, 2002) and does not require any reference to immediate and contiguous consequences to explain avoidance. Instead, shock-reduction theory proposes that a reduction in the overall frequency of shocks received maintains avoidance. Thus, the consequence maintaining avoidance is not a discrete event but is instead extended in time and results from the transition from a situation with higher obtained shock rates (i.e., in the absence of responding) to a situation with lower obtained shock rates (i.e., in the presence of responding). Some empirical support for shock-reduction theory has been generated by experiments showing that avoidance is maintained when responding results in equal or lower overall shock frequency, but not when responding increases the overall shock frequency (Herrnstein & Hineline, 1966; Hineline, 1970; Sidman, 1962b).

Alternatives to Response Strength

As we hope our earlier review suggests, the concept of response strength is at the core of many influential, contemporary behavioral theories (e.g., the matching law, behavioral momentum theory). Despite the fact that response strength continues to shape the way behavior analysts think about reinforcement, there are reasons one may wish to look elsewhere for potential mechanisms that drive learning. First, as we described earlier, most theories of reinforcement that deal with response strength (e.g., the matching law, behavioral momentum theory) are faced with conceptual or empirical challenges that raise questions about their characterizations of response strength. Additional, more general, reasons have received extensive treatment elsewhere (Gallistel et al., 2019; Gallistel & Gibbon, 2000; Shahan, 2010, 2017), so we do not attempt to reinvent the wheel here. To provide additional context, though, we summarize the general argument against response strength offered by Shahan (2017), who provided a critique of the construct and its place (or lack thereof, as the case may be) in behavior analysis.

Strengthening a behavior by means of reinforcement implies that individual reinforcer deliveries impart some amount of strength to the behavior that accumulates with additional reinforcer deliveries. Presumably, too, response strength decumulates to some extent when organisms experience nonreinforcement. Furthermore, if response strength is taken as a fundament of learning, then in the absence of reinforcement, learning should not occur. Such accumulation–decumulation-based processes fail to account for complex behavioral outcomes such as cue-competition effects in Pavlovian conditioning and relapse processes after extinction (see, in this volume, Escobar et al., Chapter 7; Saini et al., Chapter 19). There is also substantial evidence at this point that organisms are able to learn the predictive relation between events in their environments without reinforcement.

Some alternative approaches to understanding reinforcer effects stress not the response-strengthening effects of reinforcers but instead view reinforcers as sources of information that may help organisms more successfully navigate their environments (Davison & Baum, 2006; Gallistel & Gibbon, 2000; Killeen & Jacobs, 2016; Shahan, 2010, 2017; Simon et al., 2020; Timberlake, 1988). For example, Randy Gallistel, Peter Balsam, and their colleagues (Balsam et al., 2010; Balsam & Gallistel, 2009; Gallistel et al., 2014, 2019) suggest that organisms may learn the temporal and spatial relations between biologically relevant events, and the predictive relations between those events are what guide responding. Furthermore, their approach is based on Shannon's information theory, thereby providing a concrete way of thinking about behaviorally meaningful concepts that might otherwise be somewhat fuzzy like stimulus–stimulus or response–stimulus contingency, temporal contiguity, and stimulus predictability. Full development of this approach to understanding how reinforcers affect behavior is outside the scope of this chapter. The articles cited earlier, however, are very helpful review articles that may provide interested readers with additional background.

Identification of Reinforcers in Practice

Regardless of the way one thinks about reinforcement processes, the practical importance of reinforcement for the science of behavior is immutable. From our earlier discussion, we learned that reinforcement (1) increases the future probability of behavior that produces it, (2) increases the likelihood that a specific behavior will occur relative to other behaviors that are concurrently available, and (3) enhances the persistence of behavior. All of these may be desirable outcomes, and all are also affected to some extent by the "goodness" of the conditions of reinforcement in place; that is, better conditions of reinforcement (i.e., higher rates, larger magnitudes, better qualities, and shorter delays of reinforcement) tend to be associated with higher rates, higher relative likelihoods, and greater resistance to change of behavior than worse conditions of reinforcement. When one has the goal in mind of modifying human behavior, important first steps are to identify what the relevant reinforcers are and what steps can be taken to ensure that the reinforcement conditions they arrange are sufficiently good from the perspective of the behaver to produce the desired behavioral outcome.

When it comes to human behavior, reinforcer preferences themselves are as individualized as fingerprints. The identification of reinforcers in clinical practice is therefore done on an individualized basis with *preference assessments* (for identification of reinforcers to reinforce nonestablished future behavior) and *functional behavior assessment* (for identification of reinforcers already maintaining preexisting behavior). In the sections that follow, we briefly describe these assessment procedures.

Preference Assessments

Although it is not uncommon for the topography of a stimulus to influence the use of the stimulus as a reinforcer, research has demonstrated that this type of selection method is often not ideal (Piazza et al., 2011); that is, the arbitrary selection of stimuli often falls short of identifying effective reinforcers for behavior change. For example, although Johnny may enjoy and readily consume donuts, he may not be willing to complete algebra problems to obtain access to them. A good place to start when selecting preferred stimuli may be by vocal–verbal self-report or caregiver report. Although this approach is intuitive, research has demonstrated that reported preference often does not align with observed preference (Green et al., 1988; Northup et al., 1996). Thus, direct assessment of individual preferences may be necessary through systematic identification of preferred items. There are various systematic assessment methodologies used within the field of behavior analysis to help practitioners identify preferred items that contain reinforcing properties.

The use of direct assessment of individual preference was first noted in 1985, with the introduction of the single-stimulus preference assessment (Pace et al., 1985). In a single-stimulus preference assessment, a pool of items is selected, and each item is presented, one at a time. If the individual approaches (e.g., reaches toward) the item, they are given access to the item for a brief interval (e.g., 30 seconds). Given this arrangement, the individual's preference for each item is determined based on the percentage of trials in which they approach each item. In addition to identification of preference for items, Pace and colleagues also examined the reinforcer efficacy of the selected items; that is, the researchers provided participants with access to either preferred or nonpreferred stimuli contingent on emission of specified responses. Results demonstrated that participants engaged in higher levels of responding when that response produced access to items identified as preferred in the single-stimulus preference assessment than when it produced access to nonpreferred items. These findings provided initial evidence for the relationship between preference for stimuli and the corresponding reinforcer efficacy of those stimuli.

Following the development of the single-stimulus preference assessment, several choice-based preference assessments emerged in which two or more items are available concurrently from which a participant can choose. A benefit of this concurrent arrangement is that it allows for the identification of a hierarchy of preference. Additionally, it capitalizes on and builds technology off of decades of basic research on reinforcer effects from the basic laboratory. Recall that Herrnstein (1961, 1970, 1974) demonstrated that organisms tend to allocate their behavior lawfully between competing sources of reinforcement in such a way that matches the relative values associated with those sources. Furthermore, the matching law quantified these effects; thus, when two or more reinforcers are presented, participants can be expected to spend more time engaging with whichever of those reinforcers is subjectively more valuable.

In a paired-choice preference assessment (Fisher et al., 1992), an individual is presented with two items from a larger pool of items and is asked to make a selection. Upon selecting (e.g., vocalizing) or approaching (e.g., reaching toward) one of the items, the individual is provided with brief access to the selected item. Each item is presented with every other item one time. The percentage of trials that each item is selected indicates a relative hierarchy of preference; that is, a degree of preference (e.g., high, medium, low) is observed based on the allocation of choice responses across items and trials.

The multiple-stimulus preference assessment (Windsor et al., 1994) is similar to the paired-choice preference assessment, with the exception that all items in a selected pool (e.g., six items) are concurrently presented to an individual. As in the paired-choice assessment, selection of an item produces brief access to the item. However, in each subsequent trial, all of the items are presented again for selection. Typically, several trials (e.g., 10) are presented across numerous sessions (e.g., five). Although the multiple-stimulus preference assessment may result in identification of a highly preferred item, it may not readily produce a hierarchy of preference given that all items are presented on each trial. An individual may engage with only the most valuable reinforcer in every trial. Thus, an iteration of the multiple-stimulus assessment is the multiple-stimulus without replacement (MSWO; DeLeon & Iwata, 1996) preference assessment. In an MSWO arrangement, all items are initially presented concurrently. Once an item is selected, it is not included in subsequent choice trials. This format allows for the identification of a hierarchy of preference, as the individual has to make selections from less-preferred items as the assessment progresses.

These single- and concurrent-operant arrangements rely solely on an individual's approach toward or selection of presented items. However, duration of engagement with an item is also a relevant variable in identification of preference. Conceptually, choice and preference have been defined not only in terms of *response* allocation but also as *time* allocation across competing response alternatives (see Baum & Rachlin, 1969); thus, time allocation is also thought to correspond to reinforcer value.

In a free-operant preference assessment (Roane et al., 1998) individuals can access a variety of items and engage with any, all, or none of these items during a predetermined observation interval. Preference is then determined based on the amount of time during the observation interval during which the individual engages with each available item. However, much like with single-stimulus and multiple-stimulus preference assessments, a hierarchy of preference may not emerge (e.g., if an individual only plays with the iPad). Thus, if identification of a hierarchy is a clinically relevant goal, a duration-based assessment such as the response-restriction assessment (Hanley et al., 2003) may be an option.

In a response-restriction assessment, individuals are presented with a variety of items concurrently and, as in a free-operant assessment, they can engage with all, any, or none, with duration of engagement being the primary measure of preference. However, the response-restriction assessment also incorporates a trial-based structure in which items with relatively high levels of engagement in one trial are excluded in subsequent trials. The removal of items with high levels of engagement across trials from the overall array of items provides the individual with increased opportunity to sample all available items, ultimately resulting in a hierarchy of preference.

The extant literature on preference assessments clearly demonstrates the utility of directly and systematically evaluating individual preferences. However, as noted previously, preference does not necessarily equate to reinforcer efficacy, and reinforcer efficacy may be related to many variables that are not explored in the context of preference assessments (e.g., unit price or availability of complementary or substitutable reinforcers; Madden et al., 2007a, 2007b; see also Madden et al., Chapter 21, this volume, and the earlier section "Behavior-Economics Framework"). Other approaches have taken a more applied lens to understanding and evaluating the relationship between preference and reinforcer efficacy (e.g., DeLeon & Iwata, 1996; Fisher et al., 1992; Hanley et al., 2003; Lee et al., 2010; Pace et al., 1985; Roane et al., 1998), and the relationship identified by these studies has been strong and positive. For example, Piazza et al. (1996) identified a direct relation between the levels of an individual's preference (i.e., low, medium, and high preference) for stimuli and the reinforcing effectiveness of each stimulus following a reinforcer assessment. These findings indicate that even stimuli identified as relatively low preferred may still have reinforcing qualities, although responding is likely to be less when it produces access to a low-preferred stimulus relative to a high-preferred stimulus.

Practical Considerations

Several considerations guide the selection of the most appropriate preference assessment for an individual given their personal characteristics and available resources. The assessments described earlier provide for both selection- (e.g., MSWO) and engagement-based (e.g., free-operant) measures of preference. An individual's behavioral presentation and characteristics determine, to some degree, the most appropriate measure of preference. For example, single-stimulus preference assessments or assessments that include a duration-based measure may be best suited for individuals who cannot readily make choices. For individuals who engage in challenging behavior upon removal of potentially reinforcing stimuli, a selection-based arrangement that involves removal of the selected item after a brief period may evoke challenging behavior. Thus, duration-based measures (e.g., free-operant assessment) may be more suitable.

The static or fluid nature of an individual's preferences may also be considered when selecting a preference assessment. In laboratory settings, a multitude of preferred items or activities are generally not available as they are in applied settings. Thus, if an individual's preference changes often or time to administer assessments is limited, less time-consuming assessments may be selected. For example, a limitation of both the paired-choice preference assessment (Fisher et al., 1992) and response-restriction assessment (Hanley et al., 2003) is the time needed to complete them. Thus, implementation of the paired-choice or response-restriction assessments may not be reasonable prior to daily teaching sessions and are not ideal for situations in which measures of individual preferences need to be updated frequently (e.g., when an individual readily loses motivation for items). In such situations, a more rapid assessment such as the MSWO (DeLeon & Iwata, 1996) or free-operant assessment (Roane et al., 1998) may be more practical and helpful.

Functional Behavior Assessment

Assessment of preference provides a starting place for the identification of reinforcers. These reinforcers can then be used to systematically reinforce new behaviors and teach new skills. However, while reinforcement can be programmed into a context, reinforcement also occurs when it has not been intentionally programmed. For example, a child may engage in tantrum behavior when asked to share a toy and be provided with access to comfort or a different toy, which may reinforce tantrums. In applied settings, reinforcement is often programmed to be delivered after target behaviors of social significance to the individual, such as requesting a hug from a caregiver or asking for a break from academic demands. Outside of clinical and laboratory settings, reinforcement continues to operate on behaviors that are considered desirable, as well as behaviors that are considered undesirable. As these reinforcers were not *intended* by others in the environment to reinforce specific behaviors, the reinforcers that come to maintain undesirable behaviors can be difficult to identify.

For many individuals with developmental disabilities who struggle with communication and experience skills deficits across areas of daily living, reinforcement can come to maintain behaviors that are potentially hazardous to their well-being. For example, self-injurious or aggressive behaviors such as head banging, eye gouging, hitting, biting or kicking, or destroying property may unintentionally be reinforced in the individual's home or school life. These behaviors put the individual and others around them at risk physically. They also put the individual at risk for more restrictive placements, increased likelihood of mental health disorders, and decreased opportunity for community and social engagement (e.g., Jang et al., 2011).

In the case of unintentional reinforcement of dangerous behaviors, applied interventions that identify the function of the behavior and teach replacement behaviors to help the individual meet their needs are more effective than interventions that use reinforcers that are arbitrary with respect to the individual's challenging behavior (e.g., Austin et al. 2015; Healy et al., 2014). The process of identifying consequences that reinforce and maintain challenging behavior is referred to as *functional behavior assessment* (FBA). Although the process of identifying reinforcers through FBA can be time and resource intensive, the use of functional reinforcers in treating problem behavior has demonstrated efficacy across behavior topographies, settings, and populations (Beavers et al., 2013; Healy et al., 2014; Tiger et al., 2008).

Basic research has no analogue for functional assessment of which we are aware. Thus far, most of the research on how to identify unintentional established reinforcers has taken place within the applied realm. Translational research is uniquely positioned to identify aspects of the assessment of unintentionally established reinforcers that may be modified to increase the efficiency and efficacy of these procedures. Additionally, even though coverage of functional assessment is a slight departure from the thread woven through the earlier sections, we would be remiss not to describe functional assessment in a chapter on reinforcement given the central role this process has played in identifying reinforcing stimuli in applied settings.

To identify established but unknown sources of reinforcement, FBA generally uses three levels of analysis: indirect assessment, descriptive assessment, and functional analysis (FA). Indirect analysis includes non-experimental methodology such as interviews or questionnaires (e.g., Motivation Assessment Scale [MAS]: Durand & Crimmins, 1988, 1992; Functional Analysis Screening Tool [FAST]: Iwata et al., 2013, among others).

These methods may help identify relevant stimuli to assess further but are neither observational nor experimental. Therefore, they can only provide correlational but not causational information about possible consequences that maintain problem behavior and have mixed psychometric evidence supporting their reliability and validity (e.g., Zarcone et al., 1991). These tools may be a useful starting place for identifying potential sources of reinforcement to test in later analysis (Sturmey, 1994), but the information gained rarely identifies sources of reinforcement without additional assessment.

The second level of analysis in an FBA consists of descriptive assessment (e.g., Anderson & Long, 2002; Bijou et al., 1968; Vollmer et al., 2001). Descriptive assessment has the benefit of being observational. Like indirect assessment methods, however, it does not allow for claims regarding causation, as no variables are manipulated. Descriptive assessment for the identification of reinforcement in clinical populations often takes the form of antecedent–behavior–consequence (ABC) analysis. Maintaining consequences identified by descriptive analysis, however, often have poor correspondence with those identified through functional analysis (e.g., Thompson & Iwata, 2007; St. Peter et al., 2005). While descriptive assessment provides additional information about potentially relevant reinforcement conditions, additional sources of assessment and analysis should be used to confirm hypotheses.

The final level of analysis for clinical identification of reinforcement is an FA, which is both observational and experimental. The purpose of an FA is ultimately to identify the maintaining consequences of a challenging behavior, so that a beneficial replacement skill may be taught that allows the individual to have their wants and needs met. Although multielement experimental designs were not new, Iwata's (1982) investigation of the relationship between self-injurious behavior and environmental events using operant methodology is often referenced as one of the initial FA studies. In this study, three variations of experimental conditions were systematically presented to subjects, with play materials either present or absent, experimental demands either high or low, and social attention either absent, contingent, or noncontingent. Six of the nine subjects in this experiment demonstrated higher levels of self-injury in specific conditions, suggesting a functional relationship between the condition and self-injury for that participant. Since this initial exploration, several variations of the multielement design and included conditions have been explored (see Saini et al., 2020; Hanley, 2012; Hagopian et al., 2013, for further details), but all look to identify the relationship between specific stimulus conditions and some form of challenging behavior.

The process of completing a functional analysis may be more effective if relevant conditions are first identified. For example, clinicians may wish to first identify the type of attention a child typically receives (e.g., praise, reprimands, physical comfort), the topography of demands usually present when problem behavior occurs (e.g., social demands, math worksheets), or the presence of synthesized reinforcers (e.g., escape from a classroom to a sensory room with adult attention). The information gained from indirect or descriptive assessments can be valuable in identifying and therefore programming these relevant conditions, reducing the need for multiple iterations of assessment in order to accurately identify maintaining consequences. Ultimately, the best determination of whether accurate reinforcers have been identified is treatment validity, or whether the treatment developed from an FA results effectively decreases maladaptive behavior and increases adaptive replacement behaviors. If reinforcement conditions have been identified incorrectly, treatment is unlikely to be successful.

Practical Considerations

FAs that are cumbersome, time consuming, or complex may be less likely to be used in clinical practice (Northup et al., 1991; Oliver et al., 2015). The design and procedure of an FA will, like preference assessments, depend on the characteristics of the individual needing assessment, as well as the resources that are available (e.g., time, expertise). In a study comparing efficiency of types of FAs, Saini et al. (2020) identified six primary experimental designs that utilize the principles of single-case research design and variations of test and control conditions: brief FA, trial-based FA, reversal design, multielement design, pairwise design, and synthesized-contingency analysis. A brief FA allows for shorter assessment time (Northup et al., 1991), while a trial-based FA (Sigafoos & Saggers, 1995) allows for presentation of trials within an individual's current context (e.g., classroom). Multielement designs allow clinicians to test for multiple sources of reinforcement, while pairwise FAs allow for the assessment of one form of reinforcement in a test/control arrangement (Saini et al., 2020). Synthesized contingency analyses (Hanley et al. 2014) allow for assessment of more than one function simultaneously within a single condition. Other forms include latency-based FAs (Thomason-Sassi et al., 2011), wherein latency to respond is used as a measure of problem behavior for individuals whose problem behavior is either difficult to replicate (e.g., vomiting, elopement) or too severe to allow for repetition. Regardless of the type of FA selected, the follow-up treatment generally teaches an alternative skill that allows the individual to meet their needs in an adaptive manner (e.g., Tiger et al., 2008).

Throughout the literature on FAs, numerous variations such as those described earlier have been explored. Any variation comes with potential detriments and benefits. As FA is a procedure that involves reinforcing challenging behavior, translational research provides an opportunity to explore behavioral processes without concerns for the safety or well-being of individuals. For example, Retzlaff et al. (2020) trained surrogate destructive behavior (i.e., arbitrary nondestructive behavior) maintained by predetermined consequences prior to completing traditional FAs and FAs with synthesized reinforcement contingencies. They found that traditional FAs were more effective at identifying the trained consequences. This is just one example of how translational research regarding the efficacy and potential pitfalls of FA procedures will help us to better understand and meet the needs of clients in applied settings.

Conclusions

Reinforcement is one of the most fundamental principles in the science of behavior. Behavior analysts have learned a great deal about how humans and nonhuman animals interact with and adapt to their environments through the clever application of reinforcement in laboratory settings. They have also developed a flexible, practical, and effective kit of intervention strategies that may be used to promote socially significant behavior change in the natural environment. Elaboration on all of the significant advances in behavioral science precipitated by reinforcement is beyond the scope of this chapter.

Our goals in writing this chapter were to provide an understanding of where the concept of reinforcement came from, how behavior analysts have thought about it over the years, and some fundamental assessment strategies that are critical for effective application of reinforcement in practical settings. As you read other chapters in this volume, we hope that you develop a deeper appreciation for the ubiquity of reinforcement within the field. We also hope that the material that we have presented in this chapter provides helpful context as you further explore translational perspectives on applied behavior analysis.

REFERENCES

Anderson, C., & Long, E. (2002). Use of a structured descriptive assessment methodology to identify variables affecting problem behavior. *Journal of Applied Behavior Analysis, 35*(2), 137–154.

Austin, P. C., & Stuart, E. A. (2015). Moving towards best practice when using inverse probability of treatment weighting (IPTW) using the propensity score to estimate causal treatment effects in observational studies. *Statistics in Medicine, 34*(28), 3661–3679.

Avcu, P., Fortress, A. M., Fragale, J. E., Spiegler, K. M., & Pang, K. (2019). Anhedonia following mild traumatic brain injury in rats: A behavioral economic analysis of positive and negative reinforcement. *Behavioural Brain Research, 368*, Article 111913.

Ayllon, T., & Azrin, N. H. (1964). Reinforcement and instructions with mental patients. *Journal of the Experimental Analysis of Behavior, 7*(4), 327–331.

Ayllon, T., & Azrin, N. H. (1965). The measurement and reinforcement of behavior of psychotics. *Journal of the Experimental Analysis of Behavior, 8*(6), 357–383.

Ayllon, T., & Haughton, E. (1964). Modification of symptomatic verbal behaviour of mental patients. *Behaviour Research and Therapy, 2*, 87–97.

Azrin, N. H., & Lindsley, O. R. (1956). The reinforcement of cooperation between children. *Journal of Abnormal and Social Psychology, 52*, 100–102.

Balsam, P. D., Drew, M. R., & Gallistel, C. R. (2010). Time and associative learning. *Comparative Cognition and Behavior Reviews, 5*, 1–22.

Balsam, P. D., & Gallistel, C. R. (2009). Temporal maps and informativeness in associative learning. *Trends in Neurosciences, 32*(2), 73–78.

Baron, A., & Galizio, M. (2005). Positive and negative reinforcement: Should the distinction be preserved? *Behavior Analyst, 28*(2), 85–98.

Baron, A., & Galizio, M. (2006). The distinction between positive and negative reinforcement: Use with care. *Behavior Analyst, 29*(1), 141–151.

Barrett, B. H. (1962). Reduction in rate of multiple tics by free operant conditioning methods. *Journal of Nervous and Mental Disease, 135*, 187–195.

Baum, W. M. (1973). Time allocation and negative reinforcement. *Journal of the Experimental Analysis of Behavior, 20*(3), 313–322.

Baum, W. M. (1993). Performances on ratio and interval schedules of reinforcement: Data and theory. *Journal of the Experimental Analysis of Behavior, 59*(2), 245–264.

Baum, W. M. (2002). From molecular to molar: A paradigm shift in behavior analysis. *Journal of the Experimental Analysis of Behavior, 78*(1), 95–116.

Baum, W. M., & Rachlin, H. C. (1969). Choice as time allocation. *Journal of the Experimental Analysis of Behavior, 12*(6), 861–874.

Beavers, G. A., Iwata, B. A., & Lerman, D. C. (2013). Thirty years of research on the functional analysis of problem behavior. *Journal of Applied Behavior Analysis, 46*(1), 1–21.

Bensberg, G. J., Colwell, C. N., & Cassel, R. H. (1965). Teaching the profoundly retarded self-help activities by behavior shaping techniques. *American Journal of Mental Deficiency, 69*, 674–679.

Bickel, W. K., DeGrandpre, R. J., & Higgins, S. T. (1993). Behavioral economics: A novel experimental approach to the study of drug dependence. *Drug and Alcohol Dependence, 33*(2), 173–192.

Bijou, S. W. (1955). A systematic approach to an experimental analysis of young children. *Child Development, 26*, 161–168.

Bijou, S. W. (1957). Patterns of reinforcement and extinction in young children. *Child Development, 28*, 47–54.

Bijou, S. W., Peterson, R. F., & Ault, M. H. (1968). A method to integrate descriptive and experimental field studies at the level of data and empirical concepts. *Journal of Applied Behavior Analysis, 1*, 175–191.

Blackman, D. (1968). Response rate, reinforcement frequency, and conditioned suppression. *Journal of the Experimental Analysis of Behavior, 11*, 503–516.

Boren, J. J., Sidman, M., & Herrnstein, R. J. (1959). Avoidance, escape, and extinction as functions of shock intensity. *Journal of Comparative and Physiological Psychology, 52*(4), 420–425.

Borrero, J. C., Francisco, M. T., Haberlin, A. T., Ross, N. A., & Sran, S. K. (2007). A unit price evaluation of severe problem behavior. *Journal of Applied Behavior Analysis, 40*(3), 463–474.

Cassidy, R. N., & Kurti, A. N. (2018). Behavioral economic research in addiction as an area of growth for the experimental analysis of behavior. *Behavior Analysis: Research and Practice, 18*(4), 333–339.

Catania, A. C. (1963). Concurrent performances: Reinforcement interaction and response independence. *Journal of the Experimental Analysis of Behavior, 6*(2), 253–263.

Catania, A. C. (2005). The operant reserve: A computer simulation in (accelerated) real time. *Behavioral Processes, 69*(2), 257–278.

Chance, P. (2014). *Learning and behavior* (7th ed.). Cengage Learning.

Chase, P. N. (2006). Teaching the distinction between positive and negative reinforcement. *Behavior Analyst, 29*(1), 113–115.

Christensen, C. J., Silberberg, A., Hursh, S. R., Huntsberry, M. E., & Riley, A. L. (2008). Essential value of cocaine and food in rats: Tests of the exponential model of demand. *Psychopharmacology, 198*, 221–229.

Chung, S. H., & Herrnstein, R. J. (1967). Choice and delay of reinforcement. *Journal of the Experimental Analysis of Behavior, 10*, 67–74.

Cohen, S. L. (1998). Behavioral momentum: The effects of the temporal separation of rates of reinforcement. *Journal of the Experimental Analysis of Behavior, 69*(1), 29–47.

Cohen, S. L., Riley, D. S., & Weigle, P. A. (1993). Tests of behavior momentum in simple and multiple schedules with rats and pigeons. *Journal of the Experimental Analysis of Behavior, 60*(2), 255–291.

Craig, A. R., & Shahan, T. A. (2016). Behavioral momentum theory fails to account for the effects of reinforcement rate on resurgence. *Journal of the Experimental Analysis of Behavior, 105*(3), 375–392.

Davison, M., & Baum, W. M. (2006). Do conditional reinforcers count? *Journal of the Experimental Analysis of Behavior, 86*, 269–283.

de Villiers, P. A. (1974). The law of effect and avoidance: A quantitative relationship between response rate and shock-frequency reduction. *Journal of the Experimental Analysis of Behavior, 21*(2), 223–235.

de Villiers, P. A. (1980). Toward a quantitative theory of punishment. *Journal of the Experimental Analysis of Behavior, 33*, 15–25.

DeLeon, I. G., & Iwata, B. A. (1996). Evaluation of a multiple-stimulus presentation format for assessing reinforcer preferences. *Journal of Applied Behavior Analysis, 29*, 519–533.

Delmendo, X., Borrero, J. C., Beauchamp, K. L., & Francisco, M. T. (2009). Consumption and response output as a function of unit price: Manipulation of cost and benefit components. *Journal of Applied Behavior Analysis, 42*(3), 609–625.

Deluty, M. Z. (1976). Choice and the rate of punishment in concurrent schedules. *Journal of the Experimental Analysis of Behavior, 25*, 75–80.

Dinsmoor, J., Hughes, L., & Matsuoka, Y. (1958). Escape-from-shock training in a free-response situation. *American Journal of Psychology, 2*, 325–337.

Dinsmoor, J. A., & Sears, G. W. (1973). Control of avoidance by a response-produced stimulus. *Learning and Motivation, 4*, 284–293.

Domjam, M. (2015). *The principles of learning and behavior* (7th ed.). Cengage Learning.

Durand, V. M., & Crimmins, D. B. (1988). Identifying the variables maintaining self-injurious behavior. *Journal of Autism and Developmental Disorders, 18*, 99–117.

Durand, V. M., & Crimmins, D. B. (1992). *The Motivation Assessment Scale (MAS) administration guide.* Monaco and Associates.

Fantino, E. (1969). Choice and rate of reinforcement. *Journal of the Experimental Analysis of Behavior, 12*(5), 723–730.

Ferster, C. B., & DeMyer, M. K. (1962). A method for the experimental analysis of the autistic child. *American Journal of Orthopsychiatry, 32*, 89–98.

Ferster, C. B., & Skinner, B. F. (1957). *Schedules of reinforcement.* Appleton-Century-Crofts.

Fisher, W. W., & Mazur, J. E. (1997). Basic and applied research on choice responding. *Journal of Applied Behavior Analysis, 30*(3), 387–410.

Fisher, W. W., Piazza, C. C., Bowman, L. G., Hagopian, L. P., Owens, J. C., & Slevin, I. (1992). A comparison of two approaches for identifying reinforcers for persons with severe and profound disabilities. *Journal of Applied Behavior Analysis, 25*, 491–498.

Fragale, J. E., Beck, K. D., & Pang, K. C. (2017).

Use of the exponential and exponentiated demand equations to assess the behavioral economics of negative reinforcement. *Frontiers in Neuroscience, 11*, Article 77.

Fuller, P. R. (1949). Operant conditioning of a vegetative human organism. *Journal of Psychology, 62*, 587–590.

Gallistel, C. R., Craig, A. R., & Shahan, T. A. (2014). Temporal contingency. *Behavioural Processes, 101*, 89–96.

Gallistel, C. R., Craig, A. R., & Shahan, T. A. (2019). Contingency, contiguity, and causality in conditioning: Applying information theory and Weber's Law to the assignment of credit problem. *Psychological Review, 126*(5), 761–773.

Gallistel, C. R., & Gibbon, J. (2000). Time, rate, and conditioning. *Psychological Review, 107*(2), 289–344.

Green, C. W., Reid, D. H., White, L. K., Halford, R. C., Brittain, D. P., & Gardner, S. M. (1988). Identifying reinforcers for persons with profound mental handicaps: Staff opinion versus systematic assessment of preferences. *Journal of Applied Behavior Analysis, 21*, 31–43.

Guercio, J. M. (2018). The importance of a deeper knowledge of the history and theoretical foundations of behavior analysis: 1863–1960. *Behavior Analysis: Research and Practice, 18*(1), 4–15.

Hagopian, L. P., Rooker, G. W., Jessel, J., & DeLeon, I. G. (2013). Initial functional analysis outcomes and modifications in pursuit of differentiation: A summary of 176 inpatient cases. *Journal of Applied Behavior Analysis, 46*(1), 88–100.

Hanley, G. P. (2012). Functional assessment of problem behavior: Dispelling myths, overcoming implementation obstacles, and developing new lore. *Behavior Analysis in Practice, 5*, 54–72.

Hanley, G. P., Iwata, B. A., Lindberg, J. S., & Conners, J. (2003). Response-restriction analysis: I. Assessment of activity preferences. *Journal of Applied Behavior Analysis, 36*, 47–58.

Hanley, G. P., Iwata, B. A., & McCord, B. E. (2003). Functional analysis of problem behavior: A review. *Journal of Applied Behavior Analysis, 36*(2), 147–185.

Hanley, G. P., Jin, C. S., Vanselow, N. R., & Hanratty, L. A. (2014). Producing meaningful improvements in problem behavior of children with autism via synthesized analyses and treatments. *Journal of Applied Behavior Analysis, 47*, 16–36.

Healy, O., Lydon, S., & Murray, C. (2014). Aggressive behavior. In P. Sturmey & R. Didden (Eds). *Evidence-based practice and intellectual disabilities* (pp. 103–132). Wiley-Blackwell.

Herrnstein, R. J. (1961). Relative and absolute strength of response as a function of frequency of reinforcement. *Journal of the Experimental Analysis of Behavior, 4*(3), 267–272.

Herrnstein, R. J. (1969). Method and theory in the study of avoidance. *Psychological Review, 76*(1), 49–69.

Herrnstein, R. J. (1970). On the law of effect. *Journal of the Experimental Analysis of Behavior, 13*, 243–266.

Herrnstein, R. J. (1974). Formal properties of the matching law. *Journal of the Experimental Analysis of Behavior, 21*(1), 159–164.

Herrnstein, R. J., & Hineline, P. N. (1966). Negative reinforcement as shock-frequency reduction. *Journal of the Experimental Analysis of Behavior, 9*(4), 421–430.

Hineline, P. N. (1970). Negative reinforcement without shock reduction. *Journal of the Experimental Analysis of Behavior, 14*(3), 259–268.

Hineline, P. N., & Rachlin, H. (1969). Escape and avoidance of shock by pigeons pecking a key. *Journal of the Experimental Analysis of Behavior, 12*(4), 533–538.

Hineline, P. N., & Rosales-Ruiz, J. (2013). Behavior in relation to aversive events: Punishment and negative reinforcement. In G. J. Madden, W. V. Dube, T. D. Hackenberg, G. P. Hanley, & K. A. Lattal (Eds.), *APA handbook of behavior analysis: Vol. 1. Methods and principles* (pp. 483–512). American Psychological Association.

Hursh, S. R. (1980). Economic concepts for the analysis of behavior. *Journal of the Experimental Analysis of Behavior, 34*, 219–238.

Hursh, S. R. (1984). Behavioral economics. *Journal of the Experimental Analysis of Behavior, 42*, 435–452.

Hursh, S. R. (1991). Behavioral economics of drug self-administration and drug abuse policy. *Journal of the Experimental Analysis of Behavior, 56*(2), 377–393.

Hursh, S. R., Raslear, T. G., Bauman, R., & Black, H. (1989). The quantitative analysis of economic behavior with laboratory animals. In K. G. Grunert & F. Ölander (Eds.), *Understanding economic behaviour. Theory and decision library* (Vol. 11, pp. 393–407). Springer, Dordrecht.

Hursh, S. R., Raslear, T. G., Shurtleff, D., Bauman, R. A., & Simmons, L. (1988). A cost–benefit analysis of demand for food. *Journal of the Experimental Analysis of Behavior, 50*, 419–440.

Hursh, S. R., & Roma, P. G. (2013). Behavioral economics and empirical public policy. *Journal of the Experimental Analysis of Behavior, 99*(1), 98–124.

Hursh, S. R., & Roma, P. G. (2016). Behavioral economics and the analysis of consumption and choice. *Managerial and Decision Economics, 37*(4–5), 224–238.

Hursh, S. R., & Silberberg, A. (2008). Economic demand and essential value. *Psychological Review, 115*, 186–198.

Iwata, B. A. (2006). On the distinction between positive and negative reinforcement. *Behavior Analyst, 29*(1), 121–123.

Iwata, B. A., Deleon, I. G., & Roscoe, E. M. (2013). Reliability and validity of the functional analysis screening tool. *Journal of Applied Behavior Analysis, 46*(1), 271–284.

Iwata, B. A., Dorsey, M. F., Slifer, K. J., Bauman, K. E., & Richman, G. S. (1982). Toward a functional analysis of self-injury. *Analysis & Intervention in Developmental Disabilities, 2*(1), 3–20.

Jackson Marr, M. (2006). Through the looking glass: Symmetry in behavioral principles? *Behavior Analyst, 29*(1), 125–128.

Jang, J., Dixon, D. R., Tarbox, J., & Granpeesheh, D. (2011). Symptom severity and challenging behavior in children with ASD. *Research in Autism Spectrum Disorders, 5*, 1028–1032.

Johnson, M. W., & Bickel, W. K. (2006). Replacing relative reinforcing efficacy with behavioral economic demand curves. *Journal of the Experimental Analysis of Behavior, 85*(1), 73–93.

Kamin, L. J. (1957). The effects of termination of the CS and avoidance of the US on avoidance learning: An extension. *Canadian Journal of Psychology/Revue Canadienne De Psychologie, 11*(1), 48–56.

Keller, F. S., & Schoenfeld, W. N. (1950). *Principles of psychology: A systematic text in the science of behavior*. Appleton-Century-Crofts.

Kelsey, J. E. (1977). Escape acquisition following inescapable shock in the rat. *Animal Learning and Behavior, 5*, 83–92.

Killeen, P. R. (1988). The reflex reserve. *Journal of the Experimental Analysis of Behavior, 50*(2), 319–331.

Killeen, P. R., & Hall, S. S. (2001). The principal components of response strength. *Journal of the Experimental Analysis of Behavior, 75*(2), 111–134.

Killeen, P. R., & Jacobs, K. W. (2016). Coal is not black, snow is not white, food is not a reinforcer: The roles of affordances and dispositions in the analysis of behavior. *Behavior Analyst, 40*(1), 17–38.

Lattal, K. A. (1989). Contingencies on response rate and resistance to change. *Learning and Motivation, 20*(2), 191–203.

Lattal, K. (1998). A century of effect: Legacies of E. L. Thorndike's Animal Intelligence Monograph. *Journal of the Experimental Analysis of Behavior, 70*(3), 325–336.

Lattal, K. A. (2013). The five pillars of the experimental analysis of behavior. In G. J. Madden, W. V. Dube, T. D. Hackenberg, G. P. Hanley, & K. A. Lattal (Eds.), *APA handbook of behavior analysis: Vol. 1. Methods and principles* (pp. 33–63). American Psychological Association.

Lattal, K. A., & Lattal, A. D. (2006). And yet . . . : Further comments on distinguishing positive and negative reinforcement. *Behavior Analyst, 29*(1), 129–134.

Lee, M. S. H., Yu, C. T., Martin, T. L., & Martin, G. L. (2010). On the relation between reinforcer efficacy and preference. *Journal of Applied Behavior Analysis, 43*, 95–100.

Mace, F. C., & Belfiore, P. (1990). Behavioral momentum in the treatment of escape-motivated stereotypy. *Journal of Applied Behavior Analysis, 23*, 507–514.

Mace, F. C., Hock, M. L., Lalli, J. S., West, B. J., Belfiore, P., Pinter, E., & Brown, D. K. (1988). Behavioral momentum in the treatment of noncompliance. *Journal of Applied Behavior Analysis, 21*(2), 123–141.

Mace, F. C., McComas, J. J., Mauro, B. C., Progar, P. R., Taylor, B., Ervin, R., & Zangrillo, A. N. (2010). Differential reinforcement of alternative behavior increases resistance to extinction: Clinical demonstration, animal modeling, and clinical test of one solution. *Journal of the Experimental Analysis of Behavior, 93*(3), 349–367.

Madden, G. J. (2000). A behavioral economics primer. In W. K. Bickel & R. E. Vuchinich (Eds.), *Reframing health behavior change with behavioral economics* (pp. 3–26). Erlbaum.

Madden, G. J., Smethells, J. R., Ewan, E. E., & Hursh, S. R. (2007a). Tests of behavioral-economic assessments of relative reinforcer efficacy: Economic substitutes. *Journal of the Experimental Analysis of Behavior, 87*(2), 219–240.

Madden, G. J., Smethells, J. R., Ewan, E. E., & Hursh, S. R. (2007b). Tests of behavioral-economic assessments of relative reinforcer efficacy II: Economic complements. *Journal of the Experimental Analysis of Behavior, 88*(3), 355–367.

Mazur, J. E. (1987). An adjusting procedure for studying delayed reinforcement. In M. L. Commons, J. E. Mazur, J. A. Nevin, & H. Rachlin (Eds.), *The effect of delay and of intervening events on reinforcement value* (pp. 55–73). Erlbaum.

McDowell, J. J. (1988). Matching theory in natural human environments. *Behavior Analyst, 11*, 95–109.

McDowell, J. J. (1989). Two modern developments in matching theory. *Behavior Analyst, 12*, 153–166.

McLean, A. P., Grace, R. C., & Nevin, J. A. (2012). Response strength in extreme multiple schedules. *Journal of the Experimental Analysis of Behavior, 97*(1), 51–70.

Michael, J. (1975). Positive and negative reinforcement: A distinction that is no longer necessary, or a better way to talk about bad things. *Behaviorism, 3*, 33–44.

Michael, J. (2006). Comment on Baron and Galizio (2005). *Behavior Analyst, 29*(1), 117–119.

Morris, E. K., Altus, D. E., & Smith, N. G. (2013). A study in the founding of applied behavior analysis through its publications. *Behavior Analyst, 36*(1), 73–107.

Nevin, J. A. (1974). Response strength in multiple schedules. *Journal of the Experimental Analysis of Behavior, 21*, 389–408.

Nevin, J. A. (2012). Resistance to extinction and behavioral momentum. *Behavioural Processes, 90*(1), 89–97.

Nevin, J. A., Craig, A. R., Cunningham, P. J., & Podlesnik, C. A. (2017). Quantitative models of persistence and relapse from the perspective of behavioral momentum theory: Fits and misfits. *Behavioural Processes, 141*(1), 92–99.

Nevin, J. A., & Grace, R. C. (2000). Behavioral momentum and the law of effect. *Behavioral and Brain Sciences, 23*, 73–90.

Nevin, J. A., & Mandell, C. (2017). Comparing positive and negative reinforcement: A fantasy experiment. *Journal of the Experimental Analysis of Behavior, 107*(1), 34–38.

Nevin, J. A., Mandell, C., & Atak, J. R. (1983). The analysis of behavioral momentum. *Journal of the Experimental Analysis of Behavior, 39*(1), 49–59.

Nevin, J. A., & Shahan, T. A. (2011). Behavioral momentum theory: Equations and applications. *Journal of Applied Behavior Analysis, 44*, 877–895.

Nevin, J. A., Tota, M. E., Torquato, R. D., & Shull, R. L. (1990). Alternative reinforcement increases resistance to change: Pavlovian or operant contingencies? *Journal of the Experimental Analysis of Behavior, 53*(3), 359–379.

Northup, J., George, T., Jones, K., Broussard, C., & Vollmer, T. R. (1996). A comparison of reinforcer assessment methods: The utility of verbal and pictorial choice procedures. *Journal of Applied Behavior Analysis, 29*, 201–212.

Northup, J., Wacker, D., Sasso, G., Steege, M., Cigrand, K., Cook, J., & DeRaad, A. (1991). A brief functional analysis of aggressive and alternative behavior in an outclinic setting. *Journal of Applied Behavior Analysis, 24*(3), 509–522.

Oliver, A. C., Pratt, L. A., & Normand, M. P. (2015). A survey of functional behavior assessment methods used by behavior analysts in practice. *Journal of Applied Behavior Analysis, 48*, 817–829.

Pace, G. M., Ivancic, M. T., Edwards, G. L., Iwata, B. A., & Page, T. J. (1985). Assessment of stimulus preference and reinforcer value with profoundly retarded individuals. *Journal of Applied Behavior Analysis, 18*, 249–255.

Piazza, C. C., Fisher, W. W., Hagopian, L. P., Bowman, L. G., & Toole, L. (1996). Using a choice assessment to predict reinforcer effectiveness. *Journal of Applied Behavior Analysis, 29*, 1–9.

Piazza, C. C., Roane, H. S., & Karsten, A. (2011). Identifying and enhancing the effectiveness of positive reinforcement. In W. W. Fisher, C. C. Piazza, & H. S. Roane (Eds.), *Handbook of applied behavior analysis* (pp. 151–164). Guilford Press.

Plaud, J. J., & Gaither, G. A. (1996). Human behavioral momentum: Implications for applied behavior analysis and therapy. *Journal of Behavior Therapy and Experimental Psychiatry, 27*(2), 139–148.

Powell, R. A., Honey, L., & Symbaluk, D. G. (2017). *Introduction to learning and behavior* (5th ed.). Cengage Learning.

Pritchard, D., Hoerger, M., & Mace, F. C. (2014).

Treatment relapse and behavioral momentum theory. *Journal of Applied Behavior Analysis, 47*, 814–833.

Rachlin, H. (1971). On the tautology of the matching law. *Journal of the Experimental Analysis of Behavior, 15*(2), 249–251.

Rachlin, H. C., Kagel, J. H., & Battalio, R. C. (1980). Substitutability in time allocation. *Psychological Review, 87*(4), 355–374.

Reed, D. D., Niileksela, C. R., & Kaplan, B. A. (2013). Behavioral economics: A tutorial for behavior analysts in practice. *Behavior Analysis in Practice, 6*(1), 34–54.

Rescorla, R. A. (1969). Conditioned inhibition of fear resulting from negative CS–US contingencies. *Journal of Comparative and Physiological Psychology, 67*(4), 504–509.

Retzlaff, B. J., Fisher, W. W., Akers, J. A., & Greer, B. D. (2020). A translational evaluation of potential iatrogenic effects of single and combined contingencies during functional analysis. *Journal of Applied Behavior Analysis, 53*(1), 67–81.

Roane, H. S., Call, N. A., & Falcomata, T. S. (2005). A preliminary analysis of adaptive responding under open and closed economies. *Journal of Applied Behavior Analysis, 38*(3), 335–348.

Roane, H. S., Lerman, D. C., & Vorndran, C. M. (2001). Assessing reinforcers under progressive schedule requirements. *Journal of Applied Behavior Analysis, 34*(2), 145–167.

Roane, H. S., Vollmer, T. R., Ringdahl, J. E., & Marcus, B. A. (1998). Evaluation of a brief stimulus preference assessment. *Journal of Applied Behavior Analysis, 31*, 605–620.

Romani, P. W., Ringdahl, J. E., Wacker, D. P., Lustig, N. H., Vinquist, K. M., Northup, J., . . . Carrion, D. P. (2016). Relations between rate of negative reinforcement and the persistence of task completion. *Journal of Applied Behavior Analysis, 49*(1), 122–137.

Roscoe, E. M., Iwata, B. A., & Kahng, S. (1999). Relative versus absolute reinforcement effects: Implications for preference assessments. *Journal of Applied Behavior Analysis, 32*, 479–493.

Saini, V., Fisher, W. W., Retzlaff, B. J., & Keevy, M. (2020). Efficiency in functional analysis of problem behavior: A quantitative and qualitative review. *Journal of Applied Behavior Analysis, 53*, 44–66.

Schwartz, L. P., Silberberg, A., Casey, A. H., Paukner, A., & Suomi, S. J. (2016). Scaling reward value with demand curves versus preference tests. *Animal Cognition, 19*(3), 631–641.

Shahan, T. A. (2010). Conditioned reinforcement and response strength. *Journal of the Experimental Analysis of Behavior, 93*(2), 269–289.

Shahan, T. A. (2017). Moving beyond reinforcement and response strength. *The Behavior Analyst, 40*(1), 107–121.

Shahan, T. A., & Craig, A. R. (2017). Resurgence as choice. *Behavioural Processes, 141*(Pt. 1), 100–127.

Shahan, T. A., & Sweeney, M. M. (2011). A model of resurgence based on behavioral momentum theory. *Journal of the Experimental Analysis of Behavior, 95*(1), 91–108.

Sidman, M. (1953a). Avoidance conditioning with brief shock and no exteroceptive warning signal. *Science, 118*, 157–158.

Sidman, M. (1953b). Two temporal parameters of the maintenance of avoidance behavior by the white rat. *Journal of Comparative and Physiological Psychology, 46*(4), 253–261.

Sidman, M. (1962a). Classical avoidance without a warning stimulus. *Journal of the Experimental Analysis of Behavior, 5*(1), 97–104.

Sidman, M. (1962b). Reduction of shock frequency as reinforcement for avoidance behavior. *Journal of the Experimental Analysis of Behavior, 5*(2), 247–257.

Sidman, M. (1989). *Coercion and its fallout*. Authors Cooperative.

Sigafoos, J., & Saggers, E. (1995). A discrete-trial approach to the functional analysis of aggressive behavior in two boys with autism. *Australian and New Zealand Journal of Developmental Disabilities, 20*, 287–297.

Simon, C., Bernardy, J. L., & Cowie, S. (2020). On the "strength" of behavior. *Perspectives on Behavior Science, 43*(4), 677–696.

Skinner, B. F. (1938). *The behavior of organisms: An experimental analysis*. Appleton-Century.

Skinner, B. F. (1948). "Superstition" in the pigeon. *Journal of Experimental Psychology, 38*(2), 168–172.

Skinner, B. F. (1953a). *Science and human behavior*. Macmillan.

Skinner, B. F. (1953b). Some contributions of an experimental analysis of behavior to psychology as a whole. *American Psychologist, 8*(2), 69–78.

Spiegler, K. M., Fortress, A. M., & Pang, K. (2018). Differential use of danger and safety signals in an animal model of anxiety vulnerability: The behavioral economics of avoidance. *Progress in Neuro-Psychopharmacology and Biological Psychiatry, 82,* 195–204.

St. Peter, C. C., Vollmer, T. R., Bourret, J. C., Borrero, C. S. W., Sloman, K. N., & Rapp, J. T. (2005). On the role of attention in naturally occurring matching relations. *Journal of Applied Behavior Analysis, 38,* 429–443.

Sturmey P. (1994). Assessing the functions of aberrant behaviors: A review of psychometric instruments. *Journal of Autism and Developmental Disorders, 24*(3), 293–304.

Thomason-Sassi, J. L., Iwata, B. A., Neidert, P. L., & Roscoe, E. M. (2011). Response latency as an index of response strength during functional analyses of problem behavior. *Journal of Applied Behavior Analysis, 44,* 51–67.

Thompson, R. H., & Iwata, B. A. (2007). A comparison of outcomes from descriptive and functional analyses of problem behavior. *Journal of Applied Behavior Analysis, 40,* 333–338.

Thorndike, E. L. (1898). Animal intelligence: An experimental study of the associative processes in animals. *Psychological Review: Monograph Supplements, 2*(4), i–109.

Thorndike, E. L. (1911). *Animal intelligence: Experimental studies.* Macmillan.

Thorndike, E. L. (1932). Reward and punishment in animal learning. *Comparative Psychology Monographs, 8*(4; Whole No. 39).

Thorndike, E. L., & Columbia University, Institute of Educational Research, Division of Psychology. (1932). *The fundamentals of learning.* Teachers College Bureau of Publications.

Tiger, J. H., Hanley, G. P., & Bruzek, J. (2008). Functional communication training: A review and practical guide. *Behavior Analysis in Practice, 1*(1), 16–23.

Timberlake, W. (1988). The behavior of organisms: Purposive behavior as a type of reflex. *Journal of the Experimental Analysis of Behavior, 50*(2), 305–317.

Vollmer, T. R., Borrero, J. C., Wright, C. S., Camp, C. V., & Lalli, J. S. (2001). Identifying possible contingencies during descriptive analyses of severe behavior disorders. *Journal of Applied Behavior Analysis, 34,* 269–287.

Wacker, D. P., Harding, J. W., Berg, W. K., Lee, J. F., Schieltz, K. M., Padilla, Y. C., Nevin, J. A., & Shahan, T. A. (2011). An evaluation of persistence of treatment effects during long-term treatment of destructive behavior. *Journal of the Experimental Analysis of Behavior, 96*(2), 261–282.

Windsor, J., Piche, L. M., & Locke, P. A. (1994). Preference testing: A comparison of two presentation methods. *Research in Developmental Disabilities, 15,* 439–455.

Wolf, M., Risley, T., & Mess, H. (1964). Application of operant conditioning procedures to the behaviour problems of an autistic child. *Behaviour Research and Therapy, 1,* 305–312.

Zarcone, J. R., Rodgers, T. A., Iwata, B. A., Rourke, D. A., & Dorsey, M. F. (1991). Reliability analysis of the Motivation Assessment Scale: A failure to replicate. *Research in Developmental Disabilities, 12*(4), 349–360.

Zuriff, G. E. (1970). A comparison of variable-ratio and variable-interval schedules of reinforcement. *Journal of the Experimental Analysis of Behavior, 13*(3), 369–374.

Zuj, D. V., Xia, W., Lloyd, K., Vervliet, B., & Dymond, S. (2020). Negative reinforcement rate and persistent avoidance following response-prevention extinction. *Behaviour Research and Therapy, 133,* Article 103711.

CHAPTER 10

Punishment

Rusty W. Nall
Tara A. Fahmie
Amanda N. Zangrillo

Punishment is a naturally occurring process that influences behavior in the everyday environment. For example, ingesting a particular berry may make a bird ill, resulting in a decreased likelihood of eating that berry in the future. A child may break a toy by playing with it in a rough manner, rendering the toy inoperable and reducing the likelihood of roughly operating toys in the future. These are processes in our everyday world by which behavior is altered; thus, as students of the processes that govern behavior, it is essential that we understand the punishment process. It is equally important to recognize that the term *punishment* carries a societal and perceptual weight that often biases perceptions of punishment toward the negative. We will discuss ethical concerns that give merit to some of these perceptions while contextualizing the use of punishment in basic and clinical research.

Much like its counterpart reinforcement, punishment is a basic process by which a consequence that follows behavior influences the future likelihood of that behavior. As such, *punishment* occurs when a consequence that follows behavior results in a decrease in the future likelihood of that behavior. In addition to defining punishment, we focus in this chapter on how punishment has been used in the basic lab and clinic; factors that influence punishment efficacy (called *dimensions* of punishment); and discuss considerations for maximizing ethical, effective, and safe implementation of punishment throughout. By the end of this chapter, the reader will be familiar with these concepts and be able to describe how each affects the use and perception of punishment as a procedure.

Terminology and Types of Punishment

As discussed earlier, *punishment* describes the process by which a stimulus change following a behavior results in a decrease in the future likelihood of that behavior (Azrin & Holz, 1966). *Punishment* can be further defined by whether decreases in behavior are the result of stimulus presentation (*positive punishment*) or stimulus removal (*negative punishment*; Fox, 1982). These definitions are akin to those of positive and negative reinforcement, which describe an increase in the future likelihood of behavior when a stimulus is added (positive reinforcement) or removed (negative reinforcement) following that behavior (Michael, 2004). We discuss examples of punishment from the basic laboratory and clinic later using these definitions.

While punishment refers to a behavioral deceleration procedure, the term *punisher* refers to the specific stimulus that results in that behavioral change. Punishers can be classified as unconditioned or conditioned. An *unconditioned punisher* refers to a stimulus that is innately punishing; that is, unconditioned punishers are stimuli that do not need to be paired with another stimulus to serve a punishing function. Examples of unconditioned punishers include physical pain, illness, intense lights and sounds, extreme temperatures, social isolation, and so forth. Like unconditioned reinforcers, these tend to be stimuli that have importance for the species and should serve as punishers for all members of that species (Baum, 1994). Alternatively, *conditioned punishers* are stimuli that serve as punishers because they have been paired with other unconditioned or conditioned punishing stimuli (Hake & Azrin, 1965). For example, a tone that previously did not alter behavior can be paired with an unconditioned punisher such as electric shock. Through this pairing, the tone can become a conditioned punisher and serve to reduce behaviors that result in presentation of the tone. Like conditioned reinforcers, conditioned punishers that are repeatedly presented in the absence of the unconditioned punishers with which they were paired can lose efficacy. To continue the example, if the tone is continually presented in the absence of shock, it may eventually fail to serve as a punisher for the behavior that precedes it. Importantly, this pairing requirement is not the case for unconditioned punishers, which maintain their efficacy without any need for pairing with other stimuli. A previously neutral stimulus that has been paired with many punishers may come to serve as a *generalized conditioned punisher* and maintain its efficacy over long periods without being paired with an unconditioned punisher. For example, for many people, verbal reprimands and disapproving glances have been paired with a long history of different punishers (e.g., loss of privileges, social isolation). These types of punishers may serve to reduce the behavior they follow under most conditions.

Now that some basic terms have been defined, we can begin to examine how knowledge about punishment has been derived. Through the combined work of basic scientists and clinical therapists, much has been revealed about the factors that influence punishment efficacy (i.e., dimensions of punishment), the most ethical approaches for using punishment to change socially relevant behaviors, and some potential concerns for using punishment. Before we discuss these, it will be useful to understand some specifics of how punishment is used in the basic science laboratory and the behavior clinic. We review those methods next.

Punishment in the Basic Laboratory

The basis for much of what we know about punishment was first explored in the basic laboratory. Punishment is used in the basic laboratory both as a model for studying how parameters (e.g., punishment intensity, rate/schedule, immediacy) affect the efficacy of punishment and in translational models designed to understand how punishment controls behavior in society. Importantly, punishment is a behavioral deceleration procedure, meaning there must be an ongoing baseline of behavior prior to implementing punishment. In both human and nonhuman animal laboratory studies, arbitrary responses are often used to determine how some factor will influence punishment. Before reviewing how punishment has been implemented in the basic lab, we discuss how the approval process for lab research ensures that any punishment procedures are conducted minimally and ethically.

Ethics of Punishment in the Basic Laboratory

The appropriate use of punishment in the basic research laboratory is regulated by institutional animal care and use committees and internal review boards that operate under the guidance of organizations such as the National Academy of Sciences, the Department of Health and Human Services, and the Food and Drug Administration. To use punishment procedures, researchers must provide evidence of having searched for alternative approaches to answer the research question and provide justification for the use of punishment. In addition, they must provide detailed information on how they will minimize the amount of distress to which subjects are exposed, minimize the number of subjects, and clearly detail how punishment will be implemented. After these requirements are met, the institutional animal care and use committees and internal review boards must weigh the potential benefits of the study against the proposed methods and may offer alternatives to further minimize animal distress. The use of punishment in research always involves a detailed review of the proposed procedures to ensure that research is conducted ethically, efficiently, and such that it minimizes distress to subjects.

Positive Punishment

Electric Shock

Perhaps most common form of punishment to be used in the basic laboratory is the application of mild electric shock. Researchers have used shock to study punishment effects on the behavior exhibited by rats (Azrin & Holz, 1966), pigeons (Wesp et al., 1977), primates (Bergman & Johanson, 1981), and even fish (Kuroda et al., 2019). While punishment has been investigated across a wide range of species, the most frequent participants in punishment studies have been rodents. For rodents, a mild electric current (i.e., most often < 1 milliamp) is briefly passed through the floor bars of the experimental chamber on which the rodents stand. Foot shock in rodents has been used in translational models of compulsive drug seeking (Marchant et al., 2019; Nall & Shahan, 2020), punishment-based behavioral interventions (Nall et al., 2019), and many basic studies on punishment effects (e.g., Azrin & Holz, 1966). These models have been essential for discovering important features of punishment such as factors that influence punishment efficacy (e.g., intensity, rate/schedule, immediacy), environmental factors (e.g., alternative reinforcement availability; Nall & Shahan 2020), neurobiological mechanisms underlying compulsive drug use (e.g., relapse of punished responses; Marchant et al., 2019), and basic punishment effects such as negative contrast (Nation et al., 1975). As such, these animal models have been useful tools for discovering how punishment affects behavior in humans.

Interoceptive Punishers

Another punishment method in the basic laboratory involves ingestion of unpleasant-tasting agents or infusion of agents that lead to physical malaise. These types of punishers are often used in translational animal models of addiction to simulate the adverse consequences of substance use. In an early example of this, Wolffgramm (1991) added the bitter tastant quinine to alcohol solutions and found that it reduced alcohol drinking in rats considered "controlled" drinkers but not in alcohol-dependent rats. This model highlights the tendency for individuals with substance use disorders to continue drug use despite aversive consequences, a property called *compulsive drug use*. Similar results have also been found in mice (Lesscher et al., 2010) and with other drugs of abuse (Galli & Wolffgramm, 2004; Heyne & Wolffgramm, 1998). Relatedly, adding histamine (which produces an irritating, internal itching sensation) to drug mixtures in animal intravenous self-administration models provides a means for studying compulsive use of injectable drugs (e.g., Holtz et al., 2013).

Auditory Cues

Sound, under certain conditions, can also effectively reduce behavior when used in punishment paradigms. For example, Reed and Yoshino (2001, 2008) found that relatively brief, relatively loud tones delivered immediately following an operant response can be an effective means to reduce responding, at least when the reinforcement schedule that maintains responding is relatively lean. Another interesting stimulus occasionally used in punishment procedures in rats is 22-kHz rat vocalizations. Rats emit these vocalizations in anticipation of aversive events, in response to predator presence, and in aggressive altercations with dominant animals of the same species, making it likely that these vocalization patterns serve as a phylogenetic warning signal to other rats (Portfors, 2007). Indeed, when recordings of 22-kHz rat vocalizations are played back, locomotion of other rats is significantly reduced (Brudzynski & Chiu, 1995). This effect may be specific to actual recordings of rat vocalizations, however, as pure 22-kHz tones are not more effective than 1-kHz tones (which are not known to be phylogenetically important to rats) when used as punishers (Friedel et al., 2017). However, no studies to date have examined the potential punishing effects on rat behavior of 22kHz vocalizations emitted by other animals.

Negative Punishment

Response Cost

Response cost procedures are widely used in basic human experiments on punishment (e.g., Okouchi, 2015; Pietras et al., 2010), likely to avoid any threat of physical harm to participants and to better emulate the negative punishment procedures more commonly used in clinical settings and society (where positive punishment is less common). Most often, participants perform an arbitrary operant response to earn money or points that can be exchanged for reinforcers during a baseline phase, and then punishment is implemented by removing money or points contingent upon a particular response (e.g., Okouchi, 2015; Pietras et al., 2010). Additionally, response cost procedures have also been developed for pigeons (Pietras & Hackenberg, 2005; Raiff et al., 2008) and monkeys (Seo & Lee, 2009), allowing for the use of negative punishment in the basic animal laboratory. This is commonly achieved by first establishing a token economy in which subjects earn stimuli (e.g., tokens) that can be exchanged for reinforcers (e.g., food). Then, punishment is implemented by contingently removing tokens following specific behaviors. For example, Pietras and Hackenberg (2005) trained pigeons to respond for stimulus lights that could be "exchanged" for food. During the punishment phase, responding resulted in the removal of these token stimuli, effectively reducing the target behavior.

Time-Out from Positive Reinforcement

In addition to response cost, time-out from positive reinforcement has also been used with some success in the basic laboratory. Time-out, or *time-out from reinforcement*, describes the removal of access to reinforcers contingent upon a target behavior that results in decreased future likelihood of that behavior. Thus, time-out is a negative punishment procedure, because the contingent removal of access to reinforcers following a behavior results in a decrease in the future likelihood of that behavior. For example, Ferster showed that stimuli signaling that responding will produce a time-out from ongoing reinforcement reduce responding in both pigeons (Ferster et al., 1962) and monkeys (Ferster, 1960). In an interesting set of translational experiments, time-out punishment was used to simulate the loss of resources experienced by gamblers in a rat model. Rats earned as many food pellets as possible in 30-minute sessions by allocating responses to four different options associated with different reinforcer amounts and different probabilities and durations of time-out. Most importantly, the options with the greatest reinforcer amounts were also those that produced the most reliable and longest-duration time-out periods. Using these methods, researchers found that rats that most often choose the "risky" options (i.e., large reward, high probability for long time-out) do so because they are not as sensitive to the time-out punishers as other rats (Langdon et al., 2019), and that these choice patterns had serotonergic and dopaminergic neurobiological correlates (Zeeb et al., 2009). A general finding with laboratory models of time-out is that response suppression occurs gradually with continued exposure (Holz et al., 1963), and direct comparisons with shock has shown that time-out produced less response recovery and longer-lasting suppression (McMillan, 1967). It is perhaps because of these reasons that time-out has not been more widely used in animal models of punishment.

The procedures discussed in this section have been useful for informing our basic understanding of punishment, and some have been used in translational models to better understand socially relevant problems involving punishment. Thanks to these foundational experiments, and the continued work in the basic laboratory, understanding of punishment continues to evolve. One area that has been shaped by the data provided by these procedures is the clinical use of punishment. We explore punishment in the clinic next.

Punishment in the Clinic

Ethical considerations must be at the forefront of conversations about punishment in the clinic. In fact, behavioral clinicians are ethically obligated to use the least restrictive means to reduce target behaviors (Behavior Analyst Certification Board [BACB], 2020). This obligation involves using reinforcement rather than punishment procedures when possible, using reinforcement for alternative behaviors when punishment is implemented, increasing attention and oversight (e.g., human rights review committee) to cases involving the use of punishment, and always including a plan to discontinue punishment when it is no longer necessary (BACB, 2020). Critical conversations about the use of punishment in both clinical research and practice have occurred for decades and have recently ignited increased attention with respect to the use of contingent electric skin shock to reduce severely challenging behavior. Many of the field's leading researchers in the area of severe behavior disorders have denounced the use of contingent electric skin shock (Fisher et al., 2023), and a position statement by the *Association for Behavior Analysis International (ABAI)* strongly opposed the procedure, under any condition. In addition, recent calls to action have been made opposing the use of punishment to reduce socially stigmatized behaviors, such as non-harmful stereotypies and gender-non-conforming behavior (e.g., Conine et al., 2022).

These few examples show how broader conversations about the use of punishment in clinical practice have evolved in recent years. Published research on punishment, and the ethical guidelines associated with it, may not yet reflect contemporary views of the place for punishment in clinical practice. Thus, we encourage the reader to be mindful of these research-to-practice gaps in the remainder of the chapter. We also begin our coverage of punishment in the clinic with a description of current ethical guidelines for its use and a general warning that these guidelines themselves are likely to evolve as critical conversations continue.

Ethics of Punishment in Clinical Settings

Reinforcement-based strategies (e.g., functional communication training [FCT]) have garnered a strong empirical basis, have continued to increase in efficacy, and have minimized the conditions under which punishment need be considered (Ghaemmaghami et al., 2021). However, in the applied setting, behavior analysts may encounter situations in which implementation of reinforcement-based procedures alone may seem contraindicated. Specifically, levels of target behavior may persist despite application of reinforcement-based strategies, or the intensity of the target behavior may necessitate immediate intervention to achieve reduction. Even under these circumstances, the use of punishment is a decision that must be weighed carefully with respect to several ethical guidelines, as detailed below.

When to Consider Punishment

All individuals receiving behavioral services have a right to effective treatment (Bannerman et al., 1990; Van Houten et al., 1988), which must be balanced by the behavior analyst's ethical code to "do no harm" (BACB, 2020). Thus, when deciding whether punishment should be included in a behavior reduction plan, behavior analysts must consider both the known efficacy of punishment procedures and their potential for unanticipated effects (detailed later). The decision to include punishment in a behavior plan is made on a case-by-case basis and in consideration of several variables related to the direct recipient of the service (i.e., the "client"), as well as the environments and people the client encounters daily.

One of the first considerations is how to define appropriate treatment goals for a client, which dictates whether rapid behavioral reduction via punishment should be explored further. As is customary in the goal selection process, the behavior targeted for change must constitute a socially significant behavior for the client (Cooper et al., 2020); specific to the consideration of punishment, there must be substantial value in its immediate reduction to the client. Clinicians and researchers must maintain a keen focus on direct benefit to the client or participant and avoid selection of procedures to affect change for the benefits of other stakeholders in care (BACB, 2020). For example, behaviors that are causing a high degree of harm and injury to the client or others (e.g., severe self-injury or aggression; Hagopian et al., 2015), that are greatly impacting the functioning level of the client (e.g., interfering with feeding or self-care; Volkert et al., 2011), or that are posing an immediate threat to members of society (e.g., inappropriate sexual behavior; Falligant & Pence, 2020) and risking the client's freedom are likely candidates for rapid suppression. However, this distinction alone does not constitute a default to punishment procedures. Even under these extreme circumstances, clinicians and researchers are obligated to refrain from using punishment when possible.

A functional assessment of the behavior revealing the environmental variables contributing to the maintenance of the target behavior will assist in first evaluating whether environmental manipulations (e.g., changing the way in which caregivers set up the environment and react to target behavior), teaching procedures (e.g., teaching an alternative communication response), or both may be effective without the addition of punishment. If the behavior remains insensitive to these less intrusive procedures, and continues to pose a substantial threat, the addition of punishment may be warranted (e.g., Fisher et al., 1993; Hagopian et al., 1998; Hanley et al., 2005). Behavior analysts are continuously improving methods for the function-based assessment and reinforcement-based treatment (i.e., skills-based treatment) of target behavior (Ghaemmaghami et al., 2021); therefore, these crucial initial steps in treatment planning often provide many avenues to prevent the use of punishment procedures altogether (Campbell, 2003; Pelios et al., 1999). Recent calls for trauma-informed therapy endorse these alternative avenues (Rajaraman et al., 2022).

Several additional considerations should be made if programmatic punishment is indicated as a treatment option. First, clients or their caregivers should be apprised of the proposed procedures and any alternative options during a thorough informed consent process. Clinicians should take care to inform clients or guardians of potential risks and benefits particular to the punishment procedure. In addition, ongoing oversight of the punishment procedure (e.g., regular peer review, specialized training and supervision; Luiselli, 2011; Reed et al., 2013) helps to ensure that the procedure is being implemented as intended and consented, is producing behavior change in the predicted direction, and is not causing undue harm or unforeseen risk to the client. Any undesirable effects of the punishment procedure should be documented and remedied in an efficient manner. To establish social validity of the punishment procedure, client and stakeholder preference should be systematically and continuously assessed. For some clients and stakeholders, interviews and questionnaires may be sufficient, but for individuals who do not use vocal-verbal language (as is the case for many recipients of behavioral services), other considerations must be made.

One option is to conduct a concurrent choice preference assessment between treatments including and excluding punishment (Hanley, 2010). For example, Hanley et al. (2005) was one of the first to document a client's preference for a punishment component in FCT using a modified concurrent chains arrangement. The authors exposed their two participants to FCT with and without punishment using discriminative stimuli (colored microswitches) to signal the conditions. After exposure to both conditions, participants could select among the conditions, demonstrating a direct indicator of preference. FCT with punishment was both more efficacious and preferred for both participants. This procedure, although maximally responsive to client autonomy, requires exposure to punishment ahead of the preference assessment, may be lengthy and laborious, and has not been replicated widely in behavior reduction research (Morris et al., 2021). Thus, another option in consideration of client preference is to use alternative assent-affirming practices, such as the enhanced choice model described by Rajaraman et al. (2022). This procedure included a continuous choice between treatment or no-treatment conditions that required the participants to make a simple request or move between rooms. Providing clients with the opportunity to withdraw assent from treatment in this manner represents a promising approach to assessing the social validity of punishment procedures and would benefit from replication in cases where punishment is otherwise warranted. In sum, all punishment procedures should have a process for both informed consent and client assent.

If caregivers are expected to implement the punishment procedure, factors that may influence caregiver adherence (e.g., effort) must also be addressed. Some punishment procedures (e.g., a response cost in a token reinforcement program) are equally or even sometimes less effortful to implement than alternative reinforcement procedures. However, other procedures (e.g., programmatic restraint) may require substantially more effort and come with additional concerns to safety of the implementer. At times, these procedures may be explicitly banned from some settings, like schools. Therefore, training strategies should be tailored to the punishment procedure, as well as the capabilities of the caregiver in maintaining the procedure in the typical environment with high fidelity. A clear plan for fading the punishment procedure should be established from the beginning of the program and reevaluated continuously as data are collected.

As clinicians evaluate procedures and stimuli for use as programmatic punishers, we offer some additional considerations to maximize safety, ethical use, and long-term benefit to the individual. Current practices suggest that positive punishment practices require specialized training and supervision. Similarly, it is recommended that this specialized training and supervision be extended to care providers implementing the procedures. It is also recommended that practitioners include external review from an expert panel to further ensure safe and ethical consideration for, implementation of, and plans for fading use of punishment (Luiselli, 2011; Reed et al., 2013).

Selecting a Potential Punisher

Research on the use of punishment procedures in applied settings is relatively less developed than research on the use of reinforcement procedures. Nevertheless, the research that exists on punishment provides guidelines for reducing risk and increasing benefit to both the client and their support system. One guideline is to systematically assess the potential punisher(s) that are considered for use prior to implementation (i.e., preassessments). Assessments may involve client or caregiver interviews, formal or informal observations, or experimental evaluations. A preassessment to identify a punisher can be beneficial for enhancing ecological and social validity and improving efficacy and efficiency of the procedure. Lydon et al. (2015) reviewed punishment research and identified 31 articles describing a pretreatment assessment of the punisher, of which 18 (58.1%) articles included an experimental assessment. Examples of experimental assessments documented in the extant literature include the stimulus avoidance assessment (i.e., assessment of relative avoidance or aversiveness of various stimuli; Fisher, Piazza, Bowman, Hagopian, et al., 1994; Fisher, Piazza, Bowman, Kurtz, et al., 1994), punisher assessment (Verriden & Roscoe, 2019), choice assessments (i.e., assessment of relative preference between treatment alternatives; Hanley et al., 1997; Hanley et al., 2005), and activity assessments (i.e., contingent application of low-probability activities following the target behavior; Krivacek & Powell, 1978). Conducting an experimental assessment should enhance the decision making involved in selecting the most appropriate punisher (Lydon et al., 2015).

For example, Verriden and Roscoe (2019) modified the stimulus avoidance assessment described by Fisher, Piazza, Bowman, Kurtz, et al. (1994) to evaluate reinforcement-based interventions prior to punishment-based interventions, assess punishment in the context of a reinforcement-based intervention, and measure several additional dependent variables (e.g., appropriate item engagement). Their progressive approach aligned evidence-based assessment procedures with current professional and ethical guidelines. Similarly, Simmons et al. (2022) extended this research by including caregivers as therapists in the stimulus avoidance assessment and treatment evaluation to optimize the impact of social and ecological validity of the assessment. Results indicated that caregivers could implement the procedures with high levels of fidelity and that social acceptability ratings of stimuli shifted following their own implementation. These results highlight the importance of the dynamic interplay among efficacy, acceptability, and feasibility when selecting treatment components.

Unanticipated Effects on Target and Nontarget Behaviors

Punishment-induced increases in undesirable behaviors, decreases in desirable behaviors, and escape behaviors present a challenge in applied settings. Of particular concern is the implementation of punishment in the absence of an understanding of the function of the target behavior. In these cases, the punishing stimulus may accidentally reinforce the target behavior instead of reduce it. For example, reprimands may increase behavior maintained by attention, and time-outs may increase behavior maintained by escape from demands. This underscores the importance of evaluating punishment based on its effect on behavior rather than any topographical characteristic of the stimulus change, per se. Additional unanticipated effects could include decreases in nontargeted undesirable behaviors and increases in sensitivity to reinforcement for desirable behaviors. The suggestion that punishment may increase escape behaviors and affect other nontarget behaviors has received some scrutiny. Escape from the punishing stimulus can certainly present a problem for maintenance of treatment integrity, but appropriately designed punishment protocols should minimize the opportunity for escape. Furthermore, refraining from the behavior that produces punishment could be conceptualized as avoidance behavior and would be considered a desirable outcome of punishment. All these effects have been noted in applied settings, but little research has examined the conditions under which punishment produces advantageous or disadvantageous nontarget effects (for detailed discussion, see Fontes & Shahan, 2020; Lerman & Vorndran, 2002). Finally, the short-term impact of punishment-based procedures on client–therapist rapport, and the long-term impact on client wellness, have not been established. Thus, while it is difficult to accurately predict the effects of punishment on nontargeted behavior, it is wise to consider that adverse effects are possible.

Negative Reinforcement of the Punishment Contingency for the Punishing Agent

Before reviewing types of punishment used in the clinic, we offer a final caution when considering punishment procedures. Targeted behaviors decrease when punishment is administered. This can create a negative reinforcement contingency in which the target behavior is serving as an aversive stimulus for the individual implementing punishment, and punishment removes that aversive stimulus. This is an issue that must be considered when applying punishment, as use of punishment could increase if it serves a negative reinforcement contingency for the individual applying punishment. Thompson et al. (2011) demonstrated a related effect in the context of infant caregiving. The authors arranged a laboratory simulation in which a baby doll's crying was terminated by various caregiving responses (e.g., rocking, feeding, playing). Results showed an increase in the caregiving response that reliably terminated crying, and the authors suggested that this negative reinforcement relation in its extreme form may account for some forms of physical abuse (e.g., shaken baby syndrome); that is, when suppression of behavior is a reinforcing event, the use of punishment may be negatively reinforcing and subject to misuse by the implementer.

Types of Punishment in Clinical Settings

In this section, we review punishment procedures that have been used in clinical or classroom settings, describe other procedures that have punishment-like effects, and discuss relevant terminology and examples of these procedures.

Positive Punishment

There exist examples of the use of physical positive punishers in applied contexts across visual, auditory, tactile, and gustatory modalities, as well as other external agents that impact the biological status in the body (e.g., inducing nausea; Jørgensen et al., 2011). Early applied research regarding positive punishment used punishers such as electric shock (e.g., Powell & Azrin, 1968), oral administration of lemon juice (e.g., Sajwaj et al., 1974), and water-mist sprays (e.g., Dorsey et al., 1980). The focus of much of this research was to decrease severe challenging behavior such as self-injurious behavior (SIB). For example, Lovaas and Simmons (1969) and Corte et al. (1971) demonstrated that contingent electric skin shock successfully reduced SIB exhibited by participants to near-zero levels. However, their results did not generalize across settings and only showed limited generalization across implementers. In addition, many of the ethical guidelines described before were not documented, as these research applications predated them. As function-based approaches to intervention emerged in the 1980s, the use of punishers such as electric skin shock waned, and researchers shifted their focus to reinforcement-based procedures and (when required) less intrusive punishers such as tones (e.g., WetStop® Device or urine alarm; Hanney et al., 2013), reprimands, and restraint (e.g., Pokorski & Barton, 2021), further detailed below. In 2010, *ABAI* adopted a position statement in strong opposition to the inappropriate and/or unnecessary use of restraints; in 2022, *ABAI* adopted a position in strong opposition to the use contingent electric skin shock. As such, many of the clinical studies and procedures described in this chapter are included for historical perspective and should not be viewed as current common practices in the clinic.

Reprimands

As described earlier, verbal reprimands come to serve as a generalized conditioned punisher of behavior in many humans. Indeed, reprimands are perhaps the most widely used form of punishment in everyday life. Generally, a *verbal reprimand* is broadly defined as a verbalization of displeasure, accusation, or criticism in the form of speaking, yelling, pleading, or reasoning. Other nonverbal gestures such as crossed arms, eye-rolling, stern looks, and sighing can also function as reprimands. For example, teachers often use reprimands when students misbehave, individuals often use subtle reprimands when a peer is engaging in undesirable conversation, employers may use reprimands to correct tardiness in employees, and parents often use reprimands to guide behavior in their children. Importantly, for a reprimand to function as a punisher, a reprimand must follow behavior and result in a decrease in the future likelihood of that behavior. As with all stimuli, it is possible for reprimands to have the opposite effect and increase the future likelihood of behavior. In fact, the use of reprimands following challenging behavior may be at least partially responsible for the over 50% of published outcomes showing evidence of attention as a reinforcer (Melanson & Fahmie, 2023). Perhaps for this reason, among others, reprimands are rarely included in behavior intervention plans for challenging behavior.

Blocking (Physical and Mechanical)

Blocking refers to the physical interruption of a behavior that prevents completion of the behavior and engagement with the reinforcer controlling the behavior. For example, a therapist might place his hand between the hand and mouth of an individual with pica, preventing foreign objects from entering the mouth and precluding automatic reinforcement that placing objects in the mouth may provide. Blocking may be employed using person-to-person contact (physical) or with use of a device (mechanical; e.g., body suit). It is not entirely clear what mechanism produces reductions in target behavior, but research to determine whether blocking operates via punishment or extinction processes mostly supports the conclusion that blocking operates via punishment. Lerman and Iwata (1996) determined the effects of varying schedules of blocking on hand-mouthing responses. They found that hand mouthing occurred fairly infrequently when blocking occurred on 25–100% of trials, and that blocking a greater proportion of trials resulted in further decreased hand mouthing. This finding led them to conclude that blocking served a punishing function, as continued reinforcement on 25–75% of trials (i.e., fixed-ratio [FR] 1.3–4 schedule of reinforcement) should have maintained responding and does not constitute extinction. Their conclusion that blocking serves a punishing function is consistent with a similar study (Mazaleski et al., 1994). However, counterexamples exist in the literature (Smith et al., 1999).

Overcorrection

Overcorrection refers more to a class of multicomponent positive punishment interventions than to a specific intervention. The first component of overcorrection procedures is based on the Premack principle (Premack, 1959), which states that low-probability behaviors made contingent upon high-probability behaviors may reduce the high-probability behavior. This principle is enacted in overcorrection procedures by requiring the individual to overcorrect the disruptive effects of the behavior. This component is also called *restitutional overcorrection*, because it requires the individual to return the disrupted situation to a state better than it was prior to the behavior occurring. In an early example, Azrin and Wesolowski (1974) implemented overcorrection to reduce stealing among residents of an institution. As a comparison of treatment procedures, the researchers required residents who stole other residents' snacks to either return the stolen item (i.e., simple correction) or return the stolen item and acquire a similar item to give the victim of the theft (i.e., overcorrection). Overcorrection was shown to suppress stealing to a greater extent than simple correction, though the study lacked an adequate experimental design. More modern applications of overcorrection can be found in toilet training and stereotypy research, though the necessity and ethical defensibility of those applications have come under recent scrutiny (e.g., Bacotti et al., 2023). Overcorrection procedures may also involve *positive practice*, which requires the individual to engage in an appropriate behavior directly related to the target behavior. Obviously, the restitutional component is only applicable to behaviors that produced a change in the environment that can be corrected. However, overcorrection broadly refers to procedures using restitutional overcorrection, positive practice, or both components.

Response Interruption and Redirection

Response interruption and redirection (RIRD) is a combined procedure in which a target behavior is interrupted and individuals are required to complete a high-probability response. This procedure has been used to reduce stereotypic behaviors (again, a practice recently viewed as having only individualized necessity), and involves interrupting the ongoing response, while issuing a demand for a high-probability appropriate response. For example, Hagopian et al. (2011) used an RIRD procedure to reduce pica in two children with autism. When a child began to engage in the earliest step of the behavioral chain leading to pica (i.e., picking up bated items), a therapist would physically block later steps of the chain (e.g., placing the bated item in the mouth) and redirect the participant to discard the item. This procedure was assessed only after blocking alone and competing stimuli alone were proven ineffective, and it was implemented in conjunction with noncontingent access to competing stimuli and reinforcement for the alternative response (discarding the item). The RIRD package produced a reduction in pica for both individuals. Like overcorrection, RIRD is not clearly defined as a punishment procedure, as interrupting the response precludes the reinforcer (which may be automatic). In a similar study to Lerman and Iwata (1996), discussed earlier, Ahrens et al. (2011) found that RIRD maintained similarly low levels of both vocal and motor stereotypy despite varying the proportion of responses intervened upon, indicating that RIRD may function as a punishment procedure.

Restraint (Physical and Mechanical)

In general, *restraint* is defined as contingent application of procedures to immobilize an individual's voluntary movement (Luiselli et al., 2015). Restraint applications in the clinic may be *emergent* (in response to crisis) and/or *programmatic* (e.g., as a punishment component of a behavior intervention plan). Programmatic restraint is applied contingent on a specific target behavior (e.g., self-injury) resulting in decreased instances of the target behavior in the future. Restraint procedures may be applied using person-to-person contact (physical) or a device (mechanical; e.g., splints). Forms of physical restraint exist along a continuum ranging from hand holding to prevent elopement into unsafe locations to standing, chair, or supine restraints involving multiple care providers to prevent ongoing self-injury. Similarly, mechanical restraint devices are applied to immobilize movement of appendages, body parts, or muscle groups. Devices may have fixed levels of immobilization (e.g., Posey® Strap) or be designed with varying levels of programmable immobilization (e.g., splints with adjustable stays; DeRosa et al., 2015). Readers are referred to the ABAI position statement mentioned earlier for guidance on identifying the "rare occasions" potentially necessitating restraint and the "meticulous clinical oversight and controls" required for its use.

Negative Punishment

Time-Out

Another oft debated punishment procedure in applied settings (e.g., home and school) is time-out (Barkin et al., 2007). To reiterate, time-out is a negative punishment procedure in which access to reinforcers is removed contingently upon a behavior, resulting in a decrease in the future likelihood of that behavior. Time-out can be further differentiated by specifying the location, duration, release, and mode of administration (verbal or physical; Donaldson et al., 2013) and is often termed exclusionary, nonexclusionary, or seclusion time-out (Harris, 1984). *Nonexclusionary time-out* (sometimes also referred to as *contingent observation*; Porterfield et al., 1976) refers to a decrease in the future likelihood of a behavior following the removal from positive reinforcers while the individual remains in the reinforcing environment (i.e., room with reinforcers) and may maintain visual and auditory feedback from the reinforcers or from others engaging with the reinforcers. *Exclusionary time-out* refers to a decrease in the future likelihood of a behavior following the removal of the individual from the reinforcers and restricting feedback from the environment (i.e., a room with reinforcers, but child is positioned in a corner facing away from the reinforcers). Alternatively, *seclusion time-out* (sometimes referred to as *isolation*) refers to a decrease in the future likelihood of a behavior following the removal of the individual from the reinforcers and the reinforcing environment. For example, a child causing a disruption during a recess activity at school may be sent to the sidelines for a brief time period while they watch the rest of the class continue their game of soccer (*nonexclusionary time-out*), may be sent to sit in a time-out chair next to the teacher facing toward a corner for a brief time period while still outside with their class (*exclusionary time-out*), or may be sent to a barren time-out room next to the principal's office for a brief time period while under adult supervision (*seclusion timeout*). All variations of time-out result in the removal of the child's access to the reinforcing stimuli (e.g., social reinforcement from peers), but vary in the degree to which removal from the reinforcing environment occurs. The comparative efficacy of the procedures is largely unknown; however, general guidance favors the less-restrictive inclusionary time-out when possible (Foxx & Shapiro, 1978; Wolf et al., 2006).

Clinicians may weigh a number of factors when selecting the type of time-out appropriate for a given individual. Available resources (e.g., extra personnel to monitor the individual, physical space, location), regulatory guidelines (e.g., school districts that ban seclusion), control of external reinforcers and the time-in environment (e.g., social reinforcement from peers), feasibility (e.g., duration of procedure, release strategy [time-based vs. contingency-based], mode of implementation [verbal or physical]), and safety of the individual and clinician (e.g., response topography) should all be fully evaluated and adjusted to optimize safety and efficacy of the punishment procedure. In addition, ruling out a negative reinforcement function of the targeted behavior is an important first step to ensure that the time-out procedure is not countertherapeutic.

Response Cost

Another form of punishment that has been used in the clinic is the response cost procedure. *Response cost* refers to the removal of a specified amount of reinforcer contingent upon a behavior, resulting in decreased future likelihood of that behavior. This means that response cost is also a negative punishment procedure, because a stimulus is removed following a behavior, resulting in a decrease in the future likelihood of that behavior. Common stimuli removed include specific toys, tokens, or money (i.e., fines). For example, Silva and Wiskow (2020) compared two versions of the Good Behavior Game (a group contingency to decrease disruptive behavior in classrooms) involving either the loss of tokens for disruptive behavior (i.e., response cost) or the addition of tokens for disruptive behavior (i.e., positive punishment). In the response cost condition, teams of classroom students had access to a set number of tokens, the removal of which was contingent on breaking a classroom rule. Both versions were effective, and preference probes suggested that the students and teachers preferred the response cost version of the game.

Dimensions of Punishment

Like reinforcement, there are dimensions of punishment that influence the efficacy of punishment procedures. These dimensions are intensity, rate/schedule, immediacy, availability of alternative reinforcement, and stimulus effects. In the following subsections we explore exactly what each of these dimensions is, and discuss how they influence punishment effects.

Intensity

It might seem that the most compassionate way to introduce punishment would be to gradually increase punishment frequency and intensity, starting with infrequent low-intensity punishers and increasing only when necessary. However, one of the foundational findings in punishment research is that gradual introduction of punishment may reduce sensitivity to the punisher. For example, Miller (1960) trained two groups of rats to run to the end of a maze to receive food. The Gradual group began to receive foot shock at increasing intensities (125–335 V), as well as food for reaching the end of the maze. Alternatively, the Sudden group received shock at the maximum intensity (335 V). When comparing running rate at the maximum intensity (335 V) for both groups, Miller found that the Gradual group ran the maze faster than the Sudden group. In other words, the same punishment intensity was *less* effective when introduced gradually than when it was when introduced suddenly (see also, Azrin & Holz, 1966; Powell & Morris, 1969). This is important because the goal of punishment is often to reduce behavior to some low-level criterion. If gradual introduction of punishment reduces efficacy, then it becomes necessary to expose the individual to punishment longer and with greater intensity than if more-intense punishment was used initially.

While this method of introducing punishment may seem counterintuitive, the basic effect of punishment intensity is predictable: More intense punishment tends to reduce behavior more effectively than less intense punishment. This finding is supported by basic literature in which increases in intensity of shock (Azrin et al., 1963), time-out (Kaufman & Baron, 1968), and loud tones (Reed & Yoshino, 2008) produce greater suppression of behavior across a broad range of species. Thus, when manipulated in isolation, punishment intensity is positively correlated with response suppression. However, one of the guidelines for the effective and ethical use of punishment is to use the least restrictive procedure possible. Although it is important to select an intensity of punishment that effectively reduces the target behavior but is no more restrictive than necessary, limited guidance exists toward this goal (see Lerman & Vorndran, 2002, for an extended discussion). Thus, clinicians may base selections of intensities of punishment on existing literature or contingency-based criteria (e.g., calm criteria to release from a restraint or time-out) to inform this parameter. Punishment programs that leverage the other dimensions of punishment to maximize punishment efficacy can help achieve a balance of therapeutic benefit, compassion, and safety. We explore these other dimensions next.

Rate/Schedule

Punishment can be delivered continuously or intermittently according to a variety of punishment schedules. Classic studies from the basic laboratory indicate that punishment is most effective when delivered continuously following a response (i.e., following each instance of the target behavior). For example, Pietras et al. (2010) asked adults to press buttons to earn money in a three-component multiple schedule. In the reinforcement component, money was earned for pressing the button. In the punishment component, responding continued to produce money but also produced money losses (i.e., a response cost procedure). In the third component, participants received either reinforcers (i.e., yoked reinforcement component) or punishers (i.e., yoked punishment component) at the same rate as in the punishment component. In the yoked reinforcement component, responding was similar to the reinforcement component. In the yoked punishment component, responding was reduced relative to the reinforcement component, but not as suppressed as responding in the punishment component. Furthermore, they found that the rate of punishment directly affected response suppression, with more-frequent punishment suppressing responding more than less-frequent punishment. Altogether, this study demonstrated that punishment effects are not simply the product of reduced reinforcement rate, and that punishment rate directly influences suppression of targeted responses (also see Critchfield et al., 2003; Ferraro, 1967).

Clinical data using punishment to reduce target behavior have shown more mixed results, however, with intermittent punishment schedules sometimes suppressing behavior to a level similar to continuous punishment. This difference from the basic studies discussed earlier is likely due to other factors (e.g., punishment modality, concurrent use of extinction, availability of alternative reinforcement, and schedules of reinforcement). Foreman et al. (2021) evaluated the use of an intermittent time-out procedure on the aggressive behavior of two children in an alternative-education public school. Using a series of descriptive observations, the authors first identified that teachers in the school were unlikely to implement time-out on a continuous schedule. The authors next conducted an experimental comparison of continuous and intermittent time-out, in which the intermittent schedule was matched to that naturally occurring in the classroom (time-out was implemented at less than 25% integrity). Results showed that the intermittent punishment schedule resulted in decreases in aggressive behavior comparable to that achieved by the continuous schedule (also see Clark et al., 1973).

In a review of punishment literature, Lerman and Vorndran (2002) pointed out that several studies showing effective suppression of target behavior using intermittent punishment may have confounded punishment effects with concurrent use of extinction or other nonprogrammed aversive stimuli (e.g., verbal reprimands). This is an important finding, as classic studies from the basic laboratory have shown that combined punishment and extinction generally suppresses behavior more effectively than punishment alone (Azrin & Holz, 1966), and as we discuss below, reinforcement for alternative behavior can enhance suppression by punishment.

Finally, the reinforcement schedule maintaining the behavior to be reduced by punishment can influence punishment efficacy. Reinforcement schedules control characteristic response patterns: VI and variable-ratio (VR) schedules produce constant-rate behavior (though VR produces higher-rate responding), FI schedules produce accelerations of behavior toward the end of the interval (i.e., "scalloped" responding), and fixed-ratio (FR) schedules produce a postreinforcement pause followed by high-rate behavior (i.e., "break-and-run" responding; Ferster & Skinner, 1957). Adding punishment to an ongoing VI, VR, or FI reinforcement schedule reduces the overall rate of behavior without changing the characteristic response patterns, but punishment under FR schedules increases the postreinforcement pause, with little effect on the high-rate "break" portion of the characteristic response pattern (Azrin & Holz, 1966).

Immediacy

The immediacy of punishment following a behavior is also critical for punishment efficacy. The sooner punishment follows a response, the more effective it is. Research with both humans and animals clearly shows this effect (for reviews see Azrin & Holz, 1966; Lerman & Vorndran, 2002), and basic research indicates that there is indeed a gradient from most suppression when punishment is immediate to least suppression when punishment is delayed (Kamin, 1959). However, immediate punishment may be difficult to achieve in the natural environment, where target behaviors may occur mostly in the absence of the caregiver, be delayed by other behaviors that occur in anticipation of punishment (e.g., escape), and be delayed by physical distance of the caregiver when the target behavior occurs (Lerman & Vorndran, 2002). Because of this, and as reviewed in detail by Meindl and Casey (2012), five strategies to bridge the gap between the target behavior and delayed punishment have proven effective: presenting punishment-paired stimuli immediately following behavior (Altman & Krupsaw, 1983; Tedford, 1969); increasing the intensity of the delayed punisher (Myer & Ricci, 1968); explicitly explaining the response–punishment contingency (Jackson et al., 1981; Verna, 1977); providing punishment after replaying a recorded instance of the behavior (Coppage & Meindl, 2017; Rolider & Van Houten, 1985); and providing immediate punishment after having the individual reenact the behavior (Van Houten & Rolider, 1988). These methods provide promise for applications in which immediate punishment may be difficult to achieve due to the reasons discussed earlier.

Availability of Alternative Reinforcement

It is well documented that punishment suppression is enhanced when an alternative behavior is reinforced, both in clinical (DeRosa et al., 2016; Fisher et al., 1993; Hagopian et al., 1998; Hanley et al., 2005; Rooker et al., 2013) and basic studies (Herman & Azrin, 1964; Leitenberg et al., 1975; Nall et al., 2019; Nall & Shahan, 2020; Pelloux et al., 2015). In one example of a combined punishment and reinforcement procedure, DeRosa et al. (2016) assessed the ability of a facial screen (a blocking procedure) or noncontingent reinforcement to reduce severe rumination. They found that neither procedure alone meaningfully reduced rumination, but when the procedures were combined, rumination was reduced by more than 95% compared to baseline. A related study in rats showed that while foot-shock punishment reduced ongoing lever pressing for food, lever pressing was more suppressed when reinforcement was made available for an alternative response (Nall et al., 2019). Thus, these examples demonstrate that combined alternative reinforcement and punishment can suppress behavior more effectively than punishment or alternative reinforcement alone. Furthermore, because combinations of punishment and alternative reinforcement are more effective at suppressing the target behavior, they also reduce the amount of punishment that is administered and allow lower intensities of punishment to effectively suppress the target behavior. For this reason, the Professional and Ethical Compliance Code for Behavior Analysts requires that alternative reinforcement is provided whenever punishment is used in the clinic (BACB, 2020).

Enhancement of Punishment Effects by Stimuli

A stimulus that is differentially associated with punishment (*punishment discriminative stimulus*, or S^{Dp}) can come to suppress behavior even when punishment is not in place. For example, Piazza et al. (1996) used verbal reprimands and blocking to suppress cigarette pica in an individual with autism spectrum disorder. Importantly, they provided reprimands and blocks in the presence of a purple card (i.e., the S^{Dp}). During later tests of stimulus control, they found that pica was reduced in the presence of the purple card relative to a neutral stimulus (i.e., a yellow card). Similarly, McKenzie et al. (2008) established wristbands as an S^{Dp} for verbal reprimands used to reduce automatically reinforced eye poking in an individual with intellectual and developmental delays. After training, they observed that eye poking was reduced in both training and novel environments relative to a control condition. Maglieri et al. (2000) established stickers as an S^{Dp} for verbal reprimands used to reduce food stealing in an individual with Prader–Willi syndrome. After training, stickers successfully suppressed food stealing even when it was not directly observed by clinicians (i.e., clinicians weighed containers with stickers before and after the individual had an opportunity to steal food). Together, these studies highlight the ability of discriminative stimuli associated with punishers to suppress behavior in novel environments (e.g., eye-poking study) and in the absence of the punishing agent (e.g., refraining from food stealing when the clinician is absent). Also, it is noteworthy that using S^{Dp} can provide a means to reduce the use of actual punishers, as behavior can be suppressed by their presence alone. Finally, a recent study in pigeons has shown that presenting an S^D associated with extinction contingent upon a target behavior can effectively punish the target behavior (Bland et al., 2018). This innovation could provide a means to establish a punishment contingency without having ever provided positive or negative punishment.

Summary and Conclusion

In this chapter we have aimed to provide an equal-handed review of the punishment process, with the goals of understanding punishment in the natural world and considering factors that influence the use punishment in application. Just as with reinforcement-based procedures, understanding and informing the responsible and ethical use of punishment is paramount to its effective application. In this chapter, we acknowledge substantial research-to-practice gaps that highlight how much we still must learn about such a basic process. More research is warranted to (1) inform the processes by which clinicians translate basic principles to applied practice, (2) develop contemporary guidelines for the use and fading of punishment as part of a behavior intervention plan, (3) establish systems to evaluate client assent to punishment procedures, and (4) continue to educate ourselves and those around us regarding safety and ethical concerns about the use of punishment.

REFERENCES

Ahrens, E. N., Lerman, D. C., Kodak, T., Worsdell, A. S., & Keegan, C. (2011). Further evaluation of response interruption and redirection as treatment for stereotypy. *Journal of Applied Behavior Analysis, 44*(1), 95–108.

Altman, K., & Krupsaw, R. (1983). Suppressing aggressive–destructive behavior by delayed overcorrection. *Journal of Behavior Therapy and Experimental Psychiatry, 14*(4), 359–362.

Azrin, N. H., & Holz, W. C. (1966). Punishment. In W. K. Honig (Ed.), *Operant behavior: Areas of research and application* (pp. 380–447). Appleton-Century-Crofts.

Azrin, N. H., Holz, W. C., & Hake, D. F. (1963). Fixed-ratio punishment. *Journal of the Experimental Analysis of Behavior, 6*, 141–148.

Azrin, N. H., & Wesolowski, M. D. (1974). Theft reversal: An overcorrection procedure for eliminating stealing by retarded persons. *Journal of Applied Behavior Analysis, 7*(4), 577–1581.

Bacotti, J. K., Perez, B. C., & Vollmer, T. R. (2023). Reflections and critical directions for toilet training in applied behavior analysis. *Perspectives on Behavior Science*, 1–12.

Bannerman, D. J., Sheldon, J. B., Sherman, J. A., & Harchik, A. E. (1990). Balancing the right to habilitation with the right to personal liberties: The rights of people with developmental disabilities to eat too many doughnuts and take a nap. *Journal of Applied Behavior Analysis, 23*(1), 79–89.

Barkin, S., Scheindlin, B., Ip, E. H., Richardson, I., & Finch, S. (2007). Determinants of parental discipline practices: A national sample from primary care practices. *Clinical Pediatrics, 46*(1), 64–69.

Baum, W. M. (1994). *Understanding behaviorism: Science, behavior, and culture*. HarperCollins College Division.

Bergman, J., & Johanson, C. E. (1981). The effects of electric shock on responding maintained by cocaine in rhesus monkeys. *Pharmacology, Biochemistry and Behavior, 14*, 423–426.

Bland, V. J., Cowie, S., Elliffe, D., & Podlesnik, C. A. (2018). Does a negative discriminative stimulus function as a punishing consequence? *Journal of the Experimental Analysis of Behavior, 110*(1), 87–104.

Behavior Analyst Certification Board. (2020). *Ethics code for behavior analysts*. Retrieved fom *https://bacb.com/wp-content/ethics-code-for-behavior-analysts*.

Brudzynski, S. M., & Chiu, E. M. (1995). Behavioural responses of laboratory rats to playback of 22 kHz ultrasonic calls. *Physiology and Behavior, 57*(6), 1039–1044.

Campbell, J. M. (2003). Efficacy of behavioral interventions for reducing problem behavior in persons with autism: A quantitative synthesis of single-subject research. *Research in Developmental Disabilities, 24*(2), 120–138.

Clark, H. B., Rowbury, T., Baer, A. M., & Baer, D. M. (1973). Timeout as a punishing stimulus in continuous and intermittent schedules. *Journal of Applied Behavior Analysis, 6*(3), 443–455.

Conine, D. E., Campau, S. C., & Petronelli, A. K. (2022). LGBTQ+ conversion therapy and applied behavior analysis: A call to action. *Journal of Applied Behavior Analysis, 55*(1), 6–18.

Cooper, J. O., Heron, T. E., & Heward, W. L. (2020). *Applied behavior analysis.* Pearson UK.

Coppage, S., & Meindl, J. N. (2017). Using video to bridge the gap between problem behavior and a delayed time-out procedure. *Behavior Analysis in Practice, 10*, 285–289.

Corte, H. E., Wolf, M. M., & Locke, B. J. (1971). A comparison of procedures for eliminating self-injurious behavior of retarded adolescents. *Journal of Applied Behavior Analysis, 4*(3), 201–213.

Critchfield, T. S., Paletz, E. M., MacAleese, K. R., & Newland, M. C. (2003). Punishment in human choice: direct or competitive suppression? *Journal of the Experimental Analysis of Behavior, 80*, 1–27.

DeRosa, N. M., Roane, H. S., Bishop, J. R., & Silkowski, E. L. (2016). The combined effects of noncontingent reinforcement and punishment on the reduction of rumination. *Journal of Applied Behavior Analysis, 49*, 680–685.

DeRosa, N. M., Roane, H. S., Wilson, J. L., Novak, M. D., & Silkowski, E. L. (2015). Effects of arm-splint rigidity on self-injury and adaptive behavior. *Journal of Applied Behavior Analysis, 48*(4), 860–864.

Donaldson, J. M., Vollmer, T. R., Yakich, T. M., & Van Camp, C. (2013). Effects of a reduced time-out interval on compliance with the time-out instruction. *Journal of Applied Behavior Analysis, 46*(2), 369–378.

Dorsey, M. F., Iwata, B. A., Ong, P., & McSween, T. E. (1980). Treatment of self-injurious behavior using a water mist: Initial response suppression and generalization. *Journal of Applied Behavior Analysis, 13*, 343–353.

Falligant, J. M., & Pence, S. T. (2020). Interventions for inappropriate sexual behavior in individuals with intellectual and developmental disabilities: A brief review. *Journal of Applied Behavior Analysis, 53*(3), 1316–1320.

Ferraro, D. P. (1967). Response suppression and recovery under some temporally defined schedules of intermittent punishment. *Journal of Comparative and Physiological Psychology, 64*(1), 133–139.

Ferster, C. (1960). Suppression of a performance under differential reinforcement of low rates by a pre-time-out stimulus. *Journal of the Experimental Analysis of Behavior, 3*(2), 143–153.

Ferster, C., Appel, J., & Hiss, R. (1962). The effect of drugs on a fixed-ratio performance suppressed by a pre–time-out stimulus. *Journal of the Experimental Analysis of Behavior, 5*(1), 73–88.

Ferster, C. B., & Skinner, B. F. (1957). *Schedules of reinforcement.* Appleton-Century-Crofts.

Fisher, W. W., Greer, B. D., & Mitteer, D. R. (2023). Additional comments on the use of contingent electric skin shock. *Perspectives on Behavior Science*, 1–10.

Fisher, W., Piazza, C. C., Bowman, L. G., Hagopian, L. P., & Langdon, N. A. (1994). Empirically derived consequences: A data-based method for prescribing treatments for destructive behavior. *Research in Developmental Disabilities, 15*(2), 133–149.

Fisher, W. W., Piazza, C. C., Bowman, L. G., Kurtz, P. F., Sherer, M. R., & Lachman, S. R. (1994). A preliminary evaluation of empirically derived consequences for the treatment of pica. *Journal of Applied Behavior Analysis, 27*(3), 447–457.

Fisher, W. W., Piazza, C. C., Cataldo, M., Harrell, R., Jefferson, G., & Conner, R. (1993). Functional communication training with and without extinction and punishment. *Journal of Applied Behavior Analysis, 26*, 23–36.

Fontes, R. M., & Shahan, T. A. (2020). Punishment and its putative fallout: A reappraisal. *Journal of the Experimental Analysis of Behavior, 115*, 185–203.

Foreman, A. P., Peter, C. C. S., Mesches, G. A., Robinson, N., & Romano, L. M. (2021). Treatment integrity failures during timeout from play. *Behavior Modification, 45*(6), 988–1010.

Fox, R. M. (1982). *Decreasing behaviors of persons with severe retardation and autism.* Research Press.

Foxx, R., & Shapiro, S. (1978). THE timeout ribbon: A nonexclusionary timeout procedure. *Journal of Applied Behavior Analysis, 11*(1), 125–136.

Friedel, J. E., DeHart, W. B., & Odum, A. L. (2017). The effects of 100 dB 1-kHz and 22-kHz tones as punishers on lever pressing in rats. *Journal of the Experimental Analysis of Behavior, 107*, 354–368.

Galli, G., & Wolffgramm, J. (2004). Long-term voluntary D-amphetamine consumption and behavioral predictors for subsequent D-amphetamine addiction in rats. *Drug and Alcohol Dependence, 73*, 51–60.

Ghaemmaghami, M., Hanley, G. P., & Jessel, J.

(2021). Functional communication training: From efficacy to effectiveness. *Journal of Applied Behavior Analysis, 54*(1), 122–143.

Hagopian, L. P., Fisher, W. W., Sullivan, M. T., Acquisto, J., & LeBlanc, L. A. (1998). Effectiveness of functional communication training with and without extinction and punishment: A summary of 21 inpatient cases. *Journal of Applied Behavior Analysis, 31*, 211–235.

Hagopian, L. P., González, M. L., Rivet, T. T., Triggs, M., & Clark, S. B. (2011). Response interruption and differential reinforcement of alternative behavior for the treatment of pica. *Behavioral Interventions, 26*(4), 309–325.

Hagopian, L. P., Rooker, G. W., & Zarcone, J. R. (2015). Delineating subtypes of self-injurious behavior maintained by automatic reinforcement. *Journal of Applied Behavior Analysis, 48*(3), 523–543.

Hake, D., & Azrin, N. (1965). Conditioned punishment. *Journal of the Experimental Analysis of Behavior, 8*(5), 279–293.

Hanley, G. P. (2010). Toward effective and preferred programming: A case for the objective measurement of social validity with recipients of behavior-change programs. *Behavior Analysis in Practice, 3*, 13–21.

Hanley, G. P., Piazza, C. C., Fisher, W. W., Contrucci, S. A., & Maglieri, K. A. (1997). Evaluation of client preference for function-based treatment packages. *Journal of Applied Behavior Analysis, 30*, 459–473.

Hanley, G. P., Piazza, C. C., Fisher, W. W., & Maglieri, K. A. (2005). On the effectiveness of and preference for punishment and extinction components of function-based interventions. *Journal of Applied Behavior Analysis, 38*, 51–65.

Hanney, N. M., Jostad, C. M., LeBlanc, L. A., Carr, J. E., & Castile, A. J. (2013). Intensive behavioral treatment of urinary incontinence of children with autism spectrum disorders: An archival analysis of procedures and outcomes from an outpatient clinic. *Focus on Autism and Other Developmental Disabilities, 28*(1), 26–31.

Harris, K. R. (1984). Definitional, parametric, and procedural considerations in timeout interventions and research. *Exceptional Children, 51*(4), 279–288.

Herman, R. L., & Azrin, N. H. (1964). Punishment by noise in an alternative response situation. *Journal of the Experimental Analysis of Behavior, 7*, 185–188.

Heyne, A., & Wolffgramm, J. (1998). The development of addiction to D-amphetamine in an animal model: Same principles as for alcohol and opiate. *Psychopharmacology, 140*, 510–518.

Holtz, N. A., Anker, J. J., Regier, P. S., Claxton, A., & Carroll, M. E. (2013). Cocaine self-administration punished by I.V. histamine in rat models of high and low drug abuse vulnerability: Effects of saccharin preference, impulsivity, and sex. *Physiology and Behavior, 122*, 32–38.

Holz, W. C., Azrin, N. H., & Ayllon, T. (1963). Elimination of behavior of mental patients by response-produced extinction. *Journal of the Experimental Analysis of Behavior, 6*, 407–412.

Jackson, A. T., Salzberg, C. L., Pacholl, B., & Dorsey, D. S. (1981). The comprehensive rehabilitation of a behavior problem child in his home and community. *Education and Treatment of Children, 4*(3), 195–215.

Jørgensen, C. H., Pedersen, B., & Tønnesen, H. (2011). The efficacy of disulfiram for the treatment of alcohol use disorder. *Alcoholism: Clinical and Experimental Research, 35*(10), 1749–1758.

Kamin, L. J. (1959). The delay-of-punishment gradient. *Journal of Comparative and Physiological Psychology, 52*, 434–437.

Kaufman, A., & Baron, A. (1968). Suppression of behavior by timeout punishment when suppression results in loss of positive reinforcement. *Journal of the Experimental Analysis of Behavior, 11*, 595–607.

Krivacek, D., & Powell, J. (1978). Negative preference management: Behavioral suppression using Premack's punishment hypothesis. *Education and Treatment of Children, 1*, 5–13.

Kuroda, T., Mizutani, Y., Cançado, C. R. X., & Podlesnik, C. A. (2019). Predator videos and electric shock function as punishers for zebrafish (*Danio rerio*). *Journal of the Experimental Analysis of Behavior, 111*, 116–129.

Langdon, A. J., Hathaway, B. A., Zorowitz, S., Harris, C. B., & Winstanley, C. A. (2019). Relative insensitivity to time-out punishments induced by win-paired cues in a rat gambling task. *Psychopharmacology, 236*(8), 2543–2556.

Leitenberg, H., Rawson, R. A., & Mulick, J. A. (1975). Extinction and reinforcement of alternative behavior. *Journal of Comparative and Physiological Psychology, 88*, 640–652.

Lerman, D. C., & Iwata, B. A. (1996). A methodology for distinguishing between extinction and punishment effects associated with response blocking. *Journal of Applied Behavior Analysis, 29*(2), 231–233.

Lerman, D. C., & Vorndran, C. M. (2002). On the status of knowledge for using punishment implications for treating behavior disorders. *Journal of Applied Behavior Analysis, 35*(4), 431–464.

Lesscher, H. M. B., Van Kerkhof, L. W. M., & Vanderschuren, L. J. M. J. (2010). Inflexible and indifferent alcohol drinking in male mice. *Alcoholism: Clinical and Experimental Research, 34*, 1219–1225.

Lovaas, O. I., & Simmons, J. Q. (1969). Manipulation of self-destruction in three retarded children. *Journal of Applied Behavior Analysis, 2*(3), 143–157.

Luiselli, J. (2011). Therapeutic implementation of physical restraint. In J. K. Luiselli (Ed.), *Handbook of high-risk challenging behaviors in people with intellectual and developmental disability* (pp. 243–256). Brookes.

Luiselli, J. K., Sperry, J. M., & Draper, C. (2015). Social validity assessment of physical restraint intervention by care providers of adults with intellectual and developmental disabilities. *Behavior Analysis in Practice, 8*(2), 170–175.

Lydon, S., Healy, O., Moran, L., & Foody, C. (2015). A quantitative examination of punishment research. *Research in Developmental Disabilities, 36*, 470–484.

Maglieri, K. A., DeLeon, I. G., Rodriguez-Catter, V., & Sevin, B. M. (2000). Treatment of covert food stealing in an individual with Prader–Willi syndrome. *Journal of Applied Behavior Analysis, 33*(4), 615–618.

Marchant, N. J., Campbell, E. J., Pelloux, Y., Bossert, J. M., & Shaham, Y. (2019). Context-induced relapse after extinction versus punishment: Similarities and differences. *Psychopharmacology, 236*, 439–448.

Mazaleski, J. L., Iwata, B. A., Rodgers, T. A., Vollmer, T. R., & Zarcone, J. R. (1994). Protective equipment as treatment for stereotypic hand mouthing: Sensory extinction or punishment effects? *Journal of Applied Behavior Analysis, 27*, 345–355.

McKenzie, S. D., Smith, R. G., Simmons, J. N., & Soderlund, M. J. (2008). Using a stimulus correlated with reprimands to suppress automatically maintained eye poking. *Journal of Applied Behavior Analysis, 41*(2), 255–259.

McMillan, D. E. (1967). A comparison of the punishing effects of response-produced shock and response-produced time out. *Journal of the Experimental Analysis of Behavior, 10*, 439–449.

Meindl, J. N., & Casey, L. B. (2012). Increasing the suppressive effect of delayed punishers: A review of basic and applied literature. *Behavioral Interventions, 27*, 129–150.

Melanson, I. J., & Fahmie, T. A. (2023). Functional analysis of problem behavior: A 40-year review. *Journal of Applied Behavior Analysis, 56*(2), 262–281.

Michael, J. L. (2004). *Concepts and principles of behavior analysis*. Western Michigan University, Association for Behavior Analysis International.

Miller, N. E. (1960). Learning resistance to pain and fear: Effects of overlearning, exposure, and rewarded exposure in context. *Journal of Experimental Psychology, 60*(3), 137–145.

Morris, C., Detrick, J. J., & Peterson, S. M. (2021). Participant assent in behavior analytic research: Considerations for participants with autism and developmental disabilities. *Journal of Applied Behavior Analysis, 54*(4), 1300–1316.

Myer, J. S., & Ricci, D. (1968). Delay of punishment gradients for the goldfish. *Journal of Comparative and Physiological Psychology, 66*(2), 417–421.

Nall, R. W., Rung, J. M., & Shahan, T. A. (2019). Resurgence of a target behavior suppressed by a combination of punishment and alternative reinforcement. *Behavioural Processes, 162*, 177–183.

Nall, R. W., & Shahan, T. A. (2020). Resurgence of punishment-suppressed cocaine seeking in rats. *Experimental and Clinical Psychopharmacology, 28*, 365–374.

Nation, J. R., Mellgren, R. L., & Wrather, D. M. (1975). Contrast effects with shifts in punishment level. *Bulletin of the Psychonomic Society, 5*, 167–169.

Okouchi, H. (2015). Resurgence of two-response sequences punished by point-loss response cost in humans. *Mexican Journal of Behavior Analysis, 41*, 137–154.

Pelios, L., Morren, J., Tesch, D., & Axelrod, S. (1999). The impact of functional analysis methodology on treatment choice for self-injurious and aggressive behavior. *Journal of Applied Behavior Analysis, 32*(2), 185–195.

Pelloux, Y., Murray, J. E., & Everitt, B. J. (2015). Differential vulnerability to the punishment of cocaine related behaviours: Effects of locus of punishment, cocaine taking history and alternative reinforcer availability. *Psychopharmacology, 232*, 125–134.

Piazza, C. C., Hanley, G. P., & Fisher, W. W. (1996). Functional analysis and treatment of cigarette pica. *Journal of Applied Behavior Analysis, 29*(4), 437–449.

Pietras, C. J., Brandt, A. E., & Searcy, G. D. (2010). Human responding on random-interval schedules of response-cost punishment: The role of reduced reinforcement density. *Journal of the Experimental Analysis of Behavior, 93*, 5–26.

Pietras, C. J., & Hackenberg, T. D. (2005). Response-cost punishment via token loss with pigeons. *Behavioural Processes, 69*, 343–356.

Pokorski, E. A., & Barton, E. E. (2021). A systematic review of the ethics of punishment-based procedures for young children with disabilities. *Remedial and Special Education, 42*(4), 262–275.

Porterfield, J. K., Herbert-Jackson, E., & Risley, T. R. (1976). Contingent observation: an effective and acceptable procedure for reducing disruptive behavior of young children in a group setting. *Journal of Applied Behavior Analysis, 9*(1), 55–64.

Portfors, C. V. (2007). Types and functions of ultrasonic vocalizations in laboratory rats and mice emission of ultrasonic vocalizations by adult rodents. *Journal of the American Association for Laboratory Animal Science, 46*(1), 28–34.

Powell, J., & Azrin, N. (1968). The effects of shock as a punisher for cigarette smoking. *Journal of Applied Behavior Analysis, 1*, 63–71.

Powell, R. W., & Morris, G. (1969). Continuous punishment of free-operant avoidance in the rat. *Journal of the Experimental Analysis of Behavior, 12*(1), 149–157.

Premack, D. (1959). Toward empirical behavior laws: I. Positive reinforcement. *Psychological Review, 66*(4), 219–233.

Raiff, B. R., Bullock, C. E., & Hackenberg, T. D. (2008). Response-cost punishment with pigeons: Further evidence of response suppression via token loss. *Learning and Behavior, 36*, 29–41.

Rajaraman, A., Austin, J. L., Gover, H. C., Cammilleri, A. P., Donnelly, D. R., & Hanley, G. P. (2022). Toward trauma-informed applications of behavior analysis. *Journal of Applied Behavior Analysis, 55*, 40–61.

Reed, D. D., Luiselli, J. K., Miller, J. R., & Kaplan, B. A. (2013). Therapeutic restraint and protective holding. In D. D. Reed, R. F. DiGennaro, & J. K. Luiselli (Eds.), *Handbook of crisis intervention and developmental disabilities* (pp. 107–120). Springer.

Reed, P., & Yoshino, T. (2001). The effect of response-dependent tones on the acquisition of concurrent behavior in rats. *Learning and Motivation, 32*, 255–273.

Reed, P., & Yoshino, T. (2008). Effect of contingent auditory stimuli on concurrent schedule performance: An alternative punisher to electric shock. *Behavioural Processes, 78*, 421–428.

Rolider, A., & Van Houten, R. (1985). Suppressing tantrum behavior in public places through the use of delayed punishment mediated by audio recordings. *Behavior Therapy, 16*, 181–194.

Rooker, G. W., Jessel, J., Kurtz, P. F., & Hagopian, L. P. (2013). Functional communication training with and without alternative reinforcement and punishment: An analysis of 58 applications. *Journal of Applied Behavior Analysis, 46*, 708–722.

Sajwaj, T., Libet, J., & Agras, S. (1974). Lemon-juice therapy: The control of life-threatening rumination in a six-month-old infant. *Journal of Applied Behavior Analysis, 4*, 557–563.

Seo, H., & Lee, D. (2009). Behavioral and neural changes after gains and losses of conditioned reinforcers. *Journal of Neuroscience, 29*, 3627–3641.

Silva, E., & Wiskow, K. M. (2020). Stimulus presentation versus stimulus removal in the Good Behavior Game. *Journal of Applied Behavior Analysis, 53*(4), 2186–2198.

Simmons, C. A., Zangrillo, A. N., Fisher, W. W., & Zemantic, P. K. (2022). An evaluation of a caregiver-implemented stimulus avoidance assessment and corresponding treatment package. *Behavioral Development, 27*(1–2), 1–20.

Smith, R. G., Russo, L., & Le, D. D. (1999). Distinguishing between extinction and punishment effects of response blocking: A replication. *Journal of Applied Behavior Analysis, 32*(3), 367–370.

Tedford, W. H. (1969). Effect of delayed punishment upon choice behavior in the white rat. *Journal of Comparative and Physiological Psychology, 69*, 673–676.

Thompson, R. H., Bruzek, J. L., & Cotnoir-Bichelman, N. M. (2011). The role of negative reinforcement in infant caregiving: An experimental simulation. *Journal of Applied Behavior Analysis, 44*(2), 295–304.

Van Houten, R., Axelrod, S., Bailey, J. S., Favell,

J. E., Foxx, R. M., Iwata, B. A., & Lovaas, O. I. (1988). The right to effective behavioral treatment. *Journal of Applied Behavior Analysis, 21*(4), 381–384.

Van Houten, R., & Rolider, A. (1988). Recreating the scene: An effective way to provide delayed punishment for inappropriate motor behavior. *Journal of Applied Behavior Analysis, 21*, 187–192.

Verna, G. B. (1977). The effects of four-hour delay of punishment under two conditions of verbal instruction. *Child Development, 48*(2), 621–624.

Verriden, A. L., & Roscoe, E. M. (2019). An evaluation of a punisher assessment for decreasing automatically reinforced problem behavior. *Journal of Applied Behavior Analysis, 52*, 205–226.

Volkert, V. M., Vaz, P. C., Piazza, C. C., Frese, J., & Barnett, L. (2011). Using a flipped spoon to decrease packing in children with feeding disorders. *Journal of Applied Behavior Analysis, 44*(3), 617–621.

Wesp, R. K., Latral, K. A., Poling, A. D., & Lattal, K. A. (1977). Punishment of autoshaped key-peck responses of pigeons. *Journal of the Experimental Analysis of Behavior, 27*(3), 407–418.

Wolf, T. L., McLaughlin, T., & Williams, R. L. (2006). Time-out interventions and strategies: A brief review and recommendations. *International Journal of Special Education, 21*(3), 22–29.

Wolffgramm, J. (1991). An ethopharmacological approach to the development of drug addiction. *Neuroscience and Biobehavioral Reviews, 15*, 515–519.

Zeeb, F. D., Robbins, T. W., & Winstanley, C. A. (2009). Serotonergic and dopaminergic modulation of gambling behavior as assessed using a novel rat gambling task. *Neuropsychopharmacology, 34*(10), 2329–2343.

CHAPTER 11

Schedules of Reinforcement and Punishment
TRANSLATION INTO APPLICATIONS

Alec M. Bernstein
Nathan A. Call
Kennon A. Lattal
Victoria R. Verdun

An organism's behavior is largely a function of its consequences, whether reinforcing or punishing. The availability of food and the presence of predators affect the migratory patterns of birds. Peer interactions at school and children's academic performance affect truancy. Consumers' choices affect the products that vendors select when restocking their shelves. The arrangement of such reinforcers or punishers in time and in relation to behavior creates a two-term contingency or a *schedule* (Zeiler, 1984).

Researchers have long analyzed and systematized the properties of schedules of reinforcement and punishment. Schedules, however, are not esoteric constructions artificially created to investigate equally esoteric problems in laboratories. They are both ubiquitous in every environment that living organisms inhabit and fundamental to the understanding of behavior. Schedules also do not require translation into practice in any usual sense of that expression, because schedules already were there. Schedules of reinforcement or punishment, respectively, maintain or suppress bird migration, truancy, and the restocking of store shelves before a behavior analyst intervenes. Because every intervention involves a schedule of reinforcement, punishment, or both, knowledge of these schedules is essential to best practices.

In many applications, the schedule simply serves as a conduit for delivering a reinforcer following a response. Here, the practitioner has a variety of options, each of which may yield different response rates, patterns, and resistance to change. In other instances, conceptualizing a clinical problem in terms of one schedule versus another (e.g., extinction vs. alternative reinforcement) may have different implications for treatment approaches and outcomes. In still others, drawing from knowledge about schedules of reinforcement to recast a clinical problem can lead to novel applications advancing both the basic and applied science of behavior.

The questions posed in this chapter involve the relevance of reinforcement and punishment schedules. The chapter is not a compendium or taxonomy of these. It assumes readers' familiarity with the ways in which reinforcers and punishers can be arranged in what are commonly referred to as "simple schedules," and we refer those less conversant with them to any of several works that cover this topic (Catania, 2013; Pierce & Cheney, 2017). Also, this chapter is not a comprehensive survey of schedules of reinforcement in practice—the ubiquity of schedules is prohibitive of such a venture. Rather, the chapter emphasizes the theme of ubiquity by examining how basic research on schedules has and might further influence the practices of applied behavior analysts. We first review some of the core laboratory findings of schedules of reinforcement and punishment, followed by a review of some of the practices of applied behavior analysis. We next offer a more detailed review of examples of research illustrating how reinforcement and punishment schedules underpin behavior change strategies commonly used in practice. The chapter ends with a discussion of some conceptual issues regarding translational research related to schedules and their application.

Schedules of Reinforcement and Punishment

Scheduling Response-Independent Events

The simplest two-term contingency is that between a consequence and the passage of a fixed or variable amount of time (FT and VT schedules, respectively). Although the reinforcer or punisher occurs independently of responding in these arrangements, both can still affect the response it follows, albeit adventitiously. Skinner (1948) described how response-independent reinforcement shaped novel topographies of behavior, a result subsequently replicated (Neuringer, 1970; Skinner, 1953; Zeiler, 1968, 1972; for alternative interpretations, see Staddon & Simmelhag, 1971; Timberlake & Lucas, 1985). He called this behavior *superstitious* due to its nominal similarity to the pattern of responding of humans when reinforcement occurs independently of, but within close temporal proximity following, a response. Ono (1987) told college students upon entering a room that included three levers, a point counter, and a light, that they need not emit any particular behavior, but "if you do something, you may get points on the counter." Participants accrued points according to either an FT or VT 30- or 60-second schedule. Most students exhibited transient superstitious behavior (e.g., lever pulling), and three exhibited marked repetitive, stereotyped responding (e.g., climbing on and jumping off the table).

Even when reinforcement is dependent on a particular response, other responses for which there is no dependency can increase. Rats earning food by lever pressing on fixed or variable-interval (FI or VI, respectively) schedules come to drink water soon after consuming each reinforcer, which can result in consumption of almost 10 times as much water per day than when the same amount of food is presented all at once, despite reinforcement occurring independently of drinking (Falk, 1961). Other topographies of schedule-induced behavior, or *adjunctive behavior*, occur in animals when reinforcement follows an FT schedule or a specific interresponse time (IRT) according to interval or differential reinforcement of low (DRL) rate schedules (Githens et al., 1973; Yoburn & Cohen, 1979). The topography of the adjunctive behavior often depends on the structure of the environment in which it is studied. If a running wheel is present, wheel running occurs. The same is true for stimuli that evoke adjunctive aggression (Hutchinson et al., 1968), pica (Roper & Crossland, 1982), defecation (Wylie et al., 1992), and drug self-administration (Lang et al., 1977). In humans, eating (Fallon et al., 1979), drinking (Porter et al., 1982), grooming (Gray Granger et al., 1984), fidgeting (Clarke et al., 1977), pacing (Muller et al., 1979), smoking (Cherek & Brauchi, 1981), and vocalizing (Porter et al., 1982) also can be schedule-induced. Lerman et al. (1994) examined whether the delivery of edible reinforcers on different FT schedules induced stereotypy or self-injurious behavior in four individuals with developmental disabilities who engaged in both responses. Although self-injury was not schedule-induced, stereotypy increased for three individuals under at least one FT schedule, suggesting that it likely was a form of adjunctive behavior.

In both the experimental analysis of behavior and applied behavior analysis, researchers have emphasized schedules of positive reinforcement. Just as these schedules, labeled or not, occur regularly in all environments, so do schedules of punishment. Walking in the dark results in stubbed toes, parents scold children for disobedience, and graduate advisors critique poorly written papers. Whether we label such events as punishers, consequences function as such if they reduce the future probability of the response. Because we can arrange these punishing events temporally or in relation to responses, any discussion of schedules and their effects necessarily includes schedules of punishment. Azrin (1956) evaluated response-punisher dependency and punishment schedules by maintaining key pecking by pigeons on a VI schedule of reinforcement while concurrently imposing punishment on variable (VI or VT) or fixed (FI or FT) schedules. Although greater response suppression occurred when punishment was response-dependent, FT and VT schedules also still reduced responding somewhat, indicating that, as with reinforcement, punishment can affect behavior that precedes it, even when there is no dependency between them.

Scheduling Response-Dependent Events

Reinforcers and punishers delivered independently of responding can affect responding, but the effects often are erratic and unstable. Most discussions of schedules focus on response-dependent reinforcers and punishers, the simplest of which specifies that a single response produces the reinforcer or punisher. This two-term contingency is the most basic reinforcement or punishment schedule: A fixed-ratio (FR) 1 schedule, or a schedule of continuous reinforcement or punishment. A two-term contingency in effect after a specified time constitutes an *interval schedule*. That same contingency in effect after several other topographically similar responses constitutes a *ratio schedule*. Fixed and variable intervals or numbers of responses complete the prescriptions for the four most common schedules of reinforcement and punishment: Fixed-ratio (FR), variable-ratio (VR), fixed-interval (FI), and variable-interval (VI). A remarkable variety of different schedules is based on this simple algorithm of placing a two-term contingency at the end of some preceding requirement for reinforcement and by combining individual schedules into concurrent, alternating, and otherwise sequenced, more complex arrangements. Schedules of punishment are always arranged concurrently with a schedule of reinforcement, because a response must be maintained before it can be punished. Reinforcement schedules that involve combinations of single schedules often translate into *designs* in applied behavior analysis. For example, there is an alternating-treatments design (a multiple schedule), a simultaneous-treatments design (a concurrent schedule), and a changing-criterion design (a progressive schedule). There also are schedule-thinning procedures (progressive schedules), chains of events or responses (chained schedules), and tests to assess preference between two or more alternatives (also concurrent schedules) that translate directly from their basic schedule research foundation.

In the case of reinforcement, the *basic schedules* (i.e., FR, VR, FI, and VI) noted earlier each control characteristic patterns of responding. For example, ratio schedules of reinforcement produce a higher rate of responding than equivalent interval schedules (Catania et al., 1977; Killeen, 1969; Zuriff, 1970). Fixed schedules tend to produce a reliable pause after reinforcement (Ferster & Skinner, 1957), and responding tends to be more persistent when schedules get leaner during intervals relative to equivalently reinforced ratio schedules (Kuroda et al., 2018; Lattal et al., 1998). Some common characteristics of responding on schedules make them suited to certain applications. Interval schedules can allow greater control over the rate of reinforcement than ratio schedules, which is one reason that they often appear as baselines in the experimental analysis of behavior, as when holding reinforcement rates constant between baseline and conditions designed to reduce response rates (e.g., Azrin, 1960a). In contrast, reinforcement rates are a function of response rates during ratio schedules: The higher the response rate, the more frequent the reinforcement. Although FR schedules seem to be common in applied behavior analysis, it is unclear whether this is because the schedule allows the client's responding to control the rate of reinforcement or for more practical reasons, such as counting discrete responses being easier than simultaneously tracking both time and responses.

Transitions between schedules of reinforcement also often produce characteristic patterns of responding. For example, the duration of the postreinforcement pause is controlled by the previous reinforcer when transitioning between two FR components in a mixed schedule, whereas it is controlled by both the previous reinforcer and the signaled upcoming reinforcer when transitioning between the two components of a multiple FR schedule (Baron & Herpolsheimer, 1999; Perone & Courtney, 1992; Retzlaff et al., 2017; Williams et al., 2011). Similar results appear with transitions between FI schedules (e.g., Brown & Flory, 1972). Nevin (1974, Experiment 2) reinforced pecking by pigeons on a multiple VI 2-minutes VI 6-minutes schedule, before transitioning both components to extinction. During extinction, responding persisted more in the presence of the discriminative stimulus previously associated with the VI 2-minutes schedule. This pattern of responding (i.e., resistance to change) has been described as *behavioral momentum* (Nevin & Shahan, 2011; Svartdal, 2008), which suggests that resistance to change (see Craig et al., Chapter 18, this volume) is a product of the amount of reinforcement accrued in a particular context (cf. Cohen et al., 1993; Mackintosh, 1970; Zarcone et al., 1997), with such momentum a function of the different parameters of the different reinforcement schedules. These parameters include the rate of reinforcement, devaluing the reinforcer through satiation (e.g., Capaldi et al., 1981) or added reinforcers in a different context (Nevin et al., 1990), and delays to reinforcement (Podlesnik et al., 2006; Shahan & Lattal, 2005).

As previously noted, the experimental analysis of punishment requires that responding be maintained by reinforcement, positive or negative, because there must be a maintained response to punish. In many laboratory experiments on punishment, VI schedules are used to maintain responding, because they allow a relatively wide range of response rates without affecting reinforcement rate. By far the most widely used punishment schedule in both basic and applied research is FR 1, even though punishers more often occur intermittently in natural contexts. An FR 1 schedule of punishment results in greater response suppression than leaner punishment schedules given that other variables (e.g., intensity and duration) are equal (cf. Azrin, 1956; Camp et al., 1966). As the ratio requirement or the interpunisher interval increases, response rates increase proportionally relative to those occurring with FR 1 punishment. To the limited extent that punishment schedule effects have been studied, response patterns of FI and FR punishment have been characterized as the inverse of those observed under their counterpart schedules of reinforcement (see Azrin, 1956; Azrin & Holz, 1966). For example, responding maintained on a VI schedule of positive reinforcement that is simultaneously punished on an FI schedule gradually decreases as the fixed-interval elapses and approaches the next scheduled punisher. Following the punisher, the response rate is elevated, creating a mirror image of the scallop pattern associated with responding under FI schedules of reinforcement (Azrin, 1956). The fact that punishment necessarily occurs in the context of reinforcement has led some to question whether punishment is a distinct behavioral process. Instead, punishment has been suggested to be either a variable that modifies the effect of reinforcement (e.g., Baum & Rachlin, 1969) or the suppressive effect of punishment is a by-product of the negative reinforcement of responses other than the punished response (Dinsmoor, 1954).

Parameters of Reinforcement and Punishment

Patterns of responding are determined predominantly by the schedule of reinforcement, punishment, or both. Response rates are determined by the response–reinforcer dependency (Zeiler, 1968), the schedule of reinforcement (e.g., VI vs. VR or DRL vs. differential reinforcement of high [DRH] rate), and, with the schedule held constant, the parameters of the reinforcer that are arranged by the schedule. The most studied parameters of both reinforcers and punishers are rate, immediacy, magnitude (duration or amount), and quality (type or intensity). Responding is generally more frequent when reinforcement is more frequent (Lalli & Casey, 1996), immediate (as opposed to delayed; Horner & Day, 1991), of greater magnitude (Borrero et al., 2005), or of higher quality (Harzem et al., 1978). Responding also is less frequent with more frequent (Appel, 1968), immediate (as opposed to delayed; Camp et al., 1967), and intense punishers (Azrin & Holz, 1966; Church, 1969). There are exceptions and qualifications to these generalizations. For example, response rates are higher and delay-of-reinforcement gradients are less steep for signaled compared to unsignaled delays (Richards, 1981; Sizemore, 1976).

Similarly, although reinforcer magnitude can influence response allocation and response rates (e.g., Catania, 1963; Hutt, 1954; Jenkins & Clayton, 1949; Reed, 1991; Reed & Wright, 1988; Stebbins et al., 1959), there are inconsistent findings regarding the direction in which reinforcer magnitude and quality impact responding (see Bonem & Crossman, 1988, for a review). Some have found a positive relation between reinforcer duration and response rates (Bradshaw et al., 1978), whereas others have found the opposite for reinforcer quality (e.g., sucrose concentration; Harzem et al., 1978). Reed (1991) found that the effects of the number of food pellets comprising a single reinforcer for lever pressing by rats depended on the schedule of reinforcement. Increasing the quality of reinforcement, defined by the number of food pellets delivered, resulted in higher response rates on VR, concurrent VI VI, and multiple VI VI schedules, but depressed response rates on VI schedules.

Applied behavior analysts often are concerned with the quality of a reinforcer—a focus that has contributed to the development of a substantial literature on preference and reinforcer assessments (Cannella et al., 2005; Hagopian, Long, et al., 2004). Responses targeted for change by applied behavior analysts also are affected by other reinforcement parameters (Neef et al., 1994; Neef & Lutz, 2001; Perrin & Neef, 2012). For example, Athens and Vollmer (2010) arranged a concurrent schedule in which problem behavior and an appropriate alternative response each produced the reinforcer that maintained problem behavior. They then manipulated several parameters of reinforcement (i.e., duration of access, quality, immediacy, or a combination) for each response. The response associated with longer, higher-quality, and more immediate reinforcement occurred most frequently. Greater differentiation, however, occurred when they simultaneously manipulated several reinforcer parameters. Kunnavatana et al. (2018) assessed which parameters of reinforcement exerted the greater influence over arbitrary responses before manipulating these parameters during the treatment of problem behavior. Although both appropriate and problem behavior were reinforced during treatment, the reinforcer was manipulated along the dimension identified by the assessment and inversely applied to problem (e.g., decreased quality) and appropriate (e.g., increased quality) behavior, resulting in an increase and decrease of appropriate and problem behavior, respectively.

Regarding punishment, response suppression is related directly to punishment intensity (Appel, 1961; Azrin, 1960a; Azrin & Holz, 1966; Church, 1963). Azrin et al. (1963) irreversibly suppressed pigeons' responding by delivering a sudden, intense shock (80 V). In contrast, pigeons initially receiving a moderate shock (60 V) continued responding as the shock intensity gradually increased to a substantially higher intensity (130 V; cf. Miller, 1960). This effect parallels how punishment often affects responding outside the laboratory. Parents might deliver a mild reprimand following their child's annoying behavior. Continued annoying behavior may result in increasingly loud or harsh reprimands until the parent eventually screams the reprimand. Yet the findings of Azrin et al. (1963) suggested that (leaving aside the issue of whether a reinforcement-based strategy would be more effective or ethical) if the parent is going to use punishment, a moderately intense punisher may suppress responding sufficiently if delivered after the first occurrence. This reductive effect also can be durable (Azrin & Holz, 1966; Masserman, 1946). If responding recurs after the discontinuation of punishment, it often recovers to prepunishment levels; however, responding after lower-intensity punishment recovers more rapidly than after higher-intensity punishment (Filby & Appel, 1966; Hobbs et al., 1978).

Also, like reinforcement, punishment generally has the greatest effect on behavior it immediately follows (e.g., Baron et al., 1969; Camp et al., 1967; Cohen, 1968). Delays of 10–30 seconds have been shown to degrade the effects of punishment on responding by rats (Goodall, 1984) and humans (Banks & Vogel-Sprott, 1965; Trenholme & Baron, 1975). Abramowitz and O'Leary (1990) reported a similar punishment finding during a classroom-based intervention. A teacher delivered reprimands either immediately or 2 minutes after an instance of off-task behavior by first and second graders. Although both procedures decreased off-task behavior, immediate punishment reduced it more than delayed punishment. There are ways, however, to moderate the effects of delays to punishment using signals. Rolider and Van Houten (1985) audio-recorded a child's tantrums and then played those recordings for the child several hours later, delivering a punisher immediately following audio of a tantrum. The child's tantrums decreased, providing evidence that delayed punishment may still be viable from an efficacy standpoint when procedures are adopted to diminish the impact of those delays.

Schedules of Reinforcement and Punishment in Application

Schedules to applied behavior analysts are tools to achieve therapeutic goals. These goals are the functions of applied behavior analysis, the most general of which are increasing behavior that is more conducive to and decreasing behavior that conflicts with optimal functioning and sustaining behavior once it is changed in positive ways. Sometimes the changes require but a "tweaking" of schedules already in play, and other times they require a major redesign of the contingencies of living. We discuss how each of the therapeutic goals can be, and have been, impacted by schedules of reinforcement and punishment in the following sections.

Increasing Behavior

A basic request of applied behavior analysts is to establish new forms of behavior not present in the client's repertoire. *Response shaping,* or the differential reinforcement of successive approximations, is important for establishing a certain type of response before that target response type is maintained by naturally occurring reinforcement schedules. Shaping is detailed elsewhere in this book (see Falcomata & Neuringer, Chapter 20, this volume) thus, it is not considered in this review of schedules. Requiring a level equal to that of a functionally equivalent but topographically dissimilar form of behavior can increase existing forms (i.e., response differentiation). Gradually changing a topographically related form already existing at an appropriate level can produce novel forms (i.e., discriminated operants). Sometimes the form of behavior is too rigid and stereotyped, restricting the individual's optimal functioning in the relevant environment. It is the applied behavior analysts' job to increase the variability of the response under such circumstances (i.e., response variability).

Response Differentiation and Variability

Schedules of reinforcement are used to change the characteristics of previously established responses, a process of response differentiation. Ratio and interval schedules, for example, differentially reinforce shorter or longer IRTs, respectively (e.g., Morse, 1966). On a ratio schedule, each additional response brings the total number of responses closer to the one that will meet the criterion for reinforcement, regardless of the IRT. In contrast, on an interval schedule, the longer the IRT, the greater the proportion of the interval that elapses and the greater the probability that the next response will be reinforced. Thus, ratio schedules differentially reinforce (i.e., shape) shorter IRTs, whereas interval schedules shape longer ones. These naturally developing relations between responses and reinforcement are more explicit in DRL and DRH schedules in which only responses separated from one another by a required IRT are reinforced.

The DRL schedule can be arranged by making reinforcement dependent on (1) the first response after a set IRT ($IRT > t$ or *spaced-responding DRL*; Ferster & Skinner, 1957) or (2) a period during which overall response rates are lower than a predetermined criterion (*interval* or *full-session DRL*; Deitz, 1977; Deitz & Repp, 1973). The experimental analysis of behavior has almost exclusively used spaced-responding DRL to evaluate, for example, the role of response rate in producing behavioral effects (e.g., Freeman & Lattal, 1992). Combining a short DRL schedule (e.g., 3 seconds) with a VI schedule to yield a tandem VI DRL schedule can greatly reduce response rates, while allowing the experimenter to control reinforcement rates in a way not possible with a simple spaced-responding DRL arrangement (Lattal, 1989). In contrast, applied behavior analysts have relied more on full-session DRL, likely because the procedures are more easily implemented and controlled (e.g., Hagopian et al., 2009). In an exception to this tendency, Anglesea et al. (2008) decreased the rapid eating of three teenagers by matching the intervals for bites in a spaced-responding DRL to the IRTs of bites by a typically developing adult. In another, Austin and Bevan (2011) arranged a spaced-IRT DRL schedule to decrease student bids for teacher attention by setting the interval to align with class periods (i.e., 20 minutes) and the response criterion to match the rate of bids that the teacher deemed appropriate.

Although both are referred to as DRL schedules, the spaced-responding DRL can produce different patterns of responding than full-session DRL. Spaced-responding DRL maintains a low response rate because reinforcement immediately follows the first response after the predetermined criterion IRT. In a full-session DRL, reinforcement occurs at the end of an interval during which responding occurred at or below the criterion. Reinforcement, therefore, can occur following a low rate *or no instances* of responding, the latter closely resembling a differential reinforcement of other behavior (DRO) schedule (Jessel & Borrero, 2014), and resulting in a near-zero rate of responding. Although this approach may be useful for eliminating behavior without using extinction or punishment (Bonner & Borrero, 2018), the purpose of DRL often is to maintain a low level of, not eliminate, responding. The use of discriminative stimuli to signal the duration of the DRL interval might produce the low rate of responding like spaced-responding DRL (Becraft et al., 2017, 2018). For example, Piper et al. (2020) implemented spaced-responding and full-session DRL schedules in an alternating treatments design to reinforce a low level of "virtual" recycling during a computer-based game for 10 individuals with autism spectrum disorder (ASD). They included the image of an open and a closed receptacle as discriminative stimuli to signal the availability and unavailability of reinforcement, respectively, within both DRL schedules. Spaced-responding and full-session DRL schedules, which included discriminative stimuli, produced similarly low rates of responding, and full-session DRL produced a greater proportion of reinforcers earned.

Two forms of DRH include reinforcement for lower IRTs across responses (*IRT < t* or *spaced-responding DRH*) or for a minimum number of responses within a predetermined period (*interval* or *full-session DRH*). As with DRL, spaced-responding DRH is more common in the experimental analysis of behavior, and full-session DRH is more common in applied behavior analysis. Girolami et al. (2009) used a full-session DRH to increase the rate of self-eating of a 9-year-old boy receiving treatment for food refusal. Baseline mealtimes lasted 35–60 minutes, and food refusal had resulted in reliance on a gastrostomy tube for 60% of his calories. During DRH, meal completion under 30 minutes resulted in 10-minute access to a highly preferred video. The DRH rapidly increased the rate of independent bites and shorter meals, which resulted in the boy being tube-weaned at the end of an intervention. Zeiler (1970) reported similar increases in response rates when time limits for pigeons to complete an FR 25 schedule were imposed. A potential drawback to both types of DRH arrangements is that if the participant starts to miss scheduled reinforcers, the response can extinguish rapidly, resulting in what could be called a death-spiral effect. High response rates also can be generated by using a tandem VI VR schedule with a relatively small VR requirement (Lattal, 1989; Peele et al., 1984). Such an arrangement greatly reduces the likelihood of the death-spiral extinction effect just described.

Related to the DRH schedule is the reinforcement of a minimum number of responses in a specified period following the availability of a reinforcer (i.e., a *limited hold*; Ferster & Skinner, 1957; Mace et al., 1994). Such arrangement also is common in nonlaboratory settings. For example, homework can be graded only after the material is taught, but before the homework due date; bills must be paid between the first and 10th of the month to avoid late fees; and one can only board their flight between the first boarding call and 10 minutes before departure. Although not always conceptualized as DRH, limited holds are commonly used with time- or interval-based reinforcement and have been used with, for example, VI (Ferster & Skinner, 1957), FI (Black et al., 1972), and DRL (Conrad et al., 1958) schedules. Schoenfeld et al. (1970) described a strictly temporal reinforcement schedule classification system based on the limited hold. In that system, the interreinforcer interval is divided into two parts, one in which reinforcement is not available (the T period) and another in which it is (the tau period). They went on to show how varying the ratios of T and tau could mimic the behavioral effects of more conventionally taxonomized interval and ratio schedules. Although used infrequently in contemporary basic research, the limited hold has been used with DRL schedules to examine how narrowing the window of reinforcement availability affects the temporal control of responding. A difficulty with limited holds is the death-spiral effect described earlier. Tiger et al. (2007) reinforced brief latencies in answering questions by a young man diagnosed with Asperger syndrome. Each answer was reinforced (FR 1) with the restriction that answers had to be initiated before a specified period expired (i.e., the limited hold). The limited hold was set to 10% less than the mean latency to responding in the previous session. An instruction (e.g., "Answer the questions in less than X seconds to earn a reinforcer") preceded each session. Failure to meet the contingency on a trial resulted in the therapist restating the contingency (e.g., "Too slow; you need to answer in under X seconds"). Latencies decreased across easy, medium, and difficult questions. Accuracy, however, varied until responding that both met the limited hold criteria and was accurate was reinforced.

Responses also can be established through the differential reinforcement of successive approximations of a target response—response shaping—that can change both the topography and probability of a target response. Shaping begins by (1) defining the target response and (2) determining the available response repertoire from which shaping can begin. Skinner (1953) famously likened the shaping process to a sculptor forming a lump of clay into an object. With respect to shaping a key pecking response of a pigeon, for example, he observed that "we reinforce only slightly exceptional values of the behavior observed while the pigeon is standing or moving about. We succeed in shifting the whole range of heights at which the head is held, but there is nothing which can be accurately described as a 'new' response" (pp. 91–92). The shaping process involves the successive extinction of earlier approximations and the reinforcement of subsequent ones more closely resembling the target response, until the latter is achieved. Two dimensions of shaping are the time spent reinforcing and the size of the increments between each approximation of the target response. Eckerman et al. (1980) found that shaping "proceeds most efficiently with rapid, relatively large shifts in criterion performance" (p. 299; see Pear & Legris, 1987, for an example of shaping pigeon movements using a computer-controlled system).

Shaping in its usual format is a subjective process that relies on the skills and judgment of the shaper. Percentile schedules offer a more objective method of shaping that has found many uses in both basic and applied behavior analysis. Its basic method involves the reinforcement (Davis & Platt, 1983; Galbicka, 1988; Galbicka & Platt, 1989; Platt, 1973; Scott & Platt, 1985) or punishment (Arbuckle & Lattal, 1992) of a particular response relative to its recent frequency. Athens et al. (2007), for example, used a percentile schedule to increase the on-task behavior of four children by making reinforcement dependent on being on-task longer than they had been in 50% of the most recent 5, 10, or 20 trials. Similar percentile schedules were used to differentiate other clinically relevant responses, such as longer periods of smoking abstinence (Lamb et al., 2004, 2005, 2010), fluency of academic responding (Clark et al., 2016), variability in computer game playing (Miller & Neuringer, 2000), and duration of eye contact (Hall et al., 2009).

Just as schedules of reinforcement or punishment can produce differentiation in the rate or topography of a response, so, too, can it influence variability of these attributes (see Falcomata & Neuringer, Chapter 20, this volume). For example, intermittent reinforcement generally engenders more variation in response rate than does continuous reinforcement, in part because there are simply more responses comprising the sample (Boren et al., 1978). The results of other basic and applied behavior-analytic experiments have shown that variability also can be increased through extinction (Antonitis, 1951) or *lag schedules* that arrange reinforcement of an individual or a sequence of responses that differ from a predetermined number of previous responses (Joyce & Chase, 1990; Page & Neuringer, 1985; Valentino et al., 2011). Lag schedules have increased the variability of, for example, activity selection (Cammilleri & Hanley, 2005), play (Baruni et al., 2014; Lang et al., 2020), martial arts skills (Harding et al., 2004), and verbal behavior (e.g., Falcomata et al., 2017; Silbaugh & Falcomata, 2019; Susa & Schlinger, 2012). Heldt and Schlinger (2012) used a Lag 3 schedule to increase the variability of tacts for two children with disabilities. Accurate tacts of various pictures were reinforced only if they differed from those on any of the previous three trials. Variability in tacts increased and maintained during a follow-up test conducted 3 weeks after terminating the experiment. Smaller-valued lag schedules (e.g., Lag 1) can produce higher-order stereotypy like FR and extinction schedules, because reinforcement requires *alternating,* or sequencing, responding rather than true variability (Neuringer, 1991; Schwartz, 1982). This limitation can be mitigated by increasing the lag schedule requirement (Dracobly et al., 2017).

Response Variability: Developing Discriminated Operants

In addition to shaping the rate and form of a response, a significant aspect of applied behavior-analytic treatment involves bringing responses under stimulus control. Yelling, for example, is appropriate in certain contexts (e.g., a rock concert or school pep rally), but is problematic if it occurs at the wrong time or in the wrong place (e.g., the library). One circumstance where stimulus control has been used clinically is following successful treatment of problem behavior using functional communication training (FCT). In the early stages of FCT, alternative responses that replace problem behavior (e.g., mands or compliance) usually are reinforced on an FR 1 schedule, which rapidly reduces problem behavior. Rarely, however, is it practical to continue reinforcing each alternative response once problem behavior has decreased. Yet thinning the schedule of reinforcement of mands likely will increase the rate of manding. Mands typically occur in the presence of discriminative stimuli (e.g., a listener attending to the speaker). This circumstance comprises a multiple schedule in which periods of FCT (FR 1 for alternative behavior; extinction for problem behavior) alternate with periods of extinction of both problem behavior and the alternative response. Typically, each component also is correlated with distinct arbitrary (Hanley et al., 2001) or nonarbitrary (Kuhn et al., 2010) stimuli. The duration of the extinction component of the multiple schedule generally is brief at first relative to the FCT component. This duration often is set a priori. If the initial extinction component is too brief, problem behavior may not contact the absence of reinforcement (procedural extinction), whereas a long period of nonreinforcement may completely eliminate the alternative response (functional extinction) before it contacts reinforcement in the FCT component. After successfully reducing the problem behavior of five individuals, Call et al. (2018) yoked the duration of an extinction component of a multiple schedule to the mean IRT of their mands during FCT. The mands of all five participants came under the control of the stimuli associated with the extinction and reinforcement components of the multiple schedule.

One outcome of employing multiple schedules is that the behavior controlled by the different components is affected by not only by the conditions in effect in the component under consideration but also the conditions in the other components. Such interactions often are described in terms of the relations between the rates of responding in the two components (Reynolds, 1961), although the controlling relation is between response rate in the unchanged or constant component and an independent variable (as opposed to the dependent variable of response rate) in the changed one. Table 11.1 identifies the four interactions between the two components of a multiple schedule. When an alteration in the conditions of reinforcement in one component changes the rate of responding, changes in the rate of responding in the other, constant component, may occur that are in the same direction (*induction*) or in the opposite direction (*contrast*). These changes may occur despite the conditions of reinforcement in the constant component remaining unaltered. The valence (positive or negative) indicates the direction of the response rate change in the unchanged component. Halliday and Boakes (1971) illustrated the differences in the effects of response and reinforcement rate changes noted earlier by comparing transitions from a multiple VI VI schedule to either a multiple VI VT schedule or to a multiple VI extinction schedule. In the former transition, reinforcement rates in the VI to VT component were held constant, so that the only change was greatly reduced response rates during the VT component. The transition from VI to extinction resulted in both reduced response and reinforcement rates. Increased response rates—*positive behavioral contrast*—occurred in the constant VI component only when the transition in the other component was to extinction. Thus, response rate reduction by itself was insufficient to produce contrast, which occurred only when the opportunity for reinforcement was eliminated. Behavioral contrast also can occur during concurrent (Catania, 1961) and chained (Wilton & Gay, 1969) schedules of reinforcement.

TABLE 11.1. Schedule Interactions: Induction and Contrast

Change in reinforcement value	Response rate in unchanged component of schedule	
	Increase	Decrease
Increase	Positive induction	Negative contrast
Decrease	Positive contrast	Negative induction

Note. Primarily observed within a multiple schedule, changes in the schedule of reinforcement under one component of the multiple schedule can affect responding under that component and also under the unchanged component of the multiple schedule.

Schedule interactions may occur in any number of situations where a schedule of reinforcement is altered as part of a treatment in one context (e.g., a clinical setting) but not others (e.g., home). For example, Wahler et al. (2004) trained the parent of a child with oppositional behavior to place it on extinction, resulting in a reduction of such behavior at home. The child's teacher declined the same training. Even though the rate of teacher-delivered reinforcement did not change, contrast occurred in the classroom in the form of increases and decreases in the rate of oppositional behavior that were negatively correlated with his parent implementing extinction and then reversing to baseline conditions at home. Induction and contrast also have been observed in multiple schedules in which responding in one component is punished (e.g., Brethower & Reynolds, 1962; Crosbie et al., 1997; Thomas, 1968), but the controlling variables of these effects on unpunished responding remain largely uninvestigated.

Applied behavior analysts also often introduce schedule changes that are correlated with treatment setting (Craig et al., 2017; Koegel et al., 1980; Sullivan et al., 2020). For example, functional analyses (FAs) typically introduce an FR 1 schedule of reinforcement of problem behavior and are frequently conducted in a distinct assessment setting (e.g., a specially equipped clinic room). This arrangement may induce problem behavior in other settings (e.g., home or other parts of the clinic), where the problem behavior remains on a presumably intermittent schedule. Several evaluations have produced mixed results regarding whether contrast and induction occur in such situations (Call et al., 2012; Shabani et al., 2013). For example, Call et al. (2017) reinforced problem behavior on a VR 3 schedule across all of the settings in a clinic before introducing an FR 1 during an FA conducted only within a specific room. The VR 3 remained in place when participants were in any other part of the clinic. When the FA was initiated, the problem behavior of two of the six participants increased in the nonassessment settings (positive induction). Such behavior decreased for a third participant (negative contrast). Thus, induction of problem behavior in nonclinical settings may occur because of conducting an FA in a clinical one, but beneficial contrast also can result.

Decreasing Behavior

Designing schedule-based interventions for decreasing behavior that is problematic for the person or for those responsible for the person's well-being is another major activity of applied behavior analysts. This function is intertwined with establishing new forms of behavior, because reducing one class of behavior creates a vacuum that may be filled by other undesirable forms of behavior unless more useful ones replace it. Response-elimination methods can be based on schedules of reinforcement, punishment, or both together.

Time-Based Schedules

Extinction (i.e., the discontinuation of reinforcement) is perhaps the most widely used method for decreasing behavior. Time-based schedules that arrange delivery of response-independent reinforcers also have been considered a form of extinction by some (i.e., they include periods of nonreinforcement; Lattal et al., 2013; Rescorla & Skucy, 1969), but whether this is functionally equivalent to reinforcement removal is an open question. In experiments with nonhuman animals, transitioning from response-dependent to response-independent reinforcement decreases the rate of the previously reinforced response (Appel & Hiss, 1962; Lachter, 1971; Lachter et al., 1971; Lattal, 1972, 1973; Skinner, 1938; Zeiler, 1968), sometimes to zero. Lattal (1974) and Kuroda et al. (2013) delivered reinforcers after fixed or variable times. Across several conditions, the proportions of those reinforcers that were response-dependent varied from 0 to 1.0, with the remainder occurring independently of responding. Response rates were proportional to the proportion of response-dependent reinforcers. Similar results were reported by Bergmann et al. (2017) in an experimental analysis of procedural integrity. Whereas errors of *omission* are instances in which an expected consequence is not delivered when prescribed, thereby disrupting the response-reinforcer dependency similar to extinction as the discontinuation of reinforcement, errors of *commission* are instances in which the consequence is delivered but inaccurately. The experiments of Lattal (1974) and Kuroda et al. (2013) illustrated the latter in that differing proportions of the reinforcers were "uncoupled" from responding. These errors of commission are more detrimental to treatment outcomes (DiGennaro Reed et al., 2011; St. Peter et al., 2016).

The reductive effects of time-based schedules also are replicated in applied behavior analysis (Baer & Sherman, 1964; Britton et al., 2002; Hagopian et al., 1994; Lomas et al., 2010; Marcus & Vollmer, 1996; O'Reilly et al., 1999; Roscoe et al., 1998; Vollmer et al., 1995). The use of FT and VT schedules is described as *noncontingent reinforcement* (NCR; Vollmer et al., 1993). This term has been debated given that a contingent (really, dependent) relation is part of the definition of reinforcement and the fact that so-called NCR is dependent on the passage of time (e.g., Lattal & Poling, 1981; Poling & Normand, 1999). Vollmer et al. (1998) showed that FT schedules decreased the severe problem behavior of three children more rapidly than extinction (reinforcement removal) alone (cf. Thompson et al., 2003). Additionally, it has been suggested that the use of time-based schedules may be more ethical than extinction alone, because they do not require the complete elimination of reinforcement (Vollmer et al., 1993). Despite limited comparisons of the relative effects of FT and VT schedules, extant applied behavior-analytic research suggests little difference in the reductive effects of the two (Carr et al., 2001; Van Camp et al., 2000). Findings with nonhuman animals suggest that the reductive effects of FT and VT schedules depend on the schedule of response-dependent reinforcement in effect prior to removal of the response-reinforcer dependency. Using rats, Lattal (1972) showed that transitions to FT after FI resulted in considerably higher rates in the absence of the response-reinforcer dependency than was maintained by a VT schedule following the reinforcement of responding according to a VI schedule (see Zeiler, 1968, for examples of other combinations of interval and time schedule transitions). Regardless of whether the preceding schedule is VI or FI, FT schedules result in positively accelerated responding (Lattal, 1972; Zeiler, 1968), suggesting that such patterns might occur if FT schedules follow interval schedules during treatment.

The difference in reinforcement rate between the baseline schedule of reinforcement and the subsequent schedule of response-independent reinforcement also affects the rate and extent to which time-based schedules reduce responding (see Lachter et al., 1971). Hagopian et al. (1994) compared rich and lean FT schedules to treat the problem behavior of quadruplet 5-year-old girls. The former reduced that behavior more quickly and to a greater degree than did lean FT schedules. Ringdahl et al. (2001) extended Hagopian et al.'s results by also including a condition in which they yoked the rate of reinforcement in an FT condition to the rate of reinforcement in the previous baseline condition. For two of three participants, responding decreased most under a rich FT schedule, whereas responding of the third was reduced most under the leaner FT schedule. In contrast, the

FT schedule yoked to the rate of reinforcement at baseline did not reduce any participants' responding. These findings suggest that although richer time-based schedules may reduce responding more than leaner time-based schedules, the efficacy of time-based schedules in reducing responding may be a function of how much the rate of reinforcement differs from that of baseline reinforcement, regardless of whether it is richer or leaner. The possibility that relatively leaner FT schedules than the previous rate of reinforcement can have a reductive effect is clinically notable, because rich FT schedules often must be thinned to more practical levels; however, there still remains limited research on the effects of time-based schedules when comparing baseline to treatment rates of reinforcement.

A final, practical consideration of using time-based schedules to reduce behavior is that they may adventitiously reinforce problem behavior (e.g., Ono, 1987; Skinner, 1948). Vollmer et al. (1997) required the absence of problem behavior for a period just before the delivery of reinforcement on an FT schedule, which helped facilitate discrimination between response-reinforcer relations and likely prevented adventitious reinforcement. By adding this contingency, the schedule technically became a tandem time schedule followed by a DRO (cf. Craig et al., 2014; Lattal & Boyer, 1980). In that DRO and time schedules have different reductive effects, we caution interpreting DRO as a time schedule at all.

Differential Reinforcement of Other Behavior

When reinforcement depends on a period elapsing without a target response, a DRO (Reynolds, 1961) schedule is defined, although many have pointed out the conceptual problems of defining a schedule in terms of reinforcing the absence of the response (e.g., Lattal & Poling, 1981) and some have offered alternative descriptions. Kelleher (1961) described it as the differential reinforcement of pausing, and others have labeled the "O" of DRO as "omission" (Uhl & Garcia, 1969) or "zero rates" of the target response. The DRO label, like the equally questionable NCR, persists. Like many other schedules (e.g., DRL and DRH), DRO schedules can be programmed in different ways. Resetting the DRO interval immediately after the response or at the conclusion of a predetermined period has roughly equivalent effects on the rate and level of response reduction (Gehrman et al., 2017; Nighbor et al., 2020). Similarly, reinforcement can be delivered for the absence of a target behavior across a whole interval (i.e., FI and VI; Repp et al., 1983), or during a brief observation at the conclusion of an interval (i.e., momentary DRO; Lattal & Boyer, 1980). Specific momentary DROs include fixed- (FM; Hammond et al., 2011) and variable- (VM; Hamilton et al., 2020) momentary schedules. Lindberg et al. (1999) found that reinforcement delivered on FI, VI, and VM schedules within a DRO were equally effective in immediately decreasing self-injury, highlighting the utility of DRO schedules in reducing problem behavior. These results are supported by findings in the experimental analysis of behavior suggesting that the type of DRO is less important than the contingency itself (Capriotti et al., 2012; Nighbor et al., 2020). Although research suggests that they are as effective as interval-based DROs, momentary DROs require less effort to implement, because one need not monitor responding throughout the entire interval (Barton et al., 1986; Kahng et al., 2001; Toussaint & Tiger, 2012; cf. Derwas & Jones, 1993; Hammond et al., 2011).

Outcomes of comparative analyses between DRO and other response-reduction procedures are mixed regarding which produces the greatest reductions in responding (Lerman & Iwata, 1996). After maintaining lever pressing by rats on a VI 30-seconds schedule, Davis and Bitterman (1971) grouped rats in pairs with similar baseline response rates. One member of each pair then was exposed to a resetting DRO 10-seconds schedule (i.e., reinforcement occurred following the absence of lever pressing for a 10-second period, and each response restarted the interval). The other member of the pair received response-independent reinforcers yoked in frequency and temporal location to its partner. Responding was reduced more quickly and to lower levels over the 21 sessions of the experiment by the DRO than by the yoked VT schedule (cf. Zeiler, 1976). In another experiment, Topping and Ford (1975) compared DRO, extinction, and FT schedules using a multiple schedule and found that the former two schedules produced more rapid reductions in responding, but all three eventually resulted in equally low levels. Comparisons of DRO to extinction also suggest that DRO might reduce responding faster than extinction (Topping & Ford, 1974; Zeiler, 1971; cf. Rescorla & Skucy, 1969; Uhl & Garcia, 1969; Uhl & Sherman, 1971), and many have found DRO to produce more permanent reductions in responding than extinction (Uhl & Sherman, 1971; Zeiler, 1971). Thompson et al. (2003), in a comparison of the response-reducing efficacy of DRO, extinction, and FT schedules, however, found that extinction reduced responding the quickest, but also resulted in greater and quicker response recovery when the response was reinforced again in a subsequent condition.

Although DRO most often is taxonomized as a schedule of positive reinforcement, it also meets the formal definition of negative punishment: The temporary, response-dependent removal of the opportunity for reinforcement that results in suppression of the response on which the removal depends (Jessel et al., 2015; Lattal, 2013). It can therefore be categorized with two other procedures—response cost and response-dependent time-out from positive reinforcement—that share the features noted in the earlier definition of negative punishment. The difference between DRO and the other two is that in the case of DRO, the punished response does not produce an immediate stimulus change. Zeiler (1977), Lattal and Boyer (1980), and Craig et al. (2014) described how intermittent schedules of DRO punishment imposed on FI or VI schedules of reinforcement suppress behavior like schedules of positive punishment.

Punishment

The heyday of basic behavior-analytic research on the reductive effects of positive punishment (i.e., a delivered stimulus dependent on a response that results in the reduction of that response) was more than 60 years ago when Azrin and his colleagues (see, especially, Azrin & Holz, 1966) articulated many of the basic effects of punishers on operant behavior (see also Church, 1963, for a review of parallel research on basic punishment effects using group-design methods). Although there is a scattering of experimental analyses of punishment effects, including that of schedules of punishment, the experimental analysis of punishment has been largely dormant since Azrin's pioneering research. Lerman and Vorndran (2002) documented the limited amount of research on punishment in applied behavior analysis. This dearth is likely due to ethical concerns with using punishment, especially with the vulnerable populations who are frequent recipients of applied behavior-analytic interventions. Some of these concerns might derive from accounts of limitations and side effects of punishment (e.g., Sidman, 1989). Fontes and Shahan (2021; see also Leaf et al., 2019) suggested, however, that some of the widely accepted limitations and side effects of punishment might not be as prevalent, pervasive, or permanent as originally portrayed. The decreasing trend in the use of punishment in applied behavior analysis (Rico et al., 2018) still indicates little advancement despite the two decades since Lerman and Vorndran's (2002) review. Thus, the understanding of punishment in applied behavior analysis is mostly derived from findings in the experimental analysis of behavior and, as noted earlier, punishment has not been a frequent topic in that literature either, leaving many questions on punishment either unanswered or based on dated findings (e.g., Azrin, 1960b).

Although there are ethical concerns regarding the use of punishment in applied behavior analysis, as described earlier, it is inevitable in most environments. When it occurs, it does so according to a schedule. Thus, it is worthwhile for applied behavior analysts to familiarize themselves with the research on punishment and how the schedule upon which it occurs may influence how it affects behavior. For example, punishment can produce more immediate, complete, and durable reductions in behavior than either extinction or satiation (e.g., Holz & Azrin, 1963). The degree of reductive effects, however, depends at least in part on the schedule of punishment. Parke and Deur (1972) evaluated the effect of FR 1 and FR 2 punishment schedules on the aggressive behavior of young children toward a Bobo doll. Following a baseline in which aggression resulted in no programmed consequences, aggression was punished (i.e., followed by a buzzer) on either an FR 1 or FR 2 schedule for children in different groups. Aggression punished on an FR 1 decreased more from baseline than when it was punished on an FR 2. The greater suppressive effects of more consistent schedules of punishment replicated earlier basic research (e.g., Azrin et al., 1963; Zimmerman & Baydan, 1963).

As mentioned earlier, there are fewer studies on schedules of punishment than on schedules of reinforcement, and even fewer have focused on negative punishment in the experimental analysis of behavior. In some exceptions, laboratory experiments with non-human animals arranged for negative punishment in the form of loss of reinforcement for the target response (i.e., DRO). Although a DRO is often conceptualized as a schedule of reinforcement in applied behavior analysis, it also can meet the definition for negative punishment, because it involves the response-dependent, time-limited, removal of the opportunity for reinforcement. Craig et al. (2014) maintained key pecking of pigeons with a VI schedule. Operating concurrently with the VI schedule was a negative punishment procedure in the form of a tandem VT DRO 5-seconds schedule in which the first pause in responding (response suppression) after lapse of the VT period was reinforced. Thus, responding was available for both pecking and not pecking. The rate of key pecking was proportional to the number of reinforcers available for pecking relative to those available for pausing. Evaluations of negative punishment, however, are more common in applied behavior analysis, perhaps because its use is considered more ethical than positive punishment. Donaldson et al. (2014) compared two DRO 1-minute schedules to decrease the disruptive behavior of 12 students. In the first DRO schedule, students began with no tokens and could earn up to 10, one for each interval with the absence of disruption. In the second DRO schedule, students began with all 10 tokens and lost one token per interval during which disruption occurred (i.e., response cost). Both DRO schedules reduced responding equally. Participants also most often selected the DRO with response cost when the two schedules were available in a concurrent schedules arrangement. With respect to other forms of negative punishment (i.e., time-out and response cost), denser schedules of punishment suppress responding more than leaner schedules (Clark et al., 1973; Pfiffner et al., 1985).

Sustaining Behavior Changes

Once targeted behavior is established, modified, or reduced, applied behavior analysts design systems to sustain durable behavior change (Stokes & Baer, 1977). These include procedures for reducing dependence on relatively contrived interventions by substituting ones that are more natural and developing prosthetic systems for sustainability. The following sections consider the relations between all these activities of applied behavior analysts and the contributions of basic research on schedules of reinforcement and punishment.

Schedule Thinning

Applied behavior analysts, at least initially, often rely on rich schedules of reinforcement, notably FR 1. Such schedules are rarely generalizable or in a client's best long-term interests. Although transitioning a response from a richer to a leaner schedule of reinforcement often is necessary for practical purposes, intermittent schedules of reinforcement, as previously described, also engender greater resistance to disruption and can result in the same response occurring in contexts different than that during training (Stokes & Baer, 1977). Transitioning from a richer to a leaner schedule also can reduce responding, because behavior may become *strained* when sudden, large schedule transitions occur (i.e., the response requirement vastly increases but the amount of reinforcement remains constant, see Ferster & Skinner, 1957, especially Chapter 4). Strained responding is characterized by irregular and lengthy pauses, with eventual cessation of responding altogether, as when responding on a progressively incrementing response requirement (a progressive-ratio schedule) reaches a break point (e.g., Hodos, 1961). Some clinical practice guidelines and review articles suggest avoiding strain by *thinning* the schedule of reinforcement gradually across sessions (e.g., Hagopian et al., 2011), and there are many examples that such an approach works (e.g., Hagopian et al., 1994).

One method of schedule thinning is to increase the schedule by a fixed amount each session if there is no evidence of strain. For example, Hagopian et al. (1994) systematically thinned an FT 10-seconds schedule that reduced the problem behavior of quadruplets by decreasing the rate of reinforcement by one reinforcer per minute across 20-minute sessions. Across an average of 26.5 sessions, reinforcement was thinned to the terminal FT 5-minutes schedule, and a low rate of responding was maintained. Alternatively, Kahng et al. (2000) thinned an FT 10-seconds schedule of reinforcement after it had been shown to reduce the self-injurious behavior of three participants by yoking it to the IRT in the previous 15-minute session. As self-injury decreased and IRTs increased, the schedule became leaner, until it reached an FT 5-minutes schedule. In an example specific to schedules of punishment, Lerman et al. (1997) found that the self-injury of three of five adults returned to baseline levels following a transition from delivering punishment on an FR 1-second to an FI 120-second schedule. Thinning the FI schedule in increments as small as 5 or 10 seconds allowed them to reach the desired schedule of punishment while maintaining low levels of self-injury.

Although experiments on schedule thinning in applied behavior analysis often include methods for doing so gradually, there also are reports of schedule thinning that maintains responding when the schedule increases more rapidly (Hagopian et al., 2005; LeBlanc et al., 2002) or even abruptly transitioning to the terminal schedule (Hagopian, Toole, et al., 2004). In the experimental analysis of behavior, the effects of the rate of schedule thinning have been investigated largely using progressive-ratio (PR) schedules in which the response requirement increases within session each time a set number of reinforcers is delivered (Hodos & Kalman, 1963). Strain appears to be unaffected by how rapidly the PR increases, whether by the magnitude of each schedule increase (Eckerman et al., 1980; Stafford & Branch, 1998) or how frequently the schedule increases (Killeen et al., 2009). This, however, does not appear to be the case for interval schedules (Dougherty et al., 1994). Analogous progressive-interval (PI) schedules have been reported (Harzem, 1969), and Lattal et al. (1998) showed that PI schedules develop more persistent responding than do analogous PR schedules.

Manipulating other parameters of reinforcement also can decrease strain during schedule thinning. Destructive behavior of an adolescent with ASD returned as a DRO schedule was thinned after it previously had reduced target behavior when it was richer (i.e., DRO 10-seconds schedule; Roane et al., 2007). Schedule thinning was successful, however, when the magnitude of the reinforcer was yoked to the DRO, such that an increase in the DRO requirement proportionally increased reinforcer duration. Gilroy et al. (2019) extended this analysis following successful treatment of escape-maintained aggression and disruptive behavior of a 7-year-old boy in which requests produced a 30-second break (FR 1). The schedule at which compliance began to strain on a PR schedule served as an indicator of the optimal ratio between response effort and reinforcer magnitude. Compliance persisted during schedule thinning that yoked the magnitude of reinforcement to the number of tasks required, as in Roane et al. (2007).

Token Schedules

Token schedules can make the positive results of behavioral interventions more durable, because they use generalized conditioned reinforcers (i.e., tokens; Ayllon & Azrin, 1965; Nelson & Cone, 1979; Cowles, 1937; DeFulio et al., 2014; Fox et al., 1987; Kelleher, 1958, 1966; Kazdin, 1982; Phillips et al., 1971; Winkler, 1970; Wolfe, 1936). These tokens are then exchangeable for numerous backup reinforcers, decreasing their susceptibility to satiation (Russell et al., 2018; Skinner, 1953). As a result, tokens can be delivered on richer schedules than backup reinforcers, especially primary reinforcers (Scheithauer et al., 2016; Stocco & Thompson, 2015). Andrade and Hackenberg (2017) found that pigeons pecked keys associated with earning generalized tokens (i.e., those exchangeable for the choice of food or water) at a higher rate than, and to the exclusion of, keys associated with reinforcer-specific tokens (i.e., those exchangeable for either only food or only water).

A token economy is a three-component chained schedule of reinforcement (Hackenberg, 2009, 2018; McLaughlin & Williams, 1988; Kelleher, 1957). The first component schedule is the *token-production schedule*, which specifies the relation between the response and token delivery. For example, a DRO 2-minutes token-production schedule results in one token delivered for the absence of a target behavior for 2 minutes. The second is the *exchange-production schedule*, or the criteria by which the tokens become exchangeable for backup reinforcers. An FR 10 exchange-production schedule results in the availability of opportunities to exchange tokens once 10 tokens have been accrued. The third is the *token-exchange schedule*, or the schedule on which token exchange produces the backup reinforcer. A FR 1 token-exchange schedule results in each of the 10 earned tokens being exchangeable for a backup reinforcer.

Token-production (De Luca & Holborn, 1990, 1992; Repp & Deitz, 1975) and exchange-production (Bullock & Hackenberg, 2015; Foster et al., 2001; McLaughlin & Malaby, 1972; Staats et al., 1962; Webbe & Malagodi, 1978) schedules generally produce responding that is similar to the characteristic responding associated with the same basic schedule when it is not a part of a token economy. For example, Gadaire et al. (2021) observed a gradual reduction in response rates and shorter postreinforcement pauses during leaner FR token-production schedules compared to schedules arranging more frequent reinforcement or conditions in which rates of reinforcement were yoked. Some research from the experimental analysis of behavior, however, suggests that lean and rich token-production schedules might control similar response rates if the former are followed by the same token-exchange schedule (Hyten et al., 1994; Jackson & Hackenberg, 1996); that is, responding appears to be under the control of the token-exchange schedules to a greater degree than the token-production schedule. Tarbox et al. (2006) demonstrated the independent effects of manipulating the three component schedules of a token economy with a 5-year-old boy with ASD. When an FR exchange-production schedule was gradually thinned, responding maintained if the token-exchange schedule remained an FR 1. Responding, however, decreased as the FT token-exchange schedule became leaner. This result is consistent with other findings indicating that conditioned reinforcers require recurring pairing with the primary (i.e., backup) reinforcer to maintain behavior (Kelleher & Gollub, 1962; Schaal & Branch, 1990). Other research directly manipulating the exchange-production schedule suggests that humans (DeLeon et al., 2014; Falligant & Kornman, 2019; Ward-Horner et al., 2017) and nonhumans (Yankelevitz et al., 2008) often select leaner exchange-production schedules if doing so produces accrual of more tokens that corresponds with greater (e.g., higher magnitude, longer duration, or better quality) reinforcement, despite this arrangement resulting in longer delays to reinforcement.

Schedules, Applications, and Translation

The valuable feature of schedules of reinforcement and punishment in application is their function, not their form, and certainly not their nomenclature. Taxonomic systems, and there are others besides the most widely used system of Ferster and Skinner (1957; e.g., Mechner, 1959; Schoenfeld & Cole, 1972), may be useful in relating seemingly disparate situations in both research and practice to one another. Other conceptualizations of reinforcement schedules have involved considering them less as entities or structures and more functionally in terms of how particular arrangements interact with behavior in the form of feedback systems (Baum, 1989; Nevin & Baum, 1980). Baum (1989) accounted for response rate differences between VI and VR schedules based on different dynamic interactions, or feedback, between responding under the two schedules. Those feedback functions are but two of many that might be arranged and in so doing provide a different conceptualization of schedules of reinforcement and punishment from any of the aforementioned taxonomic systems, with major implications for how schedules are arranged and used in both the laboratory and in application.

For applied behavior analysts, taxonomizing reinforcement schedules is useful only to the extent that it is a portal into basic or applied research related to the procedures being considered for application, thereby providing insights into how the schedule might be operating or might be changed, or what might be expected from those changes, in a contemplated intervention. Attaching a label to a particular set of contingencies in effect can help in relating the application back to its foundation in basic research, but excessive concern with a schedule's taxonomy seems just that. Whether a schedule, for example, is labeled an FI 1-minute schedule or a tandem FT 1-minute FR-1 only makes a difference if it makes a difference. Ninety-nine times out of a 100, it does not. The present suggestion is to allow parsimony to rule. If a taxonomic label is needed, the simplest and most straightforward is sufficient ("FI 1-minute" in the previous example).

The questions posed in this chapter involve the dynamic interplay between basic research and practice, as such interplay relates to schedules of reinforcement and punishment. The more conventional expression might be "translating schedules into practice," but such a use implies a unidirectionality that can be misleading (cf. Neef & Peterson, 2003), as when one changes colloquial expressions from one language into another. Moreover, and perhaps even more importantly, as suggested in the opening pages of this chapter, schedules do not require translation into practice in the usual sense of that expression, because schedules have been an inextricable element of practice since the first "human vegetative organism" (Fuller, 1949) was freed from immobility by using an FR 1 schedule of reinforcement to affect the change. Perhaps a more useful way of thinking about the relation of schedules to practice is to consider schedules as the common ground between the two major areas of behavior analysis. It is a well-verified assumption that all operant behavior—virtually all human behavior—is maintained by reinforcement and punishment. In turn, all reinforcers and punishers are arranged by schedules, either by nature or by human design. It follows, then, that almost every human behavior problem can be reduced to a problem of what and how consequences occur. Sometimes a behavior problem bears a direct, straightforward relation to a schedule, as when attention is provided intermittently for inappropriate behavior. At other times, the connection may be less apparent, as when a child is having difficulty reading—a problem in stimulus control that in turn reduces to a problem of interest in the realm of multiple schedules of reinforcement.

We have reviewed here some of the ways schedules of reinforcement and punishment impact the work of applied behavior analysts. Neef and Peterson (2003) suggested a matrix of interactions between basic science, applied science, and technology, emphasizing multifaceted, dynamic relations among the three domains. The ubiquity of schedules in application and the sheer volume of schedule research (at least with reinforcement, but, unfortunately, less so with punishment) has facilitated the passage of schedule research from "lab to life," providing applied behavior analysts both tools and conceptual frameworks for understanding problems in living. Neef and Peterson's observation of the relatively small impact of applied research and practice on basic research certainly is true in the case of schedules of reinforcement and punishment. The applications of schedules reviewed in this chapter raise as many questions as they answer, providing basic researchers with the opportunity to reverse what has been largely a unidirectional flow of ideas from the basic to the applied realm into a far more valuable bidirectional one with respect to these most important behavioral processes.

REFERENCES

Abramowitz, A. J., & O'Leary, S. G. (1990). Effectiveness of delayed punishment in an applied setting. *Behavior Therapy, 21*(2), 321–239.

Andrade, L. F., & Hackenberg, T. D. (2017). Substitution effects in a generalized token economy with pigeons. *Journal of the Experimental Analysis of Behavior, 107*(1), 123–135.

Anglesea, M. M., Hoch, H., & Taylor, B. A. (2008). Reducing rapid eating in teenagers with autism: Use of a pager prompt. *Journal of Applied Behavior Analysis, 41*(1), 107–111.

Antonitis, J. J. (1951). Response variability in the white rat during conditioning, extinction, and reconditioning. *Journal of Experimental Psychology, 42*(4), 273–281.

Appel, J. B. (1961). Punishment in the squirrel monkey *Saimiri sciurea. Science, 133*(3445), Article 36.

Appel, J. B. (1968). Fixed-interval punishment. *Journal of the Experimental Analysis of Behavior, 11*(6), 803–808.

Appel, J. B., & Hiss, R. H. (1962). The discrimination of contingent from noncontingent reinforcement. *Journal of Comparative and Physiological Psychology, 55*(1), 37–39.

Arbuckle, J. L., & Lattal, K. A. (1992). Molecular contingencies in schedules of intermittent punishment. *Journal of the Experimental Analysis of Behavior, 58*(2), 361–375.

Athens, E. S., & Vollmer T. R. (2010). An investigation of differential reinforcement of alternative behavior without extinction. *Journal of Applied Behavior Analysis, 43*(4), 569–589.

Athens, E. S., Vollmer, T. R., & Pipkin, C. C. (2007). Shaping academic task engagement with percentile schedules. *Journal of Applied Behavior Analysis, 40*(3), 475–488.

Austin, J. L., & Bevan, D. (2011). Using differential reinforcement of low rates to reduce children's requests for teacher attention. *Journal of Applied Behavior Analysis, 44*(3), 451–561.

Ayllon, T., & Azrin, N. H. (1965). The measurement and reinforcement of behavior of psychotics. *Journal of the Experimental Analysis of Behavior, 8*(6), 357–383.

Azrin, N. H. (1956). Some effects of two intermittent schedules of immediate and nonimmediate punishment. *Journal of Psychology: Interdisciplinary and Applied, 42*(1), 3–21.

Azrin, N. H. (1960a). Effects of punishment intensity during variable-interval reinforcement. *Journal of the Experimental Analysis of Behavior, 3*(2), 123–142.

Azrin, N. H. (1960b). Sequential effects of punishment. *Science, 131*(3400), 605–606.

Azrin, N. H., & Holz, W. C. (1966). Punishment. In W. K. Honig (Ed.), *Operant behavior: Areas of research and application.* Appleton-Century-Crofts.

Azrin, N. H., Holz, W. C., & Hake, D. F. (1963). Fixed-ratio punishment. *Journal of the Experimental Analysis of Behavior, 6*(2), 141–148.

Baer, D. M., & Sherman, J. A. (1964). Reinforcement control of generalized imitation in young children. *Journal of Experimental Child Psychology, 1*(1), 37–49.

Banks, R. K., & Vogel-Sprott, M. (1965). Effect of delayed punishment on an immediately rewarded response in humans. *Journal of Experimental Psychology, 70*(4), 357–359.

Baron, A., & Herpolsheimer, L. R. (1999). Averaging effects in the study of fixed-ratio response patterns. *Journal of the Experimental Analysis of Behavior, 71*(2), 145–153.

Baron, A., Kaufman, A., & Fazzini, D. (1969). Density and delay of punishment of free-operant avoidance. *Journal of the Experimental Analysis of Behavior, 12*(6), 1029–1037.

Barton, L. E., Brulle, A. R., & Repp, A. C. (1986). Maintenance of therapeutic change by momentary DRO. *Journal of Applied Behavior Analysis, 19*(3), 277–282.

Baruni, R. R., Rapp, J. T., Lipe, S. L., & Novotny, M. A. (2014). Using lag schedules to increase toy play variability for children with intellectual disabilities. *Behavioral Interventions, 29*(1), 21–35.

Baum, W. M. (1989). Quantitative prediction and molar description of the environment. *Behavior Analyst, 12*(2), 167–176.

Baum, W. M., & Rachlin, H. C. (1969). Choice as time allocation. *Journal of the Experimental Analysis of Behavior, 12*(6), 861–874.

Becraft, J. L., Borrero, J. C., Davis, B. J., Mendres-Smith, A. E., & Castillo, M. I. (2018). The role of signals in two variations of differential-reinforcement-of-low-rate procedures. *Journal of Applied Behavior Analysis, 51*(1), 3–24.

Becraft, J. L., Borrero, J. C., Mendres-Smith, A. E., & Castillo, M. I. (2017). Decreasing excessive bids for attention in a simulated early education classroom. *Journal of Behavioral Education, 26*(4), 371–393.

Bergmann, S. C., Kodak, T. M., & LeBlanc, B. A. (2017). Effects of programmed errors of omission and commission during auditory–visual conditional discrimination training with typically developing children. *Psychological Record, 67*, 109–119.

Black, R. E., Walters, G. C., & Webster, C. D. (1972). Fixed-interval limited-hold avoidance with and without signaled reinforcement. *Journal of the Experimental Analysis of Behavior, 17*(1), 75–81.

Bonem, M., & Crossman, E. K. (1988). Elucidating the effects of reinforcement magnitude. *Psychological Bulletin, 104*(3), 348–362.

Bonner, A. C., & Borrero, J. C. (2018). Differential reinforcement of low rate schedules reduces severe problem behavior. *Behavior Modification, 42*(5), 747–764.

Boren, J. J., Moerschbaecher, J. M., & Whyte, A. A. (1978). Variability of response location on fixed-ratio and fixed-interval schedules of reinforcement. *Journal of the Experimental Analysis of Behavior, 30*(1), 63–67.

Borrero, C. S. W., Vollmer, T. R., Borrero, J. C., & Bourret, J. (2005). A method for evaluating parameters of reinforcement during parent–child interactions. *Research in Developmental Disabilities, 26*(6), 577–592.

Bradshaw, C. M., Szabadi, E., & Bevan, P. (1978). Frequency in variable-interval schedules: The effect of concentration of sucrose reinforcement. *Journal of the Experimental Analysis of Behavior, 29*(3), 447–452.

Brethower, D. M., & Reynolds, G. S. (1962). A facilitative effect of punishment on unpunished behavior. *Journal of the Experimental Analysis of Behavior, 5*(2), 191–199.

Britton, L. N., Carr, J. E., Landaburu, H. J., & Romick, K. S. (2002). The efficacy of noncontingent reinforcement as treatment for automatically reinforced stereotypy. *Behavioral Interventions, 17*(2), 93–103.

Brown, T. G., & Flory, R. K. (1972). Schedule-induced escape from fixed-interval reinforcement. *Journal of the Experimental Analysis of Behavior, 17*(3), 395–403.

Bullock, C. E., & Hackenberg, T. D. (2015). The several roles of stimuli in token reinforcement. *Journal of the Experimental Analysis of Behavior, 103*(2), 269–287.

Call, N. A., Clark, S. B., Lomas Mevers, J. L., Parks, N. A., Volkert, V. M., & Scheithauer, M. C. (2018). An individualized method for establishing and thinning multiple schedules of reinforcement following functional communication training. *Learning and Motivation, 62,* 91–102.

Call, N. A., Findley, A. J., & Reavis, A. R. (2012). The effects of conducting a functional analysis on problem behavior in other settings. *Research in Developmental Disabilities, 33*(6), 1990–1995.

Call, N. A., Reavis, A. R., Clark, S. B., Parks, N. A., Cariveau, T., & Muething, C. S. (2017). The effects of conducting a functional analysis on problem behavior in other settings: A descriptive study on potential interaction effects. *Behavior Modification, 41*(5), 609–625.

Cammilleri, A. P., & Hanley, G. P. (2005). Use of a lag differential reinforcement contingency to increase varied selections of classroom activities. *Journal of Applied Behavior Analysis, 38*(1), 111–115.

Camp, D. S., Raymond, G. A., & Church, R. M. (1966). Response suppression as a function of the schedule of punishment. *Psychonomic Science, 5,* 23–24.

Camp, D. S., Raymond, G. A., & Church, R. M. (1967). Temporal relationship between response and punishment. *Journal of Experimental Psychology, 74*(1), 114–123.

Cannella, H. I., O'Reilly, M. F., & Lancioni, G. E. (2005). Choice and preference assessment research with people with severe to profound developmental disabilities: A review of the literature. *Research in Developmental Disabilities, 26*(1), 1–15.

Capaldi, E. D., Myers, D. E., & Davidson, T. L. (1981). A comparison of resistance to satiation and resistance to extinction. *Animal Learning and Behavior, 9,* 108–114.

Capriotti, M. R., Brandt, B. C., Ricketts, E. J., Espil, F. M., & Woods, D. W. (2012). Comparing the effects of differential reinforcement of other behavior and response-cost contingencies on tics in youth with Tourette syndrome. *Journal of Applied Behavior Analysis, 45*(2), 251–263.

Carr, J. E., Kellum, K. K., & Chong, I. M. (2001). The reductive effects of noncontingent reinforcement: Fixed-time versus variable-time schedules. *Journal of Applied Behavior Analysis, 34*(4), 505–509.

Catania, A. C. (1961). Behavioral contrast in a multiple and concurrent schedule of reinforcement. *Journal of the Experimental Analysis of Behavior, 4*(4), 335–342.

Catania, A. C. (1963). Concurrent performances: A baseline for the study of reinforcement magnitude. *Journal of the Experimental Analysis of Behavior, 6*(2), 299–300.

Catania, A. C. (2013). *Learning* (5th ed.). Sloan.

Catania, A. C., Matthews, T. J., Silverman, P. J., & Yohalem, R. (1977). Yoked variable-ratio and variable-interval responding in pigeons. *Journal of the Experimental Analysis of Behavior, 28*(2), 155–161.

Cherek, D. R., & Brauchi, J. T. (1981). Schedule-induced cigarette smoking behavior during fixed-interval monetary reinforced responding. In C. M. Bradshaw, E. Szabadi, & C. F. Lowe (Eds.), *Quantification of steady-state operant behavior* (pp. 389–392). Elsevier/North-Holland Biomedical Press.

Church, R. M. (1963). The varied effects of punishment on behavior. *Psychological Review, 70*(5), 369–402.

Church, R. M. (1969). Response suppression. In B. A. Campbell & R. M. Church (Eds.), *Punishment and aversive behavior* (pp. 111–156). Apple-Century-Crofts.

Clark, A. M., Schmidt, J. D., Mezhoudi, N., & Kahng, S. (2016). Using percentile schedules to increase academic fluency. *Behavioral Interventions, 31*(3), 283–290.

Clark, H. B., Rowbury, T., Baer, A. M., & Baer, D. M. (1973). Timeout as a punishing stimulus in continuous and intermittent schedules. *Journal of Applied Behavior Analysis, 6*(3), 443–455.

Clarke, J., Gannon, M., Hughes, I., Keogh, C., Singer, G., & Wallace, M. (1977). Adjunctive behavior in humans in a group gambling situation. *Physiology and Behavior, 18*(1), 159–161.

Cohen, P. S. (1968). Punishment: The interactive effects of delay and intensity of shock. *Journal of the Experimental Analysis of Behavior, 11*(6), 789–799.

Cohen, S. L., Riley, D. S., & Weigle, P. A. (1993). Tests of behavior momentum in simple and multiple schedules with rats and pigeons. *Journal of the Experimental Analysis of Behavior, 60*(2), 255–291.

Conrad, D. G., Sidman, M., & Herrnstein, R. J. (1958). The effects of deprivation upon temporally spaced responding. *Journal of the Experimental Analysis of Behavior, 1*(1), 59–65.

Cowles, J. T. (1937). Food-tokens as incentives for learning by chimpanzees. *Comparative Psychology Monographs, 23*, 1–92.

Craig, A. R., Browning, K. O., & Shahan, T. A. (2017). Stimuli previously associated with reinforcement mitigate resurgence. *Journal of the Experimental Analysis of Behavior, 108*(2), 139–150.

Craig, A. R., Lattal, K. A., & Hall, E. G. (2014). Pausing as an operant: Choice and discriminated responding. *Journal of the Experimental Analysis of Behavior, 101*(2), 230–245.

Crosbie, J., Williams, A. M., Lattal, K. A., Anderson, M. M., & Brown, S. M. (1997). Schedule inductions involving punishment with pigeons and humans. *Journal of the Experimental Analysis of Behavior, 68*(2), 161–175.

Davis, E. R., & Platt, J. R. (1983). Contiguity and contingency in the acquisition and maintenance of an operant. *Learning and Motivation, 14*(4), 487–512.

Davis, J., & Bitterman, M. E. (1971). Differential reinforcement of other behavior (DRO): A yoked-control comparison. *Journal of the Experimental Analysis of Behavior, 15*(2), 237–241.

DeFulio, A., Yankelevitz, R., Bullock, C., & Hackenberg, T. D. (2014). Generalized conditioned reinforcement with pigeons in a token economy. *Journal of the Experimental Analysis of Behavior, 102*(1), 26–46.

Deitz, S. M. (1977). An analysis of programming DRL schedules in educational settings. *Behaviour Research and Therapy, 15*(1), 103–111.

Deitz, S. M., & Repp, A. C. (1973). Decreasing classroom misbehavior through the use of DRL schedules of reinforcement. *Journal of Applied Behavior Analysis, 6*(3), 457–463.

DeLeon, I. G., Chase, J. A., Frank-Crawford, M. A., Carreau-Webster, A. B., Triggs, M. M., Bullock, C. E., & Jennett, H. K. (2014). Distributed and accumulated reinforcement arrangements: Evaluations of efficacy and preference. *Journal of Applied Behavior Analysis, 47*(2), 293–313.

De Luca, R. V., & Holborn, S. W. (1990). Effects of fixed-interval and fixed-ratio schedules of token reinforcement on exercise with obese and nonobese boys. *Psychological Record, 40*, 67–82.

De Luca, R. V., & Holborn, S. W. (1992). Effects of a variable-ratio reinforcement schedule with changing criteria on exercise in obese and nonobese boys. *Journal of Applied Behavior Analysis, 25*(3), 671–679.

Derwas, H., & Jones, R. S. P. (1993). Reducing stereotyped behavior using momentary DRO: An experimental analysis. *Behavioral Interventions, 8*(1), 45–53.

DiGennaro Reed, F. D., Reed, D. D., Baez, C. N., & Maguire, H. (2011). A parametric analysis of errors of commission during discrete-trial training. *Journal of Applied Behavior Analysis, 44*(3), 611–615.

Dinsmoor, J. A. (1954). Punishment: I. The avoidance hypothesis. *Psychological Review, 61*(1), 34–46.

Donaldson, J. M., DeLeon, I. G., Fisher, A. B., & Kahng, S. (2014). Effects of and preference for conditions of token earn versus token loss. *Journal of Applied Behavior Analysis, 47*(3), 537–548.

Dougherty, D. M., Cherek, D. R., & Roache, J. D. (1994). The effects of smoked marijuana on progressive-interval schedule performance in humans. *Journal of the Experimental Analysis of Behavior, 62*(1), 73–87.

Dracobly, J. D., Dozier, C. L., Briggs, A. M., & Juanico, J. F. (2017). An analysis of procedures that affect response variability. *Journal of Applied Behavior Analysis, 50*(3), 600–621.

Eckerman, D. A., Hienz, R. D., Stern, S., & Kowlowitz, V. (1980). Shaping the location of a pigeon's peck: Effect of rate and size of shaping steps. *Journal of the Experimental Analysis of Behavior, 33*(3), 299–310.

Falcomata, T. S., Muething, C. S., Silbaugh, B. C., Adami, S., Hoffman, K., Shpall, C., & Ringdahl, J. E. (2017). Lag schedules and functional communication training: Persistence of mands and relapse of problem behavior. *Behavior Modification, 42*(3), 314–334.

Falk, J. L. (1961). Production of polydipsia in normal rats by an intermittent food schedule. *Science, 133*(3447), 195–196.

Falligant, J. M., & Kornman, P. T. (2019). Preferences for accumulated and distributed token exchange-production schedules: A behavior-economic analysis. *Behavior Analysis: Research and Practice, 19*(4), 373–378.

Fallon, J. H., Allen, J. D., & Butler, J. A. (1979). Assessment of adjunctive behaviors in humans using a stringent control procedure. *Physiology and Behavior, 22*(6), 1089–1092.

Ferster, C. B., & Skinner, B. F. (1957). *Schedules of reinforcement*. Appleton-Century-Crofts.

Filby, Y., & Appel, J. B. (1966). Variable-interval punishment during variable-interval reinforcement. *Journal of the Experimental Analysis of Behavior, 9*(5), 521–527.

Fontes, R. M., & Shahan, T. A. (2021). Punishment and its putative fallout: A reappraisal. *Journal of the Experimental Analysis of Behavior, 115*(1), 185–203.

Foster, T. A., Hackenberg, T. D., & Vaidya, M. (2001). Second-order schedules of token reinforcement with pigeons: Effects of fixed- and variable-ratio exchange schedules. *Journal of the Experimental Analysis of Behavior, 76*(2), 159–178.

Fox, D. K., Hopkins, B. L., & Anger, W. K. (1987). The long-term effects of a token economy on safety performance in open-pit mining. *Journal of Applied Behavior Analysis, 30*(3), 215–224.

Freeman, T. J., & Lattal, K. A. (1992). Stimulus control of behavioral history. *Journal of the Experimental Analysis of Behavior, 57*(1), 5–15.

Fuller, P. (1949). Operant conditioning of a vegetative human organism. *American Journal of Psychology, 62*(4), 587–590.

Gadaire, D. M., Senn, L., Albert, K. M., Robinson, T. P., Passage, M., Shaham, Y., & Topcuoglu, B. (2021). Differential effects of token production and exchange on responding of children with developmental disabilities. *Learning and Motivation, 73*, Article 101694.

Galbicka, G. (1988). Differentiating the behavior of organisms. *Journal of the Experimental Analysis of Behavior, 50*(2), 343–354.

Galbicka, G., & Platt, J. R. (1989). Response-reinforcer contingency and spatially defined operants: Testing an invariance property of phi. *Journal of the Experimental Analysis of Behavior, 51*(1), 145–162.

Gehrman, C., Wilder, D. A., Forton, A. P., & Albert, K. (2017). Comparing resetting to non-resetting DRO procedures to reduce stereotypy in a child with autism. *Behavioral Interventions, 32*(3), 242–247.

Gilroy, S. P., Ford, H. L., Boyd, R. J., O'Connor, J. T., & Kurtz, P. F. (2019). An evaluation of operant behavioural economics in functional communication training for severe problem behaviour. *Developmental Neurorehabilitation, 22*(8), 553–564.

Girolami, K. M., Kahng, S. W., Hilker, K. A., & Girolami, P. A. (2009). Differential reinforcement of high rate behavior to increase the pace of self-feeding. *Behavioral Interventions, 24*(1), 17–22.

Githens, S. H., Hawkins, T. D., & Schrot, J. (1973). DRL schedule-induced alcohol ingestion. *Physiological Psychology, 1*(4), 397–400.

Goodall, G. (1984). Learning due to the response-shock contingency in signaled punishment. *Quarterly Journal of Experimental Psychology Section B, 36*(3), 259–279.

Gray Granger, R., Porter, J. H., & Christoph, N. L. (1984). Schedule-induced behavior in children as a function of inter reinforcement interval length. *Physiology and Behavior, 33*(1), 153–157.

Hackenberg, T. D. (2009). Token reinforcement: A review and analysis. *Journal of the Experimental Analysis of Behavior, 91*(2), 257–286.

Hackenberg, T. D. (2018). Token reinforcement: Translational research and application. *Journal of Applied Behavior Analysis, 51*(2), 393–435.

Hagopian, L. P., Boelter, E. W., & Jarmolowicz, D. P. (2011). Reinforcement schedule thinning following functional communication training: Review and recommendations. *Behavior Analysis in Practice, 4*(1), 4–16.

Hagopian, L. P., Fisher, W. W., & Legacy, S. M. (1994). Schedule effects of noncontingent reinforcement on attention-maintained destruction behavior in identical quadruplets. *Journal of Applied Behavior Analysis, 27*(2), 317–325.

Hagopian, L. P., Kuhn, D. E., Strother, G. E., & Van Houten, R. (2009). Targeting social skill deficits in an adolescent with pervasive developmental disorder. *Journal of Applied Behavior Analysis, 42*(4), 907–911.

Hagopian, L. P., Kuhn, S. A., Long, E. S., & Rush, K. S. (2005). Schedule thinning following communication training: Using competing stimuli to enhance tolerance to decrements in reinforcer density. *Journal of Applied Behavior Analysis, 38*(2), 177–193.

Hagopian, L. P., Long, E. S., & Rush, K. S. (2004). Preference assessment procedures for individuals with developmental disabilities. *Behavior Modification, 28*(5), 668–677.

Hagopian, L. P., Toole, L. M., Long, E. S., Bowman, L. G., & Lieving, G. A. (2004). A comparison of dense-to-lean and fixed lean schedules of alternative reinforcement and extinction. *Journal of Applied Behavior Analysis, 37*(3), 323–338.

Hall, S. S., Maynes, N. P., & Reiss, A. L. (2009). Using percentile schedules to increase eye contact in children with Fragile X syndrome. *Journal of Applied Behavior Analysis, 42*(1), 171–176.

Halliday, M. S., & Boakes, R. A. (1971). Behavioral contrast and response independent reinforcement. *Journal of the Experimental Analysis of Behavior, 16*(3), 429–434.

Hamilton, K. M., Clay, C. J., & Kahng, S. (2020). Examining the effectiveness of a variable momentary differential reinforcement of other behavior procedure on reduction and maintenance of problem behavior. *Current Developmental Disorders Reports, 7,* 14–22.

Hammond, J. L., Iwata, B. A., Fritz, J. N., & Dempsey, C. M. (2011). Evaluation of fixed momentary DRO schedules under signaled and unsignaled arrangements. *Journal of Applied Behavior Analysis, 44*(1), 69–81.

Hanley, G. P., Iwata, B. A., & Thompson, R. H. (2001). Reinforcement schedule thinning following treatment with functional communication training. *Journal of Applied Behavior Analysis, 34*(1), 17–38.

Harding, J. W., Wacker, D. P., Berg, W. K., Rick, G., & Lee, J. F. (2004). Promoting response variability and stimulus generalization in martial arts training. *Journal of Applied Behavior Analysis, 37*(2), 185–195.

Harzem, P. (1969). Temporal discrimination. In R. M. Gilbert & N. S. Sutherland (Eds.), *Animal discrimination learning* (pp. 299–334). Academic Press.

Harzem, P., Lowe, C. F., & Priddle-Higson, P. J. (1978). Inhibiting function of reinforcement: Magnitude effects on variable-interval schedules. *Journal of the Experimental Analysis of Behavior, 30*(1), 1–10.

Heldt, J., & Schlinger, H. D. (2012). Increased variability in tacting under a lag 3 schedule of reinforcement. *Analysis of Verbal Behavior, 28,* 131–136.

Hobbs, S. A., Forehand, R., & Murray, R. G. (1978). Effects of various durations of timeout on the noncompliant behavior of children. *Behavior Therapy, 9*(4), 652–656.

Hodos, W. (1961). Progressive ratio as a measure of reward strength. *Science, 134*(3483), 943–944.

Hodos, W., & Kalman, G. (1963). Effects of increment size and reinforcer volume on progressive ratio performance. *Journal of the Experimental Analysis of Behavior, 6*(3), 387–392.

Holz, W. C., & Azrin, N. H. (1963). A comparison of several procedures for eliminating behavior. *Journal of the Experimental Analysis of Behavior, 6*(3), 399–406.

Horner, R. H., & Day, H. M. (1991). The effects of response efficiency on functionally equivalent competing behaviors. *Journal of Applied Behavior Analysis, 24*(4), 719–732.

Hutchinson, R. R., Azrin, N. H., & Hunt, G. M. (1968). Attack produced by intermittent reinforcement of a concurrent operant response. *Journal of the Experimental Analysis of Behavior, 11*(4), 489–495.

Hutt, P. J. (1954). Rate of bar pressing as a function of quality and quantity of food reward. *Journal of Comparative and Physiological Psychology, 47*(3), 235–239.

Hyten, C., Madden, G. J., & Field, D. P. (1994). Exchange delays and impulsive choice in adult humans. *Journal of the Experimental Analysis of Behavior, 62*(2), 225–233.

Jackson, K., & Hackenberg, T. D. (1996). Token reinforcement, choice, and self-control in pigeons. *Journal of the Experimental Analysis of Behavior, 66*(1), 29–49.

Jenkins, W. O., & Clayton, F. L. (1949). Rate of responding and amount of reinforcement. *Journal of Comparative and Physiological Psychology, 42*(3), 174–181.

Jessel, J., & Borrero, J. C. (2014). A laboratory comparison of two variations of differential-reinforcement-of-low-rate procedures. *Journal of Applied Behavior Analysis, 47*(2), 314–324.

Jessel, J., Borrero, J. C., & Becraft, J. L. (2015). Differential reinforcement of other behavior increases untargeted behavior. *Journal of Applied Behavior Analysis, 48*(2), 402–416.

Joyce, J. H., & Chase, P. N. (1990). Effects of response variability on the sensitivity of rule-governed behavior. *Journal of the Experimental Analysis of Behavior, 54*(3), 251–262.

Kahng, S. W., Abt, K. A., & Schonbachler, H. E. (2001). Assessment and treatment of low-rate high-intensity problem behavior. *Journal of Applied Behavior Analysis, 34*(2), 225–228.

Kahng, S., Iwata, B. A., DeLeon, I. G., & Wallace, M. D. (2000). A comparison of procedures for programing noncontingent reinforcement schedules. *Journal of Applied Behavior Analysis, 33*(2), 223–231.

Kazdin, A. E. (1982). The token economy: A decade later. *Journal of Applied Behavior Analysis, 15*(3), 431–445.

Kelleher, R. T. (1957). Conditioned reinforcement in chimpanzees. *Journal of Comparative and Physiological Psychology, 50*(6), 571–575.

Kelleher, R. T. (1958). Fixed-ratio schedules of conditioned reinforcement with chimpanzees. *Journal of the Experimental Analysis of Behavior, 1*(3), 281–289.

Kelleher, R. T. (1961). Schedules of conditioned reinforcement during experimental extinction. *Journal of the Experimental Analysis of Behavior, 4*(1), 1–5.

Kelleher, R. T. (1966). Conditioned reinforcement in second-order schedules. *Journal of the Experimental Analysis of Behavior, 9*(5), 475–485.

Kelleher, R. T., & Gollub, L. R. (1962). A review of positive conditioned reinforcement. *Journal of the Experimental Analysis of Behavior, 5*(S4), 543–597.

Killeen, P. (1969). Reinforcement frequency and contingency as factors in fixed-ratio behavior. *Journal of the Experimental Analysis of Behavior, 12*(3), 391–395.

Killeen, P. R., Posadas-Sanchez, D., Johansen, E. B., & Thrailkill, E. A. (2009). Progressive ratio schedules of reinforcement. *Journal of Experimental Psychology: Animal Behavior Processes, 35*(1), 35–50.

Koegel, R. L., Egel, A. L., & Williams, J. A. (1980). Behavioral contrast and generalization across settings in the treatment of autistic children. *Journal of Experimental Child Psychology, 30*(3), 422–437.

Kuhn, D. E., Chirighin, A. E., & Zelenka, K. (2010). Discriminated functional communication: A procedural extension of functional communication training. *Journal of Applied Behavior Analysis, 43*(2), 249–264.

Kunnavatana, S. S., Bloom, S. E., Samaha, A. L., Slocum, T. A., & Clay, C. J. (2018). Manipulating parameters of reinforcement to reduce problem behavior without extinction. *Journal of Applied Behavior Analysis, 51*(2), 283–302.

Kuroda, T., Cançado, C. R. X., Lattal, K. A., Elcoro, M., Dickson, C. A., & Cook, J. E. (2013). Combinations of response-reinforcer relations in periodic and aperiodic schedules. *Journal of the Experimental Analysis of Behavior, 99*(2), 199–210.

Kuroda, T., Cook, J. E., & Lattal, K. A. (2018). Baseline response rates affect resistance to change. *Journal of the Experimental Analysis of Behavior, 109*(1), 164–175.

Lachter, G. D. (1971). Some temporal parameters of non-contingent reinforcement. *Journal of the Experimental Analysis of Behavior, 16*(2), 207–217.

Lachter, G. D., Cole, B. K., & Schoenfeld, W. N. (1971). Response rate under varying frequency of non-contingent reinforcement. *Journal of the Experimental Analysis of Behavior, 15*(2), 233–236.

Lalli, J. S., & Casey, S. D. (1996). Treatment of multiply controlled problem behavior. *Journal of Applied Behavior Analysis, 29*(3), 391–395.

Lamb, R. J., Kirby, K. C., Morral, A. R., Galbicka, G., & Iguchi, M. Y. (2010). Shaping smoking cessation in hard-to-treat smokers. *Journal of Consulting and Clinical Psychology, 78*(1), 62–71.

Lamb, R. J., Morral, A. R., Galbicka, G., Kirby, K. C., & Iguchi, M. Y. (2005). Shaping reduced smoking in smokers without cessation plans. *Experimental and Clinical Psychopharmacology, 13*(2), 83–92.

Lamb, R. J., Morral, A. R., Kirby, K. C., Iguchi, M. Y., & Galbicka, G. (2004). Shaping smoking cessation using percentile schedules. *Drug and Alcohol Dependence, 76*(3), 247–259.

Lang, R., Muharib, R., Lessner, P., Davenport, K., Ledbetter-Cho, K., & Rispoli, M. (2020).

Increasing play and decreasing stereotypy for children with autism on a playground. *Advances in Neurodevelopmental Disorders, 4,* 146–154.

Lang, W. J., Latiff, A. A., McQueen, A., & Singer, G. (1977). Self-administration of nicotine with and without a food delivery schedule. *Pharmacology Biochemistry and Behavior,* 7(1), 65–70.

Lattal, K. A. (1972). Response-reinforcer independence and conventional extinction after fixed-interval and variable-interval schedules. *Journal of the Experimental Analysis of Behavior,* 18(1), 133–140.

Lattal, K. A. (1973). Response-reinforcer dependence and independence in multiple and mixed schedules. *Journal of the Experimental Analysis of Behavior,* 20(2), 265–271.

Lattal, K. A. (1974). Combinations of response-reinforcer dependence and independence. *Journal of the Experimental Analysis of Behavior,* 22(2), 357–362.

Lattal, K. A. (1989). Contingencies on response rate and resistance to change. *Learning and Motivation,* 20(2), 191–203.

Lattal, K. A. (2013). The five pillars of the experimental analysis of behavior. In G. J. Madden, W. V. Dube, T. D. Hackenberg, G. P. Hanley, & K. A. Lattal (Eds.), *APA handbook of behavior analysis, Vol. 1. Methods and principles* (pp. 33–63). American Psychological Association.

Lattal, K. A., & Boyer, S. S. (1980). Alternative reinforcement effects on fixed-interval performance. *Journal of the Experimental Analysis of Behavior,* 34(3), 285–296.

Lattal, K. A., & Poling, A. D. (1981). Describing response-event relations: Babel revisited. *Behavior Analyst,* 4(2), 143–152.

Lattal, K. A., Reilly, M. P., & Kohn, J. P. (1998). Response persistence under ratio and interval reinforcement schedules. *Journal of the Experimental Analysis of Behavior,* 70(2), 165–183.

Lattal, K. A., St. Peter, C., & Escobar, R. (2013). Operant extinction: Elimination and generation of behavior. In G. J. Madden, W. V. Dube, T. D. Hackenberg, G. P. Hanley, & K. A. Lattal (Eds.), *APA handbook of behavior analysis: Vol. 2. Translating principles into practice* (pp. 77–107). American Psychological Association.

Leaf, J. B., Townley-Cochran, D., Cihon, J. H., Mitchell, E., Leaf, R., Taubman, M., & McEachin, J. (2019). Descriptive analysis of the use of punishment-based techniques with children diagnosed with autism spectrum disorder. *Education and Training in Autism and Developmental Disabilities,* 54(2), 107–118.

LeBlanc, L. A., Hagopian, L. P., Maglieri, K. A., & Poling, A. (2002). Decreasing the intensity of reinforcement-based interventions for reducing behavior: Conceptual issues and a proposed model for clinical practice. *Behavior Analyst Today,* 3(3), 289–300.

Lerman, D. C., & Iwata, B. A. (1996). Developing a technology for the use of operant extinction in clinical settings: An examination of basic and applied research. *Journal of Applied Behavior Analysis,* 29(3), 345–382.

Lerman, D. C., Iwata, B. A., Shore, B. A., & DeLeon, I. G. (1997). Effects of intermittent punishment on self-injurious behavior: An evaluation of schedule thinning. *Journal of Applied Behavior Analysis,* 30(2), 187–201.

Lerman, D. C., Iwata, B. A., Zarcone, J. R., & Ringdahl, J. (1994). Assessment of stereotypic and self-injurious behavior as adjunctive responses. *Journal of Applied Behavior Analysis,* 27(4), 715–728.

Lerman, D. C., & Vorndran, C. M. (2002). On the status of knowledge for using punishment: Implications for treating behavior disorders. *Journal of Applied Behavior Analysis,* 35(4), 431–464.

Lindberg, J. S., Iwata, B. A., Kahng, S., & DeLeon, I. G. (1999). DRO contingencies: An analysis of variable-momentary schedules. *Journal of Applied Behavior Analysis,* 32(2), 123–136.

Lomas, J. E., Fisher, W. W., & Kelley, M. E. (2010). The effects of variable-time delivery of food items and praise on problem behavior reinforced by escape. *Journal of Applied Behavior Analysis,* 43(3), 425–435.

Mace, F. C., Neef, N. A., Shade, D., & Mauro, B. C. (1994). Limited matching on concurrent-schedule reinforcement of academic behavior. *Journal of Applied Behavior Analysis,* 27(4), 585–596.

Mackintosh, N. J. (1970). Distribution of trials and the partial reinforcement effect in the rat. *Journal of Comparative and Physiological Psychology,* 73(2), 341–348.

Marcus, B. A., & Vollmer, T. R. (1996). Combining noncontingent reinforcement and differential reinforcement schedules as treatment for aberrant behavior. *Journal of Applied Behavior Analysis,* 29(1), 43–51.

Masserman, J. H. (1946). *Principles of dynamic psychiatry.* Saunders.

McLaughlin, T. F., & Malaby, J. (1972). Intrinsic reinforcers in a classroom token economy. *Journal of Applied Behavior Analysis, 5*(3), 263–270.

McLaughlin, T. F., & Williams, R. L. (1988). The token economy. In J. C. Witt, S. N. Elliot, & F. M. Gresham (Eds.), *Handbook of behavior therapy in education* (pp. 469–487). Springer.

Mechner, F. (1959). A notation system for the description of behavioral procedures. *Journal of the Experimental Analysis of Behavior, 2*(2), 133–150.

Miller, N. E. (1960). Learning resistance to pain and fear: Effects of overlearning, exposure, and rewarded exposure in context. *Journal of Experimental Psychology, 60*(3), 137–145.

Miller, N., & Neuringer, A. (2000). Reinforcing variability in adolescents with autism. *Journal of Applied Behavior Analysis, 33*(2), 151–165.

Morse, W. H. (1966). Intermittent reinforcement. In W. K. Honig (Ed.), *Operant behavior: Areas of research and application* (pp. 52–108). Appleton-Century-Crofts.

Muller, P. G., Crow, R. E., & Cheney, C. D. (1979). Schedule-induced locomotor activity in humans. *Journal of the Experimental Analysis of Behavior, 31*(1), 83–90.

Neef, N. A., & Lutz, M. N. (2001). Assessment of variables affecting choice and application to classroom interventions. *School Psychology Quarterly, 16*(3), 239–252.

Neef, N. A., & Peterson, S. M. (2003). Developmental disabilities. In K. A. Lattal & P. N. Chase (Eds.), *Behavior theory and philosophy* (pp. 369–389). Springer.

Neef, N. A., Shade, D., & Miller, M. S. (1994). Assessing influential dimensions of reinforcers on choice in students with serious emotional disturbance. *Journal of Applied Behavior Analysis, 27*(4), 575–583.

Nelson, G. L., & Cone, J. D. (1979). Multiple-baseline analysis of a token economy for psychiatric inpatients. *Journal of Applied Behavior Analysis, 12*(2), 255–271.

Neuringer, A. (1991). Operant variability and repetition as functions of interresponse time. *Journal of Experimental Psychology: Animal Behavior Processes, 17*(1), 3–12.

Neuringer, A. J. (1970). Superstitious key pecking after three peck-produced reinforcements. *Journal of the Experimental Analysis of Behavior, 13*(2), 127–134.

Nevin, J. A. (1974). Response strength in multiple schedules. *Journal of the Experimental Analysis of Behavior, 21*(3), 389–408.

Nevin, J. A., & Baum, W. M. (1980). Feedback functions for variable-interval reinforcement. *Journal of the Experimental Analysis of Behavior, 34*(2), 207–217.

Nevin, J. A., & Shahan, T. A. (2011). Behavioral momentum theory: Equations and applications. *Journal of Applied Behavior Analysis, 44*(4), 877–895.

Nevin, J. A., Tota, M. E., Torquato, R. D., & Shull, R. L. (1990). Alternative reinforcement increases resistance to change: Pavlovian or operant contingencies? *Journal of the Experimental Analysis of Behavior, 53*(3), 359–379.

Nighbor, T. D., Cook, J. E., Oliver, A. C., & Lattal, K. A. (2020). Does DRO type matter?: Cycle versus resetting contingencies in eliminating responding. *Behavioural Processes, 181*, 104257.

Ono, K. (1987). Superstitious behavior in humans. *Journal of the Experimental Analysis of Behavior, 47*(3), 261–271.

O'Reilly, M., Lancioni, G., & Taylor, I. (1999). An empirical analysis of two forms of extinction to treat aggression. *Research in Developmental Disabilities, 20*(5), 315–325.

Page, S., & Neuringer, A. (1985). Variability is an operant. *Journal of Experimental Psychology: Animal Behavior Processes, 11*(3), 429–452.

Parke, R. D., & Deur, J. L. (1972). Schedule of punishment and inhibition of aggression in children. *Developmental Psychology, 7*(3), 266–269.

Pear, J. J., & Legris, J. A. (1987). Shaping by automated tracking of an arbitrary operant response. *Journal of the Experimental Analysis of Behavior, 47*(2), 241–247.

Peele, D. B., Casey, J., & Silberberg, A. (1984). Primacy of interresponse-time reinforcement in accounting for rate differences under variable-ratio and variable-interval schedules. *Journal of Experimental Psychology: Animal Behavior Processes, 10*(2), 149–167.

Perone, M., & Courtney, K. (1992). Fixed-ratio pausing: Joint effects of past reinforcer magnitude and stimuli correlated with upcoming magnitude. *Journal of the Experimental Analysis of Behavior, 57*(1), 33–46.

Perrin, C. J., & Neef, N. A. (2012). Further analysis of variables that affect self-control with aversive events. *Journal of Applied Behavior Analysis, 45*(3), 299–313.

Pfiffner, L. J., O'Leary, S. G., Rosen, L. A., & Sanderson, W. C. (1985). A comparison of the effects of continuous and intermittent response cost and reprimands in the classroom. *Journal of Clinical Child Psychology, 14*(4), 348–352.

Phillips, E. L., Phillips, E. A., Fixsen, D. L., & Wolf, M. M. (1971). Achievement Place: Modification of the behaviors of pre-delinquent boys within a token economy. *Journal of Applied Behavior Analysis, 4*(1), 45–59.

Pierce, W. D., & Cheney, C. D. (2017). *Behavior analysis and learning: A biobehavioral approach* (6th ed.). Routledge.

Piper, A., Borrero, J. C., & Becraft, J. L. (2020). Differential reinforcement-of-low-rate procedures: A systematic replication with students with autism spectrum disorder. *Journal of Applied Behavior Analysis, 53*(2), 1058–1070.

Platt, J. R. (1973). Percentile reinforcement: Paradigms for experimental analysis of response shaping. *Psychology of Learning and Motivation, 7,* 271–296.

Podlesnik, C. A., Jimenez-Gomez, C., Ward, R. D., & Shahan, T. A. (2006). Resistance to change of responding maintained by unsignaled delays to reinforcement: A response-bout analysis. *Journal of the Experimental Analysis of Behavior, 85*(3), 329–347.

Poling, A., & Normand, M. (1999). Noncontingent reinforcement: An inappropriate description of time-based schedules that reduce behavior. *Journal of Applied Behavior Analysis, 32*(2), 237–238.

Porter, J., Brown, R., & Goldsmith, P. (1982). Adjunctive behavior in children on fixed interval food reinforcement schedules. *Physiology and Behavior, 28*(4), 609–612.

Reed, P. (1991). Multiple determinants of the effects of reinforcement magnitude on free-operant response rates. *Journal of the Experimental Analysis of Behavior, 55*(1), 109–123.

Reed. P., & Wright, J. E. (1988). Effects of magnitude of food reinforcement on free-operant response rates. *Journal of the Experimental Analysis of Behavior, 49*(1), 75–85.

Repp, A. C., Barton, L. E., & Brulle, A. R. (1983). A comparison of two procedures for programming the differential reinforcement of other behaviors. *Journal of Applied Behavior Analysis, 16*(4), 435–445.

Repp, A. C., & Deitz, S. M. (1975). A comparison of fixed-ratio and variable-ratio token-production schedules with human subjects. *Psychological Record, 25*(1), 131–137.

Rescorla, R. A., & Skucy, J. C. (1969). Effect of response-independent reinforcers during extinction. *Journal of Comparative and Physiological Psychology, 67*(3), 381–389.

Retzlaff, B. J., Parthum, E. T., Pitts, R. C., & Hughes, C. E. (2017). Escape from right-to-

lean transitions: Stimulus change and timeout. *Journal of the Experimental Analysis of Behavior, 107*(1), 65–84.

Reynolds, G. S. (1961). Behavioral contrast. *Journal of the Experimental Analysis of Behavior, 4*(1), 57–71.

Richards, R. W. (1981). A comparison of signaled and unsignaled delay of reinforcement. *Journal of the Experimental Analysis of Behavior, 35*(2), 145–152.

Rico, V. V., de Carvalho Neto, M. B., Silveira, M. V., & da Silva Barros, R. (2018). Aversive control in behavior analysis: An analysis of *JEAB* and *JABA* publications (1958–2018). *Brazilian Journal of Behavior Analysis, 14*(2), 199–206.

Ringdahl, J. E., Vollmer, T. R., Borrero, J. C., & Connell, J. E. (2001). Fixed-time schedule effects as a function of baseline reinforcement rate. *Journal of Applied Behavior Analysis, 34*(1), 1–15.

Roane, H. S., Falcomata, T. S., & Fisher, W. W. (2007). Applying the behavioral economics principle of unit price to DRO schedule thinning. *Journal of Applied Behavior Analysis, 40*(3), 529–534.

Rolider, A., & Van Houten, R. (1985). Suppressing tantrum behavior in public places through the use of delayed punishment maintained by audio recordings. *Behavior Therapy, 16*(2), 181–194.

Roper, T. J., & Crossland, G. (1982). Schedule-induced wood-chewing in rats and its dependence on body weight. *Animal Learning and Behavior, 10*(1), 65–71.

Roscoe, E. M., Iwata, B. A., & Goh, H. (1998). A comparison of noncontingent reinforcement and sensory extinction as treatment for self-injurious behavior. *Journal of Applied Behavior Analysis, 31*(4), 635–646.

Russell, D., Ingvarsson, E. T., Haggar, J. L., & Jessel, J. (2018). Using progressive ratio schedules to evaluate tokens as generalized conditioned reinforcers. *Journal of Applied Behavior Analysis, 51*(1), 40–52.

Schaal, D. W., & Branch, M. N. (1990). Responding of pigeons under variable-interval schedules of signaled-delayed reinforcement: Effects of delay-signal duration. *Journal of the Experimental Analysis of Behavior, 53*(1), 103–121.

Scheithauer, M. Cariveau, T., Call, N. A., Ormand, H., & Clark, S. (2016). A consecutive case review of token systems used to reduce socially maintained challenging behavior in individuals with intellectual and developmental delays. *International Journal of Developmental Disabilities, 26*(3), 157–166.

Schoenfeld, W. N., & Cole, B. K. (1972). *Stimulus schedules: The T-[tau] systems.* Harper-Collins.

Schoenfeld, W. N., Farmer, J., & Vickery, C. (1970). Effects of varying probability of a response-pause requirement on a regular reinforcement baseline. *Psychonomic Science, 18*(3), 177–179.

Schwartz, B. (1982). Failure to produce response variability with reinforcement. *Journal of the Experimental Analysis of Behavior, 37*(2), 171–181.

Scott, G. K., & Platt, J. R. (1985). Model of response-reinforcer contingency. *Journal of Experimental Psychology: Animal Behavior Processes, 11*(2), 152–171.

Shabani, D. B., Carr, J. E., Pabico, R. S., Sala, A. P., Lam, W. Y., & Oberg, T. L. (2013). The effects of functional analysis test sessions on subsequent rates of problem behavior in the natural environment. *Behavioral Interventions, 28*(1), 40–47.

Shahan, T. A., & Lattal, K. A. (2005). Unsignaled delay of reinforcement, relative time, and resistance to change. *Journal of the Experimental Analysis of Behavior, 83*(3), 201–219.

Sidman, M. (1989). *Coercion and its fallout.* Authors Cooperative.

Silbaugh, B. C., & Falcomata, T. S. (2019). Effects of a lag schedule with progressive time delay on sign mand variability in a boy with autism. *Behavior Analysis in Practice, 12,* 124–132.

Sizemore, O. J. (1976). *The relation of response-reinforcer dependency and contiguity to signaled and unsignalled delay of reinforcement* [Unpublished doctoral dissertation]. West Virginia University.

Skinner, B. F. (1938). *The behavior of organisms.* Appleton-Century-Crofts.

Skinner, B. F. (1948). "Superstition" in the pigeon. *Journal of Experimental Psychology, 38*(2), 168–172.

Skinner, B. F. (1953). *Science and human behavior.* Macmillan.

St. Peter, C. C., Byrd, J. D., Pence, S. T., & Foreman, A. P. (2016). Effects of treatment-integrity failures on a response-cost procedure. *Journal of Applied Behavior Analysis, 49*(2), 308–328.

Staats, A. W., Staats, C. K., Schutz, R. E., & Wolf, M. (1962). The conditioning of textual responses using "extrinsic" reinforcers. *Journal of the Experimental Analysis of Behavior, 5*(1), 33–40.

Staddon, J. E., & Simmelhag, V. L. (1971). The "superstition" experiment: A reexamination of its implications for the principles of adaptive behavior. *Psychological Review, 78*(1), 3–43.

Stafford, D., & Branch, M. N. (1998). Effects of step size and break-point criterion on progressive-ratio performance. *Journal of the Experimental Analysis of Behavior, 70*(2), 123–138.

Stebbins, W. C., Mead, P. B., & Martin, J. M. (1959). The relation of amount of reinforcement to performance under a fixed-interval schedule. *Journal of the Experimental Analysis of Behavior, 2*(4), 351–355.

Stocco, C. S., & Thompson, R. H. (2015). Contingency analysis of caregiver behavior: Implications for parent training and future directions. *Journal of Applied Behavior Analysis, 48*(2), 417–435.

Stokes, T. F., & Baer, D. M. (1977). An implicit technology of generalization. *Journal of Applied Behavior Analysis, 10*(2), 349–367.

Sullivan, W. E., Saini, V., DeRosa, N. M., Criag, A. R., Ringdahl, J. E., & Roane, H. S. (2020). Measurement of nontargeted problem behavior during investigations of resurgence. *Journal of Applied Behavior Analysis, 53*(1), 249–264.

Susa, C., & Schlinger, H. D. (2012). Using a lag schedule to increase variability of verbal responding in an individual with autism. *Analysis of Verbal Behavior, 28,* 125–130.

Svartdal, F. (2008). Reverse PREE under multiple schedules: Exploration of a modulation hypothesis. *Learning and Motivation, 39*(1), 45–57.

Tarbox, R. S., Ghezzi, P. M., & Wilson, G. (2006). The effects of token reinforcement on attending in a young child with autism. *Behavioral Interventions, 21*(3), 155–164.

Thomas, J. R. (1968). Fixed-ratio punishment by timeout of concurrent variable-interval behavior. *Journal of the Experimental Analysis of Behavior, 11*(5), 609–616.

Thompson, R. H., Iwata, B. A., Hanley, G. P., Dozier, C. L., & Samaha, A. L. (2003). The effects of extinction, noncontingent reinforcement, and differential reinforcement of other behavior as control procedures. *Journal of Applied Behavior Analysis, 36*(2), 221–238.

Tiger, J. H., Bouxsein, K. J., & Fisher, W. W. (2007). Treating excessively slow responding of a young man with Asperger syndrome using differential reinforcement of short response latencies. *Journal of Applied Behavior Analysis,* *40*(3), 559–563.

Timberlake, W., & Lucas, G. A. (1985). The basis of superstitious behavior: Chance contingency, stimulus substitution, or appetitive behavior? *Journal of the Experimental Analysis of Behavior, 44*(3), 279–299.

Topping, J. S., & Ford, T. W. (1974). Response elimination with DRO and extinction: A within-subject comparison. *Psychological Record, 24*(4), 563–568.

Topping, J. S., & Ford, T. W. (1975). A within-subject comparison of three response-elimination procedures in pigeons. *Bulletin of the Psychonomic Society, 6*(3), 257–260.

Toussaint, K. A., & Tiger, J. H. (2012). Reducing covert self-injurious behavior maintained by automatic reinforcement through a variable momentary DRO procedure. *Journal of Applied Behavior Analysis, 45*(1), 179–184.

Trenholme, I. A., & Baron, A. (1975). Immediate and delayed punishment of human behavior by loss of reinforcement. *Learning and Motivation, 6*(1), 62–79.

Uhl, C. N., & Garcia, E. E. (1969). Comparison of omission with extinction in response elimination in rats. *Journal of Comparative and Physiological Psychology, 69*(3), 554–562.

Uhl, C. N., & Sherman, W. O. (1971). Comparison of combinations of omission, punishment, and extinction methods in response elimination in rats. *Journal of Comparative and Physiological Psychology, 74*(1, Pt. 1), 59–65.

Valentino, A. L., Shillingsburg, M. A., Call, N. A., Burton, B., & Bowen, C. N. (2011). An investigation of extinction-induced vocalizations. *Behavior Modification, 35*(3), 284–298.

Van Camp, C. M., Lerman, D. C., Kelley, M. E., Contrucci, S. A., & Vorndran, C. M. (2000). Variable-time reinforcement schedules in the treatment of socially maintained problem behavior. *Journal of Applied Behavior Analysis, 33*(4), 545–557.

Vollmer, T. R., Iwata, B. A., Zarcone, J. R., Smith, R. G., & Mazaleski, J. L. (1993). The role of attention in the treatment of attention-maintained self-injurious behavior: Noncontingent reinforcement and differential reinforcement of other behavior. *Journal of Applied Behavior Analysis, 26*(1), 9–21.

Vollmer, T. R., Marcus, B. A., & Ringdahl, J. E. (1995). Noncontingent escape as treatment for self-injurious behavior maintained by negative reinforcement. *Journal of Applied Behavior Analysis, 28*(1), 15–26.

Vollmer, T. R., Progar, P. R., Lalli, J. S., Van Camp, C. M., Sierp, B. J., Wright, C. S., . . . Eisenschink, K. J. (1998). Fixed-time schedules attenuate extinction-induced phenomena in the treatment of severe aberrant behavior. *Journal of Applied Behavior Analysis, 31*(4), 529–542.

Vollmer, T. R., Ringdahl, J. E., Roane, H. S., & Marcus, B. A. (1997). Negative side effects of noncontingent reinforcement. *Journal of Applied Behavior Analysis, 30*(1), 161–164.

Wahler, R. G., Vigilante, V. A., & Strand, P. S. (2004). Generalization in a child's oppositional behavior across home and school settings. *Journal of Applied Behavior Analysis, 37*(1), 43–51.

Ward-Horner, J. C., Muehlberger, A. O., Vedora, J., & Ross, R. K. (2017). Effects of reinforcer magnitude and quality on preference for response-reinforcer arrangements in young children with autism. *Behavior Analysis in Practice, 10*(2), 183–188.

Webbe, F. M., & Malagodi, E. F. (1978). Second-order schedules of token reinforcement: Comparisons of performance under fixed-ratio and variable-ratio exchange schedules. *Journal of the Experimental Analysis of Behavior, 30*(2), 219–224.

Williams, D. C., Saunders, K. J., & Perone, M. (2011). Extended pausing by humans on multiple fixed-ratio schedules with varied reinforcer magnitude and response requirements. *Journal of the Experimental Analysis of Behavior, 95*(2), 203–220.

Wilton, R. N., & Gay, R. A. (1969). Behavioral contrast in chained schedules. *Journal of the Experimental Analysis of Behavior, 12*(6), 905–910.

Winkler, R. C. (1970). Management of chronic psychiatric patients by a token reinforcement system. *Journal of Applied Behavior Analysis, 3*(1), 47–55.

Wolfe, J. B. (1936). Effectiveness of token rewards for chimpanzees. *Comparative Psychology Monographs, 12,* 1–72.

Wylie, A. M., Springis, R., & Johnson, K. S. (1992). Schedule-induced defecation: No-food and massed-food baselines. *Journal of the Experimental Analysis of Behavior, 58*(2), 389–397.

Yankelevitz, R. L., Bullock, C. E., & Hackenberg, T. D. (2008). Reinforcer accumulation in a token-reinforcement context with pigeons. *Journal of the Experimental Analysis of Behavior, 90*(3), 283–299.

Yoburn, B. C., & Cohen, P. S. (1979). Assessment of attack and drinking in White King pigeons on response-independent food schedules. *Journal of the Experimental Analysis of Behavior, 31*(1), 91–101.

Zarcone, T. J., Branch, M. N., Hughes, C. E., & Pennypacker, H. S. (1997). Key pecking during extinction after intermittent or continuous reinforcement as a function of the number of reinforcers delivered during training. *Journal of the Experimental Analysis of Behavior, 67*(1), 91–108.

Zeiler, M. D. (1968). Fixed and variable schedules of response-independent reinforcement. *Journal of the Experimental Analysis of Behavior, 11*(4), 405–411.

Zeiler, M. D. (1970). Time limits for completing fixed ratios. *Journal of the Experimental Analysis of Behavior, 14*(3), 275–286.

Zeiler, M. D. (1971). Eliminating behavior with reinforcement. *Journal of the Experimental Analysis of Behavior, 16*(3), 401–405.

Zeiler, M. D. (1972). Reinforcement of spaced responding in a simultaneous discrimination. *Journal of the Experimental Analysis of Behavior, 18*(3), 443–451.

Zeiler, M. D. (1976). Positive reinforcement and the elimination of reinforced responses. *Journal of the Experimental Analysis of Behavior, 26*(1), 37–44.

Zeiler, M. D. (1977). Elimination of reinforced behavior: Intermittent schedules of not-responding. *Journal of the Experimental Analysis of Behavior, 27*(1), 23–32.

Zeiler, M. D. (1984). The sleeping giant: Reinforcement schedules. *Journal of the Experimental Analysis of Behavior, 42*(3), 485–493.

Zimmerman, J., & Baydan, N. T. (1963). Punishment of responding of humans in conditional matching to sample by time-out. *Journal of the Experimental Analysis of Behavior, 6*(4), 589–597.

Zuriff, G. E. (1970). A comparison of variable-ratio and variable-interval schedules of reinforcement. *Journal of the Experimental Analysis of Behavior, 13*(3), 369–374.

CHAPTER 12

Extinction

Kelly M. Schieltz
Karen M. Lionello-DeNolf
Jennifer J. McComas

The fundamental goals of any treatment program are for problem behaviors not to recur and for a variety of desired behaviors to persist during and following treatment. For example, in medicine, medications or physical therapy exercises that often involve novel behaviors are prescribed, at least short term, to change the behavior (e.g., those causing pain) currently experienced to a more desired state. The most common expectation is that these treatments will be reduced or eliminated when the desired state is achieved, and that the desired state will continue indefinitely. Thus, the goal of successful treatment is the durability of the effects of treatment even in the absence or reduction of prescribed treatments. This is the same goal many clients and care providers have for reinforcement-based treatment programs; that is, problem behavior does not recur and desired behavior persists. Given that most behavioral treatment programs rely on the behavioral mechanism of reinforcement, the process of reinforcement clearly plays a role in achieving the goals of intervention. However, what is perhaps less clear is the role that extinction plays during both initial treatment outcomes and maintenance. This uncertainty may be, at least in part, because our terminology (e.g., the label, differential reinforcement treatment programs) does not specify the role of other variables, including extinction. As both a process and procedure, extinction underlies many reinforcement-based programs for problem behavior. In this chapter, we describe how extinction functions to facilitate the short- and long-term effects of reinforcement-based treatment programs, as we rarely recommend that extinction be used in the absence of reinforcement.

In behavior analysis, there exists a balance between considering behavioral mechanisms as procedures (most often in applied behavior analysis) and behavioral mechanisms as processes. The distinction between a behavioral procedure and a behavioral process is often based on its purpose or use; they are not mutually exclusive. The evaluation of a mechanism as a process can extend our understanding of its use as a procedure; understanding the mechanism assists us in modifying our interventions; thus, translational analyses of mechanisms can provide information that maximizes the effects and, therefore, the outcomes of interventions for those we serve. To illustrate, we use reinforcement as the example, because we know more about its procedures and processes than we do about extinction. For decades, applied researchers evaluated the effects of differential reinforcement on problem behavior (as a procedure; for a review, see Petscher et al., 2009, and Agnew et al., Chapter 9, this volume), with the results often evaluated within reversal designs (i.e., decreases in problem behavior with reinforcement of alternative behavior present, increases in problem behavior with reinforcement of alternative behavior absent). The results of these studies led many applied behavior analysts to conclude that differential reinforcement of alternative behavior (DRA) programs, such as functional communication training (FCT; Carr & Durand, 1985), was both a necessary and sufficient treatment procedure for treating problem behavior. However, subsequent translational evaluations then focused specifically on how the effects of reinforcement, as a process, influenced behavior (e.g., Mace et al., 2010). These studies increased our understanding of the specific impact of reinforcement (e.g., increasing the persistence of all behaviors within the same response class within a specific context), and provided an explanation for the common occurrence of treatment relapse. These translational studies resulted in findings that may improve the effects of differential reinforcement treatment, specifically in regard to the maintenance of treatment effects (Nevin & Wacker, 2013). In this example, evaluation decisions were based on the basic studies that evolved from behavioral momentum theory (BMT; Nevin & Grace, 2000), which provides a quantitative framework for understanding the occurrence, or lack thereof, of behavioral persistence (for discussion of resistance to change, see Craig et al., Chapter 18, this volume). By basing more applied evaluations on BMT, translational researchers have begun to develop a bridge to continue advancing our understanding of the impact of reinforcement as it relates to the long-term maintenance of treatment outcomes (e.g., Suess et al., 2020).

As redefined by Nevin and Wacker (2013) and discussed more recently by Greer and Shahan (2019), *maintenance* occurs when the prevailing conditions of treatment are challenged and the following two conditions are met: (1) problem behavior fails to relapse and (2) adaptive behavior persists. With this definition, the two dependent variables of interest are problem behavior (its relapse) and adaptive behavior (its continued occurrence). Basic BMT research has demonstrated that the rate of reinforcement influences relapse. The higher the overall rate of reinforcement is for a behavior, the more resistant that behavior is to change when challenged, thus resulting in higher levels of relapse (Nevin et al., 1990). Similarly, applied research has demonstrated that when the reinforcement-based treatment program is removed (i.e., returned to baseline conditions), problem behavior often quickly recurs (e.g., Berg et al., 2015). As we have now learned, both the relapse of problem behavior and continued occurrence of adaptive behavior are issues of behavioral persistence; that is, problem behavior relapses when it persists and adaptive behavior persists when it continues to occur. Thus, these behavioral outcomes simply do not covary with one replacing the other. Rather, they are correlated with one influencing the other, whereby the value of each response is determined by the current and historical variables in place for each response (Shahan & Craig, 2017). Maintenance, then, is a function of the persistence of both dependent variables, and one cannot treat one without considering the other.

The translational studies on the effects of reinforcement on behavioral persistence (relapse of problem behavior and continued occurrence of adaptive behavior) have benefited from the bidirectional relationship between basic and applied researchers; they highlight the integration of our science and move us toward a better understanding of how to more effectively treat and maintain the achieved treatment effects via the reinforcement schedules implemented in specific contexts (e.g., Mace et al., 2010; Ringdahl et al., 2018; Shahan & Craig, 2017; Suess et al., 2020; Wacker et al., 2011). We often refer to DRA programs, such as FCT, as simply "reinforcement-based treatments." Although the current literature largely focuses on the role of reinforcement, and rightly so, reinforcement is rarely the only component in any treatment program and is never the only component in DRA programs; that is, other components, such as extinction, also play a critical role in behavior change programs and the maintenance of treatment but are much less frequently studied than reinforcement. To further our understanding of how treatment programs such as differential reinforcement result in persistence of treatment effects, every component of the treatment package, such as extinction, needs to be evaluated on both a procedural and process level.

Extinction Defined

As an effect, *extinction* refers to an observed decline in response rate of a target behavior when that behavior is no longer reinforced. Extinction is considered a basic principle of behavior and has been observed across species (e.g., rats, pigeons, humans) and settings (natural, experimental, applied) and in both Pavlovian and operant conditioning (Lattal et al., 2013). As a procedure, extinction refers to withholding the unconditioned stimulus (US) upon presentation of the conditioned stimulus (CS; in Pavlovian conditioning) or the reinforcer when the response occurs (in operant conditioning). Thus, one could say that the behavior was "put on extinction." Extinction has also been referred to as the discontinuation of the response–reinforcer contingency (Rescorla & Skucy, 1969), such as when noncontingent reinforcement (NCR) procedures are used to decrease a target behavior (e.g., Phillips et al., 2017). In either case, the organism is not prevented from making the target response; rather, the response no longer produces the consequence.

Procedure

The *procedure of extinction* is an active component of many interventions based on both Pavlovian and operant conditioning. For example, extinction is often used as part of a treatment package to reduce anxiety or other conditioned emotional responses that are elicited by a CS (e.g., Hoffman & Smits, 2008; for more discussion of Pavlovian conditioning and anxiety, see Thrailkill et al., Chapter 6, and Brewer et al., Chapter 8, respectively, this volume). In this situation, the procedure of extinction involves repeated presentations of the CS without the pairing of a US or other CS. In operant conditioning, extinction is a common component of treatment packages involving differential reinforcement. For instance, many FCT programs teach a socially acceptable response (e.g., requesting attention by saying, "play") to compete with a functionally equivalent inappropriate response (e.g., self-injury that produces attention). Here, the learner is taught the appropriate communication response using reinforcement and prompting procedures, while instances of self-injury are placed on extinction. Extinction is, therefore, a critical component of FCT.

The procedure of extinction takes on many forms, and the first procedural consideration is to ensure that its form matches the function of target behavior (Iwata et al., 1994). This demonstration was shown by Iwata et al. with three children with moderate to severe intellectual disabilities who engaged in self-injury maintained by different behavioral functions. For one child, self-injury was shown to be maintained by automatic reinforcement. Following this analysis of behavioral function, extinction variations were implemented in each condition. For example, during an alone condition, extinction was conducted to remove the sensory consequences of the self-injury (i.e., helmet placed on the head of the child), whereas during an escape condition, extinction was conducted by either removing the sensory consequences (as already described) or eliminating the negative reinforcement consequence (i.e., tasks remained present when self-injury occurred). Results showed that across all conditions, self-injury reduced only when the extinction procedure eliminated the sensory consequences, which was consistent with the automatic function. For the other two children, similar results of the reductions of self-injury were obtained only when the extinction procedure matched the function of target behavior. Therefore, from a procedural perspective, one cannot simply ignore the occurrence of problem behavior and expect that it will decrease via extinction, because, in some cases, the simple act of ignoring behavior may not be removing the reinforcement contingency responsible for the behavior's occurrence.

A second consideration is to determine how the procedure of extinction will be implemented, which is typically based on the reinforcement strategy used. For example, when using NCR, reinforcers are typically provided on continuous or dense, fixed-time schedules. Because reinforcers are provided independent of responding, extinction is considered a component of this reinforcement strategy when the response–reinforcer contingency is eliminated (Vollmer et al., 1995; see Lalli et al., 1997, for a comparison between NCR with and without extinction). Relative to differential reinforcement procedures, reinforcers are provided contingent on the omission of target behavior in differential reinforcement of other behavior (DRO) programs and the display of a specific alternative behavior in DRA programs (Vollmer & Iwata, 1992). In DRO programs, extinction is implemented with an interval resetting procedure when the target behavior occurs; that is, if target behavior occurs in the programmed interval (fixed or variable), the reinforcer is withheld and the interval resets. Thus, the goal in most DRO programs is to decrease a target response with any other neutral to desired response that may occur in its place. In DRA programs, extinction is implemented for the occurrence of every behavior except the specified alternative behavior. Thus, in most DRA programs, the goal is to replace a target behavior with a predefined acceptable response. Local extinction occurs in lag reinforcement schedules, where reinforcers are provided for responses that differ from a specified number of prior responses, which is noted in the schedule. For example, in a Lag 3 schedule, only a response that differs in form from the three responses that occurred immediately prior to its occurrence produces reinforcement. Thus, all responses that do not differ from the previous three responses result in extinction (Lee et al., 2002). The most common goal of treatment programs that use lag schedules is to produce varied, or diverse, responding. Across studies in which one or more of these different reinforcement schedules are implemented with extinction, positive effects have been shown in reducing target behavior (e.g., Schlichenmeyer et al., 2015; Lalli et al., 1997; Vollmer et al., 1993, 1995), increasing a specific adaptive response (DRA; e.g., Carr & Durand, 1985), or in increasing alternative (DRO; e.g., Kodak et al., 2003) or varied (lag schedules; e.g., Lee et al., 2002) responding.

Process

The *process of extinction* refers to the observed change in behavior when an extinction procedure is put in place; functionally, the process of operant extinction begins when the organism first encounters the absence of the reinforcer following the target behavior (Katz & Lattal, 2021). The rate of behavior may decrease to its pre-reinforcement levels, or it may decrease to zero occurrences.

The effects of extinction as a process can be quite complicated. Multiple aspects of behavior can be affected, and reductions in target behavior are not necessarily permanent. The primary effect of an extinction procedure is the decline in responding of the previously reinforced response, but this outcome is not necessarily a rapid process. The reduction in target responding can often be gradual, and the rate of reduction depends on the similarity between the reinforcement and extinction context (Lattal & Lattal, 2012). Extinction procedures can also increase behavior. The most common example in applied behavior analysis is often labeled as an extinction burst (Holton, 1961; Keller & Schoenfeld, 1950; Lerman et al., 1999; Woods & Borrero, 2019), which is a temporary acceleration of responding when extinction procedures are implemented. Extinction bursts have also been reported when extinction is implemented after different types of schedules, but sometimes does not occur (for discussion, see Katz & Lattal, 2021; Nist & Shahan, 2021). In addition, extinction procedures can generate other response topographies that are related to the target response (Eckerman & Lanson, 1969), completely new behaviors (Neuringer et al., 2001), and aggressive and emotional behavior (extinction induced variability; Azrin et al., 1966).

It is important to note that new behaviors generated by extinction procedures do not replace the target behavior, and extinction does not cause "unlearning" to occur (Bouton et al., 2021). Behavior submitted to an extinction procedure does not reduce to zero permanently (see Podlesnik & Kelley, 2015, for discussion), nor does it reduce globally. In other words, behavior is reduced locally within the context in which it had been previously reinforced, and it can return under a variety of circumstances or contextual conditions. The classic example of the return of extinguished behavior is the phenomenon of *spontaneous recovery* (Keller & Schoenfeld, 1950), or the return of the extinguished response when reintroduced to the extinction context after a period away from that context (e.g., Lattal et al., 2013). Instances of spontaneous recovery are typically limited if the extinction procedure remains in effect (i.e., the behavior is not inadvertently reinforced). The extinguished response can also recur when its maintaining reinforcer is delivered noncontingently (reinstatement), when there is a change within the context (renewal), and when additional behaviors related to the same reinforcer are put on extinction (resurgence) (see Lattal & Wacker, 2015, for a discussion).

As the previous description illustrates, extinction is more than simply a procedure to reduce or eliminate a behavior. It also has a critical role in the generation of new behavior (i.e., behavioral variability; see Falcomata & Neuringer, Chapter 20, this volume), which can be capitalized on within intervention programs. When used to reduce unwanted behavior, long-term maintenance of behavior reduction is a goal. Resurgence can be thought of as the return of an extinguished response, and the likelihood that resurgence occurs is influenced by a host of variables, including whether extinction is the sole intervention or used as part of a treatment package. Therefore, an increased understanding of both the procedure of extinction and the process of extinction is needed to facilitate the success of treatment. Although some effects of extinction may appear to be distinct, they, in fact, exist along the same continuum. In the remaining sections of this chapter, we consider the process (underlying mechanism) of extinction within the basic literature and the procedure (application) of extinction within the applied and translational literatures related to two "distinct" effects of extinction: (1) the durability (maintenance) of the effects of treatment, and (2) the variability (response generalization) of responding. We focus on these two effects because, as noted by Baer et al. (1968), generality of behavioral change occurs when that change demonstrates durability over time or across contexts, and/or spreads to other related behaviors, which are all important goals for applied treatment programs.

Effects and Implications of Extinction on Durability

Durability refers to the robustness of the treatment effects and is often assessed during periods of extinction, which are a routine part of daily life (e.g., because reinforcement schedules in daily life are most often intermittent). When a behavioral response recurs (e.g., previously extinguished response) or continues (e.g., most recently trained response), those responses are said to be durable (Wong & Amsel, 1976). Ideally, in most applied situations, we want the desired behaviors (often the most recently trained response) to show durability rather than the behavior previously reduced via extinction. Durability is the focus of this section of the chapter.

Basic Mechanism of Extinction and Its Relation to Durability

We consider the factors that affect response durability first from the perspective of the persistence (continued occurrence) of desired responding under extinction (resistance to extinction), followed by the perspective of the recurrence of reduced or eliminated responding over time (resurgence of responding during extinction).

Continued Occurrence of Responding and Its Resistance to Extinction

Durability of behavior can be measured as persistence of a response during extinction; behavior that persists at high rates during extinction procedures is said to be resistant to extinction. Persistence can be measured in several ways (e.g., response rate during extinction relative to response rate during reinforcement, the total number of responses emitted until an extinction criterion has been met, the total amount of time until a criterion is reached), and sometimes different conclusions can be drawn depending on the method used (Mowrer & Jones, 1945). Moreover, there are several variables that can affect behavioral persistence during an extinction procedure, and these can interact with each other in complex ways. Separating the effects of different variables, such as rate and overall amount of reinforcement, can be quite complicated, because doing so requires holding one variable (e.g., amount) constant while manipulating the other variable (e.g., rate), which then may result in other differences between the conditions (e.g., the number of reinforced responses). As a result, the use of extinction in an intervention requires careful consideration of many factors.

First, the most well-known factor contributing to resistance to extinction is the schedule of reinforcement that had been used during reinforcement of the behavior (e.g., Capaldi, 1966; Hug & Amsel, 1969; Nevin, 1988; Rescorla, 1999; Robbins, 1971). It is often reported that behavior that has been reinforced on a continuous schedule (i.e., fixed-ratio [FR] 1) is less persistent under extinction than behavior that has been reinforced on an intermittent schedule, a phenomenon known as the *partial reinforcement extinction effect* (PREE; e.g., Capaldi, 1966; De Meyer et al., 2019; Nevin, 1988). For example, De Meyer et al. (2019) compared responding in extinction after training a simple discrimination task under conditions of continuous (FR 1), partial (variable-ratio [VR] 5), and reinforcement schedule thinning (i.e., gradually increasing the VR requirement across trials) in both children without known disabilities and children with attention-deficit/hyperactivity disorder (ADHD) in a group design. Following training, correct responses were reinforced according to the programmed reinforcement schedule until the training criterion was met (20 reinforcers earned), whereby all responses were then placed on extinction. Results showed no differences between children with and without ADHD. However, during extinction, the children in the FR-1 group made significantly fewer responses than those in the other two groups, and the proportion of responding to the previously reinforced stimulus was higher in the VR-5 and ratio-thinning groups than the FR-1 group. Thus, greater durability of the target response was achieved when training occurred under more intermittent reinforcement schedules. This difference in durability may occur because training under intermittent schedules produces conditions that are more similar to those of extinction than does training under continuous reinforcement, which supports greater generalization of responding under extinction conditions (Capaldi, 1966). In other words, organisms that experience intermittent schedules sometimes receive reinforcement for making a response when the most recent prior response was not reinforced; thus, they experience reinforcement for continuing to respond under conditions of nonreinforcement. By contrast, organisms that experience continuous schedules do not learn to respond under conditions of nonreinforcement. Thus, studies investigating the PREE have shown that resistance to extinction is not solely a function of the prior number of reinforced responses, as experiencing nonreinforcement (i.e., extinction) is an important contributor to persistence.

Second, reinforcement rate and magnitude of reinforcement for the target response are factors known to contribute to resistance to extinction (Nevin, 1974; Shettleworth & Nevin, 1965) in free-operant preparations involving multiple schedules. *Rate* refers to the frequency of reinforcement in a session (or a component of a multiple schedule), whereas *magnitude* refers to the size of the reinforcer delivered. For example, Shettleworth and Nevin (1965) trained pigeons on a two-component multiple schedule in which the rate of reinforcement was the same but the magnitude differed (e.g., responses were reinforced on a VI 2-seconds schedule in each component, but in one component pigeons had 1-second access to the food hopper and in the other they had 9-second access). In a subsequent extinction session, there was greater persistence of responding in the component associated with the larger magnitude reinforcer than the smaller magnitude reinforcer. Furthermore, Nevin (1974, Experiment 2) showed that greater reinforcement rates can lead to greater resistance to extinction. In this study, pigeons were exposed to a multiple schedule in which responding in one (green) component was reinforced on a VI 2 minutes schedule and responding in the other (red) component was reinforced on a VI 6 minutes schedule for an extended number of sessions. During the final 10 sessions, extinction was in effect for both components, and the results indicated greater persistence of responding in the green component than in the red. This effect has been replicated under a variety of conditions and with different species (see Nevin & Grace, 2000, for a review).

Third, some dimensions of reinforcement (i.e., magnitude/size, quality, effort) have been shown to interact with schedules of reinforcement to influence resistance to extinction. For example, target responding displayed by rats under extinction conditions is often more persistent after (1) intermittent reinforcement schedules that provided medium to high magnitudes of reinforcement than continuous schedules that provided medium to high magnitudes of reinforcement (e.g., Roberts, 1969; Likely et al., 1971), (2) continuous reinforcement schedules that provided low magnitudes of reinforcement than intermittent schedules that provided low magnitudes of reinforcement (e.g., Roberts, 1969), and (3) continuous reinforcement schedules that provided high magnitudes of a relatively higher-quality reinforcer than continuous schedules that provided high magnitudes of a relatively lower-quality reinforcer (e.g., Likely et al., 1971). Additionally, responses that are less effortful tend to show more persistence during extinction (Capehart et al., 1958; Solomon, 1948), such as when Capehart et al. exposed rats to extinction procedures after reinforcement for bar pressing in which different amounts of force (low, intermediate, and high) were required to activate the bar. Results showed that persistence of bar pressing declined as the amount of force required to respond increased.

Fourth, durability of responding in an extinction procedure can be affected by motivating operations (Greer & Shahan, 2019). Typically, if an establishing operation is in effect for the reinforcer, behavior will persist longer in extinction than when the establishing operation is not in effect. However, motivating operations can also interact with other variables, such as reinforcement schedules. For example, Mikula and Pavlik (1966) studied the effects of level of food deprivation in rats that were trained to run in a straight runway under continuous or intermittent reinforcement schedules in a between-groups design. Three deprivation levels (low, intermediate, and high) were used; rats experienced four runs per day, and those in the continuous group received food on every trial, whereas those in the intermittent group received food on only half the trials. The results indicated faster run speeds (i.e., greater response persistence) with higher levels of deprivation, and this effect was larger in the intermittent than in the continuous reinforcement group.

Finally, prior exposure to extinction can affect resistance to extinction (e.g., Anger & Anger, 1976; Baum, 2012; Bullock & Smith, 1953; Craig et al., 2019; Mahoney et al., 2012; but for possible limitations, see Bai & Podlesnik, 2017). For instance, in baseline, Bullock and Smith (1953) reinforced rats' bar pressing 40 times and then implemented a 1-hour extinction session. This cycle was repeated across 10 days, and the results indicated that fewer total responses were emitted in the latter extinction sessions compared to the first five extinction sessions.

Resurgence of Responding during Extinction

There is a sizable literature documenting the conditions under which an extinguished response may return in both Pavlovian and operant conditioning. The classic example of this phenomenon is spontaneous recovery, or the return of the extinguished response when reintroduced to the extinction context after a period of time away from that context. For example, Rescorla (2004, Experiment 3) demonstrated spontaneous recovery in operant conditioning. Rats were trained to make two operant responses: lever pressing and chain pulling. Rats received separate sessions of training for each response, followed by extinction sessions. Rats were then given 6 days of rest in the home case, followed by a return to the experimental apparatus. For both operant responses, there was an increase in responding relative to the end of the prior extinction session.

The length of the interval between removal from and return to the extinction context influences the probability of a return of responding, with greater intervals resulting in more spontaneous recovery (Brooks & Bouton, 1993). For example, Howat and Grant (1958) exposed college students to a Pavlovian conditioning procedure in which a light was followed by a puff of air to the eye until a conditioned response (CR; an eyeblink) reliably occurred. Following this training, extinction trials were conducted in which only the CS was presented. The participants were then excused from the lab and asked to return either 20 minutes or 24 hours later. Upon return, the CS was again presented without the US. The results indicated spontaneous recovery (emission of the CR) in both groups, but the effect was greater in the group that returned after 24 hours than it was after the group that returned after 20 minutes. Moreover, if there are repeated instances of removal from and return to the extinction context, the amount of spontaneous recovery decreases with each return. Skinner (1950) suggested that stimulus cues associated with being returned to the context function as discriminative stimuli that evoke responding. Since extinction is in effect, these responses are not reinforced, and the stimulus cues become less likely to evoke responding with each removal from and return to the context.

Extinguished responding can return under circumstances other than spontaneous recovery. *Resurgence* is one such situation and is defined as the return of a previously extinguished behavior when subsequently reinforced behaviors undergo extinction (e.g., Alessandri et al., 2015; Epstein, 1983; St. Peter, 2015; Winterbauer et al., 2013). In experimental work, resurgence is investigated using a three-phase procedure. For example, Epstein (1983) reinforced and then extinguished key pecking by pigeons (Phase 1) and subsequently reinforced an alternative behavior incompatible with key pecking (e.g., head turning, wing raising; Phase 2). During Phase 3, both key pecking and the alternative behavior were placed on extinction. Results indicated that as the rate of the alternative behavior approached zero, key pecking returned. Generally, evidence for resurgence is strong and has been demonstrated across species (e.g., rats, pigeons, fish, mice, and humans) and response topographies (e.g., lever pressing, key pecking, nose poking, treadle pushing, and more complex behavioral sequences; for a review, see St. Peter, 2015). Although we focus our discussion here on resurgence, other circumstances whereby extinguished responding returns include reinstatement (Bouton & Bolles, 1979; Bouton & Peck, 1989; Doughty et al., 2004; Franks & Lattal, 1976; Rescorla & Heth, 1975) and renewal (Bouton & Bolles, 1979; Bouton & Peck, 1989; Bouton et al., 2011; Nakajima et al., 2000).

As mentioned previously, BMT research has suggested that resurgence is influenced by higher overall reinforcement rates within a context prior to extinction. Although BMT has provided a good framework for understanding resurgence, it has some limitations. The resurgence as choice (RaC) model proposed by Shahan and Craig (2017) potentially offers a more complete quantitative and theoretical model of factors that influence resurgence. The overarching model suggests that resurgence is a function of the relative value of a target behavior, which is influenced by its historic and current reinforcement history and the historic and current reinforcement history of alternative behavior (Greer & Shahan, 2019). Factors accounted for in this model include those that affect resistance to extinction: the rate of reinforcement, other reinforcement dimensions such as quality, magnitude, immediacy, and effort, and motivating operations. Any one of, or a combination of, these factors can influence the value of, and thus the engagement in, one behavior versus another behavior. Consideration of all these factors is necessary for potentially mitigating resurgence; that is, making adjustments to one or more of these factors may result in maintenance (lack of recurrence) of responding that has been placed on extinction, which is a primary goal in applied treatment programs (for additional discussion on relapse, see Saini et al., Chapter 19, this volume).

Application of Extinction and Its Relation to Durability

In behavior analysis, we use the term *covariation* to describe the relation of two behaviors. For example, in FCT programs, when the alternative or replacement communication response increases and problem behavior decreases, or vice versa, we say that the two behaviors covary; that is (in this example), as one behavior goes up, the other behavior must go down to show covariation (note that covariation is also said to occur when a nontarget behavior changes by increasing or decreasing as a function of changes in a target behavior; for an example of this, see Schieltz et al., 2011). However, using the label covariation for these behavioral observations, while accurate, does not describe the underlying process that contributes to these behavioral occurrences, thereby reducing our overall understanding of when outcomes such as resurgence occurs (e.g., when problem behavior again occurs despite the occurrence of appropriate communication). By analyzing the occurrence of these behaviors through the lens of behavioral processes, we may begin to understand which factors, such as extinction, contribute to or result in durability, leading then to alterations in how to improve behavioral treatments to promote behavioral durability.

Resurgence of Responding during Extinction

As previously mentioned, understanding how behavioral processes, in the applied context, contribute to the durability of behavioral responses was demonstrated by Mace et al. (2010), who specifically evaluated the effects of a differential reinforcement program on the resurgence of problem behavior that had been successfully reduced via DRA. However, despite the initial success of DRA, these researchers showed that resurgence was more likely to occur following DRA treatment conditions than following baseline extinction conditions, thus demonstrating that the durability of problem behavior was directly related to the reinforcement received during treatment. In this case, then, maintenance of treatment effects was compromised by the preceding condition in which the participants received more rather than less reinforcement. They further showed that resurgence could be reduced by implementing DRA in a context separate from the context historically associated with the reinforcement of problem behavior, a finding replicated across species (pigeons, humans) by Craig et al. (2018) and Suess et al. (2020), respectively. Thus, resurgence was reduced by altering the way in which DRA was implemented. A second option for reducing resurgence, shown by Wacker et al. (2011), was to continue to provide extinction for problem behavior for much longer periods of time than is typical in more applied studies; that is, FCT with extinction was alternated with periods of extinction alone, and these combined procedures were implemented across months (up to 18 months). This applied finding was consistent with basic studies demonstrating that prior exposures to extinction contributed to reduced levels of resurgence over time (Shahan et al., 2020; Sweeney & Shahan, 2013).

Both Mace et al. (2010) and Wacker et al. (2011) provided options for improving the maintenance (lack of resurgence of reduced responding) of differential reinforcement treatments by further evaluating the mechanisms responsible for durability. The provision of extinction prior to (baseline extinction conditions; Mace et al., 2010) and during (alternating periods of reinforcement and extinction; Wacker et al., 2011) treatment was based on the process of extinction (programming for responses to encounter the absence of reinforcement), which was shown to actively contribute to maintenance in the form of less resurgence. Subsequent applied and translational research has continued to focus on variables other than reinforcement schedules that influence maintenance. For example, the presence of discriminative stimuli (Fisher et al., 2020; Kimball et al., 2018; Shvarts et al., 2020) and preference for specific alternative responses (Berg et al., 2015, Ringdahl et al., 2018) have been shown to influence the persistence of desired responding.

The influence of these variables on resurgence has led to alternative theories such as the development of RaC as discussed earlier (see Greer & Shahan, 2019, for a discussion). However, the role that extinction plays with obtaining durability of target responding, although included within the RaC model, remains largely unknown.

Implications for the Next Translational Steps

Because applied and translational researchers, as well as practitioners, almost exclusively focus on the role of reinforcement (and rightly so), little is known about the role extinction plays in the durability of behavioral responses. However, as mentioned previously, Mace et al. (2010) and Wacker et al. (2011) showed that extinction may be an active variable in long-term maintenance.

Schieltz et al. (2017) conducted a retrospective study to determine the role of extinction on behavioral persistence, specifically on the maintenance of reduced or eliminated responding. In this study, data from five of the children in the Wacker et al. (2011) study were evaluated to determine the correlation between the number of FCT treatment sessions needed to reach stable 90% reductions in problem behavior (no resurgence) when treatment was challenged with extinction. Results of this study showed a strong negative correlation (–.87; although not reported in the article, results approached significance at $p < .10$), whereby when more FCT sessions (that each contained extinction for problem behavior) were needed to reach a stable 90% reduction in problem behavior during the FCT phases, less resurgence occurred. In contrast, when the stable reduction in problem behavior occurred more quickly in FCT, more resurgence occurred. The authors hypothesized that these differences occurred because of the different exposures to extinction during the FCT treatment; that is, problem behavior was likely exposed to more extinction during treatment when treatment effects took longer to obtain. These results suggested that extinction plays a role in behavioral persistence, such that exposures to extinction weaken or reduce the value of problem behavior. However, if exposures to extinction do not occur within the treatment phases, maintenance, and specifically the lack of resurgence, may take much longer to obtain.

Comparable results were reported by Brown et al. (2020), who compared the effects of DRA without extinction and DRA with extinction plus NCR on the resurgence of target responding displayed by two children with autism spectrum disorder (Experiment 1) and 10 rats (Experiment 2). Results showed that higher levels of resurgence occurred in the DRA without extinction condition, suggesting that when target responding results in exposures to extinction during DRA treatment, resurgence is less likely to occur when treatment is challenged. Similar results were shown by Saini et al. (2017) with NCR schedules (see also Epstein, 1983; Trask et al., 2015 for alternative explanations). Similar to Schieltz et al. (2017), neither Brown et al. (2020) nor Saini et al. (2017) specifically accounted for the number of exposures to extinction across the conditions, and so a logical next step is to equate the number of extinction encounters across treatment procedures and to further evaluate the influence of extinction on maintenance.

The implications of previous studies have potential clinical implications for applied behavior analysts. For example, differential reinforcement treatment programs are often arranged, at least initially, to reduce the likelihood that problem behavior will encounter extinction; the emphasis of early treatment is often on increasing encounters with reinforcement, such as manipulating various dimensions of reinforcement such as programming for no delay to reinforcement (e.g., Athens & Vollmer, 2010). Although arranging the treatment programs in these ways often makes good clinical sense and can substantially improve the effects of early treatment, these arrangements may inadvertently reduce long-term maintenance because of reduced levels of extinction. In terms of BMT and RaC, these procedures reduce the opportunity of extinction to disrupt or reduce the value of problem behavior.

Effects and Implications of Extinction on Variability

Variability refers to the generality of behavioral responses and, interestingly (given that variability is often considered the opposite of durability), is also evaluated by removing the conditions of treatment and conducting extinction sessions. When a behavioral response occurs in different ways, or occurs as different forms of the response, those responses are said to be variable (Neuringer, 2004). As shown often in the applied literature, extinction can induce or generate novel response variations of the same response (e.g., increased rate), and displays of the same response across novel stimulus conditions. In an applied situation, it is often ideal to observe variability in desired responses, because this is an indication that the effects of treatment have generalized across responses and/or stimulus conditions. We have focused on this aspect of extinction within this section of the chapter because generalization, like maintenance, is a key outcome of treatment and may often be correlated with improved maintenance. To illustrate, we briefly return to our original medical example: If the patient learned to produce multiple adaptive behaviors to avoid a return to painful conditions, this may be more related to long-term maintenance of the physical therapy program than if the patient only learned one adaptive behavior that must be repeated over and over again for maintenance to occur.

Although the outcomes of behavioral persistence and behavioral variability are often considered to be distinctly different when considered as outcomes, when we consider the behavioral mechanism(s) responsible, such as extinction, we begin to view them as being less different and instead as existing along a continuum. The process of extinction influences both durability and variability to greater or lesser degrees across target behaviors, stimulus contexts, and reinforcement schedules. In the next section, we focus on variability.

Basic Mechanism of Extinction and Its Relation to Variability

Evidence for *behavioral* (operant) *variability*, or the display of novel or other forms of the behavior that could potentially result in the reinforcer, is well established in the basic literature (e.g., Antonitis, 1951; Kinloch et al., 2009; Pear, 1985) and can be measured in several ways. One type of extinction-induced variability is the emergence of new response topographies that are related to a previously reinforced response (Antonitis, 1951; Kinloch et al., 2009; Eckerman & Lanson, 1969; Morgan & Lee, 1996). For example, Eckerman and Lanson (1969) demonstrated variability of response topographies by pigeons under extinction following a period of continuous reinforcement. Pigeons were trained to peck a 10-inch-wide rectangular response key; over the course of five baseline sessions, pecking was localized to the center of the key. In the subsequent extinction sessions, variation in response location increased and exceeded that observed during the initial training in most cases. Similarly, Morgan and Lee (1996) demonstrated increased variability of interresponse times (IRTs) by college students trained to press the spacebar on a computer keyboard on different differential reinforcement of low rate (DRL) schedules.

In addition to producing new response topographies related to the trained behavior, extinction procedures can result in the display of completely novel behavior (Neuringer et al., 2001). For instance, Neuringer et al. (Experiment 1) trained rats to make sequences of responses across three response manipulanda (two levers and a response key). The reinforcement criteria included that the sequence emitted be different from previously emitted sequences. Training was followed by four extinction sessions, resulting in the rats displaying a greater number of novel sequences in the extinction sessions than in the training sessions. Additionally, the number of novel sequences increased across extinction sessions. Extinction procedures can also result in the return of behavior that had previously been extinguished (i.e., resurgence; Epstein, 1983), which can be considered an instance of behavioral variability. For example, Lieving and Lattal (2003) first trained pigeons to peck a key for food reinforcement. In a second phase, key pecking was placed on extinction and a different response, treadle pushing, was reinforced. In a final phase, treadle pushing was placed on extinction. With both the treadle and response key available in this final extinction session, Lieving and Lattal observed a return of key pecking when treadle pushing was placed on extinction.

Another type of response variability associated with extinction procedures is the demonstration of aggressive and emotional behavior (Azrin et al., 1966; Kelly & Hake, 1970; Thompson & Bloom, 1966; Zeiler, 1971). For example, Azrin et al. (1966) reported instances of pigeons attacking other pigeons as a result of an extinction procedure (see Thompson & Bloom, 1966, for a related study in rats). Pigeons were tested in an apparatus that included a restrained "target" subject (a live or a stuffed pigeon) that allowed objective measures of attack behavior. During baseline measures, the pigeons did not peck at the target pigeon. The pigeons were exposed to alternating periods of continuous reinforcement for key pecking and extinction. The results indicated that pigeons pecked at the response key during reinforcement and pecked at the target pigeon with enough force to cause tissue damage during extinction. Attacks were the most frequent during transitions from the reinforcement to the extinction periods. Kelly and Hake (1970) replicated this finding in humans in which aggressive responses were defined as making a forceful response to an inanimate object. Nine adolescent boys worked on a knob-pulling task in which responses were reinforced with money. Periodically during the task, a 68-decibel tone was presented. The tone could be avoided or escaped from by making one of two concurrently available responses: pushing a button that required a low amount of force or punching a pad that required a high amount of force. The latter was defined as an aggressive response due to the higher force requirement. After stable response rates were reached, knob-pulling was put on extinction, but the tone was still presented. The results indicated that the participants frequently made the button-pushing (low force) response to avoid or terminate the tone when knob-pulling was reinforced and they rarely made the punching (high force) response. However, when knob-pulling was placed on extinction, button pushing decreased and punching increased. Azrin et al. (1966) hypothesized that because intermittent reinforcement schedules include periods of extinction, aggression should be observed under these types of schedules as well, and the literature supports this idea (e.g., Frederiksen & Peterson, 1977).

Application of Extinction and Its Relation to Variability

In applied behavior analysis, extinction has most often been employed to weaken the response–reinforcer relation supporting problem behavior. As expected given the findings in the basic literature, when extinction procedures are used to reduce the occurrence of target behavior, instances of response variability have been frequently reported in the applied literature. These instances of response variability, as mentioned previously, are often described as part of an "extinction burst" (Keller & Schoenfeld, 1950; Lerman et al., 1999) and in many cases involve negative findings that can include aggression (e.g., Goh & Iwata, 1994) and emotional behavior (e.g., Hammerschmidt-Snidarich et al., 2019). Given these results, we agree that caution is needed, and as we suggested previously, extinction should rarely, if ever, be conducted as the only treatment component. Even when extinction is combined with reinforcement, from a translational perspective, the relative effects of alternative reinforcement and extinction in differential reinforcement schedules are unclear. As described in the previous section, extinction can be related to positive treatment outcomes, thus warranting further study of the process of extinction as a procedural component in treatment programs.

For example, translational research has shown that extinction can be a procedure used for occasioning appropriate responses, such as creativity (Neuringer, 2004). Procedures used to obtain these varied or novel appropriate responses have included the use of DRA (e.g., Grow et al., 2008), DRO (e.g., Cengher et al., 2020; Duker & van Lent, 1991; Goetz & Baer, 1973; Harding et al., 2004; Lalli et al., 1994; Sellers et al., 2016), and lag (e.g., Lee et al., 2002; Neuringer et al., 2000; Pryor et al., 1969) reinforcement schedules. Specifically, within a DRA schedule, researchers have observed the emergence of desired behavior when problem behavior contacts extinction (e.g., Cagliani et al., 2017, 2019; Grow et al., 2008). For example, Grow et al. conducted an investigation with three boys, ages 8–15 years, diagnosed with autism and limited vocal behavior, who required intervention for problem behavior including whining and aggression. Following baseline reinforcement contingent on problem behavior, experimenters implemented extinction for target behavior and reinforced the first appropriate response that emerged. The first response that emerged for the three participants included "don't," "no," and reaching for an item, which became the extinction-induced responses that were selected through differential reinforcement procedures. These findings demonstrated that extinction resulted in reduced occurrences of problem behavior and induced appropriate response topographies that could be selected for retention in the individuals' repertoires. This study also provides a good example of combining extinction with reinforcement.

In DRO reinforcement schedules, reinforcement is provided for any response other than the target response. When promoting varied and novel responses, this procedure can be used as a lag schedule by reinforcing any response that is varied from any previous response. Thus, when a response occurs and is reinforced, that response and any reinforced response prior to its occurrence contacts extinction if it occurs again in the future. Research has demonstrated that novel desirable responses may emerge when appropriate behavior is placed on extinction using this type of procedure (e.g., Duker & van Lent, 1991). Examples of novel desirable behavior emerging under extinction conditions reported in the applied literature include but are not limited to novel forms of toy play of neurotypical preschoolers (Goetz & Baer, 1973) and young children with mild intellectual disabilities (Lalli et al., 1994), varied punching and kicking techniques during martial arts drills and sparring sessions (Harding et al., 2004), and communication responses of individuals with autism (Cengher et al., 2020; Contreras & Betz, 2016; Sellers et al., 2016). To illustrate, Harding and colleagues (2004) worked with two martial arts students to increase the variability of punching and kicking responses to instructor attacks. Following a baseline in which instructors did not provide any verbal feedback for student performance, instructors introduced differential reinforcement of varied responses during drill sessions. During differential reinforcement drills, instructors only provided verbal feedback contingent on responses that were different than any other response they demonstrated in the session; all responses that the student had previously demonstrated contacted extinction. For both students, response variability increased with differential reinforcement in the drill sessions and generalized to sparring sessions in which no verbal feedback was provided. More recently, Cengher and colleagues (2020) examined the effects of extinction on aggression, one-word mands (e.g., "Lunch!"), and mands with autoclitic frames (e.g., "I want" and "please" surrounding "lunch") of a 16-year-old girl diagnosed with autism. In this study, researchers differentially reinforced mands with autoclitic frames when aggression and one-word mands were placed on extinction. Results showed that both responses (i.e., aggression, one-word mands) decreased and mands with autoclitic frames emerged, suggesting that extinction-induced variability can be capitalized on for selecting a response for retention in the girl's communication repertoire.

Lag schedules of reinforcement have been specifically used by translational researchers to study the effects of extinction on response variability. These schedules explicitly arrange reinforcement contingent on a response that differs from previous responses and extinction for repetitive or similar responses to those previously emitted. The number following the schedule designation (i.e., Lag) indicates the number of previous responses a response must differ from to produce reinforcement. For example, a Lag 2 schedule specifies that a response must differ from the two previously emitted responses to produce reinforcement. Accordingly, responses that are the same or sufficiently similar to the two previous responses result in extinction. Thus, lag schedules capitalize on the evocative effect of extinction to induce varied responses (Neuringer, 2012). Lag schedules have resulted in varied and novel behavior in nonhuman animals (e.g., porpoises: Pryor et al., 1969; rats: Neuringer et al., 2000), and individuals with autism (Lee et al., 2002). To illustrate, Lee et al. examined the effects of a Lag 1 schedule on novel and varied responses on vocal responses to questions with three individuals with autism who had previously engaged in a restricted vocal repertoire of responses to questions. Experimenters alternated DRA (any appropriate response) and Lag 1 schedules in a reversal design and observed varied and novel responses during the Lag 1 schedule but not during the DRA schedule with two of the three participants. Furthermore, varied and novel responses were also observed with the same two participants in untrained settings and with untrained communication partners during the Lag 1 conditions. These results and others (Cengher et al., 2020; Harding et al., 2004; Sellers et al., 2016) show that the behavior-evoking effect of extinction increases the likelihood of reinforceable varied responses and therefore expands the repertoire of desirable behavior.

Implications for Next Translational Steps

The behavior-evoking effects of extinction have implications for future research. There is growing empirical evidence that extinction bursts do not always consist of response topographies that are related to the target (problem) response (Eckerman & Lanson, 1969) or aggressive and emotional behavior (Azrin et al., 1966); rather, extinction can evoke completely new responses (Grunow & Neuringer, 2002), at least some of which may be highly desirable responses that produce reinforcement. When combined with reinforcement, as in differential reinforcement or lag schedules, the extinction component provides an opportunity for a varied response to occur (i.e., within an extinction burst) and then contact reinforcement. This procedure can strengthen an existing but infrequently occurring behavior or establish a novel behavior (e.g., Lee et al., 2002) or sequence of responses (e.g., Pryor et al., 1969). These effects warrant further study to determine how to best arrange for extinction plus reinforcement conditions in treatment programs. For example, Schieltz et al. (2017) wondered if the ratio of extinction to reinforcement encounters might be a critical variable in producing long-term maintenance of the effects of treatment. Analysis of extinction warrants further translational studies, using both basic and applied preparations, and quantitative as well as single case analyses of obtained response-extinction and response-reinforcement contacts.

Summary and Connection between Durability and Variability

The concept of bridge studies was first discussed by Hake (1982) as constituting a connection between basic and applied behavioral research. At the far ends of the basic-applied continuum, basic research seeks to advance our knowledge relative to behavioral processes, whereas applied research seeks to demonstrate the immediate usefulness of behavioral procedures to matters of social significance. In between these endpoints exists the category of bridge studies, which often include applications of basic findings to applied populations and areas of concern for the purpose of determining if the findings from basic research continue to "hold" in less controlled contexts. In consideration of this continuum and the link between the two endpoints, Wacker (2000) depicted this concept as a U-shaped curve and discussed increasing the frequency of bridge studies in both directions, basic-applied and applied-basic, as a means for further integrating our science (Wacker, 2003; see also McIlvane et al., 2011). Conducting bridge studies advances our understanding of behavioral processes and leads to the emergence of new behavioral procedures; thus, bridge studies inform both sides of the behavioral continuum.

Historically, we have most often viewed the U-shaped curve as constituting the link between basic and applied research. Another way to view the U-shaped curve is based on the continuum between dependent variables. Applied research often considers different dependent variables as being distinct. For example, the occurrence of problem behavior displayed by a child with autism is considered to be distinct from the performance of a science student on a math test or the maze running of a rat. Yet this distinction is often not the case when considering translational research. If the endpoints of the U-shaped curve include dependent variables that are typically considered distinct, studies, both basic and applied, conducted between them will serve as a bridge (i.e., we learn that reinforcement affects all behaviors along the continuum), because translational studies tie processes to procedures, and vice versa. Translational studies, then, can provide links between dependent variables, showing which variables exist along the same continuum, and where on the continuum each variable is located.

In this chapter, we have discussed two "distinct" dependent variables, durability and variability, in relation to the procedures and processes of extinction. Both dependent variables are important parts of successful treatment programs, but the best ways to incorporate extinction into ongoing treatment programs is still unknown. Further studies on the role of extinction in treatment programs will likely elevate our understanding of the processes that underlie extinction and the procedures needed to improve clinical outcomes. For example, Galizio et al. (2020), evaluated the durability of response variability in college students by reinforcing target and alternative responding (drawing rectangles with variation in size or location depending on the study phase) within a resurgence paradigm. Extinction was selected as the procedure during the resurgence phase. Results showed durability of varied target responding in the majority of participants, thus, supporting a resurgence effect. However, with some participants, varied alternative responding continued or increased in the resurgence phase. These results were discussed by the authors as being consistent with extinction-induced response variability but also are not inconsistent with a resurgence effect, whereby absolute alternative responding was shown to occur at higher rates than target responding (e.g., Sweeney & Shahan, 2013). Thus, this study showed that extinction directly impacted both durability and variability.

Although more research is needed to tease out the integrative roles of reinforcement and extinction in promoting durability and variability of responses, studies such as Galizio et al. (2020) and Mace et. al. (2010) begin to inform changes in clinical practice from responses being considered mutually exclusive to responses existing along a continuum of behavioral mechanisms as both processes and procedures; that is, by viewing behavioral responses as existing along this continuum, we begin to shift focus on how to obtain both durability of responding (i.e., persistence of adaptive behavior, maintenance of reduced or eliminated problem behavior) and variability of adaptive responses when environmental changes occur (i.e., long-term maintenance). We also begin to better understand the underlying mechanism (or process) of variables such as extinction and how to best implement these variables as procedures to improve clinical practice.

REFERENCES

Alessandri, J., Lattal, K. A., & Cançado, C. R. X. (2015). The recurrence of negatively reinforced responding of humans. *Journal of the Experimental Analysis of Behavior, 104*(3), 211–222.

Anger, D., & Anger, K. (1976). Behavior changes during repeated eight-day extinctions. *Journal of the Experimental Analysis of Behavior, 26*(2), 181–190.

Antonitis, J. J. (1951). Response variability in the white rat during conditioning, extinction, and reconditioning. *Journal of Experimental Psychology, 42*(4), 273–281.

Athens, E. S., & Vollmer, T. R. (2010). An investigation of differential reinforcement of alternative behavior without extinction. *Journal of Applied Behavior Analysis, 43*(4), 569–589.

Azrin, N. H., Hutchinson, R. R., & Hake, D. F. (1966). Extinction-induced aggression. *Journal of the Experimental Analysis of Behavior, 9*(3), 191–204.

Baer, D. M., Wolf, M. M., & Risley, T. R. (1968). Some current dimensions of applied behavior analysis. *Journal of Applied Behavior Analysis, 1*(1), 91–97.

Bai, J. Y. H., & Podlesnik, C. A. (2017). No impact of repeated extinction exposures on operant re-

sponding maintained by different reinforcer rates. *Behavioural Processes, 138*, 29–33.

Baum, W. M. (2012). Extinction as discrimination: The molar view. *Behavioural Processes, 90*(1), 101–110.

Berg, W. K., Ringdahl, J. E., Ryan, S. E., Ing, A. D., Lustig, N., Romani, P., . . . Durako, E. (2015). Resurgence of mands following functional communication training. *Mexican Journal of Behavior Analysis, 41*(2), 166–186.

Bouton, M. E., & Bolles, R. C. (1979). Contextual control of the extinction of conditioned fear. *Learning and Motivation, 10*(4), 445–466.

Bouton, M. E., Maren, S., & McNally, G. P. (2021). Behavioral and neurobiological mechanisms of Pavlovian and instrumental extinction learning. *Physiological Reviews, 101*(2), 611–681.

Bouton, M. E., & Peck, C. A. (1989). Context effects on conditioning, extinction, and reinstatement in an appetitive conditioning preparation. *Animal Learning and Behavior, 17*(2), 188–198.

Bouton, M. E., Todd, T. P., Vurbic, D, & Winterbauer, N. E. (2011). Renewal after the extinction of free operant behavior. *Learning and Behavior, 39*(1) 57–67.

Brooks, D. C., & Bouton, M. E. (1993). A retrieval cue for extinction attenuates spontaneous recovery. *Journal of Experimental Psychology: Animal Behavior Processes, 19*(1), 77–89.

Brown, K. R., Greer, B. D., Craig, A. R., Sullivan, W. E., Fisher, W. W., & Roane, H. S. (2020). Resurgence following differential reinforcement of alternative behavior implemented with and without extinction. *Journal of the Experimental Analysis of Behavior, 113*(2), 449–467.

Bullock, D. H., & Smith, W. C. (1953). An effect of repeated conditioning-extinction upon operant strength. *Journal of Experimental Psychology, 46*(5), 349–352.

Cagliani, R. R., Ayres, K. M., Ringdahl, J. E., & Whiteside, E. (2019). The effect of delay to reinforcement and response effort on response variability for individuals with autism spectrum disorder. *Journal of Developmental and Physical Disabilities, 31*, 55–71.

Cagliani, R. R., Ayres, K. M., Whiteside, E., & Ringdahl, J. E. (2017). Picture exchange communication system and delay to reinforcement. *Journal of Developmental and Physical Disabilities, 29*, 925–939.

Capaldi, E. J. (1966). Partial reinforcement: A hypothesis of sequential effects. *Psychological Review, 73*(5), 459–477.

Capehart, J., Viney, W., & Hulicka, I. M. (1958). The effect of effort upon extinction. *Journal of Comparative and Physiological Psychology, 51*(4), 505–507.

Carr, E. G., & Durand, V. M. (1985). Reducing behavior problems through functional communication training. *Journal of Applied Behavior Analysis, 18*(2), 111–126.

Cengher, M., Ramazon, N. H., & Strohmeier, C. W. (2020). Using extinction to increase behavior: Capitalizing on extinction-induced response variability to establish mands with autoclitic frames. *Analysis of Verbal Behavior, 36*, 102–114.

Contreras, B. P., & Betz, A. M. (2016). Using lag schedules to strengthen intraverbal repertoires of children with autism. *Journal of Applied Behavior Analysis, 49*, 3–16.

Craig, A. R., Cunningham, P. J., Sweeney, M. M., Shahan, T. A., & Nevin, J. A. (2018). Delivering alternative reinforcement in a distinct context reduces its counter-therapeutic effects on relapse. *Journal of the Experimental Analysis of Behavior, 109*(3), 492–505.

Craig, A. R., Sweeney, M. M, & Shahan, T. A. (2019). Behavioral momentum and resistance to extinction across repeated extinction sessions. *Journal of the Experimental Analysis of Behavior, 112*(3), 290–390.

De Meyer, H., Beckers, T., Tripp, G., & van der Oord, S. (2019). Reinforcement contingency learning in children with ADHD: Back to the basics of behavior therapy. *Journal of Abnormal Child Psychology, 47*(12), 1889–1902.

Doughty, A. H., Reed, P., & Lattal, K. A. (2004). Differential reinstatement predicted by preextinction response rate. *Psychonomic Bulletin and Review, 11*(6), 1118–1123.

Duker, P. C., & van Lent, C. (1991). Inducing variability in communicative gestures used by severely retarded individuals. *Journal of Applied Behavior Analysis, 24*(2), 379–386.

Eckerman, D. A., & Lanson, R. M. (1969). Variability of response location for pigeons responding under continuous reinforcement, intermittent reinforcement, and extinction. *Journal of the Experimental Analysis of Behavior, 12*(1), 73–80.

Epstein, R. (1983). Resurgence of previously reinforced behavior during extinction. *Behavior Analysis Letters, 3*(6), 391–397.

Fisher, W. W., Fuhrman, A. M., Greer, B. D., Mitteer, D. R., & Piazza, C. C. (2020). Mitigating resurgence of destructive behavior using the discriminative stimuli of a multiple schedule. *Journal of the Experimental Analysis of Behavior, 113*(1), 263–277.

Franks, G. J., & Lattal, K. A. (1976). Antecedent reinforcement schedule training and operant response reinstatement in rats. *Animal Learning and Behavior, 4*(4), 374–378.

Frederiksen, L. W., & Peterson, G. L. (1977). Schedule-induced aggression in humans and animals: A comparative parametric review. *Aggressive Behavior, 3*(1), 57–75.

Galizio, A., Friedel, J. E., & Odum, A. L. (2020). An investigation of resurgence of reinforced behavioral variability in humans. *Journal of the Experimental Analysis of Behavior, 114*(3), 381–393.

Goetz, E. M., & Baer, D. M. (1973). Social control of form diversity and the emergence of new forms in children's block-building. *Journal of Applied Behavior Analysis, 6*(2), 209–217.

Goh, H., & Iwata, B. A. (1994). Behavioral persistence and variability during extinction of SIB maintained by escape. *Journal of Applied Behavior Analysis, 27*(1), 173–174.

Greer, B. D., & Shahan, T. A. (2019). Resurgence as choice: Implications for promoting durable behavior change. *Journal of Applied Behavior Analysis, 52*(3), 816–846.

Grow, L. L., Kelley, M. E., Roane, H. S., & Shillingsburg, M. A. (2008). Utility of extinction induced response variability for the selection of mands. *Journal of Applied Behavior Analysis, 41*(1), 15–24.

Grunow, A., & Neuringer, A. (2002). Learning to vary and varying to learn. *Psychonomic Bulletin and Review, 9*(2), 250–258.

Hake, D. F. (1982). The basic-applied continuum of the possible evolution of human operant social and verbal research. *Behavior Analyst, 5*(1), 21–28.

Hammerschmidt-Snidarich, S., McComas, J., & Simonson, G. (2019). Individualized goal setting during repeated reading: Accelerating growth with struggling readers using data based decisions. *Preventing School Failure, 63*(4), 334–344.

Harding, J. W., Wacker, D. P., Berg, W. K., Rick, G., & Lee, J. F. (2004). Promoting response variability and stimulus generalization in martial arts training. *Journal of Applied Behavior Analysis, 37*(2), 185–195.

Hoffman, S. G., & Smits, J. A. (2008). Cognitive-behavioral therapy for adult anxiety disorders: A meta-analysis of randomized placebo-controlled trials. *Journal of Clinical Psychiatry, 69*(4), 621–632.

Holton, R. B. (1961). Amplitude of an instrumental response following the cessation of reward. *Child Development, 32*, 107–116.

Howat, G., & Grant, D. A. (1958). Influence of inertia interval during extinction on spontaneous recovery of conditioned eyelid responses. *Journal of Experimental Psychology, 56*(1), 11–15.

Hug, J. J., & Amsel, A. (1969). Frustration theory and partial reinforcement effects: The acquisition-extinction paradox. *Psychological Review, 76*(4), 419–421.

Iwata, B. A., Pace, G. M., Edwards Cowdery, G., & Miltenberger, R. G. (1994). What makes extinction work: An analysis of procedural form and function. *Journal of Applied Behavior Analysis, 27*(1), 131–144.

Katz, B. R., & Lattal, K. A. (2021). What is an extinction burst?: A case study in the analysis of transitional behavior. *Journal of the Experimental Analysis of Behavior, 115*(1), 129–140.

Keller, F. S., & Schoenfeld, W. N. (1950). *Principles of psychology*. Copley.

Kelly, J. F., & Hake, D. F. (1970). An extinction-induced increase in an aggressive response

with humans. *Journal of the Experimental Analysis of Behavior, 14*(2), 153–164.

Kimball, R. T., Kelley, M. E., Podlesnik, C. A., Forton, A., & Hinkle, B. (2018). Resurgence with and without an alternative response. *Journal of Applied Behavior Analysis, 51*(4), 854–865.

Kinloch, J. M., Foster, T. M., & McEwan, J. S. A. (2009). Extinction-induced variability in human behavior. *Psychological Record, 59*(3), 347–370.

Kodak, T., Miltenberger, R. G., & Romaniuk, C. (2003). The effects of differential negative reinforcement of other behavior and noncontingent escape on compliance. *Journal of Applied Behavior Analysis, 36*(3), 379–382.

Lalli, J. S., Casey, S. D., & Kates, K. (1997). Noncontingent reinforcement as treatment for severe problem behavior: Some procedural variations. *Journal of Applied Behavior Analysis, 30*(1), 127–137.

Lalli, J. S., Zanolli, K., & Wohn, T. (1994). Using extinction to promote response variability in toy play. *Journal of Applied Behavior Analysis, 27*(4), 735–736.

Lattal, K. A., St. Peter, C., & Escobar, R. (2013). Operant extinction: Elimination and generation of behavior. In G. J. Madden, W. V. Dube, T. D. Hackenberg, G. P. Hanley, & K. A. Lattal (Eds.), *APA handbook of behavior analysis: Vol. 2. Translating principles into practice* (pp. 77–107). American Psychological Association.

Lattal, K. A., & Wacker, D. P. (2015). Some dimensions of recurrent operant behavior. *Mexican Journal of Behavior Analysis, 41*(2), 1–13.

Lattal, K. M., & Lattal, K. A. (2012). Facets of Pavlovian and operant extinction. *Behavioural Processes, 90*(1), 1–8.

Lee, R., McComas, J., & Jawar, J. (2002). The effects of differential reinforcement on varied verbal responding by individuals with autism to social questions. *Journal of Applied Behavior Analysis, 35*(4), 391–402.

Lerman, D. C., Iwata, B. A., & Wallace, M. D. (1999). Side effects of extinction: Prevalence of bursting and aggression during the treatment of self-injurious behavior. *Journal of Applied Behavior Analysis, 32*(1), 1–8.

Lieving, G. A., & Lattal, K. A. (2003). Recency, repeatability, and reinforcer retrenchment: An experimental analysis of resurgence. *Journal of the Experimental Analysis of Behavior, 80*(2), 217–233.

Likely, D., Little, L., & Mackintosh, N. J. (1971).

Extinction as a function of magnitude and percentage of food or sucrose reward. *Canadian Journal of Psychology, 25*(2), 130–137.

Mace, F. C., McComas, J. J., Mauro, B. C., Progar, P. R., Taylor, B., Ervin, R., & Zangillo, A. N. (2010). Differential reinforcement of alternative behavior increases resistance to extinction: Clinical demonstration, animal modeling, and clinical test of one solution. *Journal of the Experimental Analysis of Behavior, 90*(3), 349–367.

Mahoney, A., Durgin, A., Poling, A., Weetjens, B., Cox, C., Tewelde, T., & Gilbert, T. (2012). Mine detection rats: Effects of repeated extinction on detection accuracy. *Journal of ERW and Mine Action, 16*(3), Article 22.

McIlvane, W. J., Dube, W. V., Serna, R., Lionello-DeNolf, K. M., Barros, R. S., & Galvão, O. F. (2011). Some current dimensions of translational behavior analysis: From laboratory research to intervention for persons with autism spectrum disorders. In E. A. Mayville & J. A. Mulick (Eds.), *Behavioral foundations of effective autism treatment* (pp. 155–181). Sloan.

Mikula, P. J., & Pavlik, W. B. (1966). Deprivation level, competing responses, and the PRE. *Psychological Reports, 18*(1), 95–102.

Morgan, D. L., & Lee, K. (1996). Extinction-induced response variability in humans. *Psychological Record, 46*(1), 145–159.

Mowrer, O. H., & Jones, H. (1945). Habit strength as a function of the pattern of reinforcement. *Journal of Experimental Psychology, 35*(4), 293–311.

Nakajima, S., Tanaka, S., & Urushihara, H. I. (2000). Renewal of extinguished lever-press responses upon return to the training context. *Learning and Motivation, 31*(4), 416–431.

Neuringer, A. (2004). Reinforced variability in animals and people: Implications for adaptive action. *American Psychologist, 59*(9), 891–906.

Neuringer, A. (2012). Reinforcement and induction of operant variability. *Behavior Analyst, 35*(2), 229–235.

Neuringer, A., Deiss, C., & Olson, G. (2000). Reinforced variability and operant learning. *Journal of Experimental Psychology: Animal Behavior Processes, 26*(1), 98–111.

Neuringer, A., Kornell, N., & Olufs, M. (2001). Stability and variability in extinction. *Journal of Experimental Psychology: Animal Behavior Processes, 27*(1), 79–94.

Nevin, J. A. (1974). Response strength in multiple schedules. *Journal of the Experimental Analysis of Behavior, 21*(3), 389–408.

Nevin, J. A. (1988). Behavioral momentum and the partial reinforcement effect. *Psychological Bulletin, 103*(1), 44–56.

Nevin, J. A., & Grace, R. C. (2000). Behavioral momentum and the law of effect. *Behavioral and Brain Sciences, 23*(1), 73–130.

Nevin, J. A., Tota, M. E., Torquato, R. D., & Shull, R. L. (1990). Alternative reinforcement increases resistance to change: Pavlovian or operant contingencies? *Journal of the Experimental Analysis of Behavior, 53*(3), 359–379.

Nevin, J. A., & Wacker, D. P. (2013). Response strength and persistence. In G. J. Madden, W. V. Dube, T. D. Hackenberg, G. P. Hanley, & K. A. Lattal (Eds.), *APA handbook of behavior analysis: Vol. 2. Translating principles into practice* (pp. 109–128). American Psychological Association.

Nist, A. N., & Shahan, T. A. (2021). The extinction burst: Impact of reinforcement time and level of analysis on measured prevalence. *Journal of the Experimental Analysis of Behavior, 116*(2), 131–148.

Pear, J. J. (1985). Spatiotemporal patterns of behavior produced by variable-interval schedules of reinforcement. *Journal of the Experimental Analysis of Behavior, 44*(2), 217–231.

Petscher, E. S., Rey, C., & Bailey, J. S. (2009). A review of empirical support for differential reinforcement of alternative behavior. *Research in Developmental Disabilities, 3*(3), 409–425.

Phillips, C. L., Iannaccone, J. A., Rooker, G. W., & Hagopian, L. P. (2017). Noncontingent reinforcement for the treatment of severe problem behavior: An analysis of 27 consecutive applications. *Journal of Applied Behavior Analysis, 50*(2), 357–376.

Podlesnik, C. A., & Kelley, M. E. (2015). Translational research on the relapse of operant behavior. *Mexican Journal of Behavior Analysis, 41*(2), 226–251.

Pryor, K. W., Haag, R., & O'Reilly, J. (1969). The creative porpoise: Training for novel behavior. *Journal of the Experimental Analysis of Behavior, 12*(4), 653–661.

Rescorla, R. A. (1999). Partial reinforcement reduces the associate change produced by nonreinforcement. *Journal of Experimental Psychology: Animal Behavior Processes, 25*(4), 403–414.

Rescorla, R. A. (2004). Spontaneous recovery varies inversely with the training-extinction interval. *Learning and Behavior, 32*(4), 401–408.

Rescorla, R. A., & Heth, C. D. (1975). Reinstatement of fear to an extinguished conditioned stimulus. *Journal of Experimental Psychology: Animal Behavior Processes, 1*(1), 88–96.

Rescorla, R. A., & Skucy, J. C. (1969). Effect of response independent reinforcers during extinction. *Journal of Comparative and Physiological Psychology, 67*(3), 381–389.

Ringdahl, J. E., Berg, W. K., Wacker, D. P., Crook, K., Molony, M. A., Vargo, K. K., . . . Taylor, C. J. (2018). Effects of response preference on resistance to change. *Journal of the Experimental Analysis of Behavior, 109*(1), 265–280.

Robbins, D. (1971). Partial reinforcement: A selective review of the alleyway literature since 1960. *Psychological Bulletin, 76*(6), 415–431.

Roberts, W. A. (1969). Resistance to extinction following partial and consistent reinforcement with varying magnitudes of reward. *Journal of Comparative and Physiological Psychology, 67*(3), 395–400.

Saini, V., Fisher, W. W., & Pisman, M. D. (2017). Persistence during and resurgence following noncontingent reinforcement implemented with and without extinction. *Journal of Applied Behavior Analysis, 50*(2), 377–392.

Schieltz, K. M., Wacker, D. P., Harding, J. W., Berg, W. K., Lee, J. F., Padilla Dalmau, Y. C., . . . Ibrahimović, M. (2011). Indirect effects of functional communication training on nontargeted disruptive behavior. *Journal of Behavioral Education, 20*, 15–32.

Schieltz, K. M., Wacker, D. P., Ringdahl, J. E., & Berg, W. K. (2017). Basing assessment and treatment of problem behavior on behavioral momentum theory: Analyses of behavioral persistence. *Behavioural Processes, 141*(1), 75–84.

Schlichenmeyer, K. J., Dube, W. V., & Vargas-Irwin, M. (2015). Stimulus fading and response elaboration in differential reinforcement for alternative behavior. *Behavioral Interventions, 30*(1), 51–64.

Sellers, T. P., Kelley, K., Higbee, T. S., & Wolfe, K. (2016). Effects of simultaneous script training on use of varied mand frames by preschoolers with autism. *Analysis of Verbal Behavior, 32*(1), 15–26.

Shahan, T. A., Browning, K. O., & Nall, R. W. (2020). Resurgence as choice in context: Treatment duration and on/off alternative reinforcement. *Journal of the Experimental Analysis of Behavior, 113*(1), 57–76.

Shahan, T. A., & Craig, A. R. (2017). Resurgence as choice. *Behavioural Processes, 141*(1), 100–127.

Shettleworth, S., & Nevin, J. A. (1965). Relative rate or response and relative magnitude of reinforcement in multiple schedules, *Journal of the Experimental Analysis of Behavior, 8*(4), 199–202.

Shvarts, S., Jimenez-Gomez, C., Bai, J. Y. H., Thomas, R. R., Oskan, J. J., & Podlesnik, C. A. (2020). Examining stimuli paired with alternative reinforcement to mitigate resurgence in children diagnosed with autism spectrum disorder and pigeons. *Journal of the Experimental Analysis of Behavior, 113*(1), 214–231.

Skinner, B. F. (1950). Are theories of learning necessary? *Psychological Review, 57*(4), 193–216.

Solomon, R. L. (1948). Effort and extinction rate: A confirmation. *Journal of Comparative and Physiological Psychology, 41*(2), 93–101.

St. Peter, C. C. (2015). Six reasons why applied behavior analysts should know about resurgence. *Mexican Journal of Behavior Analysis, 41*(2), 252–268.

Suess, A. N., Schieltz, K. M., Wacker, D. P., Detrick, J., & Podlesnik, C. A. (2020). An evaluation of resurgence following functional communication training conducted in alternative antecedent contexts via telehealth. *Journal of the Experimental Analysis of Behavior, 113*(1), 278–301.

Sweeney, M. M., & Shahan, T. A. (2013). Effects of high, low, and thinning rates of alternative reinforcement on response elimination and resurgence. *Journal of the Experimental Analysis of Behavior, 100*(1), 102–116.

Thompson, T., & Bloom, W. (1966). Aggressive behavior and extinction-induced response-rate increase. *Psychological Science, 5*(9), 335–336.

Trask, S., Schepers, S. T., & Bouton, M. E. (2015). Context change explains resurgence after the extinction of operant behavior. *Revista Mexicana de Analisis de al Conducta, 41*(2), 187–210.

Vollmer, T. R., & Iwata, B. A. (1992). Differential reinforcement as treatment for behavior disorders: Procedural and functional variations. *Research in Developmental Disabilities, 13*(4), 393–417.

Vollmer, T. R., Iwata, B. A., Zarcone, J. R., Smith,

R. G., & Mazaleski, J. L. (1993). The role of attention in the treatment of attention-maintained self-injurious behavior: Noncontingent reinforcement and differential reinforcement of other behavior. *Journal of Applied Behavior Analysis, 26*(1), 9–21.

Vollmer, T. R., Marcus, B. A., & Ringdahl, J. E. (1995). Noncontingent escape as treatment for self-injurious behavior maintained by negative reinforcement. *Journal of Applied Behavior Analysis, 28*(1), 15–26.

Wacker, D. P. (2000). Building a bridge between research in experimental and applied behavior analysis. In J. C. Leslie & D. Blackman (Eds.), *Experimental and applied analysis of human behavior* (pp. 205–212). Context Press.

Wacker, D. P. (2003). Bridge studies in behavior analysis: Evolution and challenges in *JABA*. *Behavior Analyst Today, 3*(4), 405–411.

Wacker, D. P., Harding, J. W., Berg, W. K., Lee, J. F., Schieltz, K. M., Padilla, Y. C., . . . Shahan, T. A. (2011). An evaluation of persistence of treatment effects during long-term treatment of destructive behavior. *Journal of the Experimental Analysis of Behavior, 96*(2), 261–282.

Winterbauer, N. E., Lucke, S., & Bouton, M. E. (2013). Some factors modulating the strength of resurgence after extinction of an instrumental behavior. *Learning and Motivation, 44*(1), 60–71.

Wong, P. T. P., & Amsel, A. (1976). Prior fixed ratio training and durable persistence in rats. *Animal Learning and Behavior, 4*, 461–466.

Woods, J. N., & Borrero, C. S. W. (2019). Examining extinction bursts in the treatment of pediatric food refusal. *Behavioral Interventions, 34*(3), 307–322.

Zeiler, M. D. (1971). Eliminating behavior with reinforcement. *Journal of the Experimental Analysis of Behavior, 16*(3), 401–405.

CHAPTER 13

Translational Approaches to Differential Reinforcement

Brian D. Greer

In what would become one of his final papers, and the last to be published in the *Journal of Applied Behavior Analysis*, Murray Sidman (2011) characterized how applied behavior analysts benefit from an understanding of, and an appreciation for, basic behavioral research and the translational work built atop basic research findings. However, Sidman's writings on translational work differed from that of others who have addressed the topic. Sidman distinguished between two forms of translational work that both involve applying what has been learned about behavior from the findings of basic research. He defined *translational research* as using "scientific procedures to evaluate the applicability of basic research findings, procedures, or principles in situations that we cannot control as rigorously as we do in basic research" (p. 983). In contrast, Sidman described *research translation* as the more general application of knowledge gained from basic research without using scientific procedures to test or evaluate the results. Of these two forms of translational work, translational research has received considerably more attention from researchers and funding agencies alike than has research translation. Indeed, others have conceptualized what we now call translational research as science that bridges the basic–applied continuum (e.g., Fisher & Mazur, 1997; Hake, 1982; Mace & Critchfield, 2010).

Early pioneers in applied behavior analysis were first and foremost students of basic behavioral research. Notable trailblazers include the likes of Jack Michael, Montrose Wolf, Teodoro Ayllon, Nathan Azrin, Sidney Bijou, James Sherman, Richard Malott, Israel Goldiamond, Arthur Staats, and Joseph Spradlin, in addition to Murray Sidman and others. In those early days, formal experimental designs (e.g., multiple-baseline design) and procedures (e.g., interobserver agreement) for conducting well-controlled applied research by today's standards had yet to be developed. Therefore, early pioneers in applied behavior analysis set about by testing the broad generality of basic research findings with humans, often with individuals with a neurodevelopmental disorder living in an institutional or inpatient setting (e.g., Ayllon & Michael, 1959; Wolf et al., 1963). This specific population was believed to be a suitable starting point for the "transfer from rat to man" (Fuller, 1949, p. 590), and the relatively controlled environment in which this population lived afforded some of the advantages of experimental control associated with the laboratory.

Viewing these foundational studies through the lens of Sidman (2011) suggests that the earliest examples of applied-behavior-analytic research were essentially exercises in research translation (for relevant historical analyses of early applied research, see Altus et al., 2021; Morris et al., 2013). Furthermore, because there was no field of applied behavior analysis to speak of at the time, there was also no clear publication outlet for the dissemination of applied research—the *Journal of Applied Behavior Analysis* would not come about until 1968. Many of the early research translations that were to establish the field of applied behavior analysis were in fact published in the *Journal of the Experimental Analysis of Behavior* (Mazur, 2010; see also Morris et al., 2013).

The content and focus of those early research translations differed from one another, but many were common in their approach to addressing problems of social significance. A common component across early research translations was the use of differential reinforcement (e.g., Ayllon & Michael, 1959; Azrin & Foxx, 1971; Fuller, 1949), which made for a particularly promising technology for early research translation due in part to its long-standing use in basic behavioral research and also its immediate applicability to many applied problems. Differential reinforcement as an experimental procedure in basic, behavior-analytic research dates back to at least B. F. Skinner's (1938) *The Behavior of Organisms: An Experimental Approach* and continued after Ferster and Skinner's (1957) *Schedules of Reinforcement*. Additionally, it turns out that many applied problems can be adequately addressed by a careful programming of differential reinforcement (Petscher et al., 2009), and many find differential reinforcement to be preferred over other technologies for behavior reduction, including noncontingent reinforcement and extinction (e.g., Gabor et al., 2016; Hanley et al., 1997). In other words, differential reinforcement provided a highly suitable technology for the initial application of behavior analysis to problems of social significance. Since then, differential reinforcement has become a foundational component of behavior analysis, and its continued importance in behavior-analytic research and practice cannot be overstated.

Defining Differential Reinforcement

Ferster and Skinner (1957, p. 726) defined *differential reinforcement* as "reinforcement which is contingent upon (1) the presence of a given property of a stimulus, in which case the resulting process is discrimination, (2) the presence of a given intensive, durational, or topographical property of a response, in which case the resulting process is differentiation, or (3) a given rate of responding." Ferster and Skinner's definition highlights how different procedural arrangements of differential reinforcement can produce functionally dissimilar results. Responding that is differentially reinforced in the presence of a target stimulus (e.g., a picture of a piano) when presented with alternating pictures of irrelevant stimuli (e.g., musical instruments) will produce more selections of the target stimulus (i.e., piano). Alternatively, responding may be differentially reinforced with respect to a specific property of a stimulus. For instance, differentially reinforcing responses to stimuli that more closely correspond to the color wavelength of red will produce more selections of the red stimulus than selections of other stimuli.

Jenkins and Harrison (1960) provided an instructive example of how differential reinforcement is often a necessary component for the development of stimulus discrimination. The experimenters devised two types of training—one they termed *non-differential training* and another they called *differential training*. Eight pigeons experienced four pretraining sessions in which the experimenters taught a key-peck response and then reinforced key pecks according to a variable-interval (VI) schedule of food reinforcement. Three of the eight pigeons experienced nondifferential training procedures after pretraining. During nondifferential training, an auditory tone of 1,000 cycles per second (i.e., a discriminative stimulus, or S^D) played throughout each of 25 working trials per session. The remaining five pigeons experienced differential training procedures after pretraining. Differential training procedures were identical to the nondifferential training procedures except that the 25 working trials were divided into two randomly alternating component types. In one component, reinforcers were available for key pecks according to the same VI schedule used with the other group, and the same S^D remained present. In the other component, key pecks resulted in extinction, and the auditory tone was absent (i.e., no tone or S^Δ). Across sessions, the number of components with extinction in place with the absence of the tone (S^Δ) increased from 25 to 125 per session, while the number of components with reinforcement in place with the tone (S^D) remained at 25 per session for this group. Following training, the experimenters tested all pigeons under extinction in the presence of a variety of different tones, including the 1,000-cycles-per-second tone used in training (S^D) and no tone (S^Δ).

Figure 13.1 shows results of the study by Jenkins and Harrison (1960), separated by the two experimental groups. Pigeons that experienced nondifferential training prior to generalization testing failed to show stimulus discrimination with respect to the frequency

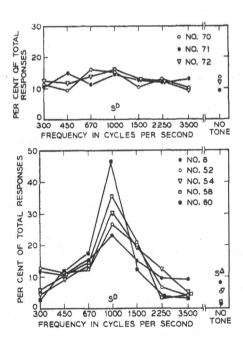

FIGURE 13.1. Generalization gradients of tonal frequency following different training histories. Generalization gradients of tonal frequency for two groups of pigeons trained under nondifferential training procedures (top panel) or differential training procedures (bottom panel). From Jenkins and Harrison (1960). This figure is in the public domain.

of the tone used in training (top panel), meaning that the 1,000-cycle-per-second tone (S^D) from training did not occasion more responding during generalization testing relative to the untrained tones (i.e., cycles per second other than 1,000 and no tone). Increased training time for pigeons in the nondifferential training group did not improve stimulus discrimination. In contrast to these findings, the five pigeons that experienced differential training prior to generalization testing showed an increased percentage of responses to the 1,000-cycle-per-second tone (S^D) from training, suggesting that the alternation of signaled reinforcement and extinction components in training facilitated stimulus discrimination during generalization testing. In other words, differential reinforcement in training was necessary to produce stimulus discrimination during generalization testing.

Response differentiation can be another functional outcome of differential reinforcement when the reinforcement contingencies favor certain response topographies or response attributes. Responding can be differentially reinforced along numerous dimensions, including topography (e.g., Greer et al., 2016; Randall et al., 2021), rate (e.g., Austin & Bevan, 2011; Ono & Iwabuchi, 1997), latency (e.g., Church & Carnathan, 1963; Fjellstedt & Sulzer-Azároff, 1973; Tiger et al., 2007), force (e.g., Pinkston & Libman, 2017), duration (e.g., Lejeune & Jasselette, 1987), and omission (e.g., Poling & Ryan, 1982; Vollmer et al., 1993). For example, a select response topography can be differentially reinforced, as is the case when reinforcing a specific alternative to a target response, a procedure called *differential reinforcement of alternative behavior* (DRA) or when reinforcing an alternative response incompatible with the target response, a subtype of DRA called *differential reinforcement of incompatible behavior* (DRI). Additionally, a range of response rates can be differentially reinforced by delivering reinforcers following responses separated by select interresponse times (IRTs). Differentially reinforcing IRTs shorter than 2 seconds will produce rapid responding, a procedure called *differential reinforcement of high-rate responding* (DRH). Alternatively, differentially reinforcing IRTs longer than 1 minute will produce slower responding, a procedure called *differential reinforcement of low-rate responding* (DRL). Finally, *differential reinforcement of other behavior* (DRO) arranges reinforcement for the absence of responding; however, at least some forms of DRO may be better conceptualized as negative punishment rather than positive reinforcement (Lerman & Vorndran, 2002; Rolider & Van Houten, 1990).

A nice example of response differentiation brought about by differential reinforcement was provided by Kelleher et al. (1959), who arranged a DRL 20-seconds schedule of food reinforcement for two naive rats. Following an initial training session in which the rats learned to press a lever for food, each rat earned 20 reinforcers according to a fixed-ratio 1 schedule, meaning that each lever press produced a reinforcer. For all sessions thereafter, food reinforcers were delivered only following responses separated by at least 20 seconds (i.e., DRL 20-seconds). Each session lasted 2 hours.

The two rats produced highly similar results. Therefore, Figure 13.2 displays the results for only one of the subjects. Left panels show responding in Session 1, and right panels show responding in Session 30—the final session of the experiment. The units along the x-axes in Figure 13.2 are IRTs segmented into 3-second bins (0–3 seconds plotted as an IRT of 3 seconds, 3–6 seconds plotted as an IRT of 6 seconds, etc.). In the first session of DRL 20-seconds, consecutive lever presses were often separated by short IRTs of 0–3 seconds and 3–6 seconds (top, left panel) with a decreasing percentage of responses with IRTs of 6–9 seconds or longer. However, the probability of responding across each bin of IRTs was relatively stable (bottom, left panel), meaning that of responding that could have occurred in each 3-second IRT bin, actual responding was

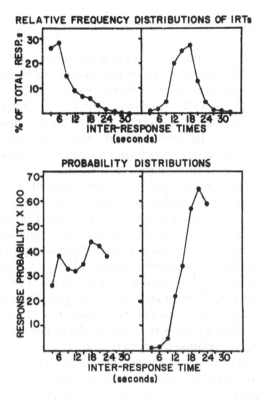

FIGURE 13.2. Development of DRL 20-seconds performance. Percentage of interresponse times that occurred within consecutive 3-second bins (top panels). Probability of responding given what could have occurred per 3-second bin (bottom panels). Left panels are from Session 1, and right panels are from Session 30. From Kelleher et al. (1959). Reprinted with permission of John Wiley & Sons, Inc.

similar across bins. In stark contrast to these results, the data from Session 30 present a markedly changed pattern of responding. Lever-pressing IRTs coalesced around 20 seconds by the end of the experiment (top, right panel), and response probabilities were highest around this same IRT (bottom, right panel). This shift in IRTs across sessions as a result of differential reinforcement produced a slowed pattern of responding such that consecutive responses were more consistently separated by greater amounts of time.

In Support of a Nuanced View of Differential Reinforcement

That IRTs can serve as the basis for differential reinforcement is theoretically interesting from the standpoint that reinforcers affect more than what is traditionally considered to be the discrete response. As the study by Kelleher et al. (1959) showed, changes in response rate under DRH or DRL schedules are brought about by affecting the temporal relation between successive responses, not aspects of the response itself. The ability to bring about IRTs of certain durations suggests that reinforcers impact behavior in more complex ways than described by traditional descriptions of reinforcement that focus explicitly on the increased future frequency of responding (e.g., Cooper et al., 2020; Michael, 2004).

A related finding involves the notion of response variability. There is a substantial body of evidence supporting the notion that responding can be differentially reinforced according to a different sort of relation with previous responses—variability (for review, see Neuringer, 2002; Falcomata & Neuringer, Chapter 20, this volume). Unlike DRH or DRL schedules that arrange reinforcers according to the amount of time that has elapsed since the last response, lag schedules of reinforcement arrange reinforcers according to whether current responding differs from a specified number of prior responses. For example, a lag-1 schedule of reinforcement sets the criterion for reinforcement such that responding must differ from that of the immediately preceding response. A sequenced response pattern of AABB would produce reinforcement so long as the immediately prior response sequence was not AABB under a lag-1 schedule. The lag number (i.e., lag X) stipulates the number of prior responses from which the current response must differ for the delivery of reinforcement. For instance, a lag-5 schedule requires the current response to differ from the preceding five responses for the delivery of reinforcement. These and related reinforcement schedules (e.g., reinforcing least-frequent IRTs across experimental conditions) produce differing levels of response variability (Blough, 1966; Page & Neuringer, 1985), and similar to DRH and DRL schedules, they do so not by increasing the future frequency of responding or by strengthening the response that precedes reinforcer delivery but by affecting the relation between responses.

My goal in providing this more nuanced view of differential reinforcement is twofold. First, to understand differential reinforcement is to first understand reinforcement, which the reader may be surprised to learn is, at best, less straightforward than often described in both introductory textbooks and in the literature, and at worst, such accounts may be fundamentally flawed. Although the concept of reinforcement as a strengthening process is implicit in most all descriptions of reinforcement in behavior analysis (Shahan, 2017), scholars within and outside the field have expressed concern over this position. Behavior analysts should consider alternative accounts of the effects of reinforcers on behavior that do not involve a reinforcement-as-strengthening conceptualization (Baum, 2012; Cowie & Davison, 2016, 2020; Gallistel & Balsam, 2014; Killeen & Jacobs, 2016; Shahan, 2010, 2017). A common view across such alternative accounts is that reinforcement as a process involves the predictability of stimuli as signals for phylogenetically important events. Thus, according to such accounts, what organisms come to learn is when, where, and how reinforcers are likely to be available based on their histories of interacting with stimuli, physical (e.g., discriminative stimuli; conditioned reinforcers) or otherwise (e.g., time, motivational states), that are predictive of future reinforcer availability. Reinforcement as a strengthening process falls somewhat short when interpreting the process by which DRH, DRL, and variability-directed schedules of reinforcement appear to operate, and this conceptualization of reinforcement has particular difficulty accounting for the seemingly powerful discriminative effects of reinforcers (see Cowie & Davison, 2016, for review).

A second benefit of characterizing differential reinforcement in this way is to help scientist-practitioners understand the broad flexibility that differential reinforcement presents as a clinical tool. A heightened focus on individual procedures is likely to convey a rigid set of technologies that may hamper the development and evaluation of novel approaches for solving intractable or persistent applied problems. However, a deeper appreciation of the commonalities that link individual differential-reinforcement procedures may promote problem solving.

Procedural Variations of Differential Reinforcement

Ferster and Skinner's (1957) definition of differential reinforcement sidesteps what has become the focus of some discussion among applied researchers. Terms such as *reinforcement* and *punishment* are widely accepted within the field as being defined functionally and not structurally, meaning that the term is not invoked unless a prescribed change in behavior has occurred. For reinforcement to have occurred, behavior must increase; for punishment to have occurred, behavior must decrease. Setting aside the question of what it means for behavior to have increased or decreased (a determination that may or may not require changes in response rate), stimulus changes that fail to bring about prescribed changes in behavior are not classified as reinforcement or punishment on account of the functional definitions of these terms. In other words, the old idiom "It's not reinforcement (or punishment) unless it works" still holds.

But should differential reinforcement be similarly defined by its outcomes? Vollmer et al. (2020) suggested that the field of applied behavior analysis has placed unnecessary emphasis on the structural characteristics of the most commonly applied form of differential reinforcement (DRA) by defining it as including extinction for other responses (e.g., target or problem behavior). As these authors point out, although arranging extinction can facilitate the efficacy of DRA-based interventions (e.g., Hagopian et al., 1998), functional changes in behavior under DRA do not always require extinction (for notable examples, see Athens & Vollmer, 2010; Briggs et al., 2019). Therefore, extinction is not a defining feature of DRA and should not be included in its definition.

Two points are relevant here. First, not only is extinction not a defining feature of DRA, but it is also not a defining feature of differential reinforcement, as differentiated responding can often occur under other differential reinforcement procedures in the absence of extinction. Second, greater emphasis on the functional outcomes of DRA and other differential-reinforcement procedures will help in better characterizing what components (or combinations of components) are and are not necessary for differential reinforcement to occur. The defining features of differential reinforcement are better understood from a functional perspective, and overemphasis on procedure or structure may stifle creative solutions when initial implementation of differential reinforcement fails to occasion its intended result. What it means to differentially reinforce is to bring about differentiated responding, and accomplishing this can be done in innumerable ways. Viewing DR(X) terms as guidelines, or perhaps goals for what behavior should look like, might be a better approach for advancing translational research.

The behavior analyst has at their disposal a vast array of concepts and principles to produce differentiated responding via differential reinforcement. For example, applied research has consistently shown that arranging differential reinforcement using the reinforcer that maintains problem behavior (i.e., the functional reinforcer) instead of an arbitrary reinforcer improves treatment efficacy (Didden et al., 1997; see also Vollmer & Iwata, 1992). However, this common finding may have less to do with the fact that problem behavior is maintained by the same reinforcer used in treatment and more to do with the robust reinforcing potency of that specific stimulus for the individual. It is true that conducting a functional analysis (Iwata et al., 1994) helps to identify the variables maintaining problem behavior, but when it comes to using that information to design a set of treatment procedures using differential reinforcement, the importance of having identified a highly reinforcing stimulus for the individual may be more important for reducing problem behavior than is the function-based nature of the treatment procedures.

Evidence that this might be true comes from studies that implemented differential reinforcement without arranging extinction for problem behavior, and studies that allowed choices between the functional and an arbitrary reinforcer for appropriate behavior. Under the former arrangement, problem behavior continues to produce its functional reinforcer (e.g., escape from nonpreferred demands), and alternative responding (e.g., compliance, requests for a break) produces either a better version of that same functional reinforcer (e.g., longer escape intervals) and/or an arbitrary reinforcer (e.g., preferred edibles). In some arrangements, alternative responding produces only an arbitrary reinforcer, and problem behavior alone produces the functional reinforcer (e.g., Lalli et al., 1999). A handful of studies has shown that when highly preferred arbitrary reinforcers are pitted against functional reinforcers, participants sometimes select the arbitrary reinforcer over the functional reinforcer by engaging in more alternative behavior than problem behavior (see Payne & Dozier, 2013, for review). When choice between an arbitrary and a functional reinforcer is made contingent on appropriate behavior or provided prior to session, fluctuations in choice tend to be driven by other schedule parameters (e.g., current or upcoming number of demands; Briggs, Akers, et al., 2018; DeLeon et al., 2001).

Functional-analysis methodology helps to ensure that the stimuli used in treatment are potent reinforcers, which likely increases the efficacy of differential-reinforcement-based interventions for problem behavior. However, selecting potent reinforcers can come from sources other than a functional analysis. Preference assessments (e.g., Fisher et al., 1992), competing stimulus assessments (e.g., Piazza et al., 1998), and evaluations of reinforcer demand (e.g., Tustin, 1994) are often helpful sources from which to select potent arbitrary reinforcers for use when treating problem behavior using differential reinforcement.

Selecting one or more potent reinforcers is not the only strategy for increasing the likelihood that differential reinforcement brings about functional changes in responding. Additional variables that may affect the efficacy of differential reinforcement can be thought of as existing along two general dimensions—manipulations that target responding and those that change aspects of the reinforcer or its schedule. Examples of the former include changing the effort associated with responding (e.g., Horner & Day, 1991; Van Camp et al., 2001) and selecting a more preferred response topography (e.g., Ringdahl et al., 2009). Alternatively, changing aspects of the reinforcer or its schedule can take many forms, including selection of a different schedule of differential reinforcement (e.g., DRA instead of DRO); changing the density of reinforcer availability (e.g., by making reinforcers available more frequently; Horner & Day, 1991); manipulating reinforcer dependency by adjusting whether, when, and how the same or functionally similar reinforcers are available outside the programmed contingency (e.g., Lattal, 1974); changing the number of responses accounted for within the programmed contingency (e.g., more than one alternative response reinforced during DRA); as well as manipulating reinforcer magnitude (e.g., Doughty & Richards, 2002), quality (e.g., Van Camp et al., 2001), and immediacy (e.g., Horner & Day, 1991).

A vast literature exists on many of these possibilities for improving the efficacy of differential reinforcement, such that each could be the subject of a devoted chapter. Rather than providing detailed explanations and examples of each, some perspective might be helpful. Conceptualizing behavior as choice under constraint (e.g., of time, resources) is often useful when designing and modifying differential-reinforcement procedures. Response and schedule parameters that comprise the differential-reinforcement contingency are variables that can be adjusted so as to bring about different response patterns. Changing the allocation of responding often requires thinking of behavior as concurrent operants and implementing procedures that tip the scales to favor the intended response or response pattern. An excellent resource on this perspective and its applied utility was published by Fisher and Mazur (1997), who also provide an accessible overview of the matching law (Herrnstein, 1961) for readers unfamiliar with the basic research findings upon which many of the previous suggestions are based.

Changing the Criterion for Reinforcement

Discussion of differential reinforcement to this point has focused on the outcomes of a predetermined arrangement of reinforcement contingencies and a brief overview of how to adjust those contingencies if the desired response pattern is not obtained. However, the criterion for reinforcement can also adjust within or across sessions, guiding behavior to new forms along the way. *Differential reinforcement of successive approximations*, or *shaping* as it is often called, establishes a criterion for reinforcement that changes as behavior closer approximates a terminal topography. Shaping is a type of differential reinforcement because only responses that approximate the terminal topography produce reinforcement; responses that are further approximations to the terminal topography are typically placed on extinction. Within or across sessions, the criterion for what constitutes a close-enough approximation to produce reinforcement changes with the goal being of guiding behavior toward the terminal topography.

Percentile schedules formalize the shaping process by setting objective criteria that determine which responses will and will not be reinforced. When using a percentile schedule, one selects a window of time from which to analyze recent behavior. The larger this temporal window is, the more instances of responding that are factored into the calculation. As additional sessions occur or time passes, the window is updated to account for new responding, and the oldest responding within the window is removed from analysis. Thus, percentile schedules update to account for only the most recent responses, and how far back in time responding is analyzed depends on the size of the window. Percentile schedules also set a criterion for reinforcement such that new responding must be within that criterion to produce reinforcement. The criterion for reinforcement in percentile schedules is set relative to responding within the temporal window (e.g., reinforcing response latencies that are within the shortest 25% of those in the window). These two elements of percentile schedules, the temporal window size and the specific criterion for reinforcement, formalize the shaping process (see Athens et al., 2007, for a demonstration of applying percentile schedules to increase student task engagement).

Resistance to Change and Relapse Susceptibility

One area of research that has generated robust translational research in recent years focuses on resistance to change and relapse susceptibility following differential reinforcement. With three children with developmental disabilities who engaged in problem behavior, Mace et al. (2010) showed that rates of problem behavior were higher and more persistent during extinction when the extinction phase was preceded by DRA than when the extinction phase was preceded by a baseline condition in which problem behavior produced its functional reinforcer. Increased and more persistent problem behavior following DRA than following baseline is troubling given DRA's frequent use when treating problem behavior (Petscher et al., 2009). The recurrence of problem behavior following

DRA and other forms of differential reinforcement is a form of relapse, called *resurgence*. Subsequent investigations by independent clinics have shown that resurgence of problem behavior is common when thinning schedules of reinforcement for alternative behavior (Briggs, Fisher, et al., 2018; Muething et al., 2021).

Concern regarding treatment relapse has brought about a considerably high amount of collaboration between basic, translational, and applied researchers. For example, translational research examining the predictive validity of behavioral momentum theory, a quantitative theory of behavior that has been extended to the phenomenon of resurgence (Shahan & Sweeney, 2011), has shown promise when procedures based on its predictions have been evaluated for the treatment of problem behavior (Fisher et al., 2018). Other resurgence-mitigation procedures based on Resurgence as Choice, another quantitative theory of resurgence (Shahan & Craig, 2017), may also hold promise for reducing this form of treatment relapse (Greer & Shahan, 2019).

Conclusion

Differential reinforcement is the most commonly used set of procedures across behavior-analytic interventions (Lennox et al., 1988; Petscher et al., 2009). It is a cornerstone technology used to treat problem behavior (Tiger et al., 2008), deliver early intensive behavioral intervention (Vladescu & Kodak, 2010), and implement contingency management (Higgins et al., 1994). Conceptualizing differential reinforcement not as a set of individual procedures but as ways to arrange the environment so as to bring about a specific response or response pattern can be facilitated by viewing behavior as choice and reinforcers as tools to guide response allocation. Applied behavior analysts have at their disposal multiple ways for improving the efficacy of treatments based on differential reinforcement, including a growing literature on strategies for mitigating resurgence following differential reinforcement.

ACKNOWLEDGMENTS

Grant Nos. 2R01HD079113, 5R01HD083214, and 5R01HD093734 from the National Institute of Child Health and Human Development provided partial support for this work.

REFERENCES

Altus, D. E., Morris, E. K., & Smith, N. G. (2021). A study in the emergence of applied behavior analysis through the referencing patterns in its founding articles. *European Journal of Behavior Analysis, 22,* 101–132.

Athens, E. S., & Vollmer, T. R. (2010). An investigation of differential reinforcement of alternative behavior without extinction. *Journal of Applied Behavior Analysis, 43*(4), 569–589.

Athens, E. S., Vollmer, T. R., & St. Peter Pipkin, C. C. (2007). Shaping academic task engagement with percentile schedules. *Journal of Applied Behavior Analysis, 40*(3), 475–488.

Austin, J. L., & Bevan, D. (2011). Using differential reinforcement of low rates to reduce children's requests for teacher attention. *Journal of Applied Behavior Analysis, 44*(3), 451–461.

Ayllon, T., & Michael, J. (1959). The psychiatric nurse as a behavioral engineer. *Journal of the Experimental Analysis of Behavior, 2*(4), 323–334.

Azrin, N. H., & Foxx, R. M. (1971). A rapid method of toilet training the institutionalized retarded. *Journal of Applied Behavior Analysis, 4*(2), 89–99.

Baum, W. M. (2012). Rethinking reinforcement: Allocation, induction, and contingency. *Jour-

nal of the Experimental Analysis of Behavior, 97(1), 101–124.

Blough, D. S. (1966). The reinforcement of least-frequent interresponse times. *Journal of the Experimental Analysis of Behavior, 9*(5), 581–591.

Briggs, A. M., Akers, J. S., Greer, B. D., Fisher, W. W., & Retzlaff, B. J. (2018). Systematic changes in preference for schedule-thinning arrangements as a function of relative reinforcement density. *Behavior Modification, 42*(4), 472–497.

Briggs, A. M., Dozier, C. L., Lessor, A. N., Kamana, B. U., & Jess, R. L. (2019). Further investigation of differential reinforcement of alternative behavior without extinction for escape-maintained destructive behavior. *Journal of Applied Behavior Analysis, 52*(4), 956–973.

Briggs, A. M., Fisher, W. W., Greer, B. D., & Kimball, R. T. (2018). Prevalence of resurgence of destructive behavior when thinning reinforcement schedules during functional communication training. *Journal of Applied Behavior Analysis, 51*(3), 620–633.

Church, R. M., & Carnathan, J. (1963). Differential reinforcement of short latency responses in the white rat. *Journal of Comparative and Physiological Psychology, 56*(1), 120–123.

Cooper, J. O., Heron, T. E., & Heward, W. L. (2020). *Applied behavior analysis* (3rd ed.). Pearson Education.

Cowie, S., & Davison, M. (2016). Control by reinforcers across time and space: A review of recent choice research. *Journal of the Experimental Analysis of Behavior, 105*(2), 246–269.

Cowie, S., & Davison, M. (2020). Generalizing from the past, choosing the future. *Perspectives on Behavior Science, 43*, 1–14.

DeLeon, I. G., Neidert, P. L., Anders, B. M., & Rodriguez-Catter, V. (2001). Choices between positive and negative reinforcement during treatment for escape-maintained behavior. *Journal of Applied Behavior Analysis, 34*(4), 521–525.

Didden, R., Duker, P. C., & Korzilius, H. (1997). Meta-analytic study on treatment effectiveness for problem behaviors with individuals who have mental retardation. *American Journal of Mental Retardation, 101*(4), 387–399.

Doughty, A. H., & Richards, J. B. (2002). Effects of reinforcer magnitude on responding under differential-reinforcement-of-low-rate schedules of rats and pigeons. *Journal of the Experimental Analysis of Behavior, 78*(1), 17–30.

Ferster, C. B., & Skinner, B. F. (1957). *Schedules of reinforcement.* Appleton-Century-Crofts.

Fisher, W. W., Greer, B. D., Craig, A. R., Retzlaff, B. J., Fuhrman, A. M., Lichtblau, K. R., & Saini, V. (2018). On the predictive validity of behavioral momentum theory for mitigating resurgence of problem behavior. *Journal of the Experimental Analysis of Behavior, 109*, 281–290.

Fisher, W. W., & Mazur, J. E. (1997). Basic and applied research on choice responding. *Journal of Applied Behavior Analysis, 30*(3), 387–410.

Fisher, W., Piazza, C. C., Bowman, L. G., Hagopian, L. P., Owens, J. C., & Slevin, I. (1992). A comparison of two approaches for identifying reinforcers for persons with severe and profound disabilities. *Journal of Applied Behavior Analysis, 25*(2), 491–498.

Fjellstedt, N., & Sulzer-Azároff, B. (1973). Reducing the latency of a child's responding to instructions by means of a token system. *Journal of Applied Behavior Analysis, 6*(1), 125–130.

Fuller, P. (1949). Operant conditioning of a vegetative human organism. *American Journal of Psychology, 62*(4), 587–590.

Gabor, A. M., Fritz, J. N., Roath, C. T., Rothe, B. R., & Gourley, D. A. (2016). Caregiver preference for reinforcement-based interventions for problem behavior maintained by positive reinforcement. *Journal of Applied Behavior Analysis, 49*(2), 215–227.

Gallistel, C. R., & Balsam, P. D. (2014). Time to rethink the neural mechanisms of learning and memory. *Neurobiology of Learning and Memory, 108*, 136–144.

Greer, B. D., Fisher, W. W., Saini, V., Owen, T. M., & Jones, J. K. (2016). Functional communication training during reinforcement schedule thinning: An analysis of 25 applications. *Journal of Applied Behavior Analysis, 49*(1), 105–121.

Greer, B. D., & Shahan, T. A. (2019). Resurgence as choice: Implications for promoting durable behavior change. *Journal of Applied Behavior Analysis, 52*(3), 816–846.

Hagopian, L. P., Fisher, W. W., Sullivan, M. T., Acquisto, J., & LeBlanc, L. A. (1998). Effectiveness of functional communication training with and without extinction and punishment: A summary of 21 inpatient cases. *Journal of Applied Behavior Analysis, 31*(2), 211–235.

Hake, D. F. (1982). The basic-applied continuum and the possible evolution of human operant social and verbal research. *Behavior Analyst, 5*(1), 21–28.

Hanley, G. P., Piazza, C. C., Fisher, W. W., Contrucci, S. A., & Maglieri, K. A. (1997). Evaluation of client preference for function-based treatment packages. *Journal of Applied Behavior Analysis, 30*(3), 459–473.

Herrnstein, R. J. (1961). Relative and absolute strength of response as a function of frequency of reinforcement. *Journal of the Experimental Analysis of Behavior, 4*, 267–272.

Higgins, S. T., Budney, A. J., & & Bickel, W. K. (1994). Applying behavioral concepts and principles to the treatment of cocaine dependence. *Drug and Alcohol Dependence, 34*(2), 87–97.

Horner, R. H., & Day, H. M. (1991). The effects of response efficiency on functionally equivalent competing behaviors. *Journal of Applied Behavior Analysis, 24*(4), 719–732.

Iwata, B. A., Dorsey, M. F., Slifer, K. J., Bauman, K. E., & Richman, G. S. (1994). Toward a functional analysis of self-injury. *Journal of Applied Behavior Analysis, 27*(2), 197–209. (Reprinted from *Analysis and Intervention in Developmental Disabilities, 2*, 3–20, 1982)

Jenkins, H. M., & Harrison, R. H. (1960). Effect of discrimination training on auditory generalization. *Journal of Experimental Psychology, 59*(4), 246–253.

Kelleher, R. T., Fry, W., & Cook, L. (1959). Interresponse time distribution as a function of differential reinforcement of temporally spaced responses. *Journal of the Experimental Analysis of Behavior, 2*(2), 91–106.

Killeen, P. R., & Jacobs, K. W. (2016). Coal is not black, snow is not white, food is not a reinforcer: The roles of affordances and dispositions in the analysis of behavior. *Behavior Analyst, 40*(1), 17–38.

Lalli, J. S., Vollmer, T. R., Progar, P. R., Wright, C., Borrero, J., Daniel, D., . . . May, W. (1999). Competition between positive and negative reinforcement in the treatment of escape behavior. *Journal of Applied Behavior Analysis, 32*(3), 285–296.

Lattal, K. A. (1974). Combinations of response-reinforcer dependence and independence. *Journal of the Experimental Analysis of Behavior, 22*(2), 357–362.

Lejeune, H., & Jasselette, P. (1987). Differential reinforcement of pause duration (DRRD) in weanling rats: A comparison with adult subjects. *Behavioural Processes, 15*(2–3), 315–332.

Lennox, D. B., Miltenberger, R. G., Spengler, P., & Erfanian, N. (1988). Decelerative treatment practices with persons who have mental retardation: A review of five years of the literature. *American Journal of Mental Retardation, 92*(6), 492–501.

Lerman, D. C., & Vorndran, C. M. (2002). On the status of knowledge for using punishment: Implications for treating behavior disorders. *Journal of Applied Behavior Analysis, 35*(4), 431–464.

Mace, F. C., & Critchfield, T. S. (2010). Translational research in behavior analysis: historical traditions and imperative for the future. *Journal of the Experimental Analysis of Behavior, 93*(3), 293–312.

Mace, F. C., McComas, J. J., Mauro, B. C., Progar, P. R., Taylor, B., Ervin, R., & Zangrillo, A. N. (2010). Differential reinforcement of alternative behavior increases resistance to extinction: Clinical demonstration, animal modeling, and clinical test of one solution. *Journal of the Experimental Analysis of Behavior, 93*(3), 349–367.

Mazur, J. E. (2010). Editorial: Translational research in JEAB. *Journal of the Experimental Analysis of Behavior, 93*(3), 291–292.

Michael, J. L. (2004). *Concepts and principles of behavior analysis* (rev. ed.). Society for the Advancement of Behavior Analysis.

Morris, E. K., Altus, D. E., & Smith, N. G. (2013). A study in the founding of applied behavior analysis through its publications. *Behavior Analyst, 36*(1), 73–107.

Muething, C., Pavlov, A., Call, N., Ringdahl, J., & Gillespie, S. (2021). Prevalence of resurgence during thinning of multiple schedules of reinforcement following functional communication training. *Journal of Applied Behavior Analysis, 54*(2), 813–823.

Neuringer, A. (2002). Operant variability: Evidence, functions, and theory. *Psychonomic Bulletin and Review, 9*(4), 672–705.

Ono, K., & Iwabuchi, K. (1997). Effects of histories of differential reinforcement of response rate on variable-interval responding. *Journal of the Experimental Analysis of Behavior, 67*(3), 311–322.

Page, S., & Neuringer, A. (1985). Variability is an operant. *Journal of Experimental Psychology: Animal Behavior Processes, 11*(3), 429–452.

Payne, S. W., & Dozier, C. L. (2013). Positive reinforcement as treatment for problem behavior maintained by negative reinforcement. *Journal of Applied Behavior Analysis, 46*(3), 699–703.

Petscher, E. S., Rey, C., & Bailey, J. S. (2009). A review of empirical support for differential reinforcement of alternative behavior. *Research in Developmental Disabilities, 30*(3), 409–425.

Piazza, C. C., Fisher, W. W., Hanley, G. P., LeBlanc, L. A., Worsdell, A. S., Lindauer, S. E., & Keeney, K. M. (1998). Treatment of pica through multiple analyses of its reinforcing functions. *Journal of Applied Behavior Analysis, 31*, 165–189.

Pinkston, J. W., & Libman, B. M. (2017). Aversive functions of response effort: Fact or artifact? *Journal of the Experimental Analysis of Behavior, 108*(1), 73–96.

Poling, A., & Ryan, C. (1982). Differential-reinforcement-of-other-behavior schedules: Therapeutic applications. *Behavior Modification, 6*(1), 3–21.

Randall, K. R., Greer, B. D., Smith, S. W., & Kimball, R. T. (2021). Sustaining behavior reduction by transitioning the topography of the functional communication response during FCT. *Journal of Applied Behavior Analysis, 54*(3), 1013–1031.

Ringdahl, J. E., Falcomata, T. S., Christensen, T. J., Bass-Ringdahl, S. M., Lentz, A., Dutt, A., & Schuh-Claus, J. (2009). Evaluation of a pre-treatment assessment to select mand topographies for functional communication training. *Research in Developmental Disabilities, 30*(2), 330–341.

Rolider, A., & Van Houten, R. (1990). The role of reinforcement in reducing inappropriate behavior: Some myths and misconceptions. In A. C. Repp & N. N. Singh (Eds.), *Perspectives on the use of nonaversive and aversive interventions for persons with developmental disabilities* (pp. 119–127). Sycamore.

Shahan, T. A. (2010). Conditioned reinforcement and response strength. *Journal of the Experimental Analysis of Behavior, 93*(2), 269–289.

Shahan, T. A. (2017). Moving beyond reinforcement and response strength. *Behavior Analyst, 40*(1), 107–121.

Shahan, T. A., & Craig, A. R. (2017). Resurgence as choice. *Behavioural Processes, 141*, 100–127.

Shahan, T. A., & Sweeney, M. M. (2011). A model of resurgence based on behavioral momentum theory. *Journal of the Experimental Analysis of Behavior, 95*, 91–108.

Sidman, M. (2011). Can an understanding of basic research facilitate the effectiveness of prac-titioners?: Reflections and personal perspectives. *Journal of Applied Behavior Analysis, 44*(4), 973–991.

Skinner, B. F. (1938). *The behavior of organisms: an experimental analysis.* Appleton-Century.

Tiger, J. H., Bouxsein, K. J., & Fisher, W. W. (2007). Treating excessively slow responding of a young man with Asperger syndrome using differential reinforcement of short response latencies. *Journal of Applied Behavior Analysis, 40*(3), 559–563.

Tiger, J. H., Hanley, G. P., & Bruzek, J. (2008). Functional communication training: A review and practical guide. *Behavior Analysis in Practice, 1*(1), 16–23.

Tustin, R. D. (1994). Preference for reinforcers under varying schedule arrangements: A behavioral economic analysis. *Journal of Applied Behavior Analysis, 27*(4), 597–606.

Van Camp, C. M., Vollmer, T. R., & Daniel, D. (2001). A systematic evaluation of stimulus preference, response effort, and stimulus control in the treatment of automatically reinforced self-injury. *Behavior Therapy, 32*(3), 603–613.

Vladescu, J. C., & Kodak, T. (2010). A review of recent studies on differential reinforcement during skill acquisition in early intervention. *Journal of Applied Behavior Analysis, 43*(2), 351–355.

Vollmer, T. R., & Iwata, B. A. (1992). Differential reinforcement as treatment for behavior disorders: Procedural and functional variations. *Research in Developmental Disabilities, 13*(4), 393–417.

Vollmer, T. R., Iwata, B. A., Zarcone, J. R., Smith, R. G., & Mazaleski, J. L. (1993). The role of attention in the treatment of attention-maintained self-injurious behavior: Noncontingent reinforcement and differential reinforcement of other behavior. *Journal of Applied Behavior Analysis, 26*(1), 9–21.

Vollmer, T. R., Peters, K. P., Kronfli, F. R., Lloveras, L. A., & Ibañez, V. F. (2020). On the definition of differential reinforcement of alternative behavior. *Journal of Applied Behavior Analysis, 53*(3), 1299–1303.

Wolf, M., Risley, T., & Mees, H. (1963). Application of operant conditioning procedures to the behaviour problems of an autistic child. *Behaviour Research and Therapy, 1*(2–4), 305–312.

CHAPTER 14

Stimulus Control

WHAT IS IT AND WHY SHOULD WE CARE?

Sarah Cowie
Rebecca A. Sharp
Stephanie Gomes-Ng

> An adequate formulation of the interaction between an organism and its environment must always specify three things: (1) the occasion upon which a response occurs, (2) the response itself, and (3) the reinforcing consequences. The interrelations among them are the contingencies of reinforcement.
>
> —B. F. Skinner (1969, p. 7)

The same behavior that is appropriate in some situations may be inappropriate in others. Ordering a mojito is perfectly acceptable at 7:00 P.M. but may raise eyebrows at 7:00 A.M. Hugging a significant other usually results in a reciprocal hug; hugging a stranger might result in a lawsuit. The consequences that are likely to result from our behavior—and, by extension, the extent to which a behavior is desirable—depend on the context in which that behavior occurs. As a result, the likelihood of a behavior occurring usually varies depending on the stimulus context—that is, behavior comes under *stimulus control*.

As Skinner (1969) pointed out, the contingencies of reinforcement that control behavior depend not only on the relation between a response and a reinforcer but also the relation between the stimulus context and the reinforcer. This relation between stimuli, responses, and reinforcers comprises the *three-term contingency*. When the likelihood of a behavior occurring changes with the context, we say behavior is under *stimulus control*. Stimulus control allows organisms to adapt to the ever-changing world around us; our past experience with a response producing consequences in one context allows us to behave appropriately in similar contexts. In this way, stimulus control may be viewed as a fundamentally prospective process, because the control is by potential reinforcers as extrapolated from past experience in a similar environment, rather than by what has more recently been reinforced or punished (e.g., see Cowie & Davison, 2020a, 2020b, 2022). In this chapter, we explore how stimulus control develops and manifests (including division of control among different stimuli and generalization across novel stimuli), and factors that impact the extent of such control. Finally, we explore how stimulus control can contribute to inappropriate, challenging, or maladaptive behaviors.

Developing Stimulus Control

Stimulus control emerges when some stimulus is reliably present when a response produces a particular outcome. While stimulus control may be achieved by training in which responding is reinforced in the presence of one stimulus S+, and no other stimulus or consequences are experienced (e.g., Ellis, 1970; Honig et al., 1959), such *single-stimulus* training typically produces relatively weak stimulus control. Associating the S+ stimulus with reinforcers for responding, and associating another stimulus—the S− stimulus —with a different outcome (e.g., extinction), usually enhances stimulus control (e.g., Ames & Yarczower, 1965; Baron, 1973; Ghirlanda & Enquist, 2003; Ohinata, 1979). In basic research, such *discrimination training* typically uses a multiple schedule (e.g., Hanson, 1959) where responding to S+ is reinforced on a variable-interval (VI) schedule, or a choice paradigm where choices of S+ result in reinforcers and choices of S− result in extinction. The effects of S− in enhancing stimulus control require that S+ and S− be presented in close temporal succession (e.g., Honig et al., 1959). Without an overt *transition* between S+ and S−, S− no longer enhances discrimination. Such transitions need not be numerous; Ellis (1970) showed that just a single transition between S+ and S− stimuli in a session was sufficient to produce the same control as could be achieved by alternating S+ and S− many times within the same session.

Multiple schedules are also used to develop stimulus control in applied settings. Responses in the presence of one stimulus, S+, are reinforced, and responses in the presence of another, S−, are placed on extinction. Stimulus discrimination training is used to establish stimulus classes, for example, auditory–visual object identification (Carp et al., 2012), tacting olfactory stimuli (Dass et al., 2018), and emitting vocal verbal operants (Kisamore et al., 2016). Training can involve teaching simple discriminations, in which there is only one S+, or conditional discriminations, in which stimuli serve as both an S+ and an S− across trials. For example, a simple discrimination is selecting the pencil when asked to "find the pencil." Selecting the pencil is reinforced, and selecting the ruler (or any other object) is placed on extinction. By contrast, a conditional discrimination involves selecting the pencil when asked to "find the pencil" and selecting the ruler when asked to "find the ruler." In a laboratory, a simple discrimination might be "Choose the left key if the light is red," whereas a conditional discrimination might be "Choose the left key if the light is red and it appears a long time into a trial; choose the right key if the light is red and it appears a short time into a trial." There is a body of research that shows that teaching simple discriminations prior to conditional discriminations may hinder development of stimulus control; discrimination is acquired more quickly when conditional discriminations are taught without first establishing simple discriminations (e.g., Grow et al., 2011; Lin & Zhu, 2020).

Why might simple discrimination training hinder the development of conditional discriminations? While simple and conditional discriminations undoubtedly involve the same underlying learning processes (e.g., see Ploog & Williams, 2010), simple discrimination does not promote attention to specific dimensions of the stimulus, whereas conditional discrimination does. A switch from simple to conditional discrimination requires attending to specific elements of the stimulus that were not necessary to perform the simple discrimination, and learning the relation between that element and subsequent behavior-reinforcer relations. Such a change would usually be required in the absence of any obvious change in the nature of the task. Indeed, basic research has shown that detection of the change in contingencies is slower when the relation between stimulus, response, and reinforcer is changed but the ambient stimulus conditions themselves remain unchanged, relative to when both the stimulus conditions *and* the relation between stimuli, responses, and reinforcers are changed (e.g., Cowie et al., 2016a).

Stimulus control may be trained, but it may also be *transferred* to a desired discriminative stimulus. While such transfer may be explicitly trained, it also often occurs through the use of prompts (Schnell et al., 2020), instructions (textual prompts; Phillips et al., 2019), and rules (contingency-specifying verbal stimuli; Danforth et al., 1990). Methods for fading prompts include physically fading a stimulus, increasing the delay to the prompt, and stimulus transformations (the prompt gradually changes to look like the desired discriminative stimulus; Cengher et al., 2018). Touchette and Howard (1984) suggested that there are two possible mechanisms for the transfer of stimulus control using prompts; Pairing the prompt with the desired discriminative stimulus operates in a Pavlovian-like process, and producing the response in the presence of the stimulus reduces the delay to reinforcement that occurs when responding is prompted. There is a need for more applied research on the behavioral processes underpinning the transfer of stimulus control.

Divided Control

What happens if *more than one* stimulus is present when a response produces a particular outcome? In these situations, stimulus control often comes to be *divided* between the stimuli that are present. When control is divided, multiple stimuli may exert an approximately equal amount of control over behavior, or some stimuli may exert stronger control than others (Born & Peterson, 1969). Therefore, when multiple discriminative stimuli are present, stimulus control exists along a continuum ranging from complete selectivity (control by a single stimulus) to equal division.

Divided stimulus control is ubiquitous in the natural world (see, e.g., Dall et al., 2005; Munoz & Blumstein, 2012; Schmidt et al., 2010). Natural environments are multidimensional—they comprise many stimuli (often, hundreds)—and so most behaviors are probably controlled by more than one stimulus. For example, successful navigation to a goal (e.g., the location of food for a foraging animal, or to a new road-trip destination for a human) typically relies on the use of multiple landmarks, and for humans, instructions provided by a map or global positioning system (GPS; e.g., Cheng et al., 2007; Cheng & Spetch, 1998). Successful communication involves a variety of verbal and nonverbal cues, such as vocalizations and bodily mating displays in animals (e.g., Rubi & Stephens, 2016c), or words spoken and gestures or facial expressions in humans. Successful *concept formation* (i.e., the ability to categorize objects into different categories, such as "animal," "plant," or "vehicle") depends on the ability to recognize the characteristics that collectively define a concept from those that do not. More generally, divided stimulus control is implicated in social, communicative, emotional, linguistic, academic, cognitive, and behavioral development (for reviews, see Lovaas et al., 1979; Ploog, 2010).

The earliest studies of divided stimulus control arranged a *go/no-go* discrimination, in which responses to a multidimensional (compound) "S+" stimulus were reinforced and responses to a different compound "S−" stimulus were not reinforced. In the first of such studies, Reynolds (1961) reinforced two pigeons' key pecks to a white triangle superimposed on a red background, whereas pecks to a white circle on a green background were never reinforced. After the pigeons had learned the discrimination, Reynolds assessed the degree of control exerted by the color and form dimensions by presenting, and measuring responding to, each stimulus element individually (i.e., red, green, triangle, circle). One pigeon responded at a high rate to the red stimulus, at a low rate to the green stimulus, and at equally low rates to the triangle and circle stimuli. Thus, this pigeon's responding appeared to be controlled by the color, but not form, dimension. The reverse appeared to be true for the other pigeon, for which response rates were differential to the form stimuli and nondifferential to the color stimuli (see also e.g., Birkimer, 1969; Born & Peterson, 1969; Born & Snow, 1970; Ploog, 2011; Sutherland & Holgate, 1966). These findings were later replicated in children with intellectual or developmental disabilities (IDDs) by Lovaas et al. (1971), who arranged a go/no-go discrimination with compound stimuli that comprised four dimensions—visual (colored light), auditory (white noise), tactile (an inflatable blood-pressure cuff), and temporal (duration of stimulus presentation). Children with IDD showed control by only one or at most two dimensions, whereas typically developing children demonstrated control by at least three dimensions. These findings demonstrate that the presence of multiple stimuli does not necessarily imply that divided control will occur, or that it will involve only the stimuli relevant to a discrimination, in experimental and applied settings. Instead, stimulus control may be selective, or control may be divided between relevant and irrelevant stimuli, or even between multiple irrelevant stimuli (e.g., Gomes-Ng et al., 2019, 2020; Koegel & Rincover, 1976; Pinto et al., 2017; Pinto & Machado, 2017; Reynolds, 1961; Rincover, 1978; Rincover & Koegel, 1975; Schreibman et al., 1982; Williams et al., 2020)!

More recent research uses the *delayed matching-to-sample* (DMTS) procedure to study divided stimulus control (Maki & Leith, 1973; Maki & Leuin, 1972). In the DMTS task, subjects are presented with a compound "sample" stimulus for a limited period of time, and then report the identity of one of its elements by choosing an identically or symbolically matching "comparison" stimulus from among several comparisons. Choice of the matching comparison is reinforced and implies control by that element's dimension. For example, Dube and McIlvane (1997) examined divided control between stimuli that had been previously associated with a high or low rate of reinforcers in a DMTS task with individuals with IDDs. During the comparison phase, participants chose between two stimuli previously associated with the same reinforcer rate, or between two stimuli previously associated with different reinforcer rates. In general, participants were more likely to choose the correct (i.e., matching) comparison when both comparisons were associated with high reinforcer rates, compared with when both were associated with low reinforcer rates. When the comparison stimuli were associated with different reinforcer rates, participants preferred the high-rate comparison, regardless of whether it matched the sample stimulus. One interpretation of these results, suggested by Dube and McIlvane, is that stimuli associated with higher reinforcer rates exert relatively stronger control over behavior. However, alternatively, these results may have nothing to do with divided stimulus control; instead, participants may simply have been more *motivated* to choose high-rate comparisons regardless of the sample-stimulus elements (cf. Lamb, 1991; Wasserman & Miller, 1997). This illustrates the importance of considering how processes unrelated to stimulus control, such as motivation to respond, may influence the apparent division of control between multiple stimuli.

Furthermore, although divided stimulus control is important for the success of many behavioral interventions, there are cases in which divided control can negatively affect learning and behavior. Control by incidental, irrelevant stimuli can prevent acquisition, maintenance, or generalization of behavior (e.g., Rincover & Koegel, 1975). However, such irrelevant stimuli may not always be incidental, as in prompt-fading procedures in which an additional prompt, such as a verbal or pictorial cue, is used to help promote correct responding (Cengher et al., 2018). This prompt has no impact on the actual intervention contingencies; that is, although it is deliberately included to increase correct responding, the prompt is not the stimulus relevant to the behavior being taught. As treatment progresses, the prompt is gradually faded out. But what happens if stimulus control is divided between the prompt and the relevant stimulus? When this occurs, control by the prompt interferes with control by the relevant stimulus, and so fading the prompt may impact behavioral performance (see, e.g., Koegel & Rincover, 1976). Therefore, in addition to considering how to enhance divided stimulus control, behavior analysts also need to consider how to reduce the likelihood that such divided control involves stimuli that are irrelevant to the discrimination. There are several strategies available to clinicians to reduce prompt dependency (i.e., control by irrelevant stimuli), the effectiveness of which differs across individuals. For example, Gorgan and Kodak (2019) compared differential reinforcement (during which higher-quality reinforcers were delivered for unprompted over prompted responses), systematic prompt fading, and an extended interval in which participants could respond. They found that for three adolescents with autism spectrum disorder (ASD) or IDDs, these strategies were differentially effective and efficacious in increasing correct, unprompted responding. Transfer of stimulus control to desired discriminative stimuli can also be achieved by combining differential reinforcement and prompt fading (i.e., ensuring that prompted responses are never reinforced).

What other considerations can researchers and clinicians make to establish or enhance divided control by the desired stimuli? Some applied research suggests that divided stimulus control can be established by arranging discriminative stimuli that differ *minimally*—that is, in only one or two aspects. This is because the discrimination can only be learned if all aspects of the stimuli control behavior. In contrast, if discriminative stimuli differ from each other in multiple aspects, then these differences are *redundant*, and the discrimination can be learned based on any of these differences. For example, Birnie-Selwyn and Guerin (1997) used minimal- and multiple-difference training to reduce spelling errors in six elementary-age children, using a DMTS task. The sample stimuli were spoken words, the comparison stimuli were written words, and participants matched the written word to its spoken equivalent. In the minimal-difference condition, the comparison stimuli differed by only one or two letters, whereas in the multiple-difference condition, all letters differed between the comparison stimuli. Accuracy was higher, and fewer spelling errors occurred, in the minimal-difference condition (see also Allen & Fuqua, 1985); that is, divided stimulus control was more likely when the discriminative stimuli differed in only one or two aspects, whereas it was less likely to occur (and selective control was more likely) with stimuli that were very different from each other. This example illustrates one way that clinicians can design discriminative stimuli to enhance divided stimulus control.

Generalization

Stimulus control is usually not specific to the exact stimuli in the presence of which the stimulus–response–reinforcer relation was learned (i.e., those with which we already have experience). When we behave similarly under slightly different stimulus contexts—falling silent when a familiar lecturer begins speaking, and also falling silent when a new lecturer begins speaking—we say there is *generalization*. Generalization is adaptive; it means we do not have to have exposure to every single stimulus for the stimulus context to affect our behavior. Imagine, for example, if your behavior of stopping failed to generalize across red traffic lights, so that you stopped only at those red traffic lights you had encountered with your driving instructor, and ignored those you had never before encountered. *Discrimination*—behaving differently as the stimulus conditions change—is the opposite of generalization. Discrimination allows us to change our behavior as the likelihood of it producing a particular consequence changes—again, without having had to experience the exact stimulus context in question. For example, you might stop at a red traffic light, but not a red "OPEN" sign on a shop. Often, stimulus control from one's learning history may be relevant to navigating new or changed environmental conditions. In this case, making the current conditions more similar to those that have previously exerted stimulus control will facilitate transfer of control to current environmental conditions (e.g., see Sharp et al., 2019). Generalization is a fundamental behavioral phenomenon whose basic characteristics appear universal across species and stimulus dimensions (see, for a review, Ghirlanda & Enquist, 2003).

Some behaviors should generalize widely across contexts (e.g., stopping at red lights, being polite), while others should be much more context specific (hugging and kissing, being loud, using behavior-analytic jargon). The extent and nature of generalization depends in part on our experience with stimuli and their associated response-consequence relations (i.e., the training conditions). Typically, reinforcers are delivered for responses in the presence of S+; programming an S− in the presence of which responses are never reinforced (*discrimination* training) tends to enhance discrimination. In a lab setting, behavior is usually reinforced on a VI schedule to promote a high, constant rate of responding that is relatively resistant to extinction (allowing for further testing). A generalization test may be conducted once responding has stabilized, by varying the stimulus across one dimension (e.g., color, or brightness, or size), and recording the amount of responding in the presence of each stimulus. Generalization tests are usually conducted in extinction to ensure responding is made on the basis of what was learned during training rather than as a result of new learning during testing. A *generalization gradient* plots a measure of responding as a function of the different stimuli used in the generalization test; this gives a measure of the extent of generalization across stimuli. The steeper the gradient, the greater the change in responding as the stimulus changes, and hence the less generalization (and the more discrimination). Panel A in Figure 14.1 shows the sort of generalization gradient we would expect in an experiment in which responding to a 2.5-inch circle (S+) was reinforced during training, then a range of circle sizes were presented during generalization testing. The peak of the generalization gradient in Panel A is at the stimulus associated with reinforcers during training (S+); the more different the circle size, the lower the rate of responding. The solid-line function is steeper than the dashed-line function, reflecting a greater change in responding as the stimulus becomes more different from S+, and hence less generalization. Although the data in Figure 14.1 are hypothetical, they reflect a commonly observed pattern. For example, Lady Bay, a horse trained by Dougherty and Lewis (1991) to respond for grain reinforcers in the presence of a 2.5-inch circle (S+ stimulus), showed a similar pattern of generalization.

The peak in responding at the training stimulus shown in Panel A of Figure 14.1 is common but not ubiquitous. Perceptual abilities sometimes mean the maximum response rate—the peak of the generalization gradient—occurs close to, but not exactly at, the original S+ stimulus from training (e.g., Hearst et al., 1964). The shape of the generalization gradient also depends critically on the type of training an organism experiences. Discrimination training with S+ and S− stimuli that differ on the same dimension

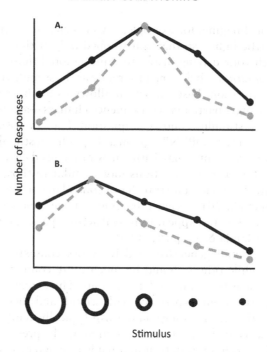

FIGURE 14.1. Generalization gradients. Panel A shows an example of a generalization gradient from an experiment in which responding to a 2.5-inch circle was reinforced during training. Panel B shows an example of a generalization gradient from a similar experiment, in which responding to a 2.5-inch circle was reinforced and responding to a smaller circle was not reinforced.

(e.g., colors, intensity, length, diameter) tends to produce *peak shift,* where the greatest amount of responding in the generalization test occurs at a stimulus different from S+, in the opposite direction from S−, and the least amount of responding occurs away from S−. Panel B of Figure 14.1 shows generalization gradients we would expect if training included the same circle stimulus as S+ *and* a smaller circle as S−. After this sort of experience, organisms often make the greatest number of responses to a novel stimulus—in this case, a circle that was larger than the original S+ used in training. As in Panel A, the solid-line generalization gradient in Panel B is steeper than the dashed-line one, and hence the solid-line gradient would indicate less generalization than the green one. Peak shift is common across species and different stimuli. For example, Köhler (1939) showed chickens trained with light gray as the S+ and dark gray as the S− chose a card that was even lighter than the S+ over the S+ itself, and Dougherty and Lewis's (1991) horse Lady Bay showed similar peak shift after discrimination training with a larger circle as S+ and a smaller circle as S−.

Peak shift is less likely to occur when the S+ and S− stimuli are more different from each other (i.e., further apart on the same dimension). Hanson (1959) found that a group of pigeons trained with a 550-nanometer S+ responded the most during a generalization test in the presence of a 550-nanometer stimulus, whereas a group trained on a multiple schedule with the same S+ and a 555-nanometer S− showed the most responding in the presence of a 540-nanometer stimulus. The more similar the S+ and S− (i.e., the closer they fall on a dimension), the further the peak in the generalization gradient is from S+, and the greater the amount of responding relative to responding in S+ (e.g., Hearst, 1968: line-tilt, pigeon; Ohinata, 1979: wavelength, goldfish; Baron, 1973: tone frequency, humans; Cheng et al., 1997: spatial location, pigeon). Using two or more S+ stimuli in training often enhances generalization, though the exact pattern of generalization still depends on the relation between those stimuli—if the stimuli are sufficiently close on one dimension, stimuli intermediate to those S+ stimuli will often maintain more responding than the S+ stimuli (see also Wagner, 1971; Weiss, 1972; Kehoe, 1986; Rosch et al., 1976; Homa et al., 1981; Shanks, 1995); but if the S+ stimuli are distant, intermediate stimuli may result in less responding (Ghirlanda & Enquist, 2003). Thus, while using S+ and S− in training can facilitate stimulus control, it may also lead to unexpected patterns of generalization in the form of increased responding in the presence of a novel stimulus from the same dimension.

Generalization of responding maintained by reinforcers appears to follow a similar pattern to generalization of *suppression* of responding by punishers; the effect of the stimulus on behavior reduces as the stimulus becomes more different. For example, Brush et al. (1952) showed similarly shaped generalization gradients for pigeon key pecks maintained by reinforcers, and for pigeon key pecks that were suppressed with electric shock.

Generalization is not a guaranteed outcome of training and must be considered in designing a training program in applied settings. There are a number of methods to promote generalization in clinical practice based on Stokes and Baer's (1977) seminal paper (e.g., varying training stimuli along noncritical dimensions). However, it has been suggested that applied approaches to generalization may lack consideration of the underpinning behavioral processes and consider generalization topographically; simply desirable responding to untrained stimuli (Song et al., 2021). For example, a tactic described by Stokes and Baer (1977) is to *program common stimuli*, which involves incorporating stimuli likely to be encountered in natural settings into training conditions. This can be useful when the target behavior carries risk (e.g., teaching people to cross a simulated road; Batu et al., 2004) and is sensible with regard to establishing stimulus control. However, applied studies infrequently determine or describe systematically the underpinning behavioral process. Kirby and Bickel (1988) identified the possible behavioral processes for generalization tactics, suggesting that programming common stimuli may function either to establish stimulus control of desired S+s, or by reducing the risk of unwanted stimulus control by irrelevant stimuli or of incompatible behaviors. Evaluating the behavioral process aligns more closely with the evaluation of stimulus generalization in basic research. Therefore, the applied use of the term *stimulus generalization* is often incorrect; it is used to describe untrained behavior change rather than the process of responding under similar stimuli to the training stimuli measured in extinction as described in 1956 by Guttman and Kalish (Johnston, 1979). Additionally, Cuvo (2003) identified that some applied studies reporting generalization data obtain those data in conditions involving prompts and reinforcement rather than extinction. As a result, he called for behavior analysts to evaluate whether responding to each new member of a stimulus class is due to training (e.g., reinforcement, prompting) or generalization (tested in extinction).

Testing for generalization in applied research and practice tends to involve evaluating whether untrained responding occurred in a narrow range of conditions (e.g., a novel location or to a novel person) rather than evaluating responding along a dimension of a stimulus in extinction. Therefore, applied examples of generalization gradients are scarce. However, generalization gradients have been demonstrated to be useful as an assessment method to determine the S+ under which responding occurs and subsequently design an intervention. Lalli et al. (1998) showed rates of the self-injurious behavior (SIB) of a girl with IDDs decreased with decreased proximity to an adult (the S+). They found that 65% of the SIB occurred to the S+ and most similar S− to the S+. This information was used to determine the distance for an adult to stand near the child during an intervention without occasioning SIB. The stimulus dimension of proximity is discriminable and able to be varied systematically. However, many stimuli in applied settings to which generalized responding may be desirable may not lend themselves to a continuum for generating a gradient (in teaching cutting with scissors, assessing behavior with novel scissors is unlikely to involve scissors that vary along a continuum of size, color, etc.) Furthermore, there is no guarantee that control by the size, color, or other specific features of the scissors will actually develop; elements of a stimulus that all correlate to the same degree with reinforcer availability do not necessarily all develop control (e.g., Reynolds, 1961).

Determinants of Stimulus Control, Its Division, and Generalization

The development and division of stimulus control, and the extent to which such control generalizes, depends on the characteristics of the stimuli, the consequences associated with the stimuli, and the organism's learning history. Indeed, we have already seen how arranging minimal versus multiple differences between stimuli in applied interventions affects divided stimulus control in Birnie-Selwyn and Guerin's (1997) study. Here, we further explore the factors that contribute to stimulus control.

Discriminability

In lab settings, control by a variety of stimulus modalities—including light intensity, tone frequency, size, color, flash duration, and the passage of time—appears to conform to the same set of rules. Differences in stimulus control hinge instead on how the organism experiences the stimuli. Where an organism's perceptual abilities mean it *cannot* detect a difference between stimuli, such stimuli will not exert differential control over behavior (i.e., the same behavior will occur in the presence of different stimuli)—regardless of how different associated reinforcer conditions are. *Stimulus discriminability*—the difference in stimulus conditions necessary to produce a difference in behavior (Lashley & Wade, 1946)—will in part determine the extent to which responding varies as the stimulus and associated reinforcer conditions differ (e.g., Chase & Heinemann, 1972; Davison & Nevin, 1999; Dinsmoor, 1995; Johnson & Cumming, 1968; White, 1986). When different reinforcer conditions are associated with highly disparate stimuli, those stimuli exert strong control; as the disparity between those stimuli reduces, so too will stimulus control (and indeed, reinforcer effects on responding). For example, Alsop and Davison (1991) showed that when different schedules of reinforcers were associated with different stimulus conditions, differences in responding in the two stimulus contexts were greater when the stimuli were more different (see also Miller et al., 1980; for discussion, see Davison & Nevin, 1999). Differences in reinforcers for responding in the two stimulus contexts had no impact on behavior when the stimulus conditions were not detectably different. Hannula et al. (2020) similarly reported that stimuli more obviously different in color were associated with fewer errors in responding in children with ASD. Where contingencies are signaled by a compound stimulus requiring a conditional discrimination, the same rules apply. Where just one element is not highly discriminable, stimulus control will be relatively weak, regardless of discriminability of other relevant elements (e.g., Miranda-Dukoski et al., 2014). Of course, when different elements of a compound stimulus all have the same association with reinforcers and a conditional discrimination is not required, control will often be divided more toward (or exclusive to) the more discriminable element. In short, the greater the perceptible stimulus disparity associated with a difference in reinforcers, the greater the potential for stimulus control of behavior.

Like stimulus control, generalization depends on discriminability of the relevant stimulus dimension. Where discriminability is low, generalization must necessarily be greater, since it is more difficult to detect that stimulus conditions have changed. Indeed, generalization tests using stimuli with low discriminability tend to reveal flatter gradients than to those conducted with stimuli with high discriminability—an effect demonstrated with pigeons (Honig & Urcuioli, 1981), humans (Kalish, 1958), and goldfish (Fay, 1970), to name a few species. When discriminability changes across the spectrum of a stimulus dimension, generalization gradients will be asymmetrical (e.g., Blough, 1972; Honig & Urcuioli, 1981). These effects of stimulus discriminability mean that the less discriminable the stimuli used in training, the wider the range of novel stimuli that will occasion the associated response. Of course, the training stimulus S+ and highly similar stimuli will likely maintain a lower rate of responding than would a highly discriminable S+; there is a trade-off between strong stimulus control and the occurrence of generalization.

Salience

Stimulus control is biased toward stimuli that are more intense (e.g., louder or brighter; Fields, 1978, 1979; Fields et al., 1976; Johnson, 1970; Miles & Jenkins, 1973; Pavlov, 1927)—perhaps because such stimuli command more attention, facilitating the learning of the relation between stimuli, responses, and their consequences. In extreme cases, stimulus control may be completely selective to highly salient or intense stimuli. In this regard, it is worth considering the parallels between development of operant and Pavlovian control by stimuli.

Some evidence suggests that differences in stimulus intensity contribute to selective stimulus control in individuals with ASD. Leader et al. (2009) arranged a conditional-discrimination task in which children with ASD and matched controls chose between two compound stimuli, each composed of two colored components of equal saturation (i.e., equal intensity) or unequal saturation. During training, choice of one compound was defined as correct and reinforced, whereas choice of the other compound was defined as incorrect and never reinforced. Leader et al. found that stimulus control was strongly biased toward colors of higher saturation, and greater selectivity was observed when the saturations were more unequal. Furthermore, such selective stimulus control was more prevalent in children with ASD than in matched controls. A similar effect has been demonstrated when written words are paired with pictures (e.g., Didden et al., 2000); pictures may overshadow the learning of written words. Dittlinger and Lerman (2011) found that overshadowing and blocking occurred when children with developmental disabilities were taught to identify written words. The children acquired the written words more quickly in the absence of the corresponding picture (overshadowing), and knowing the corresponding picture prior to training appeared to inhibit learning (blocking). Strategies to overcome overshadowing in applied settings include fading the overshadowing stimulus gradually to transfer stimulus control or embedding picture–text matching in teaching sessions to develop a stimulus class (Richardson et al., 2017). Additionally, control by the overshadowing stimulus can be extinguished by pairing the stimulus with a novel stimulus and reinforcing responding to the novel stimulus (Broomfield et al., 2008).

Some behaviors are deemed inappropriate because they occur in the wrong stimulus context. For these behaviors, it is useful to transfer stimulus control from inappropriate to appropriate stimuli. Altering an existing discriminative stimulus to make it more salient often facilitates transfer of control to that stimulus. For example, O'Neill et al. (1980) found that the amount of litter deposited in a trash receptacle made to look like a football helmet was twice as much as the amount of litter deposited in standard regular receptacles. Indeed, in basic research, any manipulation that enhances the discriminability of a stimulus—its potential for its presence (and absence) to be detected accurately—also enhances the degree to which behavior comes under stimulus control (e.g., Cowie et al., 2016b).

Familiarity

Some types, or dimensions, of stimuli appear to be more likely to control behavior than others in the absence of obvious differences in salience or discriminability—for example, Lovaas et al. (1971) found no evidence of control by a tactile stimulus dimension in any children with ASD, and no evidence of control by a temporal dimension in atypically or typically developing children. Such inherent biases toward some stimulus dimensions may arise due to the organism's sensory capacities, and biological or phylogenetic predispositions (Baron, 1965; Seligman, 1970). For example, humans and pigeons are both visual-dependent, and so visual stimuli tend to control behavior more readily than other kinds of stimuli for these species (e.g., Colavita, 1974; Hodos, 1993; Posner et al., 1976). Even within a sensory modality, some dimensions may tend to exert stronger control than others—in pigeons, control by color tends to overshadow control by other visual dimensions (e.g., flash duration; Cowie et al., 2020; line orientation; Kraemer & Roberts, 1985; Randich et al., 1978; Shahan & Podlesnik, 2006).

Generalization is greater along dimensions with which an organism has little experience than those that are more familiar (Peterson, 1962; Rubel & Rosenthal, 1975; Kerr et al., 1977; Mackintosh et al., 1991; Bennett et al., 1994), perhaps because such dimensions are more readily attended to, facilitating detection of changes in those dimensions. This means stimulus control will be faster to develop, and stronger, along dimensions that are familiar than along those that are relatively novel (e.g., Davison & Cowie, 2019). Perhaps this familiarity effect is what drives the need for requisite skills in discrimination training (see Pizarro et al., 2020); the more experience one has with discriminating along a particular dimension, the more likely one is to detect changes in that dimension that accompany changes in reinforcer conditions, and the more readily stimulus control will develop.

As control by training stimuli develops, and stimuli become more familiar, generalization across novel stimuli becomes less likely. Honig and Slivka (1964) trained pigeons on a multiple schedule in which responses were reinforced in all components, but in one component responses were punished as well. They ran generalization tests regularly, and found the generalization gradient became steeper—that is, generalization reduced—as the pigeons had more exposure to the relation between the different stimuli and reinforcers/punishers. These effects of experience may be particularly evident when reinforcer rates are low, or learning conditions are otherwise difficult. For example, Walker and

Branch (1998) showed generalization gradients following training on a VI 240-seconds schedule of reinforcers were steeper after approximately 40 sessions of training (at which point responding was stable) than after 10 sessions of training, but gradients following training on a VI 30-seconds schedule did not differ with training length. These differences may reflect the increased opportunities for learning about the relation between stimuli and reinforcers at higher reinforcer rates; perhaps the same effects would be visible were generalization following training on the VI 30-seconds schedule tested after an even smaller number of sessions. The length of the generalization test also matters: Peak shift can reduce over the course of a long generalization test (Crawford et al., 1980; Cheng et al., 1997; see also Blough, 1975), presumably reflecting ongoing learning and the dynamic nature of stimulus control.

Some stimuli may have preexisting control arising from biological or genetic factors, rather than learning. For example, gulls will retrieve dummy eggs, but only so long as they are not white (Baerends, 1982); gulls usually remove white objects from their nest as an antipredator defence (Tinbergen et al., 1962). It is worth noting that certain stimuli may have previous relevance to a client in a treatment setting, and this relevance may facilitate learning on a familiar dimension, or prevent new learning by eliciting or evoking behaviors that are not compatible with the target response.

Consequences

When different stimuli are associated with identical reinforcer conditions, even the most obviously different stimuli will not exert control over behavior (see Davison & Nevin, 1999); that is, stimulus control will fail to develop both when a change in ambient stimulus conditions cannot be detected, and when a change in reinforcer conditions cannot be detected. Thus, the reinforcers associated with behavior in different contexts are a fundamental determinant of the degree of stimulus control.

A substantial body of evidence suggests that relative reinforcement plays a key role in determining stimulus control. For example, stimuli or stimulus dimensions that differentially signal reinforcer availability appear to control behavior more readily in future discriminations than dimensions that have previously not signaled reinforcer availability (e.g., Cuell et al., 2012; Johnson, 1970; Johnson & Cumming, 1968; Kamin, 1969; Klosterhalfen et al., 1978; Mackintosh & Little, 1969; Uengoer & Lachnit, 2012). There is some evidence, however, that stimuli that signal extinction (i.e., S–) may be nonpreferred or aversive (e.g., Terrace, 1971). Tiger et al. (2006) compared S+/S– and S+ only multiple-schedule conditions for discriminated requests for attention in children. They found that the S+/S– condition was more preferred by the children whose responding was highly discriminated in this condition (i.e., who never responded in the presence of the S–). Children who sometimes responded in the presence of the S– preferred the S+/S– condition. However, both conditions were effective in producing discriminative responding. In addition to relative reinforcement across stimuli, when only one dimension of a compound stimulus is relevant to a discrimination, only that dimension controls behavior. When multiple dimensions are relevant, stimulus control is divided between them (e.g., Blough, 1969; Castro & Wasserman, 2014, 2016, 2017; Chase, 1968; Heinemann et al., 1968; Leith & Maki, 1975; Wagner, 1969).

Recent research suggests that stimulus control is graded according to the relative ability of each stimulus to predict future reinforcers. For example, Shahan and Podlesnik (2006) arranged a DMTS task with pigeons in which compound sample stimuli comprised a vertical or horizontal line superimposed on a blue or green background, and comparison stimuli were two lines or two colors. Across conditions, the probability of reinforcer deliveries following correct responses according to the color- and line-orientation dimensions varied. As the probability of reinforcer deliveries for the color dimension increased and the probability of reinforcer deliveries for the line-orientation dimension decreased, control by the color dimension increased and control by the line-orientation dimension decreased; that is, there was a *linear* relation between relative reinforcer rates and divided stimulus control. This finding has been replicated using a symbolic DMTS procedure and different stimulus dimensions (e.g., stimulus duration; Davison, 2018; Davison & Elliffe, 2010; Podlesnik et al., 2012; Shahan & Podlesnik, 2007; for similar findings in different experiment paradigms, see e.g., Cheng et al., 2007; Cowie et al., 2017; Delamater & Nicolas, 2015; Du et al., 2017; Gomes-Ng et al., 2018; Legge et al., 2016; Matell & Kurti, 2014; Rayburn-Reeves et al., 2017; Rubi & Stephens, 2016a, 2016b; Spetch, 1995; Spetch & Wilkie, 1994).

Considering divided stimulus control with regard to relative reinforcement has been demonstrated to be important when designing discrimination training procedures. Song et al. (2021) conducted a translational study using arbitrary matching to sample in which noncritical features of stimuli were either highly correlated with reinforcers (by using one exemplar as the S+ more often than others) or equally correlated with reinforcers (by using each exemplar as the S+ in an even number of trials). Responding in the group in which noncritical features were correlated with reinforcement took longer to show mastery and was more variable. They suggested that practitioners should therefore ensure that low mastery criteria are not masking responding that is under weak stimulus control (because noncritical features are more likely to be associated with reinforcement under lenient mastery criteria) and that noncritical features are systematically evaluated when faulty stimulus control is suspected. In skills acquisition programs, delivering delayed prompts may cause disparity in the relative reinforcer rate for prompted and unprompted responses, because the overall reinforcer density over time will be lower for prompted responses. Touchette and Howard (1984) varied the relative reinforcer ratio for prompted and unprompted responses in a numeral- and letter-identification discrimination training for children with disabilities. Although mastery was attained regardless of whether prompted or unprompted responses were reinforced on the denser schedule, stimulus control transferred more quickly to the task stimuli from the prompt when unprompted responses were reinforced on a denser schedule than prompted responses. These data showed that discrimination can be learned despite reinforcement rates, suggesting that there is more to the transfer of stimulus control from prompts to task stimuli than differential reinforcement.

In addition to relative reinforcer rates, which determine how stimulus control is divided between multiple stimuli, the *overall* reinforcement context also plays a role. Podlesnik et al. (2012) compared divided stimulus control in a DMTS task with pigeons, in a context delivering a higher overall reinforcer rate or a context delivering a lower overall reinforcer rate. Each context was signaled by a different-colored stimulus, presented before each trial. After training, Podlesnik et al. introduced a disruptor, which was either presession feeding or extinction. In sessions of disruption, accuracy for both dimensions of the compound sample stimuli was higher in the context associated with the higher overall reinforcer rate than in the context associated with the lower overall reinforcer rate. Thus, divided stimulus control appears to persist for longer in contexts associated with higher overall reinforcer rates. This suggests that after divided stimulus control is established, shifting stimulus control (e.g., from one relevant stimulus to another) may be more difficult in environments with strong reinforcement histories—as might be the case with divided control of behavior when working from home relative to the office, or in lectures about preferred topics relative to less preferred ones.

Overall reinforcer rate may also impact generalization across novel stimuli. Generalization gradients tend to be steeper following single-stimulus training with higher than lower reinforcer rates (e.g., Hearst et al., 1964; Haber & Kalish, 1963). These differences appear largely driven by differences in the rate of responding during the S+ stimulus; the effect of overall reinforcer rates on generalization becomes less apparent when generalization gradients are plotted in terms of relative, rather than absolute, responses (e.g., Eckerman, 1969; Walker & Branch, 1998). These findings suggest that programming for generalization in treatments is not dependent on reinforcer rates—reinforcer rates will place a limit on the amount of a behavior that occurs, but not the rate at which the behavior becomes less likely as the stimulus context changes.

Stimulus control and generalization are also affected by motivation for the reinforcer associated with a stimulus. Stimuli associated with more-preferred reinforcers maintain more responding than do those associated with less-preferred stimuli, even when presented at the same time as a stimulus signaling the equally likely occurrence of a less-preferred reinforcer for a different behavior (Cowie, Gomes-Ng, et al., 2020). In this way, stimulus control appears to increase as the associated reinforcers become more valuable. The effect of reinforcer value on generalization may differ. Lab experiments show that the range of novel stimuli that will occasion a response becomes wider (i.e., generalization increases) as motivation increases (e.g., Gaiardi et al., 1987; Jenkins et al., 1958; Li et al., 1995; Thomas & King, 1959; see Lotfizadeh et al., 2012, for a review). The impact of motivation and perceived reinforcer value on stimulus control has received relatively little attention, and related research is largely limited to animal models. Given the ever-changing nature of motivation in daily life, the interplay between motivation, stimulus control, and generalization may be a fruitful area for future translational research.

Antecedent versus Consequence

Although practitioners and experimenters typically work with exteroceptive, easily observable stimuli, *any* sort of stimulus can potentially develop control, provided it is discriminable and correlates with a change in reinforcer (or punisher) conditions. Behaviors, reinforcers, and punishers may thus function as discriminative stimuli (e.g., Perone & Courtney, 1992; Cowie et al., 2011; Krägeloh et al., 2005; Holz & Azrin, 1961). For example, Tiger and Hanley (2005) showed that children who learned to ask for an adult's attention under multiple-schedule conditions where the color of a floral lei worn by the teacher signaled whether the teacher would give attention to the student, another student, or no students at all, continued to ask for attention more often at times when the teacher would give them attention in the absence of such stimuli. Tiger and Hanley pointed out that while the lei was the discriminative stimulus arranged by the researchers, other environmental events such as the consequences of asking for attention, and the observed consequences of another student asking for attention, were also relatively reliable predictors of whether a subsequent request for attention would be reinforced. Indeed, in many situations, the discriminative effects of consequences (which depend on how those consequences have in the past related to other reinforcers or punishers) appear to out-weigh any nonstimulus-control effects (for discussion, see Cowie, 2018, 2019; Cowie & Davison, 2016; Cowie et al., 2011; Killeen & Jacobs, 2016, Roscoe et al., 2006; Shahan, 2017); that is, behavior becomes more likely when reinforcers and/or punishers are corre-lated with reinforcers for that behavior in the near future, and less likely when reinforcers and/or punishers are correlated with punishers or no more reinforcers in the near future. Thus, the discriminative effects of reinforcers and punishers might be the best predictors of what impact those consequences will have on behavior.

Consequences and behaviors are discrete events whose relation to subsequent behavior–reinforcer contingencies persists even when the stimulus itself is no longer present. Stimuli that are brief sometimes exert weaker control over responding than do stimuli that are extended in time, but likely only because brief stimuli may be forgot-ten, obscuring the relation between stimulus, response, and reinforcer (see Cowie et al., 2017). Indeed, where such brief events may be artificially extended through memory aids, their control is typically at least as strong as control by an extended stimulus (e.g., Cowie et al., 2011; Cowie & Davison, 2020b); that is, stimulus control depends heavily on how readily the *relation* between stimuli, responses, and their consequences is detected.

Faulty Stimulus Control

Some inappropriate behaviors may be conceptualized as failures of stimulus control; the problem is often with the context in which the behavior occurs rather than the topog-raphy of the behavior itself. Henceforth, we term stimulus control that promotes inap-propriate or maladaptive behaviours *faulty* stimulus control. In this section, we explore several causes of faulty stimulus control.

Adventitious Stimulus Control

Morse and Skinner (1957) described control by stimulus changes that coincided with but did not in fact predict a change in reinforcer conditions. While these effects are almost certainly transient, they underscore the importance of the *apparent* relation between stimuli and reinforcers in the development of stimulus control. Indeed, while practitio-ners and experimenters may arrange a specific stimulus to signal appropriate behavior, such stimuli do not always develop perfect control over behavior. Often, where some other stimulus also changes in approximate accordance with differences in which behav-ior produces reinforcers, control is divided among these different stimuli—for example, the instruction from the therapist *and* the way their hand is positioned. The stimulus that exerts primary control over behavior is not always the one that is arranged to be the most reliable predictor of which behavior will produce a reinforcer (e.g., see Davison & Cowie, 2019; Rayburn-Reeves et al., 2011). Where control is divided, adaptation to changes in the relation between stimuli and responses is often slower (e.g., Cowie et al., 2016b)—that is, transfer of control may be attenuated. Where control is divided among dimensions that are not good predictors of reinforcer availability, this control might be thought of as being faulty. Such faulty control may arise because of error in detecting the relation between stimuli, responses, and reinforcers (e.g., see Bai et al., 2017; Cowie et al., 2011, 2013, 2014, 2016b; Cowie, Gomes-Ng, et al., 2016)—that is, where one stimulus is difficult to detect, discriminate, or remember, other stimuli that are comparatively easier to detect, discriminate, or remember, may *appear* more reliable predictors, and hence may exert relatively stronger control over behavior.

Stimulus Overselectivity

Some stimulus-control failures may result from overselective stimulus control, in that control that is usually divided among different elements of a stimulus is exerted by just one element of a stimulus, leading to a failure to emit (or inhibit) behaviors appropriately. Imagine, for example, trying to locate your red Toyota in a crowded parking lot by looking for a red car—this control by one element of the stimulus (color) would likely result in many attempts to unlock other people's cars. A successful search would require control by multiple dimensions—the color, make, model, and the presence–absence of fluffy dice hanging in the front window. Lovaas et al. (1971) were the first to show selective stimulus control (i.e., stimulus overselectivity) in a clinical population. Since then, many other studies have shown stimulus overselectivity in clinical populations, particularly in individuals with intellectual or developmental disabilities such as ASD (see Lovaas et al., 1979; Ploog, 2010). Other populations in which overselectivity has been found include preschool- and kindergarten-age children (Bickel et al., 1984; Eimas, 1969), older adults ages 60 to 89 (Kelly et al., 2016; McHugh & Reed, 2007; McHugh et al., 2010), individuals with traumatic brain injury (Wayland & Taplin, 1982), and typically developing individuals under high cognitive load (Reed & Gibson, 2005; Reed et al., 2011, 2012).

The failure of behavior to come under the control of multiple stimuli has been linked to deficits across a range of developmental domains, including social, communicative, linguistic (reading, writing, verbal), academic, cognitive, and behavioral development (see Ploog, 2010, for a review). Furthermore, and more generally, the successful acquisition, maintenance, and generalization of behavior depends on control by relevant stimuli and little to no control by irrelevant stimuli. To illustrate, Rincover and Koegel (1975) taught 10 children with ASD a new behavior in a treatment room, and found that the behavior only transferred to a novel context for six of the children because it was under the control of incidental (irrelevant) stimuli in the treatment room, such as the therapist's gestures or furniture (see also Koegel & Rincover, 1976). Thus, selective stimulus control poses a significant challenge for behavior analysts, particularly when interventions require control by multiple stimuli (e.g., in conditional-discrimination tasks such as matching to sample, behavior must be controlled by both the sample and comparison stimuli). Given the potential negative implications of selective stimulus control for the success of behavioral interventions, the applied literature tends to focus less on divided stimulus control per se, and more on the causes and consequences of selective stimulus control.

Research on stimulus overselectivity has proposed two potential theories of overselectivity. The *attention-deficit* account suggests that overselectivity arises because the subject or participant failed to observe and attend to all of the relevant stimuli during discrimination training (e.g., Dube, 2009; Dube & McIlvane, 1999; Dube et al., 1999; Lovaas et al., 1971; Lovaas & Schreibman, 1971). As a result, only the stimuli that were attended to control behavior. According to such an account, overselectivity can be remediated using interventions that encourage or increase attention to all of the stimuli that are relevant to a discrimination. One such intervention involves introducing contingencies for observing.

Dube and McIlvane (1999) arranged an observing intervention for three individuals with IDD, each of whom was trained using a DMTS task in which sample stimuli comprised two elements, and comparison stimuli were individual elements. Stimulus overselectivity was apparent for all three participants during baseline. Then, Dube and McIlvane introduced a differential observing requirement (DOR), whereby participants had to match the compound sample to itself prior to matching one of its elements. This requirement meant that participants had to observe and attend to both elements of the sample. Matching accuracy for all three participants increased during the DOR intervention, indicating that stimulus control was now divided between the compound sample elements. Removal of the DOR contingency resulted in a reduction of accuracy. Thus, the positive effects of the DOR intervention on divided stimulus control did not persist when the intervention was discontinued.

In a similar study, Dube et al. (2010) used an eye-tracking apparatus to measure observing in a two-sample DMTS task, and found that stimulus overselectivity in individuals with IDD was related to failures to observe, or very brief observations of, both elements of the sample stimuli. Therefore, they implemented interventions in which participants were differentially reinforced for observing each stimulus element for at least 0.5 second, or participants were prompted to observe both elements (either vocally, with gestures, or with within-stimulus changes designed to draw attention to the elements, e.g., changes in color or size). In general, these interventions successfully reduced stimulus overselectivity and enhanced control by both stimulus elements (see also Dube et al., 2003). However, whether such effects maintained over time remains unclear.

A second, alternative theory of stimulus overselectivity suggests that subjects do observe and attend to all of the relevant stimuli during training, but this is not always evident in behavioral measures, or may not be expressed behaviorally. In support of this, numerous studies with typically and atypically developing individuals have shown that behavioral control by an underselected stimulus (i.e., a stimulus exerting little to no control) emerges following extinction of the overselected stimulus. In such studies, participants are first trained to choose one compound S+ stimulus over a compound S− stimulus. Then, participants choose between individual S+ and S− elements, and choice of each element is recorded. The most frequently selected S+ element is taken as the overselected element, while the other S+ element is the underselected element. The overselected element undergoes "revaluation" training, in which choice of that element is extinguished and choice of a novel element is reinforced instead. Thereafter, participants are given a choice between the individual elements again, to assess postrevaluation changes in choice of the S+ and S- elements. In general, choice of the overselected element decreases and choice of the underselected element increases after revaluation training, implying a decrease in control and an increase in control by the overselected and underselected elements, respectively. Because the underselected element was never revalued, the emergence of control by that element implies that participants attended to and learned about that element during discrimination training, but this learning was not expressed behaviorally until after revaluation (e.g., Broomfield et al., 2010; Kelly et al., 2015; Reed et al., 2009, 2012; Reynolds & Reed, 2018; Reynolds et al., 2012).

Interestingly, individuals with lower-functioning ASD, and older adults ages 60–89 appear not to show this revaluation effect, suggesting that there are differences in mechanisms of complex stimulus control for these populations (McHugh & Reed, 2007; Reed et al., 2009). However, further research is needed to determine whether there are any differences between clinical and nonclinical populations, or across the lifespan. In any case, it appears that interventions that target observing or attending responses to relevant stimuli, or that manipulate reinforcer contingencies, may be successful in remediating stimulus overselectivity.

Inappropriate Stimulus Generalization

In addition to training novel behaviors, there is an area of practice that addresses the problem of existing stimulus control of a behavior that is faulty or inappropriate (i.e., it is not the topography of the behavior, but the context in which the behavior occurs that is problematic). For example, Fichtner and Tiger (2015) discuss how inappropriate social interactions that are often characteristic of individuals with Angelman syndrome, such as hugging or kissing a stranger, or hugging a family member repeatedly in a short period of time, might be understood not as a problem behavior that needs to be eliminated but as a behavior under poor stimulus control (i.e., hugging and kissing in the presence of a wide range of stimuli rather than in the presence of only specific ones). Certainly, such behaviors can be brought under stronger stimulus control (e.g., Grow et al., 2010; Tiger et al., 2006), and their occurrence in the presence of appropriate stimuli (family) and not in the presence of inappropriate (strangers) transforms the behaviors from inappropriate to appropriate. In another example, Grow et al. (2010) used a multiple schedule to establish appropriate stimulus control of the responding of an adult with IDD who engaged in high-rate social approaches. They alternated between a fixed-ratio (FR) schedule and extinction signaled by the experimenter wearing a sign indicating that they were unavailable to talk. Social approach responses came under control of the visual stimulus, and the schedule was thinned by increasing the duration of the extinction component and decreasing the duration of the FR component. Multiple schedules have also been used to bring behaviors such as children's requests to teachers (Cammilleri et al., 2008), stereotypy (Anderson et al., 2010), and food stealing (Maglieri et al., 2000) under stimulus control.

A final generalization-based example of faulty stimulus control is generalization to the wrong context. Such faulty control occurs when the past context from which generalization occurs invokes behavior that is not appropriate in the present context. For example, Sharp et al. (2019) point out that components of the environment in aged-care homes (the presence of coffee and biscuits, the similarity of the furniture layout to one's own lounge) will determine the extent to which social interactions occur. The less similar the context to one in which social interactions usually occur (and the more similar the context to one in which social interactions are not acceptable), the less likely that space is to occasion social interaction. Understanding how stimulus control contributes to our behavior is fundamental to understanding why behavior occurs, and how it can be changed or maintained.

Despite the effectiveness of multiple schedules in establishing stimulus control, there is some evidence that discrimination between reinforcement and extinction components is difficult to establish in some participants. Heald et al. (2013) found little discrimination in the first 25 sessions of training on a multiple schedule for social approaches in children with Angelman syndrome. Only after a further 10–15 training sessions was discrimination obtained. However, some children did not show strongly differentiated responding. Pizarro et al. (2020) explored factors that might influence discrimination in multiple schedules, finding that color discrimination, and being able to receptively (e.g., "Touch the red card") or expressively (e.g., "What color is this?") identify stimuli were most correlated with discrimination under multiple schedules. Although there is some suggestion that the salience of stimuli might affect responding under multiple schedules (e.g., Saini et al., 2016), for participants with prerequisite discrimination skills, Pizarro et al. (2020) showed little difference in stimulus control when stimuli differed a lot (topographically dissimilar), a little (varied only in color), and when there was a discriminative stimulus but no stimulus correlated with extinction. Therefore, teaching discriminations may require an assessment of prerequisite skills such as visual scanning or the use of a tool such as the Assessment of Basic Learning Abilities (ABLA; Kerr et al., 1977). The ABLA comprises levels of increasingly more difficult discriminations and therefore predicts a person's likely ability to complete particular types of task. In addition to clients for whom discrimination between stimuli may be difficult, there are some populations with whom behavior analysts work and with whom faulty stimulus control is strongly associated with the behavioral phenotype. For example, people with Angelman syndrome often engage in a high rate of social behaviors that can put the person at risk of harm or exploitation (e.g., Fichtner & Tiger, 2015). Additionally, there is a growing body of research to suggest that some problematic behaviors or behaviors in deficit in people with dementia (now called *major neurocognitive disorder*; American Psychiatric Association, 2022) might stem from faulty stimulus control. For example, Gallagher and Keenan (2009) showed deficits in responding on matching-to-sample tasks in people for whom deficits were not detected in more commonly used cognitive tests, and Brogård-Antonsen and Arntzen (2020) showed older adults were less likely to learn conditional discriminations than younger participants. Therefore, an understanding of the behavioral processes responsible for faulty stimulus control facilitates assessment and intervention.

Assessment of Stimulus Control

In addition to identifying and correcting faulty stimulus control, many interventions require an assessment of existing stimulus control prior to implementation, and assessments themselves may benefit from the addition of carefully selected discriminative stimuli. In an experimental functional analysis (Iwata et al., 1994) in which consequences are systematically manipulated to determine their effect on responding, the addition of discriminative stimuli to signal each condition can facilitate differentiated responding across conditions (Connors et al., 2013). Assessments of stimulus control involve identifying the subset of stimuli under which responding occurs. For example, a demand assessment, in which responding to systematically varied demands is recorded, can be used to determine the stimuli under which compliance is least (and most) likely and therefore identify the factors affecting compliance (e.g., task difficulty, preference; e.g., Williams et al., 2020). Dozier et al. (2011) addressed inappropriate sexual behavior related to feet in a man with IDDs by systematically evaluating the particular stimulus characteristics under which the behavior occurred. They found stimulus control by a small subset of stimuli (a woman's foot in sandals), which allowed for a tailored intervention.

Assessments of stimulus control may also allow for a better understanding of the behavioral processes responsible for the transfer of stimulus control. Schussler and Spradlin (1991) taught young adults with IDD to request three-item sets of snacks that were visible in training sessions. They then assessed whether requesting occurred in the absence of all three snacks, in the presence of two out of three snacks, and in the presence of all three snacks. Responses occurred in the absence of one or all of the items, leading Schussler and Spradlin to suggest that stimulus control may have been transferred from initial controlling stimuli (e.g., the model prompt in training) to noncontrolling stimuli (e.g., expectant look from the teacher, sitting at the table). They also offered an alternative explanation to transfer of stimulus control by pairing; that anticipatory responses may be reinforced in the presence of initially noncontrolling stimuli that precede controlling stimuli. The resulting chain of behaviors means that stimuli remote from the terminal reinforcer may have stimulus control. This conceptualization offers an explanation for behaviors for which the antecedent is difficult to identify or that are part of a larger routine. The analysis of precursor behaviors in assessment (those that reliably precede problem behaviors in a response hierarchy and are part of the same response class; e.g., Najdowski et al., 2008) appears congruent with this conceptualization. However, precursor behaviors require more attention with regard to stimulus control.

Summary and Conclusions

Stimulus control is fundamental in determining behavior. Understanding how stimulus control develops, how it is divided among different stimuli, and how it generalizes to novel stimulus contexts is critical to understanding and predicting both appropriate and inappropriate behavior. Research demonstrates that all parts of the three-term contingency—the stimuli, the responses, and the reinforcers—are fundamental to the development of stimulus control. The more different the reinforcer conditions associated with different stimulus context, *and* the more different the stimulus contexts associated with different reinforcer conditions, the greater the potential for stimulus control (e.g., see Davison & Nevin, 1999). Yet it is not enough just to arrange highly differential stimulus conditions; the organism must *detect* the relation between stimulus conditions, responses, and reinforcers in order for such a relation to control behavior. Failures of detection will lead to faulty stimulus control—whether by stimuli that are suboptimal predictors of future reinforcer conditions, by some overly specific element of a stimulus, or by inappropriate generalization across novel stimuli. Indeed, based on the experimental and limited applied research on stimulus salience and disparity, Halbur et al. (2021) made some recommendations for clinical practice including (1) initial discrimination training should involve highly disparate stimuli; (2) verbal antecedent stimuli are also disparate, which can be achieved by removing parts of phrases common to multiple S+'s such as "Find the . . ."; (3) increase the salience of visual stimuli by considering the background; (4) teach a differential observing response to draw attention to the critical features of the S+; and (5) use stimulus fading procedures that gradually reduce over exaggerated critical features of the S+ to the naturally occurring S+. We echo these recommendations here. Stimulus control depends critically on (1) what the organism learns about the relation between stimuli, responses, and reinforcers; and (2) which reinforcers, and hence which stimuli, are valuable to the organism in the present. Stimuli whose relation with reinforcers is more readily detectable—by virtue of the intensity of the stimulus, its disparity with relation to other stimuli, and its relevance in context of the organism's learning history—will have the greatest potential to exert stimulus control over behavior. But at any given moment, control will be divided among stimuli according to how those stimuli correlate with reinforcers of present value to the organism. The greater the ability of a stimulus to signpost a future that satisfies current needs, the greater its control over behavior.

REFERENCES

Allen, K. D., & Fuqua, R. W. (1985). Eliminating selective stimulus control: A comparison of two procedures for teaching mentally retarded children to respond to compound stimuli. *Journal of Experimental Child Psychology, 39*, 55–71.

Alsop, B., & Davison, M. (1991). Effects of varying stimulus disparity and the reinforcer ratio in concurrent-schedule and signal-detection procedures. *Journal of the Experimental Analysis of Behavior, 56*(1), 67–80.

American Psychiatric Association. (2022). *Diagnostic and statistical manual of mental disorders* (5th ed., text rev.). Author.

Ames, L. L., & Yarczower, M. (1965). Some effects of wavelength discrimination on stimulus generalization in the goldfish. *Psychonomic Science, 3*, 311–312.

Anderson, C. M., Doughty, S. S., Doughty, A. H., Williams, D. C., & Saunders, K. J. (2010). Evaluation of stimulus control over a communication response as an intervention for stereotypical responding. *Journal of Applied Behavior Analysis, 43*(2), 333–339.

Baerends, G. P. (1982). The relative effectiveness of different egg-features in responses other than egg retrieval. *Behaviour, 82*(1–4), 225–246.

Bai, J. Y. H., Cowie, S., & Podlesnik, C. A. (2017). Quantitative analysis of local-level resurgence. *Learning and Behavior, 45*, 76–88.

Baron, A. (1973). Postdiscrimination gradients of human subjects on a tone continuum. *Journal of Experimental Psychology, 101*(2), 337–342.

Baron, M. R. (1965). The stimulus, stimulus control and stimulus generalization. In D. I. Mostofsky (Ed.), *Stimulus generalization* (pp. 62–71). Stanford University Press.

Batu, S., Ergenekon, Y., Erbas, D., & Akmanoglu, N. (2004). Teaching pedestrian skills to individuals with developmental disabilities. *Journal of Behavioral Education, 13*(3), 147–164.

Bennett, C. H., Wills, S. J., Wells, J. O., & Mackintosh, N. J. (1994). Reduced generalization following preexposure: Latent inhibition of common elements or a difference in familiarity. *Journal of Experimental Psychology: Animal Behavior Processes, 20*(3), 232–239.

Bickel, W. K., Stella, E., & Etzel, B. C. (1984). A reevaluation of stimulus overselectivity: Restricted stimulus control or stimulus control hierarchies. *Journal of Autism and Developmental Disorders, 14*, 137–157.

Birkimer, J. C. (1969). Control of responding by the elements of a compound discriminative stimulus and by the elements as individual discriminative stimuli. *Journal of the Experimental Analysis of Behavior, 12*, 431–436.

Birnie-Selwyn, B., & Guerin, B. (1997). Teaching children to spell: Decreasing consonant cluster errors by eliminating selective stimulus control. *Journal of Applied Behavior Analysis, 30*, 69–91.

Blough, D. S. (1969). Attention shifts in a maintained discrimination. *Science, 166*, 125–126.

Blough, D. S. (1975). Steady state data and a quantitative model of operant generalization and discrimination. *Journal of Experimental Psychology: Animal Behavior Processes, 1*(1), 3–21.

Blough, P. M. (1972). Wavelength generalization and discrimination in the pigeon. *Perception and Psychophysics, 12*, 342–348.

Born, D. G., & Peterson, J. L. (1969). Stimulus control acquired by components of two color-form compound stimuli. *Journal of the Experimental Analysis of Behavior, 12*, 437–442.

Born, D. G., & Snow, M. E. (1970). Stimulus control by relevant, irrelevant, and redundant components of complex stimuli as assessed by two testing methods. *Psychological Record, 20*, 311–319.

Brogård-Antonsen, A., & Arntzen, E. (2020). Matching-to-sample performance in older and younger adults. *European Journal of Behavior Analysis, 22*(1), 1–18.

Broomfield, L., McHugh, L., & Reed, P. (2008). Re-emergence of under-selected stimuli after the extinction of over-selected stimuli in an automated match to samples procedure. *Research in Developmental Disabilities, 29*(6), 503–512.

Broomfield, L., McHugh, L., & Reed, P. (2010). Factors impacting emergence of behavioral control by underselected stimuli in humans after reduction of control by overselected stimuli. *Journal of the Experimental Analysis of Behavior, 94*, 125–133.

Brush, F. R., Bush, R. R., Jenkins, W. O., John, W. F., & Whiting, J. W. M. (1952). Stimulus generalization after extinction and punishment: An experimental study of displacement. *Journal of Abnormal and Social Psychology, 47*(3), 633–640.

Cammilleri, A. P., Tiger, J. H., & Hanley, G. P. (2008). Developing stimulus control of young children's requests to teachers: Classwide applications of multiple schedules. *Journal of Applied Behavior Analysis, 41*(2), 299–303.

Carp, C. L., Peterson, S. P., Arkel, A. J., Petursdottir, A. I., & Ingvarsson, E. T. (2012). A further evaluation of picture prompts during auditory–visual conditional discrimination training. *Journal of Applied Behavior Analysis, 45*(4), 737–751.

Castro, L., & Wasserman, E. A. (2014). Pigeons' tracking of relevant attributes in categorization learning. *Journal of Experimental Psychology: Animal Learning and Cognition, 40*, 195–211.

Castro, L., & Wasserman, E. A. (2016). Attentional shifts in categorization learning: Perseveration but not learned irrelevance. *Behavioural Processes, 123*, 63–73.

Castro, L., & Wasserman, E. A. (2017). Feature predictiveness and selective attention in pigeons' categorization learning. *Journal of Experimental Psychology: Animal Learning and Cognition, 43*(3), 231–242.

Cengher, M., Budd, A., Farrell, N., & Fienup, D. M. (2018). A review of prompt-fading procedures: Implications for effective and efficient skill acquisition. *Journal of Developmental and Physical Disabilities, 30*(2), 155–173.

Chase, S. (1968). Selectivity in multidimensional stimulus control. *Journal of Comparative and Physiological Psychology, 66*, 787–792.

Chase, S., & Heinemann, E. G. (1972). Choices based on redundant information: An analysis of two-dimensional stimulus control. *Journal of Experimental Psychology, 92*(2), 161–175.

Cheng, K., Shettleworth, S. J., Huttenlocher, J., & Rieser, J. J. (2007). Bayesian integration of spatial information. *Psychological Bulletin, 133*, 625–637.

Cheng, K., & Spetch, M. L. (1998). Mechanisms of landmark use in mammals and birds. In S. Healy (Ed.), *Spatial representation in animals* (pp. 1–17). Oxford University Press.

Cheng, K., Spetch, M. L., & Johnston, M. (1997). Spatial peak shift and generalization in pigeons. *Journal of Experimental Psychology: Animal Behavior Processes, 23*(4), 469–481.

Colavita, F. B. (1974). Human sensory dominance. *Perception and Psychophysics, 16*, 409–412.

Conners, J., Iwata, B. A., Kahng, S., Hanley, G. P., Worsdell, A. S., & Thompson, R. H. (2000). Differential responding in the presence and absence of discriminative stimuli during multielement functional analyses. *Journal of Applied Behavior Analysis, 33*(3), 299–308.

Cowie, S. (2018). Behavioral time travel: Control by past, present, and potential events. *Behavior Analysis: Research and Practice, 18*, 174–183.

Cowie, S. (2019). Some weaknesses of a response-strength account of reinforcer effects. *European Journal of Behavior Analysis, 21*(1), 1–16.

Cowie, S., & Davison, M. (2016). Control by reinforcers across time and space: A review of recent choice research. *Journal of the Experimental Analysis of Behavior. 105*, 246–269.

Cowie, S., & Davison, M. (2020a). Generalizing from the past, choosing the future. *Perspectives on Behavior Science, 43*(2), 245–258.

Cowie, S., & Davison, M. (2020b). Being there on time: Reinforcer effects on timing and locating. *Journal of the Experimental Analysis of Behavior, 113*(2), 340–362.

Cowie, S., & Davison, M. (2022). Choosing a future from a murky past: A generalization-based model of behavior. *Behavioural Processes, 200*, Article 104685.

Cowie, S., Davison, M., Blumhardt, L., & Elliffe, D. (2016a). Does overall reinforcer rate affect discrimination of time-based contingencies? *Journal of the Experimental Analysis of Behavior, 105*, 393–408.

Cowie, S., Davison, M., Blumhardt, L., & Elliffe, D. (2016b). Learning in a changing environment: Effects of the discriminability of visual stimuli and of time. *Learning and Motivation, 56*, 1–14.

Cowie, S., Davison, M., & Elliffe, D. (2011). Reinforcement: Food signals the time and location of future food. *Journal of the Experimental Analysis of Behavior, 96*, 63–86.

Cowie, S., Davison, M., & Elliffe, D. (2014). A model for food and stimulus changes that signal time-based contingency changes. *Journal of the Experimental Analysis of Behavior, 102*, 289–310.

Cowie, S., Davison, M., & Elliffe, D. (2016). A model for discriminating reinforcers in time and space. *Behavioural Processes, 127*, 62–73.

Cowie, S., Davison, M., & Elliffe, D. (2017). Control by past and present stimuli depends on the discriminated reinforcer differential. *Journal of the Experimental Analysis of Behavior, 108*, 184–203.

Cowie, S., Elliffe, D., & Davison, M. (2013). Concurrent schedules: Discriminating reinforcer-ratio reversals at a fixed time after the previous reinforcer. *Journal of the Experimental Analysis of Behavior, 100,* 117–134.

Cowie, S., Gomes-Ng, S., Hopkinson, B., Bai, J. Y. H., & Landon, J. (2020). Stimulus control depends on the subjective value of the outcome. *Journal of the Experimental Analysis of Behavior, 114,* 216–232.

Crawford, L. L., Steele, K. M., & Malone, J. C. (1980). Gradient form and sequential effects during generalization testing in extinction. *Animal Learning and Behavior, 8,* 245–252.

Cuell, S. F., Good, M. A., Dopson, J. C., Pearce, J. M., & Horne, M. R. (2012). Changes in attention to relevant and irrelevant stimuli during spatial learning. *Journal of Experimental Psychology: Animal Behavior Processes, 38,* 244–254.

Cuvo, A. J. (2003). On stimulus generalization and stimulus classes. *Journal of Behavioral Education, 12*(1), 77–83.

Dall, S. R. X., Giraldeau, L., Olsson, O., McNamara, J. M., & Stephens, D. W. (2005). Information and its use by animals in evolutionary ecology. *Trends in Ecology and Evolution, 20,* 187–193.

Danforth, J. S., Chase, P. N., Dolan, M., & Joyce, J. H. (1990). The establishment of stimulus control by instructions and by differential reinforcement. *Journal of the Experimental Analysis of Behavior, 54*(2), 97–112.

Dass, T. K., Kisamore, A. N., Vladescu, J. C., Reeve, K. F., Reeve, S. A., & Taylor-Santa, C. (2018). Teaching children with autism spectrum disorder to tact olfactory stimuli. *Journal of Applied Behavior Analysis, 51*(3), 538–552.

Davison, M. (2018). Divided stimulus control: Which key did you peck, or what color was it? *Journal of the Experimental Analysis of Behavior, 109,* 107–124.

Davison, M., & Cowie, S. (2019). Timing or counting?: Control by contingency reversals at fixed times or numbers of responses. *Journal of Experimental Psychology: Animal Learning and Cognition, 45*(2), 222–241.

Davison, M., & Elliffe, D. (2010). Divided stimulus control: A replication and a quantitative model. *Journal of the Experimental Analysis of Behavior, 94,* 13–23.

Davison, M., & Nevin, J. A. (1999). Stimuli, reinforcers, and behavior: An integration. *Journal of the Experimental Analysis of Behavior, 71,* 439–482.

Delamater, A. R., & Nicolas, D.-M. (2015). Temporal averaging across stimuli signaling the same or different reinforcing outcomes in the peak procedure. *International Journal of Comparative Psychology, 28.*

Didden, R., Prinsen, H., & Sigafoos, J. (2000). The blocking effect of pictorial prompts on sight-word reading. *Journal of Applied Behavior Analysis, 33*(3), 317–320.

Dinsmoor, J. A. (1995). Stimulus control: Part I. *Behavior Analyst, 18,* 51–68.

Dittlinger, L. H., & Lerman, D. C. (2011). Further analysis of picture interference when teaching word recognition to children with autism. *Journal of Applied Behavior Analysis, 44*(2), 341–349.

Dougherty, D. M., & Lewis, P. (1991). Stimulus generalization, discrimination learning, and peak shift in horses. *Journal of the Experimental Analysis of Behavior, 56*(1), 97–104.

Dozier, C. L., Iwata, B. A., & Worsdell, A. S. (2011). Assessment and treatment of foot–shoe fetish displayed by a man with autism. *Journal of Applied Behavior Analysis, 44*(1), 133–137.

Du, Y., McMillan, N., Madan, C. R., Spetch, M. L., & Mou, W. (2017). Cue integration in spatial search for jointly learned landmarks but not for separately learned landmarks. *Journal of Experimental Psychology: Learning, Memory, and Cognition, 43,* 1857–1871.

Dube, W. V. (2009). Stimulus overselectivity in discrimination learning. In P. Reed (Ed.), *Behavioral theories and interventions for autism* (pp. 23–56). Nova.

Dube, W. V., Dickson, C. A., Balsamo, L. M., O'Donnell, K. L., Tomanari, G. Y., Farren, K. M., . . . McIlvane, W. J. (2010). Observing behavior and atypically restricted stimulus control. *Journal of the Experimental Analysis of Behavior, 94,* 297–313.

Dube, W. V., Lombard, K. M., Farren, K. M., Flusser, D., Balsamo, L. M., & Fowler, T. R. (1999). Eye tracking assessment of stimulus overselectivity in individuals with mental retardation. *Experimental Analysis of Human Behaviour Bulletin, 17,* 267–271.

Dube, W. V., Lombard, K. M., Farren, K. M., Flusser, D. S., Balsamo, L. M., & Fowler, T. R. (2003). Stimulus overselectivity and observing behaviour in individuals with mental retardation. In S. Soraci, K. Murata-Soraci, et al. (Eds.), *Visual information processing* (pp. 109–123). Praeger/Greenwood.

Dube, W. V., & McIlvane, W. J. (1997). Reinforcer frequency and restricted stimulus control. *Journal of the Experimental Analysis of Behavior, 68,* 303–316.

Dube, W. V., & McIlvane, W. J. (1999). Reduction of stimulus overselectivity with nonverbal differential observing responses. *Journal of Applied Behavior Analysis, 32,* 25–33.

Eckerman, C. O. (1969). Probability of reinforcement and the development of stimulus control. *Journal of the Experimental Analysis of Behavior, 12*(4), 551–559.

Eimas, P. D. (1969). Multiple-cue discrimination learning in children. *Psychological Record, 19,* 417–424.

Ellis, W. R. (1970). Role of stimulus sequences in stimulus discrimination and stimulus generalization. *Journal of Experimental Psychology, 83*(1), 155.

Fay, R. R. (1970). Auditory frequency generalization in the goldfish (Carassius auratus). *Journal of the Experimental Analysis of Behavior, 14*(3), 353–360.

Fichtner, C. S., & Tiger, J. H. (2015). Teaching discriminated social approaches to individuals with Angelman syndrome. *Journal of Applied Behavior Analysis, 48*(4), 734–748.

Fields, L. (1978). Fading and errorless transfer in successive discriminations. *Journal of the Experimental Analysis of Behavior, 30,* 123–128.

Fields, L. (1979). Acquisition of stimulus control while introducing new stimuli in fading. *Journal of the Experimental Analysis of Behavior, 32,* 121–127.

Fields, L., Bruno, V., & Keller, K. (1976). The stages of acquisition in stimulus fading. *Journal of the Experimental Analysis of Behavior, 26,* 295–300.

Gaiardi, M., Bartoletti, M., Bacchi, A., Gubellini, C., & Babbini, M. (1987). Increased sensitivity to the stimulus properties of morphine in food deprived rats. *Pharmacology Biochemistry and Behavior, 26*(4), 719–723.

Gallagher, S. M., & Keenan, M. (2009). Stimulus equivalence and the Mini Mental Status Examination in the elderly. *European Journal of Behavior Analysis, 10*(2), 159–165.

Ghirlanda, S., & Enquist, M. (2003). A century of generalization. *Animal Behaviour, 66*(1), 15–36.

Gomes-Ng, S., Elliffe, D., & Cowie, S. (2018). Environment tracking and signal following in a reinforcer-ratio reversal procedure. *Behavioural Processes, 157,* 208–224.

Gomes-Ng, S., Elliffe, D., & Cowie, S. (2019). Relative reinforcer rates determine pigeons' attention allocation when separately trained stimuli are presented together. *Learning and Behavior, 47,* 245–257.

Gomes-Ng, S., Elliffe, D., & Cowie, S. (2020). Timing compound stimuli: Relative reinforcer probabilities divide stimulus control in the multiple peak procedure. *Journal of Experimental Psychology: Animal Learning and Cognition, 46,* 124–138.

Gorgan, E. M., & Kodak, T. (2019). Comparison of interventions to treat prompt dependence for children with developmental disabilities. *Journal of Applied Behavior Analysis, 52*(4), 1049–1063.

Grow, L. L., Carr, J. E., Kodak, T. M., Jostad, C. M., & Kisamore, A. N. (2011). A comparison of methods for teaching receptive labeling to children with autism spectrum disorders. *Journal of Applied Behavior Analysis, 44,* 475–498.

Grow, L. L., LeBlanc, L. A., & Carr, J. E. (2010). Developing stimulus control of the high-rate social-approach responses of an adult with mental retardation: A multiple-schedule evaluation. *Journal of Applied Behavior Analysis, 43*(2), 285–289.

Guttman, N., & Kalish, H. I. (1956). Discriminability and stimulus generalization. *Journal of Experimental Psychology, 51*(1), 79–88.

Haber, A., & Kalish, H. I. (1963). Prediction of discrimination from generalization after variations in schedule of reinforcement. *Science, 142*(3590), 412–413.

Halbur, M. E., Caldwell, R. K., & Kodak, T. (2021). Stimulus control research and practice: Considerations of stimulus disparity and salience for discrimination training. *Behavior Analysis in Practice, 14*(1), 272–282.

Hannula, C., Jimenez-Gomez, C., Wu, W., Brewer, A. T., Kodak, T., Gilroy, S. P., . . . Podlesnik, C. A. (2020). Quantifying errors of bias and discriminability in conditional-discrimination performance in children diagnosed with autism spectrum disorder. *Learning and Motivation, 71,* Article 101659.

Hanson, H. M. (1959). Effects of discrimination training on stimulus generalization. *Journal of Experimental Psychology, 58*(5), 321–334.

Heald, M., Allen, D., Villa, D., & Oliver, C. (2013). Discrimination training reduces high rate social approach behaviors in Angelman syndrome: Proof of principle. *Research in Developmental Disabilities, 34*(5), 1794–1803.

Hearst, E. (1968). Discrimination learning as the summation of excitation and inhibition. *Science, 162*(3859), 1303–1306.

Hearst, E., Koresko, M. B., & Poppen, R. (1964). Stimulus generalization and the response-reinforcement contingency. *Journal of the Experimental Analysis of Behavior, 7*(5), 369–380.

Heinemann, E. G., Chase, S., & Mandell, C. (1968). Discriminative control of "attention." *Science, 160*, 553–554.

Hodos, W. (1993). The visual capabilities of birds. In H. P. Ziegler & H.-J. Bischof (Eds.), *Vision, brain, and behavior in birds* (pp. 63–76). MIT Press.

Holz, W. C., & Azrin, N. H. (1961). Discriminative properties of punishment 1. *Journal of the Experimental Analysis of Behavior, 4*(3), 225–232.

Homa, D., Sterling, S., & Trepel, L. (1981). Limitations of exemplar-based generalization and the abstraction of categorical information. *Journal of Experimental Psychology: Human Learning and Memory, 7*(6), 418–439.

Honig, W. K., & Slivka, R. M. (1964). Stimulus generalization of the effects of punishment. *Journal of the Experimental Analysis of Behavior, 7*(1), 21–25.

Honig, W. K., Thomas, D. R., & Guttman, N. (1959). Differential effects of continuous extinction and discrimination training on the generalization gradient. *Journal of Experimental Psychology, 58*(2), 145–152.

Honig, W. K., & Urcuioli, P. J. (1981). The legacy of Guttman and Kalish (1956): 25 years of research on stimulus generalization. *Journal of the Experimental Analysis of Behavior, 36*(3), 405–445.

Iwata, B. A., Dorsey, M. F., Slifer, K. J., Bauman, K. E., & Richman, G. S. (1994). Toward a functional analysis of self-injury. *Journal of Applied Behavior Analysis, 27*(2), 197–209.

Jenkins, W. O., Pascal, G. R., & Walker, R. W. Jr. (1958). Deprivation and generalization. *Journal of Experimental Psychology, 56*(3), 274–277.

Johnson, D. F. (1970). Determiners of selective stimulus control in the pigeon. *Journal of Comparative and Physiological Psychology, 70*, 298–307.

Johnson, D. F., & Cumming, W. W. (1968). Some determiners of attention. *Journal of the Experimental Analysis of Behavior, 11*, 157–166.

Johnston, J. M. (1979). On the relation between generalization and generality. *Behavior Analyst, 2*, 1–6.

Kalish, H. I. (1958). The relationship between discriminability and generalization: A re-evaluation. *Journal of Experimental Psychology, 55*(6), 637–644.

Kamin, L. J. (1969). Predictability, surprise, attention, and conditioning. In B. A. Campbell & R. M. Church (Eds.), *Punishment and aversive behavior* (pp. 279–296). Appleton-Century-Crofts.

Kehoe, E. J. (1986). Summation and configuration in conditioning of the rabbit's nictating membrane response to compound stimuli. *Journal of Experimental Psychology: Animal Behavior Processes, 12*(2), 186–195.

Kelly, M. P., Leader, G., & Reed, P. (2015). Stimulus over-selectivity and extinction-induced recovery of performance as a product of intellectual impairment and autism severity. *Journal of Autism and Developmental Disorders, 45*, 3098–3106.

Kelly, M. P., Leader, G., & Reed, P. (2016). Factors producing over-selectivity in older individuals. *Age, 38*, Article 63.

Kerr, N., Meyerson, L., Flora, J., Tharinger, D., Schallert, D., Casey, L., & Fehr, M. J. (1977). The measurement of motor, visual and auditory discrimination skills in mentally retarded children and adults and in young normal children. *Rehabilitation Psychology, 24*(3), 91–206.

Killeen, P. R., & Jacobs, K. W. (2016). Coal is not black, snow is not white, food is not a reinforcer: The roles of affordances and dispositions in the analysis of behavior. *Behavior Analyst, 40*, 17–38.

Kirby, K. C., & Bickel, W. K. (1988). Toward an explicit analysis of generalization: A stimulus control interpretation. *Behavior Analyst, 11*(2), 115–129.

Kisamore, A. N., Karsten, A. M., & Mann, C. C. (2016). Teaching multiply controlled intraverbals to children and adolescents with autism spectrum disorders. *Journal of Applied Behavior Analysis, 49*(4), 826–847.

Klosterhalfen, S., Fischer, W., & Bitterman, M. E. (1978). Modification of attention in honey bees. *Science, 201*, 1241–1243.

Koegel, R. L., & Rincover, A. (1976). Some detrimental effects of using extra stimuli to guide learning in normal and autistic children. *Journal of Abnormal Child Psychology, 4*, 59–71.

Köhler, W. (1939). Simple structural functions in the chimpanzee and in the chicken. In W. D. Ellis (Ed.), *A source book of Gestalt psychology* (pp. 217–227). Harcourt Brace Jovanovich.

Kraemer, P. J., & Roberts, W. A. (1985). Short-term memory for simultaneously presented visual and auditory signals in the pigeon. *Journal of Experimental Psychology: Animal Behavior Processes, 11*, 137–151.

Krägeloh, C. U., Davison, M., & Elliffe, D. M. (2005). Local preference in concurrent schedules: The effects of reinforcer sequences. *Journal of the Experimental Analysis of Behavior, 84*(1), 37–64.

Lalli, J. S., Mace, F. C., Livezey, K., & Kates, K. (1998). Assessment of stimulus generalization gradients in the treatment of self-injurious behavior. *Journal of Applied Behavior Analysis, 31*(3), 479–483.

Lamb, M. R. (1991). Attention in humans and animals: Is there a capacity limitation at the time of encoding? *Journal of Experimental Psychology: Animal Behavior Processes, 17,* 45–54.

Lashley, K. S., & Wade, M. (1946). The Pavlovian theory of generalization. *Psychological Review, 53*(2), 72–87.

Leader, G., Loughnane, A., McMoreland, C., & Reed, P. (2009). The effect of stimulus salience on over-selectivity. *Journal of Autism and Developmental Disorders, 39,* 330–338.

Legge, E. L. G., Madan, C. R., Spetch, M. L., & Ludvig, E. A. (2016). Multiple cue use and integration in pigeons (Columba livia). *Animal Cognition, 19,* 581–591.

Leith, C. R., & Maki, W. S. (1975). Attention shifts during matching-to-sample performance in pigeons. *Animal Learning and Behavior, 3,* 85–89.

Li, M., Garner, W. D., Wessinger, H. R., & McMillan, D. E. (1995). Effects off food deprivation and satiation on sensitivity to the discriminative-stimulus effects of pentobarbital in pigeons and morphine in rats. *Behavioural Pharmacology, 6*(7), 724–731.

Lin, F. Y., & Zhu, J. (2020). Comparison of two discrimination methods in teaching Chinese children with autism. *Journal of Applied Behavior Analysis, 53*(2), 1145–1152.

Lotfizadeh, A. D., Edwards, T. L., Redner, R., & Poling, A. (2012). Motivating operations affect stimulus control: A largely overlooked phenomenon in discrimination learning. *Behavior Analyst, 35,* 89–100.

Lovaas, O. I., Koegel, R. L., & Schreibman, L. (1979). Stimulus overselectivity in autism: A review of research. *Psychological Bulletin, 86,* 1236–1254.

Lovaas, O. I., & Schreibman, L. (1971). Stimulus overselectivity of autistic children in a two stimulus situation. *Behaviour Research and Therapy, 9,* 305–310.

Lovaas, O. I., Schreibman, L., Koegel, R., & Rehm, R. (1971). Selective responding by autistic children to multiple sensory input. *Journal of Abnormal Psychology, 77,* 211–222.

Mackintosh, N. J., Kaye, H., & Bennett, C. H. (1991). Perceptual learning in flavour aversion conditioning. *Quarterly Journal of Experimental Psychology B, 43*(3), 297–322.

Mackintosh, N. J., & Little, L. (1969). Intradimensional and extradimensional shift learning by pigeons. *Psychonomic Science, 14,* 5–6.

Maglieri, K. A., DeLeon, I. G., Rodriguez-Catter, V., & Sevin, B. M. (2000). Treatment of covert food stealing in an individual with Prader–Willi syndrome. *Journal of Applied Behavior Analysis, 33*(4), 615–618.

Maki, W. S., & Leith, C. R. (1973). Shared attention in pigeons. *Journal of the Experimental Analysis of Behavior, 19,* 345–349.

Maki, W. S., & Leuin, T. C. (1972). Information-processing by pigeons. *Science, 176,* 535–536.

Matell, M. S., & Kurti, A. N. (2014). Reinforcement probability modulates temporal memory selection and integration processes. *Acta Psychologica, 147,* 80–91.

McHugh, L., & Reed, P. (2007). Age trends in stimulus overselectivity. *Journal of the Experimental Analysis of Behavior, 88,* 369–380.

McHugh, L., Simpson, A., & Reed, P. (2010). Mindfulness as a potential intervention for stimulus over-selectivity in older adults. *Research in Developmental Disabilities, 31,* 178–184.

Miles, C. M., & Jenkins, H. M. (1973). Overshadowing in operant conditioning as a function of discriminability. *Learning and Motivation, 4,* 11–27.

Miller, J. T., Saunders, S. S., & Bourland, G. (1980). The role of stimulus disparity in concurrently available reinforcement schedules. *Animal Learning and Behavior, 8*(4), 635–641.

Miranda-Dukoski, L., Davison, M., & Elliffe, D. (2014). Choice, time and food: Continuous cyclical changes in food probability between reinforcers. *Journal of the Experimental Analysis of Behavior, 101*(3), 406–421.

Morse, W., & Skinner, B. F. (1957). A second type of superstition in the pigeon. *The American Journal of Psychology, 70*(2), 308–311.

Munoz, N. E., & Blumstein, D. T. (2012). Multisensory perception in uncertain environments. *Behavioral Ecology, 23,* 457–462.

Najdowski, A. C., Wallace, M. D., Ellsworth, C. L., MacAleese, A. N., & Cleveland, J. M. (2008). Functional analyses and treatment of precursor behavior. *Journal of Applied Behavior Analysis, 41*(1), 97–105.

Ohinata, S. (1979). Postdiscrimination shift of the goldfish (*Carassius auratus*) on a visual wavelength continuum. *Annual of Animal Psychology, 28*(2), 113–122.

O'Neill, G. W., Blanck, L. S., & Joyner, M. A. (1980). The use of stimulus control over littering in a natural setting. *Journal of Applied Behavior Analysis, 13*(2), 379–381.

Pavlov, I. P. (1927). *Conditioned reflexes.* Oxford University Press.

Perone, M., & Courtney, K. (1992). Fixed-ratio pausing: Joint effects of past reinforcer magnitude and stimuli correlated with upcoming magnitude. *Journal of the Experimental Analysis of Behavior, 57*(1), 33–46.

Peterson, N. (1962). Effect of monochromatic rearing on the control of responding by wavelength. *Science, 136*(3518), 774–775.

Phillips, C. L., Vollmer, T. R., & Porter, A. (2019). An evaluation of textual prompts and generalized textual instruction-following. *Journal of Applied Behavior Analysis, 52*(4), 1140–1160.

Pinto, C., Fortes, I., & Machado, A. (2017). Joint stimulus control in a temporal discrimination task. *Animal Cognition, 20*, 1129–1136.

Pinto, C., & Machado, A. (2017). Unraveling sources of stimulus control in a temporal discrimination task. *Learning and Behavior, 45*, 20–28.

Pizarro, E. M., Vollmer, T. R., & Morris, S. L. (2020). Evaluating skills correlated with discriminated responding in multiple schedule arrangements. *Journal of Applied Behavior Analysis, 54*, 334 –345.

Ploog, B. O. (2010). Stimulus overselectivity four decades later: A review of the literature and its implications for current research in autism spectrum disorder. *Journal of Autism and Developmental Disorders, 40*, 1332–1349.

Ploog, B. O. (2011). Selective attention to visual compound stimuli in squirrel monkeys (Saimiri sciureus). *Behavioural Processes, 87*, 115–124.

Ploog, B. O., & Williams, B. A. (2010). Serial discrimination reversal learning in pigeons as a function of intertrial interval and delay of reinforcement. *Learning and Behavior, 38*, 96–102.

Podlesnik, C. A., Thrailkill, E., & Shahan, T. A. (2012). Differential reinforcement and resistance to change of divided-attention performance. *Learning and Behavior, 40*, 158–169.

Posner, M. I., Nissen, M. J., & Klein, R. M. (1976). Visual dominance: An information-processing account of its origins and significance. *Psychological Review, 83*, 157–171.

Randich, A., Klein, R. M., & LoLordo, V. M. (1978). Visual dominance in the pigeon. *Journal of the Experimental Analysis of Behavior, 30*, 129–137.

Rayburn-Reeves, R. M., Molet, M., & Zentall, T. R. (2011). Simultaneous discrimination reversal learning in pigeons and humans: Anticipatory and perseverative errors. *Learning and Behavior, 39*, 125–137.

Rayburn-Reeves, R. M., Qadri, M. A. J., Brooks, D. I., Keller, A. M., & Cook, R. G. (2017). Dynamic cue use in pigeon mid-session reversal. *Behavioural Processes, 137*, 53–63.

Reed, P., Broomfield, L., McHugh, L., McCausland, A., & Leader, G. (2009). Extinction of over-selected stimuli causes emergence of under-selected cues in higher-functioning children with autistic spectrum disorders. *Journal of Autism and Developmental Disorders, 39*, 290–298.

Reed, P., & Gibson, E. (2005). The effect of concurrent task load on stimulus over-selectivity. *Journal of Autism and Developmental Disorders, 35*, 601–614.

Reed, P., Petrina, N., & McHugh, L. (2011). Over-selectivity as a learned response. *Research in Developmental Disabilities, 32*(1), 201–206.

Reed, P., Reynolds, G., & Fermandel, L. (2012). Revaluation manipulations produce emergence of underselected stimuli following simultaneous discrimination in humans. *Quarterly Journal of Experimental Psychology, 65*, 1345–1360.

Reynolds, G. S. (1961). Attention in the pigeon. *Journal of the Experimental Analysis of Behavior, 4*, 203–208.

Reynolds, G., & Reed, P. (2011). Effects of schedule of reinforcement on over-selectivity. *Research in Developmental Disabilities, 32*, 2489–2501.

Reynolds, G., & Reed, P. (2018). The effect of stimulus duration on over-selectivity: Evidence for the role of within-compound associations. *Journal of Experimental Psocyhology: Animal Learning and Cognition, 44*(3), 293–308.

Reynolds, G., Watts, J., & Reed, P. (2012). Lack of evidence for inhibitory processes in over-selectivity. *Behavioural Processes, 89*, 14–22.

Richardson, A. R., Lerman, D. C., Nissen, M. A., Luck, K. M., Neal, A. E., Bao, S., & Tsami, L.

(2017). Can pictures promote the acquisition of sight-word reading?: An evaluation of two potential instructional strategies. *Journal of Applied Behavior Analysis, 50*(1), 67–86.

Rincover, A. (1978). Variables affecting stimulus fading and discriminative responding in psychotic children. *Journal of Abnormal Psychology, 87,* 541–553.

Rincover, A., & Koegel, R. L. (1975). Setting generality and stimulus control in autistic children. *Journal of Applied Behavior Analysis, 8,* 235–246.

Rosch, E., Mervis, C. B., Gray, W. D., Johnson, D. M., & Boyes-Braem, P. (1976). Basic objects in natural categories. *Cognitive Psychology, 8*(3), 382–439.

Roscoe, E. M., Fisher, W. W., Glover, A. C., & Volkert, V. M. (2006). Evaluating the relative effects of feedback and contingent money for staff training of stimulus preference assessments. *Journal of Applied Behavior Analysis, 39*(1), 63–77.

Rubel, E. W., & Rosenthal, M. H. (1975). The ontogeny of auditory frequency generalization in the chicken. *Journal of Experimental Psychology: Animal Behavior Processes, 1*(4), 287–297.

Rubi, T. L., & Stephens, D. W. (2016a). Does multimodality per se improve receiver performance?: An explicit comparison of multimodal versus unimodal complex signals in a learned signal following task. *Behavioral Ecology and Sociobiology, 70,* 409–416.

Rubi, T. L., & Stephens, D. W. (2016b). Should receivers follow multiple signal components?: An economic perspective. *Behavioral Ecology, 27,* 36–44.

Rubi, T. L., & Stephens, D. W. (2016c). Why complex signals matter, sometimes. In M. A. Bee & C. T. Miller (Eds.), *Psychological mechanisms in animal communication* (pp. 119–135). Springer International.

Saini, V., Miller, S. A., & Fisher, W. W. (2016). Multiple schedules in practical application: Research trends and implications for future investigation. *Journal of Applied Behavior Analysis, 49*(2), 421–444.

Schmidt, K. A., Dall, S. R. X., & Van Gils, J. A. (2010). The ecology of information: An overview on the ecological significance of making informed decisions. *Oikos, 119,* 304–316.

Schnell, L. K., Vladescu, J. C., Kisamore, A. N., DeBar, R. M., Kahng, S., & Marano, K. (2020). Assessment to identify learner-specific prompt and prompt-fading procedures for children with autism spectrum disorder. *Journal of Applied Behavior Analysis, 53*(2), 1111–1129.

Schreibman, L., Charlop, M. H., & Koegel, R. L. (1982). Teaching autistic children to use extrastimulus prompts. *Journal of Experimental Child Psychology, 33,* 475–491.

Schussler, N. G., & Spradlin, J. E. (1991). Assessment of stimuli controlling the requests of students with severe mental retardation during a snack routine. *Journal of Applied Behavior Analysis, 24*(4), 791–797.

Seligman, M. E. (1970). On the generality of the laws of learning. *Psychological Review, 77,* 406–418.

Shahan, T. A. (2017). Moving beyond reinforcement and response strength. *Behavior Analyst, 40,* 107–121.

Shahan, T. A., & Podlesnik, C. A. (2006). Divided attention performance and the matching law. *Learning and Behavior, 34,* 255–261.

Shahan, T. A., & Podlesnik, C. A. (2007). Divided attention and the matching law: Sample duration affects sensitivity to reinforcement allocation. *Learning and Behavior, 35,* 141–148.

Shanks, D. R. (1995). *The psychology of associative learning.* Cambridge University Press.

Sharp, R. A., Williams, E., Rörnes, R., Lau, C. Y., & Lamers, C. (2019). Lounge layout to facilitate communication and engagement in people with dementia. *Behavior Analysis in Practice, 12*(3), 637–642.

Skinner, B. F. (1969). *Contingencies of reinforcement.* Prentice Hall.

Song, C. J., Vladescu, J. C., Reeve, K. F., Miguel, C. F., & Breeman, S. L. (2021). The influence of correlations between noncritical features and reinforcement on stimulus generalization. *Journal of Applied Behavior Analysis, 54*(1), 346–366.

Spetch, M. L. (1995). Overshadowing in landmark learning: Touch-screen studies with pigeons and humans. *Journal of Experimental Psychology: Animal Behavior Processes, 21,* 166–181.

Spetch, M. L., & Wilkie, D. M. (1994). Pigeons' use of landmarks presented in digitized images. *Learning and Motivation, 25,* 245–275.

Stokes, T. F., & Baer, D. M. (1977). An implicit technology of generalization 1. *Journal of Applied Behavior Analysis, 10*(2), 349–367.

Sutherland, N. S., & Holgate, V. (1966). Two-cue discrimination learning in rats. *Journal of Comparative and Physiological Psychology, 61*, 198–207.

Terrace, H. S. (1971). Escape from S–. *Learning and Motivation, 2*(2), 148–163.

Thomas, D. R., & King, R. A. (1959). Stimulus generalization as a function of level of motivation. *Journal of Experimental Psychology, 57*(5), 323–328.

Tiger, J. H., & Hanley, G. P. (2005). An example of discovery research involving the transfer of stimulus control. *Journal of Applied Behavior Analysis, 38*(4), 499–509.

Tiger, J. H., Hanley, G. P., & Heal, N. A. (2006). The effectiveness of and preschoolers' preferences for variations of multiple schedule arrangements. *Journal of Applied Behavior Analysis, 39*(4), 475–488.

Tinbergen, N., Kruuk, H., & Paillette, M. (1962). Egg shell removal by the black-headed gull (Larus r. ridibundus L.) II: The effects of experience on the response to colour. *Bird Study, 9*(2), 123–131.

Touchette, P. E., & Howard, J. S. (1984). Errorless learning: Reinforcement contingencies and stimulus control transfer in delayed prompting. *Journal of Applied Behavior Analysis, 17*(2), 175–188.

Uengoer, M., & Lachnit, H. (2012). Modulation of attention in discrimination learning: The roles of stimulus relevance and stimulus–outcome correlation. *Learning and Behavior, 40*, 117–127.

Wagner, A. R. (1969). Stimulus validity and stimulus selection. In W. K. Honig & N. J. Mackintosh (Eds.), *Fundamental issues in associative learning* (pp. 90–122). Dalhousie University Press.

Wagner, A. R. (1971). Elementary associations. In H. H. Kendler & J. T. Spence (Eds.), *Essays in neobehaviorism: A memorial volume to Kenneth W. Spence* (pp. 187–213). Appleton-Century-Crofts.

Walker, D. J., & Branch, M. N. (1998). Effects of variable-interval value and amount of training on stimulus generalization. *Journal of the Experimental Analysis of Behavior, 70*(2), 139–163.

Wasserman, E. A., & Miller, R. R. (1997). What's elementary about associative learning? *Annual Review of Psychology, 48*, 573–607.

Wayland, S., & Taplin, J. E. (1982). Nonverbal categorization in fluent and nonfluent anomic aphasics. *Brain and Language, 16*, 87–108.

Weiss, S. J. (1972). Stimulus compounding in free-operant and classical conditioning: A review and analysis. *Psychological Bulletin, 78*(3), 189–208.

White, K. G. (1986). Conjoint control of performance in conditional discriminations by successive and simultaneous stimuli. *Journal of the Experimental Analysis of Behavior, 45*, 161–174.

Williams, E. E., Sharp, R. A., & Lamers, C. (2020). An assessment method for identifying acceptable and effective ways to present demands to an adult with dementia. *Behavior Analysis in Practice, 13*(2), 473–478.

PART V

ADVANCED TOPICS
IN TRANSLATIONAL RESEARCH

CHAPTER 15

Motivation as a Platform
for Translational Research

Michael E. Kelley
Dana M. Gadaire
Andrew R. Craig

The term *motivation* for human behavior has deep roots in philosophy and science. As with many philosophical and scientific linchpins, it may not be surprising to learn that the Greek philosopher Aristotle proposed one of the first theories of motivation. Aristotle hypothesized that human motivation was produced by an "appetitive" function—curiously similar language to that used by B. F. Skinner (1938, 1953). Like Skinner, Aristotle suggested that motivation, or the appetitive function, operated to produce a particular outcome:

> [Appetite and mind] . . . are capable of originating local movement . . . mind, that is, which calculates means to an end . . . while appetite is in every form of it relative to an end . . . for that which is the object of appetite is the stimulant of mind practical. . . . And that which is last in the process of thinking is the beginning of the action . . . there is a justification for regarding these two as the sources of movement . . . for the object of appetite start a movement and as a result of that thought gives rise to movement, the object of appetite being a source of stimulation. (Aristotle, 350 B.C.E.)

In Aristotle's understanding of motivation, the anticipated outcome—or consequence—served as the stimulation to engage in "movement" to access or avoid the consequence. Aristotle interpreted the anticipated outcomes and subsequent movements as a dynamic interaction of mind and body. Of course, the starting point of a behavior-analytic interpretation of motivation lies in our capacity to operationally define *motivation* itself, including the conditions under which we might say that motivation is present or absent and the environmental situations that affect it. More specifically, behavior analysts are most likely to describe antecedent conditions that changed the value of some environmental event, and thus changed the frequency of behavior related to that event (Michael, 1982, 1993, 1988, 1993a, 1993b, 2000). Behavior analysts use this information primarily to predict and control future behavior.

The behavior-analytic language around motivation can be confusing without an understanding of the historical development of the terms and the relevant research. Keller and Schoenfeld (1950) and Millenson (1967) established and popularized the term *establishing operation* (EO) to describe events that affect motivation (Laraway et al., 2003). Subsequently, Jack Michael spent a substantial part of his career further refining and discussing the concept of the EO in a series of influential papers (Michael, 1982, 1993, 1988, 1993a, 1993b, 2000). Arguably, the most important conceptual development following the emergence of these EO refinements is in the clear distinction between *discriminative stimuli* (S^D; events that influence behavior as a function of correlations with particular consequences, e.g., reinforcement, punishment, and extinction) and *motivational events* (events that influence behavior as a function of changes in the value of consequences).

Michael noted that both S^{D}s and EOs alter the future probability of behavior; however, their behavioral mechanisms—the basic principles at play—are very different. Michael described the conceptual and practical differences between the discriminative and motivational nature of stimuli, which produced a sea change in how behavior analysts—especially applied behavior analysts—interpret and manipulate antecedent stimuli to either evoke or abate behavior. In a sense, Michael provided a new behavioral framework for interpreting motivational variables.

Michael (1982) described discriminative stimuli as stimuli that "(1) given the momentary effectiveness of some particular type of reinforcement (2) increases the frequency of a particularly type of response (3) because the stimulus condition has been correlated with an increase in the frequency with which that type of response has been followed by that type of reinforcement" (p. 149). Motivating operations are involved in the first part of this definition—they determine the momentary effectiveness of a reinforcer (or punisher). Discriminative stimuli signal contingencies. Motivating operations determine the extent to which those contingencies affect behavior. We do not wish to belabor the point, but we discuss various findings from the behavior-analytic literature that may be interpreted from the lens of either discrimination or motivation. It is important to convey at the outset that both of these variables are important components of the antecedent situations that give rise to operant behavior.

In summary, Michael's conceptual framework (which appears frequently in applied practice and research) involves three terms. *Establishing operation* (EO), as defined by Michael (1982), refers to the environmental events, operations, or stimulus conditions that affect an organism's behavior by altering (1) the reinforcing or punishing effectiveness of other environmental events and (2) the frequency of occurrence of that part of the organism's repertoire relevant to those events as consequences. Michael intended EO to serve as an omnibus term, and to include both operations that establish (i.e., increase) and abolish (i.e., decrease) motivation with concomitant evocative and abative effects on future behavior (Laraway et al., 2003). However, over time, clinicians, researchers, and practitioners have gravitated toward using the term *EO* in reference to operations designed to increase motivation and increase the future probability of behavior. The second important term, *abolishing operation* (AO), references operations designed to decrease motivation and decrease the future probability of behavior. Finally, the truly omnibus term *motivating operation* (MO) subsumes both EOs and AOs. The term *MO* specifies alteration of motivation and the frequency of behavior but does not imply a valence (Michael, 1982).

The general purpose of this chapter is to shed light on how both basic and applied research on motivation interact to discover basic principles, translate basic principles into practice, and establish new lines of both basic and applied research. Many authors have defined and described *translational research* and its potential value (e.g., Critchfield, 2011; DeLeon, 2011; Mace, 1994; Mace & Critchfield, 2010; Pilgrim, 2011; Podlesnik, 2013; Vollmer, 2011; Vyse, 2013), including in this text (Chapter 2, this volume), and a broad discussion of the dynamics and variations of translational research is beyond the scope of the chapter.

In this chapter, *translational research* refers to the dynamic interplay between basic and applied researchers, and includes clear potential impact of basic research on application, or application that sets the occasion for future basic research. We highlight the importance of cross-fertilized basic and applied research, and advocate for coordinated, purposeful translational research as a primary means for improving behavior analytic research and practice—in the context of motivation. Thus, in the remainder of this chapter, we (1) highlight existing relevant basic and applied motivation research, (2) discuss a path for basic and applied research to refine Michael's concept of the *conditioned motivating operation* (CMO), and (3) suggest some areas of translational research for refining conceptual systems (basic principles) and technology development (practice). Along the way, we introduce research that has been dedicated specifically to MOs and CMOs (when such research exists) and present other, related lines of research for readers to consider.

The Influence of Basic Research on Practice in Motivation

One defining factor of behavior analysis involves its use of single-subject research design in which each subject serves as their own control (Cooper et al., 2020). This is one of the first concepts taught to aspiring behavior analysts. In a general sense, this means that in many behavior-analytic experiments, there is no control group (Baer, 1977); rather, behavior analysts attempt to control behavior at the level of the response class (Johnston & Pennypacker, 1980). In a practical sense, behavior analysts first arrange at least two conditions (a test condition, with independent variable present, and a control condition, with independent variable absent), then compare the levels of responding in each condition by alternating back and forth between them. Basic researchers have used this design—the multiple schedule—in countless experimental arrangements. For example, a pairwise comparison (Henry et al., 2021; Iwata, Duncan, et al., 1994; Vollmer et al., 1995), often utilized during assessment of severe problem behavior in the context of a functional analysis (Iwata et al., 1982; Iwata, Duncan, et al., 1994), might include a test condition in which an individual is deprived of attention, with attention delivered contingent on a target behavior. In the control condition, the therapist might deliver attention on a continuous basis, or on a very rich fixed-time schedule, such as a fixed-time (FT) 15 schedule.

In the previous hypothetical example, the therapist contrived a specific motivational arrangement in each condition, each with an intended effect. In the test condition, the therapist arranged an environmental event (deprivation of attention) intended to affect the individual's behavior by increasing the reinforcing effectiveness of attention and thus the frequency of behavior relevant to attention (increased probability). In the control condition, the therapist arranged an environmental event (access to attention) intended to affect the individual's behavior by reducing the reinforcing effectiveness of attention and thus the frequency of behavior relevant to attention (decreased probability).

The pairwise arrangement described earlier is a very simple instructive example of the powerful effects of motivating operations. However, there are other examples of basic and translational research on motivation that have had profound impacts on behavior-analytic practice involving a broad range of behaviors and motivating conditions. In an early example of this research, Clark (1958) studied the effects of an MO, food-deprivation level, on food-motivated bar pressing in rats. Across different conditions, Clark arranged different variable-interval (VI) schedules, and he manipulated deprivation level by giving the rats more or less time to eat across conditions. Regardless of the reinforcement schedule that was arranged, Clark found that rates of lever pressing were negatively related to the amount of time the rats were given to eat; that is, rats pressed the lever more frequently when they were allowed to eat for short periods of time each day and pressed less frequently when they were allowed to eat for long periods of time.

This and other examples of research on motivation from the laboratory set the occasion for research exploring the effects of MOs on behavior in practice settings. Vollmer and Iwata (1991) showed how MOs (deprivation and satiation) affected engagement in arbitrarily selected behaviors for five individuals diagnosed with developmental disabilities. In general, deprivation increased responding relative to baseline, and satiation operations decreased responding relative to baseline. These data showed the power of simple environmental arrangements, in the context of either restricting or providing access to reinforcers, on arbitrarily selected responses. However, these translational data laid the groundwork for future behavior-analytic research in which behaviors of social significance can be exposed to conceptually identical operations to either increase or decrease the likelihood of behavior.

Vollmer et al. (1993) followed up on this translational research with the application of these basic principles for treating self-injurious behavior (SIB) maintained by contingent access to attention. In doing so, they linked basic results showing response suppression during time-based reinforcer delivery to clinical treatments for severe problems of social significance. Specifically, Vollmer et al. exposed SIB to both differential reinforcement of other behavior (DRO) and noncontingent reinforcement (NCR).

Vollmer et al. (1993) used the term NCR to refer to the time-based delivery of reinforcers; that is, the delivery of attention was contingent on the passage of time, not on the occurrence of behavior. As an intervention, NCR operates identically to an AO. In other words, the experimenters arranged an environmental event (access to attention) intended to affect the individual's behavior by altering the reinforcing effectiveness of attention (less effective) and thus the frequency of behavior relevant to attention (decreased probability). In application, Vollmer et al. demonstrated how an antecedent manipulation such as noncontingent access to attention could function as a powerful treatment to decrease SIB. This motivating operation, NCR, has been used in the voluminous research studies and clinical practice since 1993.

The link to basic research for the use of NCR as treatment is clear in the authors' introduction to the study; that is, Vollmer et al. (1993) invoked basic research comparing DRO and NCR, and noted that applied research also utilizes the noncontingent delivery of positive reinforcers as a contingency reversal technique for demonstrating experimental control (Azrin et al., 1968; Buell et al., 1968; Rescorla & Stucy, 1968).

Conditioned Motivating Operations

In *Concepts and Principles of Behavior Analysis,* Jack Michael (1993b) not only delineated an elegant framework for motivation, but he also elucidated how unconditioned and conditioned reinforcers could be integrated into that framework. For example, humans do not require a learning history for food, water, and air to serve as effective consequences for behavior; these stimuli are *unconditioned reinforcers*. Analogously, humans do not require a learning history for *unconditioned establishing operations* (UEOs)[1] to alter the value of reinforcers and the frequency of behavior related to those reinforcers. *Conditioned reinforcers* require a learning history for those stimuli to serve as effective consequences for reinforcing behavior. Analogously, humans require a learning history for *conditioned establishing operations* (CEOs) to alter the value of reinforcers and the frequency of behavior related to those reinforcers.

UEOs share a straightforward connection to deprivation, satiation, temperature change, and other unlearned stimuli (e.g., painful stimuli); that is, environmental events such as deprivation of water and food (unconditioned reinforcers) alter the reinforcing value of water and food, and behavior related to water and food becomes more probable.

CEOs, on the other hand, are more complex and reflect the vast influence of learning history on the establishment of conditioned reinforcers. An in-depth discussion of the provenance of conditioned reinforcers is beyond the scope of this chapter. However, to set the stage for Michael's framework for CEOs, we define *conditioned reinforcers* as previously neutral stimuli that acquire the capacity to function as reinforcers due to a learning history relative to other unconditioned or conditioned reinforcers. For example, the on-task behavior of children in a classroom may not change much if the teacher were to deliver poker chips for instances work completion, attentive listening, or instructions following. If those poker chips were paired with and exchangeable for preferred items (e.g., school supplies, small toys), however, they might come to increase on-task behavior in much the same way that delivering the preferred items themselves would.

Analogously, CEOs are previously neutral events that acquire the capacity to function as establishing operations due to a learning history relative to other unconditioned or conditioned establishing operations. Michael described three types of CEOs: *surrogate, reflexive,* and *transitive*. All three types of CMOs alter the efficacy of other stimuli or events as a function of the organism's learning history. The CMOs differ, however, in how they develop and are maintained.

Surrogate CEO

The surrogate CEO results as a function of pairing in time; that is, the previously neutral stimulus or event acquires the same motivational properties of the UEO or other CMO with which it is paired.

There are no specific instances in the published basic research literature on the development, maintenance, and elimination of the surrogate CEO (note, though, that several theses and dissertations can be found via literature searches). There also are findings from the basic laboratory that may be related to surrogate CEOs mechanistically. Pavlovian-to-instrumental transfer (PIT; Cartoni et al., 2016; Geurts et al., 2013), for example, illustrates that motivationally relevant stimuli (i.e., stimuli paired with appetitive or aversive outcomes) may alter operant response rates when they are presented.

---

[1] Michael used the terms EO, UEO, and CEO throughout *Concepts and Principles of Behavior Analysis*. Over time, as noted earlier, Laraway et al. (2003) introduced the omnibus term *motivating operation* (MO), which has extended to UMO instead of UEO, and CMO instead of CEO. For the sake of consistency with Michael's framework, we use the term CEO when referencing Michael's framework. However, when subsequent research articles utilize CMO, we reference CMO to maintain consistency with the published language.

In an early example of this research, Walker (1942) trained rats to lever-press for food reinforcers. Next, he presented discrimination training wherein the presence of a tone indicated that the rats would earn a food reinforcer for traversing a runway, and the absence of the tone indicated no reinforcement for runway traversal. Finally, Walker returned the rats to the operant chamber with extinction in effect for lever pressing and presented them with alternating periods during which the tone was on versus off. Rats lever-pressed substantially more when the tone was present than when it was absent. These findings have been interpreted through the lens of motivation: Stimuli correlated with reinforcers signal the availability of and increase motivation for those reinforcers. It is important to note, however, that one cannot separate the potential motivational and discriminative effects of the stimuli arranged in PIT procedures.

In addition, a wealth of research has evaluated the effects of reinforcer-correlated stimuli on subjective ratings of motivation for those stimuli (see, e.g., Ferguson & Shiffman, 2009; Garavan et al., 2000). This literature has grown out of research on addiction that has shown that stimuli that are correlated with substances of abuse are important contributors to the processes of substance use, treatment, and relapse (Bossert et al., 2013; Carter & Tiffany, 1999). For example, Lambert et al. (1991) evaluated the effects of presenting various chocolate-correlated stimuli on chocolate-deprived and chocolate-satiated participants' self-reported chocolate craving and subsequent chocolate consumption. Participants were exposed to three different chocolate-related stimuli (small bits of chocolate, a photograph of chocolate, or a story involving chocolate) or no stimulus. Relative to participants who were not exposed to a stimulus, those who were presented with small bits of chocolate or a chocolate-related photograph subsequently indicated increased motivation to eat chocolate. All participants, however, demonstrated comparable chocolate consumption when allowed free access to chocolate. Whether chocolate-correlated stimuli in this experiment would have resulted in more chocolate-motivated operant behavior, as one would expect if the stimuli were surrogate CEOs, is unknown.

In the applied literature, there is at least one research-based example in which a surrogate CEO interpretation may aid in explaining the relevant conceptual systems at play, and possibly affect practice. Adelenis et al. (1997) showed that an individual engaged in higher rates of SIB when in a wheelchair relative to being out of the wheelchair. Although the authors did not conduct an experimental arrangement to rule in or rule out a surrogate CEO, McGill (1999) suggested that the wheelchair (previously neutral stimulus) may have been paired with attention deprivation (UEO). Thus, the wheelchair may have acquired the same motivational properties as deprivation of attention and similarly evoked SIB as a function of that learning history.

Lanovaz et al. (2014) showed prospectively that specific pairing procedures may produce behavior consistent with a surrogate CMO. The authors consistently paired poster boards, which were shown to be neutral stimuli relative to stereotypy, with preferred stimuli. Subsequent to the pairing, three out of five participants showed evidence of increased engagement in stereotypy in the presence of the poster boards. Future research could assess whether additional pairings, or a different pairing arrangement, might produce a more reliable effect. Naturalistic observations might also help clinicians and researchers develop hypotheses about the occurrence of problem behavior that seems to maintain despite contingencies that do not favor engagement.

Thus, basic and applied researchers might focus on the conditions under which a previously neutral stimulus or event, paired in time with a UEO or another CEO, might acquire the same motivational properties as the paired events. The rationale for such research would be to discover conditions that might clarify why problem behavior occurs under certain conditions that are not explainable given the current operating contingencies; that is, imagine a situation in which a wheelchair evokes problem behavior as a function of its history with deprivation of attention. The individual in the wheelchair may continue to engage in problem behavior even when attention is delivered on a noncontingent basis, when the current contingencies do not support the occurrence of the response. However, the surrogate CEO explanation would substantiate and explain the occurrence of the problem behavior.

Basic researchers could make a profound contribution in this area, because many different arrangements could be compared in a relatively small amount of time; that is, the results of multiple iterations in a basic research laboratory could inform translational research, which might lead to a technology of assessment and intervention to improve problems of social significance. Clinicians might then attempt to assess and treat previously intractable behavior. If successful, we would have achieved a new technology. If unsuccessful, the results of applied research might inform basic researchers for altering the experimental arrangement to further clarify the conditions under which surrogate CEOs are acquired and extinguished.

In fact, basic research exists that may serve as a perfect foundation for such a collaboration. For example, Shahan (2010) reviewed research that focused on the potential strengthening effects of conditioned reinforcers (stimuli or events that are paired in some way with primary reinforcers or other conditioned reinforcers). The review of the research extended a voluminous literature debating the nature—or even the existence—of conditioned reinforcement (see Bolles, 1967; Fantino, 1977; Hendry, 1969; Kelleher & Gollub, 1962; Nevin, 1973; Wike, 1966; Williams, 1994a, 1994b). Basic researchers have also attempted to clarify the nature of conditioned reinforcement in the context of the matching law (e.g., Autor, 1969; Fantino, 1969), chain schedules (e.g., Squires & Fantino, 1971), and concurrent chain schedules (e.g., Williams & Dunn, 1991), among other methods.

The research broadly suggests that our understanding of the nature of conditioned reinforcers is at best incomplete. However, basic and applied researchers could collaborate in areas in which both sectors have a mutually solid foundation. For example, it is generally well accepted that generalized reinforcers (which by definition are conditioned reinforcers) maintain their capacity to support operation behavior due to the pairing with other reinforcers (Cooper et al., 2020). Thus, generalized reinforcers will fail to continue to support behavior if they are not ultimately exchangeable for other reinforcers.

It is also known that pairing neutral events with preferred events can produce *conditioned preferences*, reflected in increases in time allocation toward previously neutral events subsequent to pairing with preferred events or stimuli (e.g., Hanley et al., 2006). In the laboratory, for example, animals spend more time in a stimulus context that previously has been associated with appetitive stimuli such as drugs of abuse than in a neutral context (an outcome often referred to as "conditioned place preference"; Bardo & Bevins, 2000; Prus et al., 2009). Human participants also demonstrate conditioned place preferences (e.g., Childs & de Wit, 2009) and may develop preferences for stimuli of settings that are associated with preferred foods, activities, or even treatments (see Brower-Breitwieser et al., 2008).

Basic and applied researchers could collaborate to discover the conditions under which establishing conditioned preferences might also support behavior (e.g., contingent access to conditioned preferred event), thus establishing a method to support behavior through a novel conditioning procedure. Consider the relation in Adelinis et al. (1997)

suggested by McGill (1999). In that context, it is possible that mands for access to the wheelchair could be taught and supported by access to the wheelchair, but recall that the wheelchair, in this case, only functions as a reinforcer for mands due to the pairing of the wheelchair and deprivation of attention. The experimental procedures to discover such relations may seem complex, but perhaps only because these procedures have not yet been conducted.

Reflexive CEO

The reflexive CEO results as a function of some previously neutral event or stimulus systematically preceding either improvement or worsening of stimulus conditions. Behavior that occurs in the presence of the previously neutral stimulus either avoids the upcoming worsening or produces the upcoming improvement. Thus, the previously neutral stimulus or event acquires the same motivational properties as the UEO or CEO that it precedes.

The reflexive CEO differs from the surrogate CEO, then, in that the previously neutral response *precedes* the conditioned or the unconditioned motivational operation rather than simply being *paired in time*. Therefore, the reflexive CEO has *predictive* status; that is, the reflexive CEO predicts upcoming improvements or worsening, depending on the unconditioned or motivating operation with which it is paired.

Imagine a situation in which a teacher systematically precedes the delivery of instructions (aversive event) with a specific behavioral sequence (previously neutral event), such as picking up a particular book and walking toward a student. If that particular behavioral sequence systematically precedes the delivery of instructions, the student may engage in problem behavior when she sees the teacher pick up the book and start to approach her, rather than in the presence of the instructions. In this case, the previously neutral behavioral sequence serves as a warning stimulus, and the student effectively avoids the delivery of instructions by engaging in problem behavior in the presence of the behavioral sequence—if the teacher terminates the behavioral sequence, and does not deliver the instructions.

Autoshaping, a procedure that has been used to study associative learning in the basic laboratory for more than half of a century, illustrates the potency of reflexive CEOs in developing and maintaining operant behavior. In the seminal study on the topic, Brown and Jenkins (1968) exposed hungry pigeons to a learning situation wherein a response key was intermittently illuminated for 8 seconds and followed by presentation of a food reinforcer. If the pigeons pecked the key at any time when it was illuminated, the key was darkened and the reinforcer was delivered immediately. Even though reinforcers were delivered whether or not the pigeons pecked the key, each of 36 pigeons developed a key-peck response. One could contend that the key light served as a reflexive CEO in that it signaled the presentation of a food reinforcer, and presentation of the food momentary reduced food restriction, the MO for key pecking.

Some results from the literature on behavioral contrast may be viewed using the same lens. Pliskoff (1961), for example, studied the effects of signaling the transition between different contexts associated with different reinforcement conditions on rates of pigeons' key pecking. Pigeons started in a context associated with a white key and transitioned to a context associated with either a red key or a green key. Relative to the white-key context, the red and green keys were associated with either the same rate of reinforcement that was delivered in the white-key context, a higher rate, or a lower rate. The reinforcement contingencies associated with these contexts varied across conditions.

Prior to each white-to-red or white-to-green transition, a "warning signal" was presented that indicated the upcoming context. A steady house light signaled a white-to-red transition, and a blinking house light signaled a white-to-green transition. Pliskoff (1961) was interested in what would happen to pigeons' key pecking during presentations of the warning signal. He found that key pecking increased during the warning signal, relative to responding in the presence of the white key absent the warning signal, whenever the signal indicated that the upcoming component was associated with a lower rate of reinforcement. Whenever the signal indicated the upcoming component was associated with a higher rate of reinforcement, key pecking decreased. Finally, key pecking was unchanged when the upcoming component was associated with the same rate of reinforcement as the white-key component.

The outcomes just reported, termed *anticipatory contrast*, may be related to the motivational properties of the warning signals that Pliskoff (1961) presented. Specifically, the warning signals may have come to indicate impending presentation of a situation associated with increased satiation (i.e., transitioning to a high rate of reinforcement) or deprivation (i.e., transitioning to a low rate of reinforcement), thereby resulting in decreased and increased responding, respectively, in their presence; that is, the signals may have come to serve as reflexive CEOs. At this point, it is important to note that mechanisms that have been proposed to undergird outcomes such as anticipatory contrast and autoshaping are varied (see Williams, 2002; Gallistel et al., 2014, 2019), and that an MO-based interpretation of these outcomes is tentative. As with possible empirical examples of surrogate CEOs, it is difficult to clearly differentiate between the discriminative and motivational properties of the stimuli in the context of reflexive CEOs.

The potential importance of better understanding the reflexive CEO relation—and the ways Michael proposed to extinguish a reflexive CEO—lies in the potential of serving individuals who engage in problem behavior. Hanley et al. (2003) and Beavers et al. (2013) found that 34.2 and 29.7%, respectively (32.2% combined) of published functional analyses resulted in a negative reinforcement interpretation. Thus, a large percentage of individuals who engage in problem behavior have the potential to develop the reflexive CEO in advance of demand presentation, and research on the acquisition, maintenance, and extinguishing of the relation is warranted.

Kettering et al. (2018) evaluated two forms of unpairing—extinction and noncontingent—for extinguishing a reflexive CEO (Michael, 1993a, 1993b). Experimenter-provided instructions evoked escape-maintained problem behavior in four individuals diagnosed with disabilities. Problem behavior decreased for all four individuals subsequent to intervention with differential reinforcement of alternative behavior. Next, the experimenters arranged for an auditory signal to serve as a predictor of upcoming worsening; that is, the signal preceded the delivery of instructions. The individuals rapidly showed the acquisition of the reflexive CMO relationship, as the signal reliably evoked alternative behavior.

The primary goal in the remainder of the study was to evaluate whether *noncontingent unpairing* or *extinction unpairing* would facilitate extinguishing the alternative behavior in the presence of the signal. *Noncontingent unpairing* consisted of the presence of the signal, and the absence of the instructions; that is, the alternative behavior terminated the signal, but instructions no longer followed the signal, whether the alternative behavior occurred or not. *Extinction unpairing* consisted of the removal of the signal contingent on the occurrence of the alternative response; however, the experimenter delivered the programmed instructions.

Noncontingent unpairing was more effective than extinction unpairing for reducing occurrence of the alternative responses for all four individuals. Although these data were collected in the context of alternative behavior, it is reasonable to conclude that the conceptual systems would generalize to other typographies. However, these results should be interpreted with caution until other studies either replicate these results or shed light on alternative arrangements for extinguishing behavior evoked by reflexive CEO.

As with the surrogate CEO, basic researchers could help clarify, in a relatively small amount of time, the most likely candidates for experimental arrangements that would have the most applied impact. For example, Kettering et al. (2018) selected fairly arbitrary arrangements for the duration of the signal, and the amount of time that expired between each instructional delivery. Basic researchers could help inform clinicians and applied researchers about the best ways to arrange for the development or extinguishing of a reflexive CEO, depending on the clinical concern.

Transitive CEO

The transitive CEO is a previously neutral stimulus or event that acquires its motivational properties by pairing with a conditioned or unconditioned motivational event by changing the value of another event. For example, saying the word *spoon* is not particularly likely in most cases, as labeling/acquiring spoons isn't usually important or valuable. However, the delivery of a bowl of soup changes the value of spoons, and saying "spoon" becomes more probable—emitting the word *spoon* produces access to a spoon, and access to the soup.

Even a cursory observation in an early intensive behavioral intervention (EIBI) clinic provides a wide range of examples of the transitive CEO in clinical use. For example, EIBI therapists routinely arrange for the restriction of a specific item that is necessary to engage in a specific activity, thus increasing the value of the restricted item, and increasing the probability of a mand. Consider a situation in which a therapist hands a coloring book, but not crayons, to a client. The presence of a coloring book increases the value of crayons in that moment, and sets up a teachable moment for saying the word *crayons*. Alternatively, an individual may wish to go through a door to access a playground. The therapist may arrange for the door to be locked. The locked door changes the value of saying, "Open, please."

Although EIBI therapists may routinely arrange for transitive CEOs, questions remain about the conditions under which transitive CEOs develop, are maintained, and are extinguished. In fact, it is possible that EIBI therapists may not understand the underlying conceptual systems that make the transitive CEO effective as a teaching tool, and may simply engage in the behavior as a procedural iteration of a protocol.

Michael (2000) described the important role that transitive CEOs play in chained-schedule performance. A *chained schedule of reinforcement* is a complex schedule in which different discriminative-stimulus contexts (termed *links* in reference to the chained schedule) are arranged in a sequential manner, responses in each link produce access to the next link, and responses in the terminal link produce some reinforcer. Each link in the chain serves as a discriminative stimulus for the response that will produce the following link *and* as a conditioned reinforcer for behavior in the preceding link. For example, a child in an elementary school classroom may be required to complete a reading assignment to gain access to a math assignment, and he may then be required to complete the math assignment to earn praise from the teacher. In the context of the classroom, presentation of the word *READING* on a student's visual schedule may serve as a discriminative stimulus signaling that reading will be reinforced with access to the next activity on the visual schedule, math (a conditioned reinforcer). Presentation of the word *MATH* on the schedule may serve as a discriminative stimulus that signals that completing math problems will be reinforced by praise. Motivationally speaking, restricting access to teacher praise serves as an EO for completing math work, and restricted access to *MATH* on the visual schedule is a transitive CEO for reading.

Basic and applied research has shown that manipulating MOs for the final reinforcer in the chain can affect organisms' motivation to complete earlier links in the chain. For example, Malott (1966) trained hungry pigeons to peck response keys in a two-link chain schedule. Thirty-two key pecks were required in the initial link, signaled by a key with a white horizontal line projected on it, to transition into the terminal link, signaled by a key with a white vertical line projected on it. After 32 pecks in the terminal link, a food reinforcer was delivered. Malott manipulated the MO for food by giving the pigeons different amounts of food prior to sessions. Response rates decreased in both the terminal link (demonstrating a reduced MO for food) and the initial link (demonstrating a reduced transitive CMO for terminal-link access).

Similar findings have been reported in treatment settings with socially significant behavior. For example, Contrucci Kuhn et al. (2006) taught children with developmental disabilities to engage in chained communicative responding to earn food reinforcers. When those reinforcers were freely available prior to sessions, communication was reduced in the terminal link and initial link of the chain schedule, indicating a reduced MO for food and a reduced transitive CMO for terminal-link access. However, applied data that directly evaluate the effects of the transitive CEO are scant, but do exist. Belfiore et al. (2016) showed preliminary evidence of a transitive CEO in the context of assessment of stereotypical behavior. Four experimental functional analysis conditions consisted of attention, rule + attention, rule only, and control. Stereotypical behavior occurred at greater levels in conditions that included a rule suggesting the development of a transitive CEO.

Both basic and applied researchers could collaborate to determine the experimental and practical parameters for the development, maintenance, and extinguishing of the transitive CEO. Superficially, it appears that the greatest strides in transitive CEO research may be in the area of response acquisition and response performance. For example, EIBI therapists who become well acquainted with the use of transitive CEOs may become much more effective introducing acquisition and maintenance of target behaviors. However, Belfiore et al. (2016) showed the potential for transitive CEOs to develop in the context of problem behavior, suggesting that a better understanding of transitive CEOs may also improve assessment and intervention of problem behavior.

In summary, although Michael's elegant concept of MOs and CMOs has great intuitive appeal, there is a dearth of research addressing surrogate, reflexive, and transitive CEOs. This is an area of research that appears to be particularly amenable to cross-fertilized, collaborative efforts between basic and applied researchers. For example, we generally do not know the parameters under which previously neutral events are likely to acquire the motivational properties of unconditioned and conditioned motivational events. Thus, basic researchers could conduct parametric analyses under the surrogate, reflexive, and transitive MO framework. This will provide applied researchers with a foundation and starting point for potential application.

Motivation and Choice

Choice—another potentially fertile area for translational research involving motivation— refers to the allocation of behavior or time to concurrently available response/contingency options (Fisher & Mazur, 1997). Although Herrnstein (1961, 1970) did not specifically refer to everyday situations in which humans allocate behavior among dozens or hundreds of choice points and options, a systematic literature exists that guides our understanding of the factors that influence response allocation among alternatives.

The most basic method for studying the predictions of matching law (Herrnstein, 1961, 1970) includes arranging asymmetrical reinforcement schedules (e.g., VI 30 vs. VI 120) in concurrent schedules, but symmetry across other reinforcement and response parameters (i.e., equal magnitude, delay, quality, and effort). Some of the earliest extensions of the matching law, and examples of important extensions for clinical application, included research on asymmetrical arrangements that are common in everyday human choice options (e.g., options that include different response topographies, schedules, delays, qualities, magnitudes, and/or effort). For example, Horner and Day (1991) evaluated the effects of manipulating response effort, reinforcement schedule, and delay to reinforcement on functional communication training (FCT; Carr & Durand, 1985). Results showed that increasing effort, thinning the reinforcement schedule, and introducing delays to reinforcement compromised FCT; response allocation shifted away from the alternative behavior and toward problem behavior.

Researchers have also investigated the separate and combined effects of reinforcement and response parameters on choice behavior with humans in translational arrangements (e.g., Mace et al., 1994, 1996; Neef et al., 1992, 1993). Over the course of a series of studies, researchers prepared asymmetrical choice arrangements for one parameter (rate; Mace et al., 1994) or multiple parameters (e.g., effort and quality: Mace et al., 1996; rate and quality: Neef et al., 1992; rate, delay, and quality: Neef et al., 1993) to assess the effects on response allocation.

Although there are other studies in the applied behavior-analytic literature that utilized choice arrangements with asymmetrical sources of reinforcement, these studies in particular are instructive because they used concurrent interval schedules as opposed to concurrent ratio schedules. Applied interventions often use specific concurrent ratio schedules, such as fixed-ratio 1 for alternative behavior and extinction for problem behavior, to increase the likelihood of exclusive responding toward alternative behavior (Herrnstein & Loveland, 1975). Thus, the aforementioned studies serve as a bridge between basic research on asymmetrical arrangements and the potential for application to problems of social significance.

Several studies have evaluated the influence of motivational variables on response allocation in laboratory settings. For example, Balleine and Dickinson (1998) trained rats to perform two lever-press responses in a concurrent schedule. One lever-press response was associated with a salty food reinforcer, and the other was associated with a sour food reinforcer. Next, they evaluated the effects of reinforcer satiation on changes in rats' allocation of lever presses between the two levers by conducting a prefeeding assessment; that is, they presented rats with free access to one of the two reinforcers before sessions and subsequently exposed them to a concurrent extinction schedule. Rats performed the response associated with the preferred reinforcer significantly fewer times than the response associated with the nonpreferred reinforcer. These outcomes, referred to as *sensory-specific satiation* (see Havermans et al., 2009; Hetherington & Havermans, 2013), have been replicated several studies with nonhuman animals and humans and indicate that choice can be influenced in complex ways by the various MOs arranged in an individual's environment.

In application, consider the paired-choice preference assessment, developed by Fisher et al. (1992). The basic arrangement for the paired-choice preference assessment includes the repeated presentation of two different items and a therapist's prompt for an individual to "pick one." After the therapist pairs all items with all other items, the items are ranked in a hierarchy from most selected to least selected, as a percentage of trials.

Recall that an MO refers to an environmental event that changes the value of some event or stimulus as a reinforcer, and the frequency of behavior related to that event or stimulus. Imagine a scenario in which an individual had either been substantially deprived of a particular item, or had had immediate preassessment access to a particular item, prior to exposure to a paired-choice preference assessment. Substantial deprivation of a particular item may increase the value of that item and thus increase the percentage of trials that item is selected. Preassessment access to a particular item may decrease the value of that item, and thus decrease the percentage of trials that item is selected (Chappell et al., 2009; Kelley et al., 2017).

Thus, careful consideration must be given when interpreting the results of a preference assessment if preassessment access to the items isn't known or carefully controlled. Similarly, it is conceivable (and testable) that controlled MOs would have affected response allocation in the studies mentioned earlier that targeted the influence of response and reinforcement parameters. For example, presession access or deprivation to one or both qualitatively different stimuli may have affected response allocation, and may have interacted in a dynamic fashion with other manipulations, such as delays to reinforcement.

Kelley et al. (2017) conducted preference assessments (multiple-stimulus without replacement [MSWO]; DeLeon & Iwata, 1996) subsequent to motivating operations to assess the dynamic influence of both preassessment access to stimuli and the passage of time as an influence on choice behavior. After identifying highly preferred items for each participant (i.e., items selected on 100% of trials relative to other options), experimenters provided preassessment access to the most preferred item. Finally, participants were exposed to preference assessments immediately after preassessment exposure and then at standard time intervals subsequent to the preassessment exposure (5, 10, 15, and 20 minutes for all three participants, and 10, 20, 30, and 40 minutes for one of the three participants).

Results showed that the preassessment access to the preferred items disrupted baseline choice behavior for all three participants in the preference assessment that immediately followed the preassessment exposure; that is, all three participants selected a different item in the preference assessment that followed the preassessment access to the preferred items. However, over time, all three participants began to select the preferred item on an increasing percentage of trials as subsequent preference assessments were conducted.

This study complemented the existing literature on the use of MOs to affect choice behavior. The primary extension of the literature included the demonstration of the dynamic interaction between MOs and the passage of time. Applied behavior analysts typically utilize MOs on extreme ends of the motivation continuum. For example, complete deprivation of preferred items for brief periods of time is often used as a part of behavior acquisition or performance programs to increase the likelihood that those items will function as powerful reinforcers during training or maintenance sessions. On the other hand, noncontingent reinforcement is a powerful treatment for reducing or eliminating problem behavior, because it reduces the value of the reinforcer, as well as the probability of responding related to that reinforcer. The results for Kelley et al. (2017)

demonstrate a parametric procedure for affecting choice behavior across a broader continuum of motivation.

Interestingly, other published data support this notion of a dynamic interplay of motivation and choice behavior. For example, Chappell et al. (2009) conducted procedures similar to those of Kelley et al. (2017) but did not express their data in a way to show dynamic changes in behavior as a function of time. Kelley et al. regraphed their data, and showed that the response patterns across studies were similar. Finally, there are several other studies that evaluated a combination of access to food and leisure items, and the effects of that access on choices for qualitatively similar and dissimilar stimuli (e.g., Bokkers et al., 2004; Gewirtz & Baer, 1958a, 1958b; Goh et al., 2000; Gottschalk et al., 2000; Klatt et al., 2000; McAdam et al., 2005; Sy & Borrero, 2009; Zhou et al., 2002). Results across studies are somewhat mixed, as different methods across studies complicate specific interpretation at this time. However, the results of these studies all point in the same direction: Motivation interacts in a dynamic fashion with other environmental events to affect choice behavior.

Basic and applied behavioral-economic research may shed light on potential application relative to motivation and choice. For example, multiple basic and applied studies demonstrate the effects of preference for reinforcers/choice behavior as a function of access, deprivation, and changes in schedule requirements (Roane et al., 2001). Tustin (1994) conducted three experiments examining preference for qualitatively different reinforcers, the substitutability of reinforcers, and preference alterations as a function of changing schedule requirements. Results of Study 2 are particularly applicable to application with motivation. The results suggest that the demand for a specific stimulus (i.e., the extent to which the reinforcer continued to support responding as the schedule requirements increased) varied with the nature of the reinforcer; that is, response allocation was influenced in part by the relative substitutability of the reinforcers.

Substitutability (Green & Freed, 1993) refers to the extent to which reinforcers are easily exchanged due to functional similarity. For example, balls and oranges may be readily traded in the context of juggling. Other reinforcers tend to be consumed in tandem, such as pancakes and syrup, and are thus *complementary. Complementary reinforcers* are jointly consumed, generally in a specific proportion, and are not readily exchangeable. Finally, changes in price (among other parameters) for one reinforcer do not generally affect consumption of other *independent reinforcers.* Consumption of *independent reinforcers* generally does not affect consumption of others.

Substitutable reinforcers provide a straightforward pathway to strategically integrating MOs into an intervention designed to influence response allocation. For example, an individual may readily engage in a range of food selections that varies in calories and other health parameters (i.e., a range of foods that is readily exchangeable; substitutable reinforcers). Providing access to substitutable, yet healthy, options at strategic times— prior to choice points—may decrease choices for less healthy alternatives as a function of a decrease in value of food in general (Sy et al., 2009; Zhou et al., 2002).

For example, North and Iwata (2005) evaluated the separate and combined effects of repeated access to a reinforcer and meal consumption on reinforcer efficacy. In Study 1, the results suggested that repeated access to a reinforcer had a greater impact than meal consumption (presumably substitutable for the edible reinforcers) on reinforcer efficacy for some participants. In Study 2, the combination of repeated exposure to the reinforcer and meal consumption did not affect reinforcer efficacy for two participants, suggesting that the independent variable manipulation was not sufficient to affect behavior. Finally, Study 3 suggested that presession choice and varied reinforcement—but not increased breaks between sessions and intermittent reinforcement—helped to mitigate response decrements in Study 1.

These results are consistent with past research (e.g., Chappell et al., 2009; Kelley et al., 2017) that showed changes in reinforcement efficacy as a function of an MO that interacts with *different values* of another controllable environmental event (e.g., how much time passed since the MO); that is, Kelley et al. showed that choice behavior was disrupted by the MO, and that the passage of time produced response recovery. North and Iwata's (2005) results highlight that achieving universal outcomes across individuals in response to MOs may require the same conceptual manipulation at different values.

Conclusions

Motivation, defined by environmental events that change the value of some stimulus or event and the frequency of behavior related to those events, is a controllable, predictable, observable phenomenon. Applied behavior analysts routinely leverage naturally occurring motivational events and contrive motivational events while assessing and treating behavioral excesses and deficits. As noted earlier, the results of basic research have influenced clinical application for assessing and intervening for problem behavior, producing acquisition of new behavior, and maintaining response performance (e.g., Vollmer & Iwata, 1991; Vollmer et al., 1993).

This chapter has highlighted just a few areas in which basic and applied researchers could collaborate to enhance our understanding of the basic principles and potential clinical application of motivation. First, basic and applied researchers could glean from the literature examples in which application has directly benefited from basic research (e.g., Vollmer et al., 1993). Those studies may serve as a foundation for additional basic research that directly sets the occasion for application, as opposed to the surreptitious application of basic principles to clinical populations. Basic research studies that are arranged with application in mind are bound to produce more fruitful and valuable clinical use opportunities.

Second, Jack Michael provided an elegant framework for conditioned MOs. The sheer amount of research needed to support this framework requires basic researchers' involvement. It is simply not practical to conduct the breadth and depth of independent variable manipulations with humans in naturalistic settings. Basic researchers may conduct a series of parametric studies to exam features of surrogate, reflective, and transitive MOs to help clinicians develop a narrower range of independent variables for potential application. The results of these studies may spur additional basic research in the area of conditioned reinforcement, which is admittedly in need of additional research (e.g., Shahan, 2010). It is also important to appreciate that many of the behavioral outcomes that basic researchers study in the laboratory are related in spirit (and conceptually) to the way that Michael has conceptualized motivation from his MO framework. From Michael's perspective, MOs and CMOs are fundamental variables that undergird operant behavior. Throughout this chapter, we have suggested various findings from laboratory settings that may be interpreted through the lens of Michael's framework. We encourage readers to consider how the concepts of MOs and CMOs may be extended to help provide context to a variety of outcomes from a variety of research settings. Motivation is, after all, a principle that pervades the science and practice of behavior analysis.

Finally, there are many studies showing that motivational variables affect choice behavior in both single-operant and concurrent-operant arrangements. However, the vast majority of these studies involve MOs that are designed to either evoke behavior at high levels (e.g., acquisition studies) or abate behavior to produce low or zero levels of responding (e.g., treatment of problem behavior). Basic researchers are in a strong position to conduct parametric studies to assess the limits for evoking and abating behavior with both direct MOs (e.g., direct deprivation and satiation), as well as the manipulation of access to related reinforcers (e.g., substitutable and complementary). The results of these basic studies will undoubtedly aid the development of clinical application and serve as the foundation for coordinated, purposeful translational research.

REFERENCES

Adelinis, J., Piazza, C. C., Fisher, W. W., & Hanley, G. P. (1997). The establishing effects of client location on self-injurious behavior. *Research in Developmental Disabilities, 18*(5), 383–391.

Aristotle, & McKeon, R. L. (1941). *The basic works of Aristotle.* Random House.

Autor, S. M. (1969). The strength of conditioned reinforcers as a function of frequency and probability of reinforcement. In D. P. Hendry (Ed.), *Conditioned reinforcement* (pp. 127–162). Dorsey Press.

Azrin, N., Rubin, H., O'Brien, F., Ayllon, T., & Roll, D. (1968). Behavioral engineering: Postural control by a portable operant apparatus. *Journal of Applied Behavior Analysis, 1*(2), 99–108.

Baer, D. M. (1977). Perhaps it would be better not to know everything. *Journal of Applied Behavior Analysis, 10*(1), 167–172.

Balleine, B. W., & Dickinson, A. (1998). The role of incentive learning in instrumental outcome revaluation by sensory-specific satiety. *Animal Learning & Behavior, 26,* 46–59.

Bardo, M. T., & Bevins, R. A. (2000). Conditioned place preference: What does it add to our preclinical understanding of drug reward? *Psychopharmacology, 153,* 31–43.

Beavers, G. A., Iwata, B. A., & Lerman, D. C. (2013). Thirty years of research on the functional analysis of problem behavior. *Journal of Applied Behavior Analysis, 46*(1), 1–21.

Belfiore, P. J., Kitchen, T., & Lee, D. L. (2016). Functional analysis of maladaptive behaviors: Rule as a transitive conditioned motivating operation. *Research in Developmental Disabilities, 49–50,* 100–107.

Bokkers, E. A. M., Koene, P., Rodenburg, T. B., Zimmerman, P. H., & Spruijt, B. M. (2004). Working for food under conditions of varying motivation in broilers. *Animal Behaviour, 68*(1), 105–113.

Bolles, R. C. (1967). *Theory of motivation.* Harper & Row.

Bossert, J. M., Marchant, N. J., Calu, D. J., & Shaham, Y. (2013). The reinstatement model of drug relapse: Recent neurobiological findings, merging research topics, and translational research. *Psychopharmacology (Berlin), 229,* 453–476.

Brower-Breitwieser, C. M., Miltenberger, R. G., Gross, A., Fuqua, W., & Britwiesser, J. (2008). The use of concurrent operants preference assessment to evaluate choice of interventions for children diagnosed with autism. *International Journal of Behavioral Consultation and Therapy, 4,* 270–278.

Brown, P. L., & Jenkins, H. M. (1968). Autoshaping of the pigeon's key-peck. *Journal of the Experimental Analysis of Behavior, 11,* 1–8.

Buell, J., Stoddard, P., Harris, F. R., & Baer, D. M. (1968). Collateral social development accompanying reinforcement of outdoor play in a preschool child. *Journal of Applied Behavior Analysis, 1*(2), 167–173.

Carr, E. G., & Durand, V. M. (1985). Reducing behavior problems through functional communication training. *Journal of Applied Behavior Analysis, 18*(2), 111–126.

Carter, B. L., & Tiffany, S. T. (1999). Meta-analysis of cue-reactivity in addiction research. *Addiction, 94,* 327–340.

Cartoni, E., Balleine, B., & Baldassarre, G. (2016). Appetitive Pavlovian-instrumental transfer: A review. *Neuroscience and Biobehavioral Reviews, 71,* 829–848.

Chappell, N., Graff, R. B., Libby, M. E., & Ahearn, W. H. (2009). Further evaluation of the effects of motivating operations on preference assessment outcomes. *Research in Autism Spectrum Disorders, 3*(3), 660–669.

Childs, E., & de Wit, H. (2009). Amphetamine-induced place preference in humans. *Biological Psychiatry, 65,* 900–904.

Clark, F. C. (1958). The effect of deprivation and frequency of reinforcement on variable-interval responding. *Journal of the Experimental Analysis of Behavior, 1*(3), 221.

Contrucci Kuhn, S. A., Lerman, D. C., Vorndran, C. M., & Addison, L. (2006). Analysis of factors that affect responding in a two-response chain in children with developmental disabilities. *Journal of Applied Behavior Analysis, 39,* 263–280.

Cooper, J. O., Heron, T. E., & Heward, W. L. (2020). *Applied behavior analysis* (3rd ed.). Pearson.

Critchfield, T. S. (2011). To a young basic scientist, about to embark on a program of translational research. *The Behavior Analyst, 34,* 137–148.

DeLeon, I. G. (2011). The aesthetics of intervention in defense of the esoteric. *The Behavior Analyst, 34*(1), 41.

DeLeon, I. G., & Iwata, B. A. (1996). Evaluation of a multiple-stimulus presentation format for assessing reinforcer preferences. *Journal of Applied Behavior Analysis, 29*(4), 519–533.

Fantino, E. (1969). Choice and rate of reinforcement. *Journal of the Experimental Analysis of Behavior, 12*(5), 723–730.

Fantino, E. (1977). Conditioned reinforcement: Choice and information. In W. K. Honig & J. E. R. Staddon (Eds.), *Handbook of operant behavior* (pp. 313–339). Prentice Hall.

Ferguson, S. G., & Shiffman, S. (2009). The relevance and treatment of cue-induced cravings in tobacco dependents. *Journal of Substance Abuse Treatment, 36,* 235–243.

Fisher, W. W., & Mazur, J. E. (1997). Basic and applied research on choice responding. *Journal of Applied Behavior Analysis, 30*(3), 387–410.

Fisher, W., Piazza, C. C., Bowman, L. G., Hagopian, L. P., Owens, J. C., & Slevin, I. (1992). A comparison of two approaches for identifying reinforcers for persons with severe and profound disabilities. *Journal of Applied Behavior Analysis, 25*(2), 491–498.

Gallistel, C. R., Craig, A. R., & Shahan, T. A. (2014). Temporal contingency. *Behavioural Processes, 101,* 89–96.

Gallistel, C. R., Craig, A. R., & Shahan, T. A. (2019). Contingency, contiguity, and causality in conditioning: Applying information theory and Weber's law to the assignment of credit problem. *Psychological Review, 126,* 761–773.

Garavan, H., Pankiewicz, J., Bloom, A., Cho, J., Sperry, L., Ross, T. J., . . . Stein, E. A. (2000). Cue-induced cocaine craving: Neuroanatomical specificity of drug users and drug stimuli. *American Journal of Psychiatry, 157,* 1789–1798.

Geurts, D. E. M., Huys, Q. J. M., den Ouden, H. E. M., & Cools, R. (2013). Aversive Pavlovian control of instrumental behavior in humans. *Journal of Cognitive Neuroscience, 25,* 1428–1441.

Gewirtz, J. L., & Baer, D. M. (1958a). Deprivation and satiation of social reinforcers as drive conditions. *Journal of Abnormal and Social Psychology, 57*(2), 165–172.

Gewirtz, J. L., & Baer, D. M. (1958b). The effect of brief social deprivation on behaviors for a social reinforcer. *Journal of Abnormal and Social Psychology, 56*(1), 49–56.

Goh, H. L., Iwata, B. A., & DeLeon, I. G. (2000). Competition between noncontingent and contingent reinforcement schedules during response acquisition. *Journal of Applied Behavior Analysis, 33*(2), 195–205.

Gottschalk, J. M., Libby, M. E., & Graff, R. B. (2000). The effects of establishing operations on preference assessment outcomes. *Journal of Applied Behavior Analysis, 33*(1), 85–88.

Green, L., & Freed, D. E. (1993). The substitutability of reinforcers. *Journal of the Experimental Analysis of Behavior, 60*(1), 141–158.

Hanley, G. P., Iwata, B. A., & McCord, B. E. (2003). Functional analysis of problem behavior: A review. *Journal of Applied Behavior Analysis, 36*(2), 147–185.

Hanley, G. P., Iwata, B. A., & Roscoe, E. M. (2006). Some determinants of changes in preference over time. *Journal of Applied Behavior Analysis, 39*(2), 189–202.

Havermans, R. C., Jenssen, T., Giesen, J. C. A. H., Roefs, A., & Jensen, A. (2009). Food liking, food wanting, and sensory-specific satiety. *Appetite, 52,* 222–225.

Hendry, D. P. (1969). *Conditioned reinforcement.* Dorsey.

Henry, J. E., Kelley, M. E., Larue, R. H., Kettering, T. L., Gadaire, D. M., & Sloman, K. N. (2021). Integration of experimental functional analysis procedural advancements: Progressing from brief to extended experimental analyses. *Journal of Applied Behavior Analysis, 54*(3), 1045–1061.

Herrnstein, R. J. (1961). Relative and absolute strength of response as a function of frequency of reinforcement. *Journal of the Experimental Analysis of Behavior, 4*(3), 267–272.

Herrnstein, R. J. (1970). On the law of effect. *Journal of the Experimental Analysis of Behavior, 13*(2), 243–266.

Herrnstein, R. J., & Loveland, D. H. (1975). Maximizing and matching on concurrent ratio schedules. *Journal of the Experimental Analysis of Behavior, 24,* 107–116.

Hetheringtoon, M., & Havermans, R. C. (2013). Sensory-specific satiation and satiety. In J. E. Blundell & F. Bellisle (Eds.), *Satiation, satiety and the control of food intake* (pp. 253–269). Woodhead.

Horner, R. H., & Day, H. M. (1991). The effects of response efficiency on functionally equivalent competing behaviors. *Journal of Applied Behavior Analysis, 24*(4), 719–732.

Iwata, B. A., Dorsey, M. F., Slifer, K. J., Bauman, K. E., & Richman, G. S. (1982). Toward a functional analysis of self-injury. *Analysis and Intervention in Developmental Disabilities, 2*(1), 3–20.

Iwata, B. A., Duncan, B. A., Zarcone, J. R., Lerman, D. C., & Shore, B. A. (1994). A sequential, test-control methodology for conducting functional analyses of self-injurious behavior. *Behavior Modification, 18*(3), 289–306.

Johnston, J. M., & Pennypacker, H. S. (1980). *Strategies and tactics of human behavioral research.* Erlbaum.

Kelleher, R. T., & Gollub, L. R. (1962). A review of positive conditioned reinforcement. *Journal of the Experimental Analysis of Behavior, 5*(4), 543–597.

Keller, F. S., & Schoenfeld, W. N. (1950). *Principles of psychology: A systematic text in the science of behavior.* Appleton-Century-Crofts.

Kelley, M. E., Shillingsburg, M. A., & Bowen, C. B. (2017). Time since reinforcer access produces gradations of motivation. *Learning and Motivation, 57,* 61–66.

Kettering, T. L., Fisher, W. W., Kelley, M. E., & Larue, R. H. (2018). Sound attenuation and preferred music in the treatment of problem behavior maintained by escape from noise. *Journal of Applied Behavior Analysis, 51*(3), 687–693.

Klatt, K. P., Sherman, J. A., & Sheldon, J. B. (2000). Effects of deprivation on engagement in preferred activities by persons with developmental disabilities. *Journal of Applied Behavior Analysis, 33*(4), 495–506.

Lambert, K. G., Neal, T., Noyes, J., Parker, C., & Worrel, P. (1991). Food-related stimuli increase desire to eat in hungry and stated human subjects. *Current Psychology, 10,* 297–303.

Lanovaz, M. J., Rapp, J. T., Long, E. S., Richling, S. M., & Carroll, R. A. (2014). Preliminary effects of conditioned establishing operations on stereotypy. *The Psychological Record, 64,* 209–216.

Laraway, S., Snycerski, S., Michael, J., & Poling, A. (2003). Motivating operations and terms to describe them: Some further refinements. *Journal of Applied Behavior Analysis, 36*(3), 407–414.

Mace, F. C. (1994). The significance and future of functional analysis methodologies. *Journal of Applied Behavior Analysis, 27*(2), 385–392.

Mace, F. C., & Critchfield, T. S. (2010). Translational research in behavior analysis: Historical traditions and imperative for the future. *Journal of the Experimental Analysis of Behavior, 93*(3), 293–312.

Mace, F. C., Neef, N. A., Shade, D., & Mauro, B. C. (1994). Limited matching on concurrent-schedule reinforcement of academic behavior. *Journal of Applied Behavior Analysis, 27*(4), 585–596.

Mace, E. C., Neef, N. A., Shade, D., & Mauro, B. C. (1996). Effects of problem difficulty and reinforcer quality on time allocated to concurrent arithmetic problems. *Journal of Applied Behavior Analysis, 29*(1), 11–24.

Malott, R. W. (1966). The effects of prefeeding in plain and chained fixed ratio schedules of reinforcement. *Psychonomic Science, 4,* 285–286.

McAdam, D. B., Klatt, K. P., Koffarnus, M., Dicesare, A., Solberg, K., Welch, C., & Murphy, S. (2005). The effects of establishing operations on preferences for tangible items. *Journal of Applied Behavior Analysis, 38*(1), 107–110.

McGill, P. (1999). Establishing operations: Implications for the assessment, treatment, and prevention of problem behavior. *Journal of Applied Behavior Analysis, 32*(3), 393–418.

Michael, J. (1982). Distinguishing between discriminative and motivational functions of stimuli. *Journal of the Experimental Analysis of Behavior, 37*(1), 149–155.

Michael, J. (1988). Establishing operations and the mand. *Analysis of Verbal Behavior, 6,* 3–9.

Michael, J. (1993a). Establishing operations. *Behavior Analyst, 16*(2), 191–206.

Michael, J. L. (1993b). *Concepts and principles of behavior analysis.* Western Michigan University, Association for Behavior Analysis International.

Michael, J. (2000). implications and refinements of the establishing operation concept. *Journal of Applied Behavior Analysis, 33*(4), 401–410.

Millenson, J. R. (1967). *Principles of behavioral analysis.* Macmillan.

Neef, N. A., Mace, F. C., & Shade, D. (1993). Impulsivity in students with serious emotional disturbance: The interactive effects of reinforcer rate, delay, and quality. *Journal of Applied Behavior Analysis, 26*(1), 37–52.

Neef, N. A., Mace, F. C., Shea, M. C., & Shade, D. (1992). Effects of reinforcer rate and reinforcer quality on time allocation: Extensions of matching theory to educational settings. *Journal of Applied Behavior Analysis, 25*(3), 691–699.

Nevin, J. A. (1973). Conditioned reinforcement. In J. A. Nevin (Ed.), *The study of behavior: Learning, motivation, emotion, and instinct* (pp. 154–198). Scott, Foresman.

North, S. T., & Iwata, B. A. (2005). Motivational influences on performance maintained by food reinforcement. *Journal of Applied Behavior Analysis, 38*(3), 317–333.

Pilgrim, C. (2011). Translational behavior analysis and practical benefits. *The Behavior Analyst, 34*(1), 37.

Pliskoff, S. (1961). Rate-change effects during a pre-schedule—change stimulus. *Journal of the Experimental Analysis of Behavior, 4,* 383–386.

Podlesnik, C. A. (2013). The openness is there. *The Behavior Analyst, 36*(1), 151.

Prus, A. J., James, J. R., & Rosecrans, J. A. (2009). Conditioned place preference. In J. J. Buccafusco (Ed.), *Methods of behavior analysis in neuroscience* (2nd ed., pp. 59–76). CRC Press/Routledge/Taylor & Francis Group.

Rescorla, R. A., & Skucy, J. (1969). Effect of response-independent reinforcement during extinction. *Journal of Comparative and Physiological Psychology, 67,* 381–389.

Roane, H. S., Lerman, D. C., & Vorndran, C. M. (2001). Assessing reinforcers under progressive schedule requirements. *Journal of Applied Behavior Analysis, 34*(2), 145–166.

Shahan, T. A. (2010). Conditioned reinforcement and response strength. *Journal of the Experimental Analysis of Behavior, 93*(2), 269–289.

Skinner, B. F. (1938). *The behavior of organisms.* Appleton-Century.

Skinner, B. F. (1953). *Science and human behavior.* Free Press.

Squires, N., & Fantino, E. (1971). A model for choice in simple concurrent and concurrent-chains schedules. *Journal of the Experimental Analysis of Behavior, 15*(1), 27–38.

Sy, J. R., Borrero, J. C., & Zarcone, J. (2009). Parametric analysis of presession exposure to edible and nonedible stimuli. *Journal of Applied Behavior Analysis, 42*(4), 833–837.

Tustin, R. D. (1994). Preference for reinforcers under varying schedule arrangements: A behavioral economic analysis. *Journal of Applied Behavior Analysis, 27*(4), 597–606.

Vollmer, T. R. (2011). Three variations of translational research: Comments on Critchfield (2011). *The Behavior Analyst, 34*(1), 31.

Vollmer, T. R., & Iwata, B. A. (1991). Establishing operations and reinforcement effects. *Journal of Applied Behavior Analysis, 24*(2), 279–291.

Vollmer, T. R., Iwata, B. A., Zarcone, J. R., Smith, R. G., & Mazaleski, J. L. (1993). The role of attention in the treatment of attention-maintained self-injurious behavior: Noncontingent reinforcement and differential reinforcement of other behavior. *Journal of Applied Behavior Analysis, 26*(1), 9–21.

Vollmer, T. R., Marcus, B. A., Ringdahl, J. E., & Roane, H. S. (1995). Progressing from brief assessments to extended experimental analyses in the evaluation of aberrant behavior. *Journal of Applied Behavior Analysis, 28*(4), 561–576.

Vyse, S. (2013). Changing course. *The Behavior Analyst, 36,* 123–135.

Walker, K. C. (1942). The effect of a discriminative stimulus transferred to a previously unassociated response. *Journal of Experimental Psychology, 31,* 312–321.

Wike, E. L. (1966). *Secondary reinforcement: Selected experiments.* Harper & Row.

Williams, B. A. (1994a). Conditioned reinforcement: Neglected or outmoded explanatory construct? *Psychonomic Bulletin and Review, 1*(4), 457–475.

Williams, B. A. (1994b). Conditioned reinforcement: Experimental and theoretical issues. *Behavior Analyst, 17*(2), 261–285.

Williams, B. A. (2002). Behavioral contrast redux. *Animal Learning and Behavior, 30,* 1–20.

Williams, B. A., & Dunn, R. (1991). Preference for conditioned reinforcement. *Journal of the Experimental Analysis of Behavior, 55*(1), 37–46.

Zhou, L., Iwata, B. A., & Shore, B. A. (2002). Reinforcing efficacy of food on performance during pre- and postmeal sessions. *Journal of Applied Behavior Analysis, 35*(4), 411–414.

CHAPTER 16

Translational Approaches to Choice

Jennifer J. McComas
Corina Jimenez-Gomez
Shawn Gilroy

The word *choice* has a variety of different connotations. From an applied behavior-analytic perspective, when we refer to choice, we tend to focus on direct-acting contingencies, that is, contingencies for which the outcome of the response reinforces or punishes that response. Nonetheless, when verbal organisms are involved, we must also consider the influence of indirect-acting contingencies, which are those contingencies for which the outcome of the response does not reinforce or punish the response, but rather a statement or a rule controls behavior. To illustrate, in the northern part of the United States, icy streets and sidewalks are common for several months of the year. For some of us, icy sidewalks exist in a relational frame that includes danger and avoidance of danger. Therefore, an individual who wishes to avoid danger (e.g., falling on the ice) will likely choose to stay indoors rather than go for a run outdoors during winter (see Figure 16.1). Although the influence of indirect-acting contingencies is beyond the scope of this chapter, it is important to recognize that verbal behavior can influence the behavior, including choice, of verbal organisms.

Within direct-acting contingencies, one way to conceive of choice is based on the notion that every response we engage in throughout each day constitutes a choice

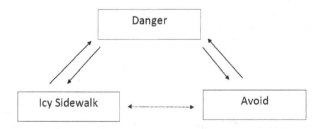

FIGURE 16.1. Relational frame depicting choice to avoid walking or running on icy sidewalks. Derived relation pertaining to avoidance of walking or running on icy sidewalks occurs within a relational frame in which icy sidewalks are dangerous and danger is to be avoided.

between that response and one or more concurrently available alternatives (Herrnstein, 1970). Even when a single alternative is intentionally arranged, for example, when a teacher instructs students to complete a math worksheet, organisms may find other options for allocating behavior, as when a student watches the birds outside the window instead of completing the worksheet. Thus, every instance of operant responding is a choice to engage in a particular response at that moment versus engaging in alternative responses. Put another way, choice is simply the emission of a particular response in lieu of others (Reed & Kaplan, 2011). Another behavior-analytic view of choice refers to an antecedent intervention involving the allocation of behavior among stimuli such as different tasks or a consequent-based intervention in which a target response results in a choice among stimuli such as small prizes or edibles. For the purposes of this chapter, we describe and discuss (1) the variables that affect choice responding (i.e., response allocation[1] across concurrently available response options) under laboratory and natural conditions, (2) choice as a behavioral strategy designed to promote specific behaviors, and (3) a behavioral-economic account of choice behavior in the context of complex and dynamic conditions (i.e., interactions existing between qualitatively different reinforcers). We provide illustrative examples of basic, translational, and applied research throughout and propose directions for future basic, translational, and applied research.

Concurrent Operants and Matching

Basic and applied researchers have typically used concurrent schedules of reinforcement to allow evaluation of the relative value of arranged alternatives based on response allocation. Concurrent-schedule research findings over the past 60 years have demonstrated a generally recognized pattern: In a two-choice situation, response allocation across alternatives roughly "matches" the reinforcement produced by those alternatives (Herrnstein, 1961).[2] The earliest research by Herrnstein examined reinforcement rate, but the effects of other variables soon followed (Catania, 2013). Often studied variables that affect response allocation in concurrent operant arrangements under laboratory and natural conditions include reinforcement rate, magnitude, quality, immediacy, and response effort (Catania, 2013). Researchers have evaluated the influence of all these variables on response allocation using one version or another of the matching law, including the concatenated generalized matching law (Baum, 1974; Baum & Rachlin, 1969; Davison & McCarthy, 1988), which posits that the ratio of responses across alternatives is a power function of the relative value of the reinforcers produced by those alternatives. Stated more simply, the relative allocation of behavior among alternatives depends on the available reinforcers' relative magnitude/rate/immediacy/quality/and so forth. Choice may be understood and accounted for by the relative reinforcement associated with each response option (e.g., pecking one of two keys, pressing a lever or pulling a chain, throwing an

---

[1]Note that we refer to response allocation broadly, as responding to a particular alternative. We do not restrict our consideration to a proportional metric but rather include counts, rates, or other dimensions of responding.

[2]Because the allocation of behavior does not perfectly match the relative proportion of reinforcers available, Baum (1974) proposed the generalized matching law to account for systematic deviations from strict matching. Our purpose in this chapter is not to provide an in-depth review of the quantitative aspects of the matching law. Interested readers may refer to existing resources on this topic (e.g., Jacobs et al., 2013; Mazur & Fantino, 2014; Podlesnik et al., 2021).

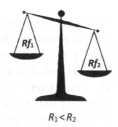

$R_1 < R_2$

FIGURE 16.2. Influence of reinforcer value on response allocation.

aluminum can in the garbage or recycling bin, problem behavior or task engagement). According to the matching law, organisms tend to allocate greater responding to the response that produces the greater reinforcement. We can picture the influence of reinforcer value (in Baum's terms) on response allocation as depicted in Figure 16.2, where Rf is reinforcement value and R is responding. Responding is generally greater for the alternative that produces greater reinforcement.

Variables Impacting Choice

As stated previously, a range of variables can influence the allocation of responding among concurrently available alternatives. In the following sections, we provide a brief description and an illustrative example of an applied study that has demonstrated the effect of the variables that contribute to "value" in the context of interventions designed to improve behavior; references to some of the basic studies, translational studies, or both that led to the featured applied study; and then suggest a research question that might follow.

Reinforcement Rate

While conducting a study with pigeons in an operant chamber, Herrnstein (1961) conceptualized the matching law. Two response keys were available for pigeons to peck, each of which produced reinforcement according to a variable-interval (VI) schedule. The concurrently available VI schedules were independent of each other; that is, pecking on one key did not affect the reinforcement schedule on the other. Herrnstein plotted the relative response rates against the relative reinforcement rates and found a nearly perfect positive correlation in which a one-unit increase in reinforcement was correlated with a one-unit increase in responding (see Figure 16.3). Accordingly, points that fall on the diagonal represent perfect matching of responses to reinforcement.

Symons et al. (2003) examined the relations between naturally occurring adult attention following self-injurious behavior (SIB) and appropriate communicative responses of a 36-year-old man diagnosed with autism spectrum disorder (ASD). The researchers conducted 29 observations (10 minutes each) of the naturally occurring interactions between the man and the staff in his residential setting. The researchers then used those descriptive data to compute sequential analyses of the rate of attention following SIB and the rate of attention following appropriate communicative responses. Next, the researchers used the generalized matching formula to determine the relative rates of SIB and appropriate

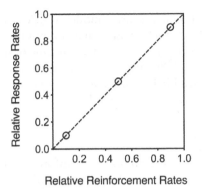

FIGURE 16.3. Example of perfect correlation between relative response rates against the relative reinforcement rates.

communicative behavior, and the relative rate of staff attention provided contingent on the two responses. Results indicated that the rate of SIB relative to appropriate communicative behavior matched the rate of staff attention for SIB relative to appropriate behavior (see Figure 16.4).

One clinical implication of this finding is that it is plausible that if staff members decreased their attention delivered contingent on SIB and instead delivered it contingent on a communicative response, one would expect that SIB would decrease and the communicative response would increase. However, it is worth noting that the effort of engaging in SIB and the communicative response may be different, which could also impact response allocation. One idea for future research would be to manipulate rate and effort in a human analogue task or an applied setting (if the target behavior does not pose harm to the client or others) and use the concatenated matching law to inform intervention based

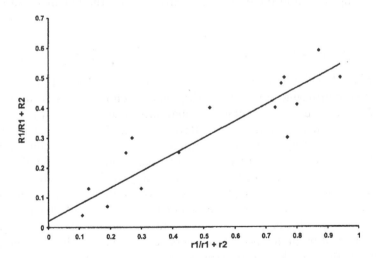

FIGURE 16.4. Correlation between relative response rates against the relative reinforcement rates. Reprinted from Symons et al. (2003) with permission from John Wiley & Sons, Inc.

on estimates derived from the quantitative model (e.g., decrease the response effort and increase the reinforcement rate for engaging in a communicative response). For example, in a classroom, when a teacher provides a dense schedule of immediate operant reinforcement contingent on prosocial behavior relative to reinforcement provided contingent on destructive behavior, prosocial behavior occurs at higher rates than destructive behavior (e.g., Bailey et al., 2002; Horner & Day, 1991).

Reinforcement Magnitude

Reinforcer magnitude refers to the amount of reinforcement, including number of reinforcers (e.g., one vs. three food pellets; Neuringer, 1967) and duration of access to reinforcement (e.g., 2-second vs. 5-second access to the food hopper; Catania, 2013; Hoch et al., 2002; Ward-Horner et al., 2014). Rogalski et al. (2020) examined the effects of three different magnitudes of negative reinforcement on problem behavior and compliance in concurrent operant arrangements with three students diagnosed with ASD, ages 5–13. The large differential magnitude of escape (240 seconds for compliance/10 seconds for problem behavior) effectively increased compliance and decreased problem behavior to low levels for all three students. The moderate differential magnitude (90 seconds/30 seconds) was only effective for one student, and for all students, problem behavior occurred at elevated rates when equivalent reinforcer magnitudes were delivered (30 seconds/30 seconds). Escape extinction was neither implemented nor required to achieve desired effects. One potential avenue for future research might be to examine the effect of differential reinforcer magnitudes on assignment completion of undergraduate students who are identified as at risk for failing one or more classes due, at least in part, to lack of assignment completion. Numerous universities have instituted academic alerts designed to quickly identify undergraduates who are at risk of poor performance in classes due to poor attendance, assignment completion, or other related issues. For students whose failure to complete sufficient course assignments triggers an academic alert, the reinforcer magnitude for completing assignments could be enhanced to increase the likelihood of assignment completion and therefore potentially increase the likelihood of student academic success.

Qualitatively Different Reinforcers

Quality is a highly subjective variable that often requires observation of the organism choosing between differing stimuli. Consider someone choosing between a chocolate bar and an apple. When we say two edibles are qualitatively different, they may differ among various dimensions (e.g., color, texture, flavor, caloric density). In this sense, *quality* represents a range of dimensions that characterize the specific stimulus and influences response allocation similar to reinforcer rate and magnitude (Cooper et al., 1999; Miller, 1976). Clay et al. (2018) conducted a multiphase study to identify relative preference and effectiveness of differing stimuli (edible, physical, vocal) on arbitrary responding (touching a card and tracing a letter) for two individuals, ages 5 and 24, diagnosed with ASD. The experimenters conducted preference assessments within stimulus sets (edible, physical, vocal), followed by preference assessments across sets (top three preferences within each set). Next, they conducted assessments to determine the reinforcing effectiveness of the stimuli on the arbitrary responses. Overall, and consistent with what one might expect based on the matching law, results indicated that the highest preferred stimuli resulted in the highest response rates across stimulus sets. Furthermore, results indicated that combining stimuli did not increase their effectiveness (i.e., no additive effect of preference was observed). One direction for future research may be to arrange qualitatively different reinforcement contingent on school attendance for individuals who refuse to attend school. For example, naturally occurring reinforcers for school refusal may be avoiding aversive variables associated with school (e.g., exposure to peers) and access to preferred activities (e.g., playing video games). School officials who provide access to preferred peers and video games contingent on appearing at school might be able to increase school attendance before gradually introducing additional response requirements beyond attendance.

Reinforcement Immediacy

Chung and Herrnstein (1967) were among the first to report the effects of reinforcement delay in the allocation of responding in concurrent schedules (see also Chung, 1965a). The inverse of reinforcement immediacy is delayed reinforcement. Austin and Tiger (2015) published an investigation aimed at addressing the aggressive behavior of a 13-year-old boy with intellectual disabilities. Assessment results suggested that positive reinforcement in the form of social attention and access to a video game (Xbox) maintained the boy's aggression. The concurrently available responses were aggression and a vocal functional communication request ("Excuse me" in the social attention conditions and "May I please play Xbox?" in the access to video game condition). Delayed access (5 minutes) to the requested reinforcer resulted in aggression. The researchers implemented delay fading, beginning at 30-second delay and increasing by 10 seconds after every two consecutive sessions with less than 0.5 aggression per minute. The researchers reduced the delay by 20 seconds after four consecutive sessions of aggression greater than 1.0 per minute. After not meeting the terminal criterion of 5 minutes without aggression during the delay to reinforcement, researchers implemented alternative reinforcers during the delay (i.e., attention during delay to Xbox condition; Xbox during delay to attention condition). Alternative reinforcement during delay resulted in meeting the delay criterion for both attention and tangible reinforcement. One potential direction for future research on the topic of delayed reinforcement might be to implement signaled delays and access to alternative reinforcers during the delay to mitigate resurgence of problem behavior during delayed reinforcement (McDevitt & Williams, 2001; Richards, 1981).

Response Effort

In concurrent operant schedules, less responding is observed on the response alternative that requires relatively greater response effort (Chung, 1965b). Fritz et al. (2017) conducted a study designed to increase recycling on a university campus by increasing the response effort to dispose of trash. Researchers removed trash cans from classrooms in university classrooms and placed the only trash cans next to the recycle bins in the hall. When trash cans were removed from classrooms, researchers observed an increase in accurate recycling. Results indicated that increased response effort to dispose of trash resulted in a decrease in the percentage of recyclable items put in the trash. These findings are consistent with previous basic research demonstrating that increased response effort for one alternative results in a decrease in responding for that alternative accompanied by an increase in the behavior allocated to other concurrently available alternatives (e.g.,

Chung, 1965b; Hunter & Davison, 1982). One direction for future research on response effort might be evaluating the effects of response effort on voting. Researchers could design a translational study that would arrange for students living in a university residence hall to vote on something related to their residential or dining plans. Researchers could arrange for half of the residents to cast their votes in a building in close proximity and the other half would be assigned a polling place on the far side of campus to cast theirs. Researchers could conduct a parametric analysis in which residents were assigned to vote at various distances away from the residence hall. Researchers would measure voter turnout at each location to evaluate the effect of response effort (distance to cast a ballot). As an additional effort manipulation, some residents would be required to wait before they could cast their vote, whereas others could cast their vote immediately. Such a study could provide important information for cities and counties regarding the effect of effort on votes cast, with the goal being to increase voter turnout.

Time and Sequence of Previous Reinforcers

Although the traditional notion of reinforcers suggests a reinforcer "strengthens" the behavior that immediately preceded it, a growing body of evidence suggests reinforcers also may serve a discriminative function (Cowie & Davison, 2016). For instance, consider the postreinforcement pause observed after reinforcer delivery to an organism responding on a fixed-ratio schedule of reinforcement. If reinforcers were merely serving as strengtheners of behavior, one would predict no pause after the reinforcer delivery. The delivery of the reinforcer may not only "strengthen" the behaviors that preceded it but also signals the immediate unavailability of another reinforcer. Krägeloh et al. (2005) arranged concurrent VI VI schedules in a manner that they could manipulate across conditions the probability of a reinforcer becoming available on the just-reinforced alternative; that is, in some conditions, staying on the alternative that recently produced a reinforcer would result in reinforcement; whereas in other conditions, switching to the other alternative would be more likely to result in reinforcement. Notably, pigeons allocated their behavior away from the just-reinforced location when the probability of reinforcement for staying on the alternative was low, supporting the notion of a discriminative function of reinforcers (see also Bolles, 1961). Cowie et al. (2021) extended this work in a translational study with children as participants. Participants engaged in a trial-based task that consisted of opening one of two drawers, one of which resulted in a reinforcer. Across conditions, researchers manipulated the probability opening the same drawer that produced the last reinforcer would result in reinforcement. Overall, and consistent with the findings of Krägeloh et al. (2005), children chose the drawer more likely to produce the next reinforcer, even when this was different than the alternative that had recently resulted in reinforcement in the previous trial (see also Jimenez-Gomez et al., 2018). Further translational and applied research is needed to elucidate the impact of the discriminative and strengthening properties of consequent stimuli, particularly when addressing challenging behaviors for which it may not be possible to easily manipulate the consequences (e.g., behaviors maintained by automatic reinforcement).

Motivating Operations

Examining response allocation allows us to evaluate the *relative* value of alternatives in not only static but also dynamic contexts. Given that motivating operations are dynamic, choice is likely also to be dynamic. Thus, it is important to consider conditional preferences. McSweeney (1974) evaluated the effects of various degrees of food deprivation on the performance of pigeons responding on concurrent VI VI schedules of reinforcement. Across conditions, researchers increased the pigeons' body weight from 85% free-feeding weight to 95% and in 5% increments to 110% free-feeding weight. As the pigeons' body weight increased and deprivation decreased, the overall response rate decreased but became more variable, demonstrating that manipulating motivating operations (e.g., food deprivation) can impact response allocation in a concurrent schedule. More recently, Lewon et al. (2019) evaluated the interaction of the motivating operations for two types of consequence, water and food, with mice as research subjects. Interestingly, manipulating the deprivation level for multiple stimuli (e.g., both food and water deprivation) influenced the reinforcing value of a single stimulus (e.g., food) and altering the motivating operation for one stimulus (e.g., food) affected the reinforcing value of multiple stimuli (e.g., food and water). Thus, the interaction between the motivating operations and reinforcing effectiveness of stimuli interact directly and indirectly, which can subsequently affect the allocation of behavior in choice situations. Consider, for instance, a child completing one task for access to a small snack (e.g., Goldfish) and a concurrently available task for access to a drink (e.g., sips of apple juice). As the session progresses, the child may become satiated on one or both the snack and the drink, which would subsequently affect the allocation of responding across tasks. In an example of conditional preference, Schieltz and colleagues (2020) demonstrated that given a choice between math and reading tasks, an 8-year-old boy chose reading. However, when provided with contingent positive reinforcement, the boy chose math over reading tasks. Future translational studies could extend the work of Lewon et al. (2019) to evaluate how to leverage changing motivating operations for available sources of reinforcement with the goal of promoting the occurrence of desirable behaviors versus concurrently available undesirable behaviors.

Choice as a Strategy for Behavior Change

Thus far, we have discussed the effects of reinforcement variables on response allocation. Choice also has been a strategy used for producing behavior change. Researchers have reported that providing the opportunity to choose among alternatives can result in increases in appropriate behavior and decreases in inappropriate behavior (e.g., Graff et al., 1998; Romaniuk & Miltenberger, 2001; Tasky et al., 2008). Ackerlund-Brandt et al. (2015) evaluated preference for the opportunity to engage in a choice and whether differential histories associated with choice and no-choice conditions resulted in changes in preference. Participants were preschool-age children who responded on a concurrent-chains procedure, where choice during the initial link led to access to terminal links associated with child choice (praise and child-selected edible), experimenter choice (praise and experimenter-selected edible), or control (praise and no-edible) outcomes. When the outcomes were identical, most participants preferred the child-choice terminal link, consistent with previous findings of preference for the opportunity to choose (e.g., Graff et al., 1998). Ackerlund-Brandt et al. (2015) also evaluated whether arranging conditioning sessions in which child or experimenter choice was paired with either high-preferred or low-preferred stimuli would result in a preference for the terminal link that had been paired with the highly-preferred stimuli. The researchers refer to the high- and low-preference stimuli as qualitatively different options, with the qualitatively superior stimulus being the highly-preferred one. Ackerlund-Brandt et al. assessed whether the quality of the terminal outcomes could affect selecting the child-choice terminal link. All participants of this study preferred the higher-quality reinforcers, even if that meant selecting the experimenter-choice terminal link. Thus, the quality of the reinforcer available was more valuable than the option to select the specific reinforcer to earn, suggesting there are conditions in which access to a choice will not function as an effective consequence for behavior change. Future translational research could further explore the interaction of reinforcer quality and the opportunity to engage in a specific choice. For instance, is it possible to leverage reinforcer quality when a choice is unavailable (e.g., when a child cannot choose which school subject is next on their daily schedule) to produce the desired allocation of behavior (e.g., task engagement and completion instead of off-task or disruptive behavior)?

In another example of access to choice as an approach to promote behavior change, Boga and Normand (2017) evaluated whether the opportunity to choose the leisure-activity context by preschool-age children impacted the level of moderate-to-vigorous physical activity (MVPA) in which they engaged. For this purpose, Boga and Normand conducted an activity-context functional analysis to identify the contexts that evoked the highest level of MVPA for each participant. Next, the researchers arranged a concurrent-chains procedure to determine whether participants preferred the activity context that evoked the most MVPA during the functional analysis or whether they preferred activity contexts that did not evoke MVPA. Participants chose MVPA contexts only, sedentary contexts only, or a combination. Boga and Normand also evaluated whether the opportunity to choose an activity context influenced MVPA beyond any possible effects of participant preference for certain activity contexts and, based on their findings, this does not appear to be the case. The authors note, however, that it is possible to choose between other aspects of physical activity, such as duration and intensity of activity, which may influence MVPA. Future research could explore how environmental variables such as context, dimensions of the target behavior/activity, and availability of alternative sources of reinforcement impact the allocation of behavior under situations similar to those evaluated by Boga and Normand.

Behavioral-Economic Account of Choice

Earlier methods for evaluating choice involved directly manipulating individual factors such as reinforcer rate, magnitude, quality, and immediacy. The goal of these earlier efforts was to explore how varying aspects of reinforcement schedules and reinforcer presentation influenced responding (i.e., matching). Although research on the matching law has suggested that it can provide a parsimonious description of response–reinforcer relations, organisms rarely allocate responding in ways that optimize reinforcer production (e.g., undermatching; Baum, 1974). Such phenomena are frequently observed across fields and populations, often labeled as "impulsive" or "suboptimal" acts. In contrast to a mainstream interpretation of "impulsivity," which explains such acts using heuristics and cognitive biases, the operant behavioral-economic approach focuses on how environmental arrangements contribute to choice (Bickel et al., 2011; see also Madden et al., Chapter 21, this volume).

The two most prevalent methodologies in the operant behavioral-economic framework are discounting and operant demand (Reed et al., 2013). *Delay discounting* (often more simply referred to as *discounting*) refers to how the immediate, subjective value of reinforcers varies as a function of its distance from the present (Ainslie, 1975); that is, it is an account of choice between reinforcers when their magnitudes and their delays differ (e.g., smaller, sooner or larger, later). Organisms typically demonstrate a preference for reinforcers with a larger magnitude over those with a smaller magnitude (i.e., matching); however, such preferences often *reverse* in the presence of delays (Kirby & Herrnstein, 1995). For instance, preference between two reinforcers often varies as one of those prospects becomes closer, and this often results in a reversal from initial preferences. Take, for example, a person asked to choose between $50 and $100 available at different points in the future, as shown in Figure 16.5. Although initially the larger, later amount is more valuable and preferred, the preference shifts toward the more immediate and smaller amount as it becomes nearer the present. Researchers have replicated this finding extensively across reinforcer types and species (Odum, 2011).

The discounting methodology has been useful for elucidating relations between reinforcer preferences and associated delays. In an applied example, Gilroy and Kaplan (2020) studied how parents make choices between behavior management strategies. When the effects of a recommended behavior change procedure (i.e., an evidence-based treatment) were either immediate or slightly delayed, parents typically endorsed a preference for the recommended approach. However, caregivers endorsed a preference for short-term and less effective strategies when the effects of recommended procedures were more delayed (e.g., giving candy to a child demonstrating a tantrum in a store rather than implementing an extinction procedure). As noted in Gilroy and Kaplan (2020), evidence-based treatments were discounted as a function of the time necessary to complete training and

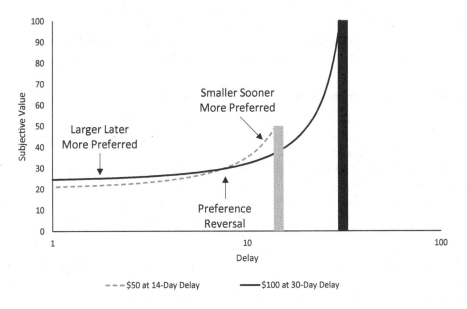

FIGURE 16.5. Delay discounting in a choice between $50 in 14 days and $100 in 30 days. The placement of vertical bars relative to the *y*-axis represents the delay to the reinforcer, in this case, the bar that is a shorter distance along the *x*-axis (lighter bar) is delayed 14 days, and the bar further along the *x*-axis (darker bar) is delayed 30 days. The height of the vertical bars indicates the magnitude of the reinforcer, in this case, the shorter (lighter) bar represents $50 and the taller (darker) bar represents $100.

implement as designed (as compared to short-term, less effective alternatives). Although the discounting framework is useful for evaluating discrete choices (e.g., concurrent chains), this approach ultimately presumes that real-world choices are dichotomous, independent, and discrete (e.g., recommended behavior strategies vs. not recommended strategies). Although direct and well-matched to experimental research, this context does not represent the range and complexity of choices that commonly occur in the natural environment (Hursh, 1980).

The operant demand framework is a methodology for evaluating reinforcers using concepts traditionally reserved for economists (Hursh, 1980). Hursh (1980, 1984) made a case for moving beyond discounting and direct extensions of matching, noting that "no simple unidimensional choice rule such as matching can account for all choice behavior" (Hursh, 1980, p. 236). For instance, investigators can use the operant demand approach to evaluate how choices can occur *together* rather than focus on relative comparisons between them (e.g., preference for choice A over choice B). This added flexibility provides researchers with a means to evaluate choices under constraints that are more analogous to the natural environment (e.g., varying costs, scarcity, availability of substitutes). For example, certain types of reinforcers may be consumed together (i.e., complementary) while others are consumed as replacements for the other (i.e., substitutes; see Reed et al., 2013, for a discussion). Viewed in this way, choice can be evaluated in the presence or absence of other prospects, each of which may be available freely or at varying costs (i.e., schedules). Revisiting caregiver choice for intervention, Gilroy et al. (2022) evaluated the relationship between caregiver consumption of evidence-based and pseudoscientific interventions, and found that caregivers, overall, indicated that they would use pseudo-scientific treatments as functional substitutes for evidence-based intervention; that is, the *relations* between the consumption of qualitatively different reinforcers can be explained functionally. Applied researchers often use the operant demand framework to explore how the relations between reinforcers influence individual choices and preferences.

Operant Behavioral Economics and Applied Behavior Analysis

The operant behavioral-economic framework has been rapidly adopted in fields such as substance misuse and abuse (Kaplan et al., 2018), though much less has been translated to applied work with children with developmental and learning issues (Gilroy et al., 2018). With respect to operant demand, various behavioral-economic concepts have strong promise for enhancing various aspects of clinical practice. For instance, knowledge of the relations that exist between reinforcers (e.g., substitutes, complements), the durability of reinforcer demand across varying schedules (i.e., price elasticity of demand), and the balance between reinforcer magnitude and schedules of reinforcement (i.e., unit price) are all relevant to designing contingencies that support desired levels of behavior. An illustration of the prototypical demand curve appears in Figure 16.6, and interested readers are directed to Gilroy et al. (2018) for a systematic review of operant demand methods and their translation into applied behavior-analytic practices.

Unit Price

Reinforcer delivery consists of the production of some magnitude of the reinforcer (e.g., 30-second access) contingent on a schedule or price (e.g., fixed-ratio 3 [FR3]). Although magnitude and schedule are useful in their own regard (see earlier sections), a

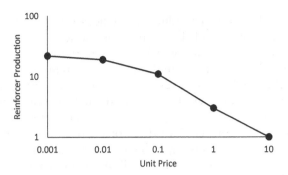

FIGURE 16.6. Example of a prototypical demand function. The typical form of the demand curve is downward sloping, with the overall reinforcer consumption/production decreasing as the price/schedule increases.

behavioral-economic approach often integrates the two by constructing a ratio of magnitude to price (Foster & Hackenberg, 2004). This concept, unit price, is a way to singularly represent the "cost" to produce a reinforcer (i.e., FR 3 30-seconds reinforcement = 30/3 = 0.1). A unit price approach has been useful for illustrating how modifying reinforcer magnitude alone alters the reinforcer–response ratio and subsequently has an effect on behavior (Borrero et al., 2007). For example, Borrero et al. retrospectively analyzed rates of severe problem behavior in terms of its unit price (i.e., response-to-reinforcer magnitude ratio). Descriptively, the data conformed to the expected shape of the demand curve and suggested that problem behavior was sensitive to changes in unit price (i.e., increasing elasticity following price increases). Apart from problem behavior, this behavioral-economic concept also has applicability to interventions predicated on work output. For instance, the process of schedule thinning is analogous to modifying the "price" to produce access to a programmed reinforcer over time (Roane et al., 2007). In a novel demonstration of unit price, Roane et al. systematically increased response requirements in a differential reinforcement of the omission of behavior (DRO) procedure using the concept of unit price. Researchers selected a unit price and thinned[3] reinforcement by increasing response requirements and simultaneously scaling reinforcer magnitude in tandem. Gilroy et al. (2019) also implemented a similar approach, though, in the context of demand fading, using unit price arrangements. Results indicated that the concept of unit price can help to guide future schedule changes and minimize the risk of ratio strain.

Price Elasticity of Demand

The *price elasticity of demand for reinforcers* refers to how relative increases in price correspond to relative decreases in reinforcer production (Gilroy et al., 2020; Lea, 1978); that is, a relative change from FR 1 to FR 2 (100% increase) is likely to have less of an impact on reinforcer production than one from FR 10 to FR 20 (100% increase). Such differential influences on reinforcer efficacy are referred to typically as *ratio strain,*

---

[3]We note here that response requirements were gradually increased in this example, but the overall unit price remained constant. In this context, "thinning" took place without progressing to a leaner schedule.

whereby responding and reinforcer production are negatively affected by lean schedules (i.e., moving to a higher price). In a behavioral-economic account of choice, this differential relation is referred to as *elasticity*, which is a quantity that varies across unit prices. Like unit price, elasticity can be useful in deciding which reinforcers to use in treatment and how to arrange them (Gilroy et al., 2019). In a study evaluating how price elasticity affects reinforcer efficacy, Gilroy et al. (2021) evaluated the effects of reinforcers with schedules drawn from the inelastic and elastic ranges, respectively. Results indicated that, overall, levels of responding tracked with the projects from a prior demand curve, and specifically, schedules considered falling in the elastic range were more associated with diminishing rates of reinforcer production overall. Behavior change procedures informed by the elasticity of demand could inform treatment regarding the effects of reinforcers, and specifically, which of the various schedule options under consideration may perform most efficiently and reliably.

Economy Type

In an operant behavioral-economic account of choice, the reinforcer *economy* directly influences reinforcer consumption. Broadly, the *reinforcer economy* refers to whether the same (or a comparable) reinforcer may be accessed elsewhere and at another price (e.g., more easily, freely). The reinforcer economy has good applied utility, because it influences the amount of work sustained by a reinforcer (e.g., Kodak et al., 2007; Roane et al., 2005). For example, Kodak et al. (2007) evaluated responding in the presence and absence of postsession reinforcement (i.e., an open and closed economy, respectively). Postsession delivery of reinforcers is analogous to an "open" economy, because a particular reinforcer is available outside of the programmed contingency, either freely or at a lower price (i.e., more dense schedule). Consistent with economic logic, Kodak et al. found that responding in open economies was much more sensitive to increases in price, and thus confirmed that reinforcers were more efficacious when used in closed economies. Regarding individual choice, research with caregiver choice of behavior therapy has also revealed similar patterns concerning preference for evidence-based therapies. Specifically, several studies have found that caregivers would choose to pursue evidence-based, parent-mediated intervention when this was the only option available (closed economy) but preferences quickly shifted when alternative options (evidence-based or not) were concurrently available at a lower price (see, e.g., Gilroy et al., 2022; Gilroy & Feck, 2022; Gilroy & Picardo, 2022).

Summary

In summary, various ecological factors such as the rate, magnitude, quality, and immediacy of reinforcers drive individual choice and preference. These factors are readily manipulated in ways that can encourage adaptive and appropriate choices while discouraging less appropriate alternatives. Even further, the presentation of alternatives (i.e., choice as an antecedent strategy) can itself serve as an effective element of behavioral programming. Aside from these strategies, recent extensions of operant behavioral economics offer the ability to reveal relations between choice options and how the schedule of one reinforcer can influence the production of others.

Despite a variety of applications using the matching law and operant behavioral economics, considerable work continues to be necessary. For instance, various areas of clinical practice may be informed by, or improved, by using quantitative methods. Regarding the demand framework, measurements of reinforcer efficacy can be used to empirically derive schedules used in treatment (Gilroy et al., 2021) guide schedule thinning and demand fading (Gilroy et al., 2019; Roane et al., 2007), and describe reinforcer performance across various contexts (Kodak et al., 2007).

REFERENCES

Ackerlund-Brandt, J. A., Dozier, C. L., Juanico, J. F., Laudont, C. L., & Mick, B. R. (2015). The value of choice as a reinforcer for typically developing children. *Journal of Applied Behavior Analysis, 48*(2), 344–362.

Ainslie, G. W. (1975). Specious reward: A behavioral theory of impulsiveness and impulse control. *Psychological Bulletin, 82*(4), 463–496.

Austin, J. E., & Tiger, J. H. (2015). Providing alternative reinforcers to facilitate tolerance to delayed reinforcement following functional communication training. *Journal of Applied Behavior Analysis, 48*(3), 663–668.

Bailey, J. J., McComas, J. J., Benavides, C., Lovascz, C., & Thompson, A. (2002). Functional assessment in a residential setting: Identifying an effective communicative replacement response for aggressive behavior. *Journal of Developmental and Physical Disabilities, 14*, 353–369.

Baum, W. M. (1974). On two types of deviation from the matching law: Bias and undermatching. *Journal of the Experimental Analysis of Behavior, 22*(1), 231–242.

Baum, W. M., & Rachlin, H. C. (1969). Choice as time allocation. *Journal of the Experimental Analysis of Behavior, 12*(6), 861–874.

Bickel, W. K., Jarmolowicz, D. P., Mueller, E. T., & Gatchalian, K. M. (2011). The behavioral economics and neuroeconomics of reinforcer pathologies: Implications for etiology and treatment of addiction. *Current Psychiatry Reports, 13*(5), 406–415.

Boga, V., & Normand, M. P. (2017). The opportunity to choose the activity context does not increase moderate-to-vigorous physical activity exhibited by preschool children. *Psychological Record, 67*(2), 189–196.

Bolles, R. C. (1961). Is the "click" a token reward? *Psychological Record, 11*(2), 163–168.

Borrero, J. C., Francisco, M. T., Haberlin, A. T., Ross, N. A., & Sran, S. K. (2007). A unit price evaluation of severe problem behavior. *Journal of Applied Behavior Analysis, 40*(3), 463–474.

Catania, A. C. (2013). *Learning* (5th ed.). Sloan.

Chung, S. H. (1965a). Effects of delayed reinforcement in a concurrent situation. *Journal of the Experimental Analysis of Behavior, 8*(6), 439–444.

Chung, S. H. (1965b). Effects of effort on response rate. *Journal of the Experimental Analysis of Behavior, 8*(1), 1–8.

Chung, S. H., & Herrnstein, R. J. (1967). Choice and delay of reinforcement. *Journal of the Experimental Analysis of Behavior, 10*(1), 67–74.

Clay, C. J., Samaha, A. L., & Bogoev, B. K. (2018). Assessing preference for and reinforcing efficacy of components of social interaction in individuals with autism spectrum disorder. *Learning and Motivation, 62*, 4–14.

Cooper, L. J., Wacker, D. P., Brown, K., Mccomas, J. J., Peck, S. M., Drew, J., . . . Kayser, K. (1999). Use of a concurrent operants paradigm to evaluate positive reinforcers during treatment of food refusal. *Behavior Modification, 23*(1), 3–40.

Cowie, S., & Davison, M. (2016). Control by reinforcers across time and space: A review of recent choice research. *Journal of the Experimental Analysis of Behavior, 105*(2), 246–269.

Cowie, S., Virués-Ortega, J., McCormack, J., Hogg, P., & Podlesnik, C. A. (2021). Extending a misallocation model to children's choice behavior. *Journal of Experimental Psychology: Animal Learning and Cognition, 47*(3), 317–325.

Davison, M., & McCarthy, D. (1988). *The matching law: A research review.* Erlbaum.

Foster, T. A., & Hackenberg, T. D. (2004). Unit price and choice in a token-reinforcement context. *Journal of the Experimental Analysis of Behavior, 81*(1), 5–25.

Fritz, J. N., Dupuis, D. L., Wu, W. L., Neal,

A. E., Rettig, L. A., & Lastrapes, R. E. (2017). Evaluating increased effort for item disposal to improve recycling at a university. *Journal of Applied Behavior Analysis, 50*(4), 825–829.

Gilroy, S. P., & Feck, C. C. (2022). Applications of operant demand to treatment selection II: Covariance of evidence strength and treatment consumption. *Journal of the Experimental Analysis of Behavior, 117*(2), 167–179.

Gilroy, S. P., Ford, H. L., Boyd, R. J., O'Connor, J. T., & Kurtz, P. F. (2019). An evaluation of operant behavioural economics in functional communication training for severe problem behaviour. *Developmental Neurorehabilitation, 22*(8), 553–564.

Gilroy, S. P., & Kaplan, B. A. (2020). Modeling treatment-related decision-making using applied behavioral economics: Caregiver perspectives in temporally-extended behavioral treatments. *Journal of Abnormal Child Psychology, 48*(5), 607–618.

Gilroy, S. P., Kaplan, B. A., & Leader, G. (2018). A systematic review of applied behavioral economics in assessments and treatments for individuals with developmental disabilities. *Review Journal of Autism and Developmental Disorders, 5*(3), 247–259.

Gilroy, S. P., Kaplan, B. A., & Reed, D. D. (2020). Interpretation(s) of elasticity in operant demand. *Journal of the Experimental Analysis of Behavior, 114*(1), 106–115.

Gilroy, S. P., & Picardo, R. (2022). Applications of operant demand to treatment selection III: Consumer behavior analysis of treatment choice. *Journal of the Experimental Analysis of Behavior, 118*(1), 46–58.

Gilroy, S. P., Waits, J. A., & Feck, C. (2021). Extending stimulus preference assessment with the operant demand framework. *Journal of Applied Behavior Analysis, 54*(3), 1032–1044.

Gilroy, S. P., Waits, J. A., & Kaplan, B. A. (2022). Applications of operant demand to treatment selection I: Characterizing demand for evidence-based practices. *Journal of the Experimental Analysis of Behavior, 117*(1), 20–35.

Graff, R. B., Libby, M. E., & Green, G. (1998). The effects of reinforcer choice on rates of challenging behavior and free operant responding in individuals with severe disabilities. *Behavioral Interventions: Theory and Practice in Residential and Community-Based Clinical Programs, 13*(4), 249–268.

Herrnstein, R. J. (1961). Relative and absolute strength of response as a function of frequency of reinforcement. *Journal of the Experimental Analysis of Behavior, 4,* 267–272.

Herrnstein, R. J. (1970). On the law of effect. *Journal of the Experimental Analysis of Behavior, 13*(2), 243–266.

Hoch, H., McComas, J. J., Johnson, L., Faranda, N., & Guenther, S. L. (2002). The effects of magnitude and quality of reinforcement on choice responding during play activities. *Journal of Applied Behavior Analysis, 35*(2), 171–181.

Horner, R. H., & Day, H. M. (1991). The effects of response efficiency on functionally equivalent competing behaviors. *Journal of Applied Behavior Analysis, 24*(4), 719–732.

Hunter, I., & Davison, M. (1982). Independence of response force and reinforcement rate on concurrent variable-interval schedule performance. *Journal of the Experimental Analysis of Behavior, 37*(2), 183–197.

Hursh, S. R. (1980). Economic concepts for the analysis of behavior. *Journal of the Experimental Analysis of Behavior, 34*(2), 219–238.

Hursh, S. R. (1984). Behavioral economics. *Journal of the Experimental Analysis of Behavior, 42*(3), 435–452.

Jacobs, E. A., Borrero, J. C., & Vollmer, T. R. (2013). Translational applications of quantitative choice models. In G. J. Madden (Ed.), *APA handbook of behavior analysis: Translating principles into practice* (Vol. 2, pp. 165–190). American Psychological Association.

Jimenez-Gomez, C., Brewer, A. L. T., & Podlesnik, C. A. (2018, May). *An automated task for evaluating the discriminative effects of reinforcers with children.* Poster presented at the annual meeting of the Society for Quantitative Analyses of Behavior, San Diego, CA.

Kaplan, B. A., Foster, R. N. S., Reed, D. D., Amlung, M., Murphy, J. G., & MacKillop, J. (2018). Understanding alcohol motivation using the alcohol purchase task: A methodological systematic review. *Drug and Alcohol Dependence, 191,* 117–140.

Kirby, K. N., & Herrnstein, R. J. (1995). Preference reversals due to myopic discounting of delayed reward. *Psychological Science, 6*(2), 83–89.

Kodak, T., Lerman, D. C., & Call, N. (2007). Evaluating the influence of postsession reinforcement on choice of reinforcers. *Journal of Applied Behavior Analysis, 40*(3), 515–527.

Krägeloh, C. U., Davison, M., & Elliffe, D. M. (2005). Local preference in concurrent schedules: The effects of reinforcer sequences. *Journal of the Experimental Analysis of Behavior, 84*(1), 37–64.

Lea, S. E. (1978). The psychology and economics of demand. *Psychological Bulletin, 85,* 441–466.

Lewon, M., Spurlock, E. D., Peters, C. M., & Hayes, L. J. (2019). Interactions between the effects of food and water motivating operations on food-and water-reinforced responding in mice. *Journal of the Experimental Analysis of Behavior, 111*(3), 493–507.

Mazur, J. E., & Fantino, E. (2014). Choice. In F. K. McSweeney & E. S. Murphy (Eds.), *The Wiley Blackwell handbook of operant and classical conditioning* (pp. 195–220). Wiley.

McDevitt, M. A., & Williams, B. A. (2001). Effects of signaled versus unsignaled delay of reinforcement on choice. *Journal of the Experimental Analysis of Behavior, 75*(2), 165–182.

McSweeney, F. K. (1974). Variability of responding on a concurrent schedule as a function of body weight. *Journal of the Experimental Analysis of Behavior, 21*(2), 357–359.

Miller, H. L. (1976). Matching-based hedonic scaling in the pigeon. *Journal of the Experimental Analysis of Behavior, 26*(3), 335–347.

Neuringer, A. J. (1967). Effects of reinforcement magnitude on choice and rate of responding. *Journal of the Experimental Analysis of Behavior, 10*(5), 417–424.

Odum, A. L. (2011). Delay discounting: I'm a k, you're a k. *Journal of the Experimental Analysis of Behavior, 96*(3), 427–439.

Podlesnik, C. A., Jimenez-Gomez, C., & Kelley, M. E. (2021). Matching and behavioral momentum. In W. W. Fisher, C. C. Piazza, & H. S. Roane (Eds.), *Handbook of applied behavior analysis* (2nd ed., pp. 94–114). Guilford Press.

Reed, D. D., & Kaplan, B. A. (2011). The matching law: A tutorial for practitioners. *Behavior Analysis in Practice, 4*(2), 15–24.

Reed, D. D., Niilleksela, C. R., & Kaplan, B. A. (2013). Behavioral economics: A tutorial for behavior analysts in practice. *Behavior Analysis in Practice, 6*(1), 34–54.

Richards, R. W. (1981). A comparison of signaled and unsignaled delay of reinforcement. *Journal of the Experimental Analysis of Behavior, 35*(2), 145–152.

Roane, H. S., Call, N. A., & Falcomata, T. S. (2005). A preliminary analysis of adaptive responding under open and closed economies. *Journal of Applied Behavior Analysis, 38*(3), 335–348.

Roane, H. S., Falcomata, T. S., & Fisher, W. W. (2007). Applying the behavioral economics principle of unit price to DRO schedule thinning. *Journal of Applied Behavior Analysis, 40*(3), 529–534.

Rogalski, J. P., Roscoe, E. M., Fredericks, D. W., & Mezhoudi, N. (2020). Negative reinforcer magnitude manipulations for treating escape-maintained problem behavior. *Journal of Applied Behavior Analysis, 53*(3), 1514–1530.

Romaniuk, C., & Miltenberger, R. G. (2001). The influence of preference and choice of activity on problem behavior. *Journal of Positive Behavior Interventions, 3*(3), 152–159.

Schieltz, K. M., Wacker, D. P., Suess, A. N., Graber, J. E., Lustig, N. H., & Detrick, J. (2020). Evaluating the effects of positive reinforcement, instructional strategies, and negative reinforcement on problem behavior and academic performance: An experimental analysis. *Journal of Developmental and Physical Disabilities, 32,* 339–363.

Symons, F. J., Hoch, J., Dahl, N. A., & McComas, J. J. (2003). Sequential and matching analyses of self-injurious behavior: A case of overmatching in the natural environment. *Journal of Applied Behavior Analysis, 36*(2), 267–270.

Tasky, K. K., Rudrud, E. H., Schulze, K. A., & Rapp, J. T. (2008). Using choice to increase on-task behavior in individuals with traumatic brain injury. *Journal of Applied Behavior Analysis, 41*(2), 261–265.

Ward-Horner, J. C., Pittenger, A., Pace, G., & Fienup, D. M. (2014). Effects of reinforcer magnitude and distribution on preference for work schedules. *Journal of Applied Behavior Analysis, 47*(3), 623–627.

CHAPTER 17

Verbal Behavior

FROM THE LABORATORY TO THE FIELD AND BACK

Anna Ingeborg Petursdottir
Einar T. Ingvarsson

B. F. Skinner's (1957) *Verbal Behavior* was a project of science translation that has few parallels in the human behavioral sciences. In *Verbal Behavior*, Skinner used principles derived from laboratory research with nonhuman animals to construct a comprehensive theory of human language and verbal cognition without any reference to uniquely human learning processes or abilities. The goal was to demystify these complex aspects of human behavior and account for them in the same scientific terms as other behavior of living organisms.

Verbal Behavior contained few references to data from human subjects, but Skinner (1957) made clear the ultimate aim was to achieve "prediction and control of verbal behavior" (p. 12). More than 60 years later, Skinner's work exerts a strong influence on behavior-analytic research and practice, particularly in the area of early language intervention. In this chapter, we summarize the major points Skinner made in *Verbal Behavior*, describe their implications for establishing language skills, and discuss additional topics of basic and applied verbal behavior research that have been prominent in the 21st century (Petursdottir, 2018).

Skinner's *Verbal Behavior*

What Is Verbal Behavior?

Skinner (1957) chose the term *verbal behavior* over *language* to describe his subject matter, as conventional usage of the latter term did not match the scope and emphasis of his work (i.e., functional relations governing the behavior of individual speakers). The "big idea" presented in *Verbal Behavior* was that verbal behavior is simply behavior, specifically, behavior under the control of operant contingencies. It follows that we should not necessarily expect a clear-cut distinction between verbal behavior and other operant behavior. After careful deliberation (Palmer, 2008), Skinner defined *verbal behavior* as behavior that has been reinforced not through its physical effects on the environment, but "through the mediation of other persons" (1957, p. 2). More precisely, Skinner added, it has been reinforced through the actions of a listener that result from the listener's own reinforcement history with respect to verbal stimuli. Verbal behavior need not be vocal behavior. At the dinner table, "May I have the bread, please?" may qualify as a verbal response whether produced vocally, in writing, or using sign language. A head nod toward the bread basket may qualify as verbal behavior as well. By contrast, reaching for and grabbing the basket is nonverbal behavior, and so is the act of physically guiding a young child to pass the bread if the child is responding simply to the physical stimulation.

It is possible to poke holes in Skinner's definition of verbal behavior if one is so inclined. For one thing, to know if particular behavior qualifies as verbal, in theory, we must know the reinforcement histories of the listeners who have reinforced it in the past, which seems impractical for classification purposes. For another, it is possible to come up with examples of behavior that qualifies as verbal according to the definition but seems unconventional to characterize at such (see Hayes et al., 2001). However, although Skinner's definition served to demarcate the general subject matter of *Verbal Behavior*, we can be fairly certain it was not intended to represent a fundamental distinction between verbal and nonverbal domains, as Skinner's big idea was exactly that no such fundamental distinction existed (Normand, 2009). Thus, if Skinner's (1957) definition does not permit definitively classifying all samples of behavior as verbal or nonverbal, it may be because Skinner saw no reason to do so.

Elementary Verbal Relations

Skinner (1957) defined his analytic unit as the *verbal operant*, consisting of a class of verbal response forms (e.g., all responses producing the auditory stimulus "water" or other stimuli to which listeners have responded similarly) that are under the functional control of a particular class of antecedents due to prior reinforcement. Skinner distinguished between different types of verbal operants based on the type of antecedent variable that controls the form or topography of the response (see Table 17.1). The most important (p. 83) verbal operant is the *tact*, in which the controlling antecedent is a discriminative stimulus originating in the physical environment outside or inside the speaker's skin. Due to the speaker's prior history, the stimulus predicts generalized social reinforcement (e.g., listener attention, acknowledgment, approval, expression of gratitude) for a particular class of responses. The tact concept, linking words and sentences to nonverbal objects and events, addresses much of what is traditionally thought of as meaning or reference.

Reinforcement histories similar to those that establish tact control can also establish discriminative control by verbal stimuli, that is, stimuli produced by other people's (or the speaker's own) verbal behavior. Skinner (1957) described several types of verbal operants in which the controlling stimuli are verbal (Table 17.1). In the *intraverbal*, the relation between the verbal stimulus and the response is formally arbitrary, such that the product of the response (e.g., the spoken word "water") differs in form from the controlling stimulus (e.g., the spoken word "swimming"). Skinner proposed adult intraverbal repertoires resulted from "hundreds of thousands of reinforcements under a great variety of inconsistent and often conflicting contingencies" (p. 74), such that a particular verbal stimulus could come to exert control over many different response forms, and a single verbal response form could be intraverbally related to many verbal antecedent stimuli. Other types of verbal operants in which the controlling antecedent is verbal are

TABLE 17.1. Elementary Verbal Relations: Antecedent Controlling Variables and Examples

Type of relation	Controlling antecedent	Example
Mand	Motivating (establishing) operation	Saying "water" as a result of water deprivation
Tact	Nonverbal discriminative stimulus	Saying "water" as a result of seeing or hearing water
Intraverbal	Verbal discriminative stimulus with no formal relation to the response product	Saying "water" as a result of hearing or seeing the word "swimming"
Echoic	Vocally produced verbal discriminative stimulus of which the vocal response product is a copy	Saying "water" as a result of hearing someone else say "water"
Copying text	Textual verbal discriminative stimulus of which the written response product is a copy	Writing or typing "water" as a result of seeing "water" written or in print
Textual behavior	Written verbal discriminative stimulus that exerts point-to-point control over a vocal response	Saying "water" as a result of seeing "water" written or in print
Transcription	Vocally produced verbal discriminative stimulus that exerts point-to-point control over a written or other nonvocal response	Writing or typing "water" as a result of hearing someone else say "water"

characterized by rigid antecedent control over the form of the verbal response, such that the formal relations between stimulus and response are either *duplic* or *codic* (Michael, 1982a). In duplic relations, the response produces a stimulus product that duplicates the controlling stimulus (echoic; copying text), whereas in codic relations, parts of the stimulus control parts of a response that differs in form from the stimulus (textual behavior; transcription), with point-to-point correspondence between stimulus and response. Of the verbal operants in which the controlling antecedent is verbal, only the intraverbal is neither duplic nor codic.

The *mand*, finally, differs from the other elementary verbal relations in that the antecedent that controls the form of the response is a motivating operation (MO)[1] rather than a discriminative stimulus. MO control results from a history of reinforcement in which the response produced a specific consequence of relevance to the MO (e.g., water under conditions of water deprivation), as opposed to producing more general reactions from listeners.

As evident from the examples in Table 17.1, any particular response form may be under the functional control of many different antecedents. "Water" can occur as a tact or a mand, a codic or a duplic, or as an intraverbal response to a variety of verbal stimuli (e.g., "H$_2$O," "wet," "faucet"). In the natural environment, controlling variables appropriate to more than one verbal operant may often contribute simultaneously to the occurrence of a particular response; for example, under conditions of water deprivation

---

[1]The term *motivating operation* postdates Skinner's passing (Laraway et al., 2003). However, Michael's (1982b, 1993) and subsequent treatments of MOs (Laraway et al., 2003) are consistent with Skinner's conceptualization of the controlling variables for the mand (Sundberg, 2013).

(controlling variable for mand), seeing particular beverages displayed in a cooler (controlling variable for tact) or reading their names on a menu (controlling variable for textual behavior) may influence which particular response occurs (e.g., "kombucha"). Skinner (1957) suggested (p. 189), in fact, that most instances of manding are jointly influenced by MOs and discriminative stimuli and are thus only partially mands (see discussion of multiple control in the next section).

In addition, Skinner (1957) noted that all verbal behavior is broadly influenced by *audience* variables; that is, the presence and characteristics of an audience influence the occurrence, form, and energy level of verbal responses under the primary control of other stimuli. For example, we may be more likely to mand for a shopkeeper's attention when the shopkeeper is not assisting another customer, and our word choices and tone of voice when talking to a close friend may differ from when we are discussing the same topic with a professional acquaintance. In some cases, the speaker serves as their own audience, as in self-talk and diary writing.

Multiple Control, Autoclitics, and Complex Verbal Behavior

After laying out his mission and introducing the elementary verbal operants as his major conceptual tools, Skinner (1957) exposed the details of his argument that functional relations of the sort he had described could fully account for the complexities of human verbal behavior. An important part of Skinner's argument revolved around combined control by multiple antecedents, or *multiple control*, setting the stage for novel verbal utterances. At any moment, a mature speaker in the natural environment is surrounded by a variety of stimuli that participate in tact relations with verbal response forms, and MOs may be present that participate in mand relations. On top of that, the environment may contain both transient and static verbal stimuli emanating from other people's speech, from text, or from the speaker's own self-talk, providing rich and dynamic sources of intraverbal control, as well as duplic and codic control. Thus, variables are continually present that are capable of evoking large numbers of different response forms. The speaker, however, is unlikely to overtly emit all of these possible responses. Instead, the probability of occurrence is influenced by the summated strength of controlling variables that are currently present. For example, the probability that the sight of a bread basket on a countertop will evoke the tact "bread" may be elevated if the speaker also is food deprived (mand control). When two or more sources of control converge on a particular response form in this manner (*convergent control*; Michael et al., 2011), the end result may be verbal behavior that appears to be novel or under novel stimulus control. A child who is asked for the first time to "name a yellow fruit" may respond with "banana" in spite of no prior history of responding to that stimulus combination (DeSouza et al., 2019) because previously established stimulus control by "yellow" and "fruit" converges on "banana." A dynamic environment rich with verbal and nonverbal stimuli continually presents novel constellations of stimuli and MOs, both public and private, resulting in utterances that appear novel or involve novel response combinations, as in sentences never previously spoken (see Michael et al., 2011, for detailed treatment).

Skinner (1957) next introduced the concept of *autoclitic* behavior to account for numerous aspects of verbal behavior, including syntax and morphology, that function to modify the effects of other verbal responses on the listener. Autoclitic behavior is reinforced because it clarifies sources of stimulus control over the speaker's other verbal behavior, which benefits the listener. The *descriptive autoclitic* "I think" in "I think it is raining" serves to tact weakness in the source of tact control over "raining," and the *qualifying autoclitic* "not" in "It is not raining" conveys that although variables are present that contribute strength to "raining" (e.g., the sound of thunder), crucial controlling variables (e.g., the sight of rain) are absent. Other types of autoclitics Skinner described included *mands upon the listener* to react to the speaker's verbal behavior in a certain way (e.g., when a speaker makes air quotes with her fingers while speaking), *quantifying autoclitics* (e.g., "all" and "some"), and *relational autoclitics*, which capture a multiplicity of grammatical (e.g., plurality, possession) and syntactical (i.e., word order) functions.

In the last several chapters of *Verbal Behavior*, Skinner applied the foregoing analysis to the production of complex verbal behavior. He began by considering sentence construction, followed by the speaker's self-editing and self-strengthening of their own verbal behavior. The book then culminated in chapters on logic, science, and thinking that provide a clear demonstration of the conceptual power of Skinner's (1957) theory.

Establishing Verbal Behavior

Skinner's conceptualization of verbal behavior implies that instructional procedures that work for nonverbal behavior should generally also be effective with verbal behavior. At the same time, certain unique practical implications follow from Skinner's functional approach. A comprehensive review of applied research and practice influenced by *Verbal Behavior* is beyond the scope of this chapter, but the following pages provide a brief overview of some of the more important considerations.

Sequence of Instruction

The logic of Skinner's conceptual analysis has implications for the sequence of intervention targets for individuals with language delays and communication deficits. Manding is an important early skill, because it allows the individual to obtain preferred and avoid nonpreferred items and activities when the relevant MOs are in place, and therefore, independently advocate for their own wants and needs (Sundberg & Michael, 2001). An echoic repertoire is also fundamental, because it allows for the recombination of echoic units into more complex responses, and it can also facilitate the acquisition of other verbal operants through transfer of function (see below).

Tacting and listener behavior (e.g., receptive identification) should generally be targeted before intraverbal behavior, because the nonverbal stimulus control characteristic of the former categories is a crucial component of "meaningful" verbal behavior. To illustrate, consider a young child who learns to say "moo" in response to the phrase "A cow says . . ." (an intraverbal). If the child had previously learned to tact and respond as a listener to a cow, the child might then be able to engage in other related behavior, such as making the sound "moo" when playing with a toy cow and pointing to a picture of a cow in a book when hearing an adult make the sound "moo." However, these outcomes would be unlikely if the tact and the listener response had not been previously established. In the latter situation, we might say that the child does not understand what he is saying, or his response is "meaningless" or "rote" (Ingvarsson et al., 2012). This observation draws attention to a key point in Skinner's analysis of verbal behavior: The meaning of words and sentences is to be found in their environmental determinants, that is, their function (Skinner, 1945).

Instructional Arrangements

Transfer of (Stimulus) Control

A common approach to teach verbal operants involves a set of procedures designed to transfer control from one antecedent to another. These procedures capitalize on specific verbal topographies already existing in the student's repertoire. For example, echoic prompts can be used to teach new tacts (Barbera & Kubina, 2005). With this procedure, the teacher presents the target antecedent stimulus (e.g., a picture of a car), while prompting the student to echo the word "car." The prompt is then faded until the picture evokes the response "car." This process results in transfer of stimulus control from the verbal stimulus "car" to the nonverbal stimulus, a picture of a car. Transfer of stimulus control can also be used to teach intraverbal responses (i.e., tact-to-intraverbal transfer or echoic-to-intraverbal transfer; Ingvarsson & Le, 2011). Transfer of control can also involve MOs (echoics to mands, mands to tacts, etc.). However, transfer-of-control procedures have the inherent limitation that the target response topography must already be in the student's repertoire under some sort of antecedent control (e.g., an echoic). With individuals who have limited or nonexistent verbal repertoires, shaping can be used to establish simple responses and chaining procedures can then be employed to combine these responses into more complex forms.

Discrete Trials and Natural Environment Training

Environmental arrangements during verbal behavior interventions can vary on a continuum from teacher-led discrete trials in highly controlled environments (Smith, 2001) to naturalistic procedures that involve following students' lead in their everyday environment (Laski et al., 1988). Discrete-trial instruction (DTI) involves a precisely defined sequence consisting of a teacher-presented antecedent, student response, and teacher-implemented consequence (reinforcement; error correction). A common natural environment teaching approach is *incidental teaching* (Hart & Risley, 1975), which involves arranging the environment to increase the likelihood of a certain response (e.g., placing preferred items in view but out of reach) and capitalizing on student initiations to prompt or shape relevant verbal responses (e.g., mands for the items). Alternatively, teachers can capitalize on naturally occurring opportunities to expand on or prompt student verbal responses.

Discrete trials allow teachers to implement a high rate of teaching opportunities and can be useful in establishing precise stimulus control through repeated and systematic presentation of multiple exemplars, each of which contains critical stimulus attributes, while noncritical stimulus attributes vary across exemplars (e.g., when teaching shapes as tacts or listener responses, the shape is a critical attribute, while color, size, background, etc. are noncritical attributes; Layng, 2019). Naturalistic teaching can facilitate generalization and maintenance by incorporating naturally occurring discriminative stimuli, MOs, and reinforcers. For this reason, Sundberg and Partington (1999) recommended that verbal behavior interventions include both approaches.

Response Modalities

Michael (1985) noted some differences between topography-based verbal behavior (e.g., speaking, writing, signing) and selection-based verbal behavior (e.g., selecting a communication card). The former involves a point-to-point correspondence between the individual's behavior and the response product, while the latter requires complex discriminations involving visual stimuli. Early research suggested topography-based verbal behavior was more easily learned than selection-based verbal behavior (e.g., Sundberg & Sundberg, 1990). Yet selection-based communication systems remain widely used. Further research is needed to elucidate the conditions under which selection-based versus topography-based verbal behavior leads to optimal outcomes for individuals with limited vocal speech (Petursdottir & Ingvarsson, 2023).

Arranging Antecedent Control

Generalization, Abstraction, and Concept Formation

Verbal behavior interventions would have limited utility if acquired responses only occurred under limited and restricted conditions that resemble the original training context. For example, when teaching a child to identify and tact a "car," the response should generalize across different types of cars (e.g., a Fiat 500, a Ford F-150, a Honda Accord). One way to achieve this is to teach using multiple exemplars, topographically diverse cars that nevertheless share the essential stimulus features that define a car (LaFrance & Tarbox, 2020). A similar principle applies to establishing abstract concepts, such as shapes and colors. For example, to teach the abstract concepts "red," "blue," and "yellow," the learner must be able to (1) discriminate between objects that are identical in every way except color, and (2) tact and identify topographically diverse objects in terms of the single stimulus property of color (an example of *stimulus abstraction*; Catania, 1998). In behavior analysis, concept formation is defined in terms of this kind of stimulus control.

Simple and Complex Stimulus Control

As noted in a previous section, an account of control by multiple antecedents is crucial to account for the complexities of verbally capable humans. However, it is also that case that in the early stages of verbal behavior interventions (as in typical development), simple stimulus control likely predominates. *Simple stimulus control* refers to uniform control over behavior exerted by a single stimulus (i.e., the stimulus control is not defined through an interaction or relation between stimuli). Thus, the learner might tact all four-legged animals as cats, and respond to any question including the word "name" by stating their own name. Therefore, an important step in verbal behavior interventions is to teach the learner to respond to more complex stimulus compounds and conditional discriminations. For example, asking a child, "Who was the first president of the USA?" (convergent multiple control) restricts the universe of intraverbal responses that will be reinforced relative to saying, "Name as many former presidents of the USA as you can" (*divergent multiple control*; Michael et al., 2011). Convergent multiple control may require teaching procedures designed to bring responding under control of all relevant aspects of the verbal antecedent (i.e., conditional or compound stimulus control). These include blocked trials (e.g., Ingvarsson et al., 2016) and differential observing responses (e.g., Kisamore et al., 2016). Establishing divergent multiple control may require additional strategies to teach the student to emit multiple responses to a single antecedent (e.g., problem solving; Sautter et al., 2011).

Joint control is a special case of multiple control, referring to convergent multiple control of two concurrent variables over a specific response topography, involving mediating responses (Lowenkron, 2006). When trying to remember a new combination to a locked door, a person may repeat it either covertly or overtly (a *self-echoic*). When the combination sequence matches the self-echoic topography, joint control (echoic and tact) occurs, setting the occasion for the response of opening the lock. Joint control has applied implications for teaching adaptive skills that involve temporal delays between an instruction and activities (Ampuero & Miklos, 2019; Sidener, 2006; Vosters & Luczynski, 2020).

Control by Multiple Verbal Operants

Another type of multiple control pertains to those common instances in which responding cannot be adequately explained by reference to a single verbal operant. As previously mentioned, simultaneous or interactive control by more than one verbal operant is likely the norm in any given verbal episode. For example, conversational exchanges include intraverbal control but may also contain elements of echoic and tact control, as well as mands for information (Palmer, 2016). Teachers can take advantage of temporary multiple control in the early stages of intervention to teach responses under simultaneous echoic and mand control. To illustrate, if being pushed on a swing is a preferred activity, the teacher waits until the child indicates they want to engage in the activity and then controls access to the activity while verbally modeling the word "push." When the child emits the word (or an approximation), the teacher pushes the child on the swing. The verbal model can then be faded until the mand occurs independently. Other situations involve more permanent combined control, such as that involved in teaching students to tact letters by name ("What's that letter called?") and by sound ("What sound does that letter make?"). The resulting performance can be thought of as a special case of an auditory–visual conditional discrimination (intraverbal–tact), in which the teacher's instructions function as a conditional stimulus, altering which responses are evoked by the letters, which function as discriminative stimuli (Axe & McCarthy-Pepin, 2021).

Minimal Repertoires, Recombinative Generalization, and Matrix Training

In the past, Skinner's analysis of verbal behavior has been criticized for failing to account for the generativity and novelty characteristic of the behavior of verbally competent humans. However, there are several well-established ways in which behavior analysts can account for generativity and novelty (e.g., stimulus equivalence, relational frame theory, naming theory, contingency adduction). One such approach, derived directly from Skinner's analysis, is the notion of minimal, or "atomic" repertoires; discrete stimulus–response units that can combine in novel ways given new permutations of environmental stimuli (Alessi, 1987; Palmer, 2012; Skinner, 1957). As an example, a robust minimal echoic repertoire (i.e., fluently echoing individual phonemes) enables the individual to echo novel combinations of phonemes (e.g., words and sentences that the individual has never heard before). These repertoires are relevant to any skill that can be conceptualized as units that involve point-to-point relations between stimuli and responses, such as echoic behavior, tacts, and textual behavior.

Matrix training refers to a set of procedures aimed at producing *recombinative generalization* by teaching strategically selected combinations of units, arranged in a matrix (Axe & Sainato, 2010). One approach involves teaching nonoverlapping combinations (i.e., *diagonal training*), such as "red ball," "blue cup," and "yellow flower," and then probing novel combinations ("red flower," "yellow cup," etc.). Alternatively, one can teach overlapping combinations, such as "red cup," "blue cup," "blue flower," "yellow flower," such that each unit occurs in at least two combinations (Curiel et al., 2020). This approach may be more appropriate when the learner has not mastered the units individually prior to matrix training (Kemmerer et al., 2021). Curiel et al. (2020) reported that in 12 studies on matrix training with individuals with autism spectrum disorder (ASD), a mean of 69% of acquired skills were the result of recombinative generalization, suggesting that matrix training can dramatically increase instructional efficiency. To determine the conditions under which matrix training can lead to highly flexible minimal or atomic repertoires, it will be necessary to further evaluate indirect effects on responding beyond the matrices used during instruction (Kemmerer et al., 2020).

Consequences That Maintain Verbal Behavior

Social Reinforcement

Previously, we noted that the definition of verbal behavior necessarily involves mediation by another person. This can mean that the social behavior of others serves as a conditioned (and possibly primary) reinforcer, or that access to nonsocial reinforcement (e.g., food) is mediated in some way by another person (e.g., as in manding for food). Importantly, tacts, intraverbals, and echoics, according to Skinner (1957), are maintained by generalized social reinforcers such as praise or other social interaction (e.g., smiling, positive affect). For some populations with whom behavior analysts frequently work (e.g., individuals with ASD), social reinforcers might be relatively weak or absent, which could explain (in part) the characteristic delays in verbal and social behavior (Gale et al., 2019). Response-contingent pairing (Lepper & Petursdottir, 2017) and discrimination training (i.e., establishing social stimuli as discriminative stimuli for responses that produce primary reinforcers; Vandbakk et al., 2019) have shown promise as procedures to condition social stimuli as reinforcers.

Automatic Reinforcement

Although reinforcement mediated by other persons is a defining characteristic of verbal behavior, automatic reinforcement may also play a role in its provenance and maintenance. The babbling of infants exemplifies the former, because it can persist independent of social interactions, and is therefore likely in part maintained by automatic reinforcement (e.g., the sound of one's own voice, sensory feedback from the speech organs). Babbling forms the foundation of early verbal behavior, because it can be deliberately or incidentally shaped into approximations to words through infant–caregiver interactions. Greater variety of sounds allow for greater flexibility in shaping of a variety of verbal topographies. However, when children do not babble, or their babbling consists solely of repetitive and restricted sounds that seem immune to environmental influences, the foundation for the development of a functional verbal repertoire is compromised. Researchers have attempted to increase babbling by pairing sounds with primary reinforcers, hoping to establish specific babbling sounds as conditioned reinforcers. The outcomes of this research have been inconsistent, but response-contingent pairing procedures (i.e., presenting a sound and a primary reinforcer together in close proximal contiguity following specific responses) may be promising (Lepper & Petursdottir, 2017).

Automatic reinforcement may also play a role in the development and maintenance of typical verbal repertoires. According to Skinner's analysis, verbal operants that are acquired through contingencies arranged by verbal communities can subsequently occur covertly (or privately), with the speaker serving as their own listener within a given verbal episode. Examples include joint control (see previous section) and covert problem solving. In both of these cases, behaving individuals emit "mediating" behavior that evokes other responses; for example, repeating to yourself the name of the item you are looking for until you see it (joint control), or listing the items you typically buy at the grocery store until you remember the one you need to get right now (problem-solving). In the moment, the responses that comprise these chains of behavior are likely automatically reinforced by the successful resolution of the task (or problem), although the resulting public behavior may also be intermittently socially reinforced. A small but growing literature focuses on teaching these covert repertoires when they are lacking (e.g., Sautter et al., 2011); however, the difficulty inherent in teaching behaviors that are not publicly observable often forces researchers to teach mediating behavior as overt behavior (e.g., Vosters & Luczynski, 2020).

Mands for Information

Teaching *manding for information* (MFI) requires specific considerations in verbal behavior interventions. In this context, *information* refers to a verbal stimulus that allows the speaker to take action, which in turn enables access to terminal reinforcers (Sundberg et al., 2001). An example is a child asking their parent for a missing TV remote. After the parent responds (e.g., "I hid it from your little brother. It's on the top bookshelf"), the child is able to access the remote, turn on the TV, and watch the show. In this example, the establishing operation (EO) is lack of access to the TV show, the MFI is the child's question, and the terminal reinforcer is watching the show. The "information" comes to function as a conditioned reinforcer due to its association with the terminal reinforcer. Furthermore, the absence of the item (the remote) functions as an EO that momentarily establishes the value of the "information" as a reinforcer.

MFIs are often taught using an interrupted chain procedure (or *behavior chain interruption*) in which one or more components of a behavior chain are made difficult or impossible to complete in order to contrive an EO for information that permits the chain to continue. In order to ensure the MFI is under the control of the appropriate EO, rather than functionally irrelevant stimuli, it is necessary to intersperse abolishing operation (AO) trials (i.e., no interruption of the chain) between EO trials (Shillingsburg et al., 2014). To facilitate generalization of the MFI across response topographies and EOs (e.g., different response chains), research suggests that teaching *mand frames* can help (e.g., "Where is the [item]?"). The mand frame comes to function as a relational autoclitic that specifies the relation between actions and environmental context (e.g., that something is missing) (Lechago et al., 2010; Skinner, 1957). A robust repertoire of mands for information under appropriate EO control has the potential for improving conversation (Landa et al., 2020) and problem-solving skills (Jessel & Ingvarsson, 2022), and can lead to the acquisition of new responses (Ingvarsson & Hollobaugh, 2010).

Functional Independence
and Emergent Stimulus Control over Verbal Operants

As previously noted, Skinner's (1957) conceptualization of the verbal operant as a unit of analysis implies that a particular response form (e.g., "water") can be a part of multiple reinforcement contingencies (e.g., a tact contingency, a mand contingency, multiple intra-verbal contingencies) that may operate independently of one another. Lamarre and Holland (1985) provided an early empirical demonstration of the functional separability of verbal operants. Through modeling and reinforcement, some participants were initially taught to tact the relative spatial location of items as "on the left" or "on the right," and others were taught to emit the same phrases to mand for the placement of items on the left and right. When tested, the former participants showed no tendency to mand using the taught phrases, and the latter did not correctly tact item locations. After these untrained functions were taught directly, a contingency reversal for tacts (i.e., reinforcing "on the left" when the target was on the right, and vice versa) did not affect manding, and a contingency reversal for manding did not affect tacting. Thus, consistent with Skinner's conceptualization of mand and tact as functionally separable units, the two were acquired separately and affected independently by contingency manipulations.

Many studies have since examined the independent acquisition of various forms of manding and tacting by children of various ages and abilities (for a review, see Gamba et al., 2015). Some studies have shown response patterns similar to Lamarre and Holland (1985), whereas in others, reinforcing a response form as a mand has produced emergent tact control or vice versa. The same is true of studies that have examined relations between other pairs of verbal operants, such as tacts and intraverbals (e.g., Partington & Bailey, 1993; May et al., 2013). From the point of view of everyday experience, it is unsurprising to find that reinforcing a response as a tact may result in the same response appearing as a mand, and so on. Such findings do not, in fact, contradict Skinner (1957), who emphasized that "a verbal response of given form sometimes seems to pass easily from one type of operant to another" (p. 188). In part, Skinner attributed such observations to the uncontrolled conditions under which verbal responses are reinforced in the natural environment. Additionally, however, he suggested that as speakers mature, they acquire mediating repertoires ("suitable behavior of transcription or translation"; p. 188) that permit a response form acquired as one verbal operant to appear under stimulus conditions that define a different operant (e.g., by creating conditions for convergent control). Thus, even though it is possible in theory to experimentally isolate controlling variables for different verbal operants, human participants may bring to the table preexisting repertoires that permit reinforcement of one verbal operant to result in the emergence of another. Without further specification of the relevant repertoires or the histories that bring them about, results of functional independence tests may be impossible to predict, and indeed, the value of such tests with respect to evaluating Skinner's (1957) account has been questioned (Fryling, 2017).

In recent years, the emphasis has shifted to examining the conditions under which reinforcement of one verbal operant yields emergent stimulus control appropriate to another, and variables that influence these outcomes. The outcome of functional independence tests for tacts and mands has been found to be influenced by the way instructions are presented in test trials. For example, in Lamarre and Holland's (1985) landmark study, the instructions presented in mand and tact probes were, respectively, "Where do you want me to put the [item]?" and "Where is the [item]?" Egan and Barnes-Holmes

(2011) found that simply adding "Which side?" to these instructions increased the occurrence of correct mands following tact instruction and vice versa. Similarly, the emergence of novel intraverbals is influenced by histories of responding to various components of the verbal stimuli presented at test. For example, in a study with elementary schoolchildren, Belloso-Díaz and Pérez-González (2015) found that after learning to intraverbally relate city names to country names, and country names to continents, correct responses to novel instructions like "Name a city in Europe" required participants to also have a history of intraverbally relating "city" to city names. In addition, teaching certain skills or repertoires may increase the probability of emergent stimulus control over verbal behavior. Consistent with one of Skinner's (1957) suggestions, Hernandez et al. (2007) showed that differential reinforcement of framed mands ("I want the [item], please") over single-word mands (i.e., "[item]") increased occurrence of novel mands in which the response form in the [item] position had previously been acquired only as a tact. Kisamore et al. (2011) found that emergent intraverbal responding as a result of learning tacts increased when children were taught to use a visual-imagining strategy when confronted with novel test questions, and Sautter et al. (2011) reported similar results of teaching children to emit existing intraverbals at test. We return to the mediating and problem-solving functions of verbal behavior in a later section.

Speaker Behavior, Listener Behavior, and Bidirectional Naming

Just as different verbal operants are products of different reinforcement contingencies in Skinner's (1957) analysis, the behavior of a listener responding to verbal stimuli is governed by reinforcement contingencies different from those that govern any particular verbal operant. The functional independence of speaker and listener behavior was illustrated by Lee (1981), who taught children to tact relative object locations, as well as to respond as listeners to instructions to place objects in particular locations. Results suggested speaker and listener behavior were acquired independently, and contingency reversals for listener behavior minimally affected tacting. As with research on the functional independence of verbal operants, and likely for the same reasons, subsequent research on the independence of speaker and listener behavior has produced variable results. In general, however, establishment of speaker behavior has been found more likely to yield emergent listener behavior than establishment of listener behavior to yield speaker behavior (e.g., Petursdottir & Carr, 2011).

Recent research on emergent speaker and listener behavior has been influenced by Horne and Lowe's (1996) proposal that early interactions between infants and caregivers result in the development of a higher-order *naming* operant (now typically referred to as *bidirectional naming* [BiN]; see Miguel, 2016) that consists of interdependent tact, listener, and echoic relations. We refer the reader to Horne and Lowe's (1996) original article for details of their account.[2] In brief, however, Horne and Lowe hypothesized that once BiN is established, reinforcement of one component of a potential new name relation (e.g., a listener response to "Hand me the spatula") may serve to also strengthen others (e.g., the tact "spatula"). Other verbal relations, such as mands and intraverbals, can also enter name relations, serving to further expand the effects of reinforcement. Horne

---

[2]See Miguel (2018) and Pohl et al. (2020) for recent perspectives. See Barnes-Holmes and Barnes-Holmes (2002) for an alternative conceptualization of a generalized naming operant.

and Lowe speculated that over time, the BiN operant comes to embed its own sources of automatic reinforcement, such that simply being exposed to a name–object pair (i.e., a modeled tact) may suffice to establish appropriate control over speaker and listener relations in the absence of social reinforcement. From this perspective, then, a BiN repertoire is indicated when the establishment of a new listener relation (e.g., responding to "Hand me the spatula") produces untaught speaker behavior (e.g., the tact "spatula") or vice versa, or when speaker and listener relations emerge from exposure to modeling alone. Hawkins et al. (2018) pointed out, however, that these outcomes do not seem to develop in unison (e.g., a child may acquire a listener relation as a result of a tact being reinforced, but not vice versa) and suggested distinguishing between subtypes of BiN based on the procedure used to assess it (see also Carnerero & Pérez-González, 2014). In turn, this may raise the question whether BiN is, in fact, a single repertoire or whether different learning histories are responsible for emergent speaker and listener behavior as a result of different experiences.

Numerous studies have evaluated interventions to induce BiN when it appears absent. One example is multiple-exemplar instruction (MEI), an intervention intended to mimic child–caregiver interactions hypothesized to contribute to the development of BiN. In the BiN literature, MEI often consists of several types of intermixed trials with a set of novel objects: tact trials, listener trials, and identity-matching trials in which the child matches identical objects while an adult names the objects. Gilic and Greer (2011) identified eight young children of typical development who did not demonstrate emergent speaker or listener behavior after exposure to names of novel objects in identity-matching trials. Following MEI with a different object set, the children demonstrated emergent tacts and listener relations with the original objects. Similar effects of MEI have been documented in studies with participants with neurodevelopmental disorders (e.g., Greer et al., 2005; Olaff et al., 2017). Other interventions that have been found to have similar effects include intensive tact instruction (e.g., Hotchkiss & Fienup, 2020) and conditioning auditory and visual stimuli as reinforcers for observing responses (Longano & Greer, 2015). These findings suggest a set of tools that can be used clinically to promote emergent stimulus control over speaker and listener behavior. It remains to be fully clarified, however, how these different interventions end up producing the same outcome, and whether that outcome, in fact, represents establishment of the complex BiN operant.

Mediating and Problem-Solving Functions of Verbal Behavior

A final area of verbal behavior research we consider here, closely related to those described in previous sections, is concerned with the mediating and problem-solving functions of verbal behavior. At heart is the issue of how to explain instances of stimulus control in humans that appear to defy principles of temporal contiguity, such as when a stimulus occasions a response hours or days after its presentation, or when a stimulus occasions a novel response in the absence of a direct learning history (i.e., emergent stimulus control). Within behavior analysis, there has long been disagreement on how to account for such phenomena in ways that are consistent with its philosophical tenets (e.g., Simon et al., 2020). One perspective (e.g., Miguel, 2018; Palmer, 2012), however, has been strongly influenced by *Verbal Behavior* and other related work of Skinner: that these apparent gaps between stimuli or responses, or gaps in learning histories, are bridged by intervening or "precurrent" behavior that occurs either overtly or covertly and generates stimuli that combine with other stimuli in the environment (i.e., convergent or joint control) to evoke effective behavior. For example, a driver who is told prior to leaving home to "turn left by the taqueria and right on the next stop sign" may behave effectively as a result of repeating this instruction overtly or covertly while scanning the environment for taquerias and stop signs.

We previously described the proposed involvement of BiN in emergent speaker and listener behavior. Horne and Lowe (1996) suggested BiN also was responsible for the ease with which other forms of emergent stimulus control are observed in humans (e.g., in stimulus equivalence tests) by way of enabling effective behavior of the sort described earlier. A number of studies have focused on the specific processes by which BiN has been proposed to mediate stimulus class formation (Horne & Lowe, 1996): *common naming* and *intraverbal naming*. Both processes involve verbal behavior that permits categorizing (i.e., grouping or matching) nonsimilar objects together in the absence of direct learning experience. In the case of common naming, novel categorization behavior occurs because the items in each category evoke a common tact (e.g., "vehicle"), to the product of which the individual responds as a listener (e.g., by matching vehicle with vehicle). In the case of intraverbal naming, novel categorization occurs because tacts evoked by particular items (e.g., "train") may evoke names of related items (e.g., "car") as intraverbal responses, again resulting in a particular listener response (e.g., looking for a car and matching it with the train). The verbal repertoires that permit common and intraverbal naming (e.g., the tact "vehicle" or the intraverbal relation between "train" and "car") may be products of deliberate teaching, but may also arise incidentally. For example, in a study by Carp and Petursdottir (2015), children learned to match visual stimuli they had previously been taught to tact; specifically, state birds, state flowers, and outline maps of the respective states. When later tested for equivalence class formation, participants who passed the test were also found to have acquired a complete set of intraverbal relations among the names of the visual stimuli. These intraverbal relations were, by contrast, not found in the repertoires of children who failed the equivalence test. Several potential explanations exist for this covariation. However, from the perspective of BiN, it could indicate that intraverbal relations among the names of the stimuli, when present, facilitated class-consistent responding on the equivalence test as described by Horne and Lowe (1996). According to this interpretation, the intraverbal relations were products of direct, incidental reinforcement that occurred during baseline match-to-sample training. Specifically, if participants consistently tacted the visual stimuli while matching them (e.g., "Virginia, cardinal, cardinal goes with Virginia"), overtly or covertly, reinforcement of correct matching responses could have simultaneously reinforced bidirectional intraverbal relations among the names of the stimuli (i.e., responding "cardinal" to "Virginia" and vice versa). On the equivalence test, when presented with novel trial types (e.g., a bird as a sample and flowers as comparisons, which never occurred during training), a tact of the sample could then have evoked intraverbal responses (e.g., "cardinal goes with Virginia and Virginia goes to dogwood"), that provided sources of stimulus control for correct stimulus selection.

Many studies on BiN and stimulus class formation have focused on deliberately building the histories that define common and intraverbal naming, and demonstrating that they produce behavior consistent with stimulus class formation. For example, Horne et al. (2004) taught young children to respond as listeners to made-up spoken names by selecting several novel objects in response to each name. On a subsequent sorting test, the experimenter presented a sample object and asked the participant to "find the others," to which a correct response consisted of selecting other objects that had been assigned the same name. Only children who demonstrated emergent tacting of the objects also passed this test. When the remaining children were directly taught to tact the objects, they went on to pass the sorting test, consistent with the proposed mechanics of the common naming process described by Horne and Lowe (1996). Moreover, some children in this and other studies have passed the sorting test only when prompted to tact the sample stimulus in each trial, supporting the notion that not only must the relevant tact and listener relations be in the repertoire but this behavior must also occur at test to provide sources of stimulus control for grouping the stimuli. Other, similar studies with children and adults (e.g., Ma et al., 2016) have focused on building intraverbal rather than common naming histories. In general, this research has produced findings consistent with the operation of these BiN-related processes in stimulus class formation. However, some inconsistencies have been noted as well. In one study (Petursdottir et al., 2015), for example, children first learned to tact several visual stimuli, next learned intraverbal relations between pairs of stimulus names (e.g., "mu goes with kibi"), and were finally tested to see if they would match the visual stimuli consistent with these intraverbal relations. Some children who passed the test failed a test for bidirectional intraverbal relations (e.g., "kibi goes with mu"), which is inconsistent with the mechanics of intraverbal naming. Such results have been hypothesized (Miguel, 2018) to potentially reflect additional sources of stimulus control that may be present at test as a result of baseline histories, such as conditioned perceptual responses, and some data are consistent with that notion. For example, using a task similar to Petursdottir et al. (2015), but with college students as participants, Cox and Petursdottir (2021) found that participants who reported covertly visualizing the absent visual stimuli while learning the intraverbal relations among their names performed better on the subsequent matching test than participants who did not report such "seeing." Moreover, participants who learned the intraverbal relations before they had learned the relevant tacts, such that they could not possibly engage in accurate visualization during intraverbal instruction, made fewer correct responses and responded more slowly than participants who learned tacts before intraverbals.

Research on mediating functions of verbal behavior has also been applied to other problem-solving situations. For example, Clough et al. (2016) found that performance in a task that involved arranging visual stimuli into sequences deteriorated when participants engaged in a concurrent task that was incompatible with proposed mediating behavior, but not when the concurrent task was compatible. Another line of research has focused on the role of verbal behavior in analogical reasoning (e.g., Meyer et al., 2019) and comparison (Diaz et al., 2020). In the applied realm, studies conducted with participants diagnosed with ASD (e.g., Vosters & Luczynski, 2020; Ribeiro & Miguel, 2020) show promise in terms of translating findings on the problem-solving functions of verbal behavior into repertoire-expanding interventions. We refer the reader to Miguel (2018) for a more thorough discussion of this topic.

Past Progress and Current Status of Research on Verbal Behavior

Much has changed since the publication of *Verbal Behavior*. Skinner's (1957) proposal that language is acquired behavior, transmitted via reinforcement contingencies embedded in human social interactions, was highly novel at the time and met with skepticism (e.g., Chomsky, 1959). Today, it is in many ways compatible with current psycholinguistic thinking (see, e.g., Tomasello, 2014). The direct influence of *Verbal Behavior* on empirical research remained minimal for decades, even within behavior analysis (Dymond et al., 2006; McPherson et al., 1984). More recently, however, research in behavior analysis has been drawing heavily on Skinner's (1957) work, with an exponential increase in verbal behavior research activity in the 21st century (Petursdottir & Devine, 2017).

Much of the recent empirical literature focuses on teaching language skills to children with language delays (Petursdottir, 2018), suggesting the increase in research activity has been in part related to the appearance of language curricula and assessments based on *Verbal Behavior* (e.g., Sundberg, 2008) and their widespread adoption in early intervention programs (Love et al., 2009). In a sense, Skinner's theory was ultimately taken straight from the animal laboratory into field application and applied research without much intervening human laboratory research to validate its principles. However, basic research on verbal behavior has also been on the rise in recent years (Petursdottir & Devine, 2017), perhaps suggesting that the success of practical applications has inspired interest in more fundamental questions about verbal behavior from the perspective of Skinner's (1957) analysis.

It has been noted that much of the applied research inspired by *Verbal Behavior* has been derived from Skinner's (1957) functional distinction between verbal operants that is presented in the first part of the book (e.g., Dixon et al., 2007). This distinction is certainly important to Skinner's (1957) analysis and its application to building verbal repertoires; however, it is the multiple control and autoclitic processes described in later sections that form the core of Skinner's argument that even the most complex aspects of human behavior are amenable to analysis in terms of behavioral principles. The relatively less empirical attention given to these parts of Skinner's analysis is perhaps, in part, a result of contingencies that have affected behavior analysis research and practice more generally—and perhaps, in part, it also represents a necessity to examine the fundamentals of Skinner's account before tackling more complex topics. In recent years, however, there has been a surge of empirical interest in both multiple control and autoclitic frames (e.g., degli Espinosa et al., 2021; DeSouza et al., 2019; Meleshkevich et al., 2021), in addition to the highly related research on emergent stimulus control and the problem-solving and mediating functions of verbal behavior that we have described in this chapter. Continued interest in these topics may serve to build a foundation upon which interventions can be developed to solve a broader range of socially significant problems.

AUTHORS' NOTE

We dedicate this chapter to the memory of Jack Michael: a teacher, a mentor, a friend, and an academic role model. Through his writings, teaching, and mentorship of influential behavior analysts, Michael was instrumental in keeping Skinner's (1957) analysis of verbal behavior alive through the decades, and inspiring present-day behavior analysts to conduct empirical research on Skinner's theory and its applications. The research discussed in this chapter is a testament to his legacy.

REFERENCES

Alessi, G. (1987). Generative strategies and teaching for generalization. *The Analysis of Verbal Behavior, 5*, 15–27.

Ampuero, M. E., & Miklos, M. (2019). The effect of joint control training on the performance of multiply controlled behavior: A systematic literature review relevant to children with autism spectrum disorder and other developmental disabilities. *The Analysis of Verbal Behavior, 35*, 149–171.

Axe, J. B., & McCarthy-Pepin, M. (2021). On the use of the term, "discriminative stimulus," in behavior analytic practice. *Behavioral Interventions, 36*(3), 667–674.

Axe, J. B., & Sainato, D. M. (2010). Matrix training of preliteracy skills with preschoolers with autism. *Journal of Applied Behavior Analysis, 43*, 635–652.

Barbera, M. L., & Kubina, R. M. (2005). Using transfer procedures to teach tacts to a child with autism. *The Analysis of Verbal Behavior, 21*, 155–161.

Barnes-Holmes, Y., & Barnes-Holmes, D. (2002). Naming, story-telling, and problemsolving: Critical elements in the development of language and cognition. *Behavioral Development Bulletin, 11*(1), 34–38.

Belloso-Díaz, C., & Pérez-González, L. A. (2015). Exemplars and categories necessary for the emergence of intraverbals about transitive reasoning in typically developing children. *The Psychological Record, 65*(3), 541–556.

Carnerero, J. J., & Pérez-González, L. A. (2014). Induction of naming after observing visual stimuli and their names in children with autism. *Research in Developmental Disabilities, 35*(10), 2514–2526.

Carp, C. L., & Petursdottir, A. I. (2015). Intraverbal naming and equivalence class formation in children. *Journal of the Experimental Analysis of Behavior, 104*(3), 223–240.

Catania, A. C. (1998). *Learning* (4th ed.). Prentice-Hall.

Chomsky, N. (1959). A review of B. F. Skinner's "Verbal Behavior." *Language, 35*, 26–58.

Clough, C., Meyer, C. S., & Miguel, C. F. (2016). The effects of blocking and joint control training on sequencing visual stimuli. *The Analysis of Verbal Behavior, 32*(2), 242–264.

Cox, R. E., & Petursdottir, A. I. (2021). Training sequence effects on emergent conditional discrimination: Replication and extension to selection-based training. *Journal of the Experimental Analysis of Behavior, 116*(2), 208–224.

Curiel, E. S., Axe, J. B., Sainato, D. M., & Goldstein, H. (2020). Systematic review of matrix training for individuals with autism spectrum disorder. *Focus on Autism and Other Developmental Disabilities, 35*, 55–64.

degli Espinosa, F., Gerosa, F., & Brocchin-Swales, V. (2021). Teaching multiply controlled tacting to children with autism. *European Journal of Behavior Analysis, 22*(2), 173–193.

DeSouza, A. A., Fisher, W. W., & Rodriguez, N. M. (2019). Facilitating the emergence of convergent intraverbals in children with autism. *Journal of Applied Behavior Analysis, 52*(1), 28–49.

Diaz, J. E., Luoma, S. M., & Miguel, C. F. (2020). The role of verbal behavior in the establishment of comparative relations. *Journal of the Experimental Analysis of Behavior, 113*(2), 322–339.

Dixon, M. R., Small, S. S., & Rosales, R. (2007). Extended analysis of empirical citations with Skinner's *Verbal Behavior*: 1984–2004. *The Behavior Analyst, 30*(2), 197–209.

Dymond, S., O'Hora, D., Whelan, R., & Donovan, A. (2006). Citation analysis of Skinner's *Verbal Behavior*: 1984–2004. *The Behavior Analyst, 29*(1), 75–88.

Egan, C. E., & Barnes-Holmes, D. (2011). Examining antecedent control over emergent mands and tacts in young children. *The Psychological Record, 61*(1), 127–140.

Fryling, M. J. (2017). The functional independence of Skinner's verbal operants: Conceptual and applied implications. *Behavioral Interventions, 32*(1), 70–78.

Gale, C. M., Eikeseth, S., & Klintwall, L. (2019). Children with autism show atypical preference for non-social stimuli. *Scientific Reports, 9*, 1–10.

Gamba, J., Goyos, C., & Petursdottir, A. I. (2015). The functional independence of mands and tacts: Has it been demonstrated empirically? *The Analysis of Verbal Behavior, 31*(1), 39–58.

Gilic, L., & Greer, R. D. (2011). Establishing naming in typically developing two-year-old children as a function of multiple exemplar speaker and listener experiences. *The Analysis of Verbal Behavior, 27*(1), 157–177.

Greer, R. D., Stolfi, L., Chavez-Brown, M., & Rivera-Valdes, C. (2005). The emergence of the listener to speaker component of naming in children as a function of multiple exemplar instruction. *The Analysis of Verbal Behavior, 21*(1), 123–134.

Hart, B., & Risley, T. R. (1975). Incidental teaching of language in the preschool. *Journal of Applied Behavior Analysis, 8*, 411–420.

Hawkins, E., Gautreaux, G., & Chiesa, M. (2018). Deconstructing common bidirectional naming: A proposed classification framework.

The Analysis of Verbal Behavior, 34(1–2), 44–61.

Hayes, S. C., Blackledge, J. T., & Barnes-Holmes, D. (2001). Language and cognition: Constructing an alternative approach within the behavioral tradition. In S. C. Hayes, D. Barnes-Holmes, & B. Roche (Eds.), *Relational frame theory: A post-Skinnerian account of human language and cognition* (pp. 3–20). Plenum Press.

Hernandez, E., Hanley, G. P., Ingvarsson, E. T., & Tiger, J. H. (2007). A preliminary evaluation of the emergence of novel mand forms. *Journal of Applied Behavior Analysis, 40*(1), 137–156.

Horne, P. J., & Lowe, C. F. (1996). On the origins of naming and other symbolic behavior. *Journal of the Experimental Analysis of Behavior, 65*(1), 185–241.

Horne, P. J., Lowe, C. F., & Randle, V. R. L. (2004). Naming and categorization in young children: II. Listener behavior training. *Journal of the Experimental Analysis of Behavior, 81*(3), 267–288.

Hotchkiss, R. M., & Fienup, D. M. (2020). A parametric analysis of a protocol to induce bidirectional naming: Effects of protocol intensity. *The Psychological Record, 70*(3), 481–497.

Ingvarsson, E. T., Cammilleri, A. C., & Macias. H. (2012). Emergent listener responses following intraverbal training in children with autism. *Research in Autism Spectrum Disorders, 6*, 654–664.

Ingvarsson, E. T., & Hollobaugh, T. (2010). Acquisition of intraverbal behavior: Teaching children with autism to mand for answers to questions. *Journal of Applied Behavior Analysis, 43*, 1–17.

Ingvarsson, E. T., Kramer, R. L., Carp, C. L., Pétursdóttir, A. I., & Macias, H. (2016). Evaluation of a blocked-trials procedure to establish complex stimulus control over intraverbal responses in children with autism. *The Analysis of Verbal Behavior, 32*, 205–224.

Ingvarsson, E. T., & Le, D. D. (2011). Further evaluation of prompting tactics for establishing intraverbal responding in children with autism. *The Analysis of Verbal Behavior, 27*, 75–93.

Jessel, J., & Ingvarsson, E. T. (2022). Teaching two children with autism to mand for known and unknown items using contrived motivating operations. *Behavioral Interventions, 37*(1), 139–152.

Kemmerer, A. R., Vladescu, J. C., Carrow, J. N., Sidener, T. M., & Deshais, M. A. (2021). A systematic review of the matrix training literature. *Behavioral Interventions, 36*(2), 473–495.

Kisamore, A. N., Carr, J. E., & LeBlanc, L. A. (2011). Training preschool children to use visual imagining as a problem-solving strategy for complex categorization tasks. *Journal of Applied Behavior Analysis, 44*(2), 255–278.

Kisamore, A. N., Karsten, A. M., & Mann, C. C. (2016). Teaching multiply controlled intraverbals to children and adolescents with autism spectrum disorders. *Journal of Applied Behavior Analysis, 49*, 826–847.

LaFrance, D. L., & Tarbox, J. (2020). The importance of multiple exemplar instruction in the establishment of novel verbal behavior. *Journal of Applied Behavior Analysis, 53*, 10–24.

Lamarre, J., & Holland, J. G. (1985). The functional independence of mands and tacts. *Journal of the Experimental Analysis of Behavior, 43*(1), 5–19.

Landa, R. K., Frampton, S. E., & Shillingsburg, M. A. (2020). Teaching children with autism to mand for social information. *Journal of Applied Behavior Analysis, 53*, 2271–2286.

Laraway, S. Snycerski, S., Michael, J., & Poling, A. (2003). Motivating operations and terms to describe them: Some further refinements. *Journal of Applied Behavior Analysis, 36*(3), 407–414.

Laski, K. E., Charlop, M. H., & Schreibman, L. (1988). Training parents to use the natural language paradigm to increase their autistic children's speech. *Journal of Applied Behavior Analysis, 21*, 391–400.

Layng, T. J. (2019). Tutorial: Understanding concepts: Implications for behavior analysts and educators. *Perspectives on Behavior Science, 42*, 345–363.

Lechago, S. A., Carr, J. E., Grow, L. L., Love, J. R., & Almason, S. M. (2010). Mands for information generalize across establishing operations. *Journal of Applied Behavior Analysis, 43*, 381–395.

Lee, V. L. (1981). Prepositional phrases spoken and heard. *Journal of the Experimental Analysis of Behavior, 35*(2), 227–242.

Lepper, T. L., & Petursdottir, A. I. (2017). Effects of response-contingent stimulus pairing on vocalizations of nonverbal children with autism. *Journal of Applied Behavior Analysis, 50*, 756–774.

Longano, J. M., & Greer, R. D. (2015). Is the source of reinforcement for naming multiple conditioned reinforcers for observing responses? *The Analysis of Verbal Behavior, 31*(1), 96–117.

Love, J. S., Carr, J. E., Almason, S. M., & Petursdottir, A. I. (2009). Early and intensive behavioral intervention for autism: A survey of clinical practices. *Research in Autism Spectrum Disorders, 3*(2), 421–428.

Lowenkron, B. (2006). An introduction to joint control. *The Analysis of Verbal Behavior, 22,* 123–127.

Ma, M. L., Miguel, C. F., & Jennings, A. M. (2016). Training intraverbal naming to establish equivalence class performances. *Journal of the Experimental Analysis of Behavior, 105*(3), 409–426.

May, R. J., Hawkins, E., & Dymond, S. (2013). Brief report: Effects of tact training on emergent intraverbal vocal responses in adolescents with autism. *Journal of Autism and Developmental Disorders, 43*(4), 996–1004.

McPherson, A., Bonem, M., Green, G., & Osborne, J. G. (1984). A citation analysis of the influence of Skinner's *Verbal Behavior. The Behavior Analyst, 7*(2), 157–167.

Meleshkevich, O., Axe, J. B., & degli Espinosa, F. (2021). Effects of time delay and requiring echoics on answering questions about visual stimuli. *Journal of Applied Behavior Analysis, 54*(2), 725–743.

Meyer, C. S., Cordeiro, M. C., & Miguel, C. F. (2019). The effects of listener training on the development of analogical reasoning. *Journal of the Experimental Analysis of Behavior, 112*(2), 144–166.

Michael, J. (1982a). Skinner's elementary verbal relations: Some new categories. *The Analysis of Verbal Behavior, 1*(1), 1–3.

Michael, J. (1982b). Distinguishing between the discriminative and motivational functions of stimuli. *Journal of the Experimental Analysis of Behavior, 37,* 149–155.

Michael, J. (1985). Two kinds of verbal behavior plus a possible third. *The Analysis of Verbal Behavior, 3,* 1–4.

Michael, J. (1993). Establishing operations. *The Behavior Analyst, 16*(2), 191–206.

Michael, J., Palmer, D. C., & Sundberg, M. L. (2011). The multiple control of verbal behavior. *The Analysis of Verbal Behavior, 27,* 3–22.

Miguel, C. F. (2016). Common and intraverbal bidirectional naming. *The Analysis of Verbal Behavior, 32*(2), 125–138.

Miguel, C. F. (2018). Problem solving, bidirectional naming, and the development of verbal repertoires. *Behavior Analysis: Research and Practice, 18*(4), 340–353.

Normand, M. P. (2009). Much ado about nothing?: Some comments on B. F. Skinner's definition of verbal behavior. *The Behavior Analyst, 32*(1), 185–190.

Olaff, H. S., Ona, H. N., & Holth, P. (2017). Establishment of naming in children with autism through multiple response-exemplar training. *Behavioral Development Bulletin, 22*(1), 67–85.

Palmer, D. C. (2008). On Skinner's definition of verbal behavior. *International Journal of Psychology and Psychological Therapy, 8*(3), 295–307.

Palmer, D. C. (2012). The role of atomic repertoires in complex behavior. *The Behavior Analyst, 35,* 59–73.

Palmer, D. C. (2016). On intraverbal control and the definition of the intraverbal. *The Analysis of Verbal Behavior, 32,* 96–106.

Partington, J. W., & Bailey, J. S. (1993). Teaching intraverbal behavior to preschool children. *The Analysis of Verbal Behavior, 11,* 9–18.

Petursdottir, A. I. (2018). The current status of the experimental analysis of verbal behavior. *Behavior Analysis: Research and Practice, 18*(2), 151–168.

Petursdottir, A. I., Carp, C. L., Peterson, S. P., & Lepper, T. L. (2015). Emergence of visual-visual conditional discriminations following intraverbal training. *Journal of the Experimental Analysis of Behavior, 103,* 332–348.

Petursdottir, A. I., & Carr, J. C. (2011). A review of recommendations for sequencing receptive and expressive language instruction. *Journal of Applied Behavior Analysis, 44*(4), 859–876.

Petursdottir, A. I., & Devine, B. (2017). The impact of *Verbal Behavior* on the scholarly literature from 2005 to 2016. *Analysis of Verbal Behavior, 33*(2), 212–228.

Petursdottir, A. I., & Ingvarsson, E. T. (2023). Revisiting topography-based and selection-based verbal behavior. *Analysis of Verbal Behavior.* [Epub ahead of print]

Pohl, P., Greer, R. D., Du, L., & Moschella, J. L. (2020). Verbal development, behavioral metamorphosis, and the evolution of language. *Perspectives on Behavior Science, 43*(1), 215–232.

Ribeiro, D. M., & Miguel, C. F. (2020). The use of multiple-tact training to produce emergent categorization in children with autism. *Journal of Applied Behavior Analysis, 53*(3), 1768–1779.

Sautter, R. A., LeBlanc, L. A., Jay, A. A., Goldsmith, T. R., & Carr, J. E. (2011). The role of problem solving in complex intraverbal repertoires. *Journal of Applied Behavior Analysis, 44*(2), 227–244.

Shillingsburg, M. A., Bowen, C. N., Valentino, A. L., & Pierce, L. E. (2014). Mands for information using "who?" and "which?" in the presence of establishing and abolishing operations. *Journal of Applied Behavior Analysis, 47*, 136–150.

Sidener, D. W. (2006). Joint control for dummies: An elaboration of Lowenkron's model of joint (stimulus) control. *The Analysis of Verbal Behavior, 22*, 119–122.

Simon, C., Bernardy, J. L., & Cowie, S. (2020). On the "strength" of behavior. *Perspectives on Behavior Science, 43*(4), 677–696.

Skinner, B. F. (1945). The operational analysis of psychological terms. *Psychological Review, 52*, 270–277.

Skinner, B. F. (1957). *Verbal behavior.* Copley.

Smith, T. (2001). Discrete trial training in the treatment of autism. *Focus on Autism and Other Developmental Disabilities, 16*, 86–92.

Sundberg, C. T., & Sundberg, M. L. (1990). Comparing topography-based verbal behavior with stimulus selection-based verbal behavior. *The Analysis of Verbal Behavior, 8*, 31–41.

Sundberg, M. L. (2008). *The Verbal Behavior Milestones Assessment and Placement Program: The VB-MAPP.* AVB Press.

Sundberg, M. L. (2013). Thirty points about motivation from Skinner's book *Verbal Behavior. The Analysis of Verbal Behavior, 29*(1), 13–40.

Sundberg, M. L., Loeb, M., Hale, L., & Eigenheer, P. (2001). Contriving establishing operations to teach mands for information. *Analysis of Verbal Behavior, 18*, 15–29.

Sundberg, M. L., & Michael, J. (2001). The benefits of Skinner's analysis of verbal behavior for children with autism. *Behavior Modification, 25*, 698–724.

Sundberg, M. L., & Partington, J. W. (1999). The need for both discrete trial and natural environment language training for children with autism. In P. M. Ghezzi, W. L. Williams, & J. E. Carr (Eds.), *Autism: Behavior analytic perspectives* (pp. 139–156). Context Press.

Tomasello, M. (Ed.). (2014). *The new psychology of language: Cognitive and functional approaches to language structure.* Psychology Press.

Vandbakk, M., Olaff, H. S., & Holth, P. (2019). Conditioned reinforcement: The effectiveness of stimulus–stimulus pairing and operant discrimination procedures. *The Psychological Record, 69*, 67–81.

Vosters, M. E., & Luczynski, K. C. (2020). Emergent completion of multistep instructions via joint control. *Journal of Applied Behavior Analysis, 53*(3), 1432–1451.

CHAPTER 18

Resistance to Change from Bench to Bedside (and Back Again)

Andrew R. Craig
Joel E. Ringdahl
William E. Sullivan

Our everyday behavior often is faced with challenges. An individual with alcohol-use disorder, for example, may be discouraged from going to the bar by his family or could experience negative collateral effects of his drinking, such as loss of friends, vocation, or health. Likewise, a cross-country runner may encounter obstacles while training, such as fatigue, injury, or inhospitable weather conditions. While writing this chapter, our writing frequently was interrupted by the unique (and many) challenges posed by the global COVID-19 pandemic. Regardless of the behavior in question or the manner by which that behavior is disrupted, a likely outcome is that the behavior will persist despite the challenges that deter it. The individual with alcohol-use disorder might continue to intermittently consume alcohol despite pleas from loved ones to stop, and the cross-country runner might continue to train in the face of adversity.

The extent to which behavior persists when faced with a disruptor is termed *resistance to change* (Nevin, 1974), and this dimension of operant behavior is important for both practical and theoretical reasons. Understanding the factors that affect resistance to change may allow practitioners to increase resistance to change when it is a desirable attribute of behavior and decrease resistance to change when it is an undesirable attribute. Moreover, resistance to change is thought to reveal information about the way that reinforcement histories are carried forward in time to affect current behavior (see Nevin & Grace, 2000; Nevin et al., 1983) and the learning factors that lead to behavioral adaptation when reinforcement conditions change over time (Gallistel, 2012).

Perhaps unsurprisingly, resistance to change has been and continues to be a highly active area of research in behavior analysis. Much of the progress in this area has been made in the basic-research laboratory. Great strides also have been made, however, in translating findings from the basic research on resistance to change into real-world applications (for discussion, see Mace & Nevin, 2017; Nevin et al., 2016; Nevin & Shahan, 2011).

Our goal in this chapter is to provide readers with a broad overview of resistance to change. First, we discuss basic-research findings on this topic. In doing so, we describe the methods that are used to study resistance to change, how it is measured, and the variables that have been shown to reliably affect it. Next, we review translational and applied research on resistance to change, including some novel findings from clinical evaluations of resistance to change in the context of assessment and treatment of severe problem behavior. Finally, we describe behavioral momentum theory (Craig et al., 2014; Nevin et al., 1983; Podlesnik & DeLeon, 2015), the most widely applied conceptual analysis of resistance to change to date. We place special emphasis on the strengths, weaknesses, and practical utility of the theory. We close by detailing recommendations for practice based on the provided overview.

Key Findings from Basic Research

Broadly speaking, resistance to change has been a topic of research within behavior analysis since its inception. Skinner (1956), for example, recounted an early empirical demonstration of operant extinction during his study of rats' lever pressing. The hopper that delivered food pellets, the consequence that maintained lever pressing, jammed. Despite the fact that lever pressing no longer produced food, the behavior did not cease immediately. Instead, rates of lever pressing gradually decreased with continued exposure to extinction contingencies (producing "a beautiful curve" on the cumulative record [Skinner, 1979, p. 95], as Skinner would later reflect in his autobiography). In this example, lever pressing initially persisted despite the fact that pressing no longer produced reinforcement, and the extent to which it persisted decreased as time in extinction increased. Examples of resistance to change like this one showed us *that* behavior resists change, but these examples told us little about *why* behavior resists change or the factors that are functionally related to resistance to change.

Nevin (1974) conducted a series of experiments that revolutionized the study of resistance to change and laid the foundation for research on this topic. In each of these experiments, Nevin studied pigeons' key pecking, and he arranged different conditions of reinforcement for key pecking using multiple schedules of reinforcement; that is, sometimes the pigeons' keys were lighted green and key pecking produced food reinforcers according to a specific schedule of reinforcement. Other times, the keys were lighted red and key pecking produced food reinforcers according to a different schedule of reinforcement. This multiple-schedule arrangement allowed Nevin to study the effects of different levels of an independent variable on behavior's resistance to change within subjects and during the same experimental condition. Nevin manipulated several variables between the multiple-schedule components across experiments, including the rate at which key pecking produced reinforcers, the overall rate of reinforcers (both response dependent and response independent), the magnitude of the reinforcer that was delivered contingently on key pecking, and the delay that separated key pecks from the reinforcers they produced. He also arranged several different tests of resistance to change, including extinction and delivery of response-independent food during the periods in between presentations of the multiple-schedule components (called *intercomponent intervals*; ICIs). Any operations that serve to change the rate at which ongoing operant behavior occurs, such as extinction, presentation of free reinforcers during ICIs, partial reinforcer satiation, and distraction from the operant task, have been termed *disruptors,* and we will provide examples of each below.

The key finding from Nevin's (1974) experiments was that resistance to change of key pecking tended to be greater in the multiple-schedule component that was associated with more valuable conditions of reinforcement. We use the word *value* here vis-à-vis the concatenated matching law (Baum, 1974; Baum & Rachlin, 1969): Higher rates of reinforcement are more valuable than lower rates, larger magnitudes of reinforcement are more valuable than smaller magnitudes, and more immediate reinforcement is more valuable than more delayed reinforcement. Thus, the multiple-schedule components that were associated with higher rates of, larger magnitudes of, or more immediate reinforcement across Nevin's experiments were also the components during which responding exhibited greater resistance to change.

This general finding, however, is by no means specific to Nevin's (1974) experiments. The effects of reinforcer *rate* on resistance to change have been particularly extensively studied, and many have replicated the positive relation between predisruption reinforcer rates and resistance to change with pigeon subjects (e.g., Bai & Podlesnik, 2017; Cohen et al., 1993; Craig et al., 2015, 2019; Nevin et al., 1990; Podlesnik & Shahan, 2009) and other nonhuman animal species including rats and fish (e.g., Blackman, 1968; Cohen, 1998; Cohen et al., 1993; Igaki & Sakagami, 2004; Pyszczynski & Shahan, 2011). As we see in the next section, these findings also have been replicated numerous times with human behavior exhibited by individuals with and without developmental disabilities. Still other studies have replicated the effects of reinforcer immediacy (e.g., Bell, 1999; Podlesnik et al., 2006) and magnitude (e.g., Harper & McLean, 1992; Rau et al., 1996; Shull & Grimes, 2006) on resistance to change in nonhuman animals, and more recent findings suggest that they are general to human behavior (e.g., McComas et al., 2008).

To understand why these variables may contribute to resistance to change, it is important to recognize that when reinforcers are delivered in a particular context, such as those arranged in multiple-schedule components, those reinforcers may have two effects. First, they may strengthen the operant response–reinforcer contingency in a manner that is consistent with the matching law (Herrnstein, 1961, 1970). Second, they may strengthen the Pavlovian stimulus–reinforcer contingency. Based on the findings so far reviewed, it is unclear which of these contingencies contributes to resistance to change. Nevin et al. (1990) conducted a series of experiments that addressed this interpretive issue.

In their Experiment 1, Nevin et al. (1990) trained pigeons to key-peck in a two-component multiple schedule across various conditions. When the key was green, key pecking produced food on average once per minute. The contingencies of reinforcement during red-key periods varied across conditions of the experiment. In one set of conditions, pecking the red key produced reinforcers, on average, once per minute; that is, the same contingencies were in place when the key was red as when it was green. In a second set of conditions, pecking the red key produced one reinforcer per minute, but additional reinforcers were delivered independently of key pecking. In a final set of conditions, the rate of peck-dependent and peck-independent reinforcer deliveries, when added together, equaled one reinforcer per minute. After each of these conditions, resistance to change of key pecking was assessed using presession feeding and extinction.

Nevin et al. (1990) reasoned that delivering peck-independent reinforcers in the red-key component should *weaken* the operant response–reinforcer contingency, because key pecks produced only a portion of the reinforcers that were delivered. Because those reinforcers were delivered in the presence of the discriminative stimulus (the red-key light), however, they should *strengthen* the Pavlovian contingency between the key light and the reinforcers that were delivered in its presence. If, on the one hand, resistance to change was a function of the response–reinforcer contingency, they expected delivery of peck-independent reinforcers in the red-key component to *reduce* the resistance to change of key pecking. On the other hand, if the stimulus–reinforcer contingency governed resistance to change, they expected delivery of peck-independent reinforcers in the red-key component to *increase* the resistance to change of key pecking. Their findings aligned with the second of these possible outcomes: Resistance to change of key pecking during extinction and presession feeding tests was higher in the red-key component when that component arranged a higher overall rate of reinforcement than the green-key component. Moreover, resistance to change was about equal between components when they arranged the same overall rate of reinforcement. Other researchers have replicated and extended the findings from Nevin et al.'s (1990) Experiment 1 by showing that delivering response-independent reinforcers in a discriminative context increases resistance to change of a behavior in that context, even when the response-independent reinforcers are qualitatively different from response-dependent reinforcers (see Craig & Shahan, 2022; Grimes & Shull, 2001; Pyszczynski & Shahan, 2011; Shahan & Burke, 2004).

In a second experiment, Nevin et al. (1990) asked whether the Pavlovian stimulus–reinforcer relation in a multiple-schedule component could be strengthened, and the resistance to change of a behavior within that component could be increased, by adding reinforcers to the component contingently on a *different* response. Nevin et al. arranged a three-component multiple schedule. In each component, both a right key (hereafter the "target" key) and a left key (hereafter the "alternative" key) were illuminated, and the authors were interested in resistance to change of target-key pecking. When both keys were green, pecking the target key produced 15 reinforcers per hour, and pecking the alternative key produced 45 reinforcers per hour (for a total of 60 reinforcers per hour). When the keys were red, pecking the target key produced 15 reinforcers per hour, and pecks to the alternative key were placed on extinction. Finally, when the keys were white, pecking the target key produced 60 reinforcers per hour, and alternative key pecks were placed on extinction. Following a baseline phase, resistance to both extinction and presession feeding was assessed. Based on their findings from Experiment 1, Nevin et al. predicted that adding reinforcers for the alternative response in the green-key component should contribute to the resistance to change of the target response in that component. Their findings aligned precisely with that prediction. Resistance to change was the lowest in the red-key component in which 15 reinforcers per hour were delivered and about equal in the green- and white-key components that both arranged a total of 60 reinforcers per hour. Thus, in terms of contributing to resistance to change, neither the source of reinforcement nor the type of reinforcer appears to matter: So long as the reinforcer is delivered in the presence of a discriminative stimulus, it may enhance resistance to change of behavior in the presence of that stimulus. The relation between reinforcement conditions and resistance to change described above is ubiquitous and has been demonstrated in dozens of articles detailing research from the basic laboratory (see Nevin, 1992; Nevin & Grace, 2000). As we describe in the following section, a growing number of translational studies using human participants has replicated these findings and extended them in important ways.

An Overview of Translational and Applied Human Research

The pipeline connecting basic-research findings to application in real-world settings sometimes is direct. For example, in 1928 while studying *Staphylococcus aureus* (a bacterium that is implicated in many common infectious diseases in humans), Alexander Fleming found that mold spores prevented growth of his cultured bacteria. He had accidentally discovered penicillin, a finding for which he would later receive the Nobel Prize in 1945 (Fleming, 1929; see also Tan & Tatsumura, 2015). Shortly after Fleming's initial discovery in 1930, penicillin was used successfully to treat infections in humans (see Wainwright & Swan, 1986). Other times and often in the case of behavior-analytic research, the pipeline connecting seminal work in the laboratory to application is indirect: Intervening research often is dedicated to verifying that findings produced in the animal laboratory are general to humans and to less-controlled settings before that work is applied to socially significant behavior (for discussion, see Mace & Critchfield, 2010; McIlvane, 2009). Resistance to change followed the second of these two trajectories in its course from bench to bedside.

Mace et al. (1990) conducted an early example of translational research on resistance to change. In a two-part experiment, these researchers examined resistance to change of behavior exhibited by two adults with developmental disabilities. Mace et al. arranged a multiple schedule by having participants sort red and green utensils, the colors of which served as discriminative stimuli for each component. In Part 1 of the experiment, sorting was reinforced by delivering a small cup of coffee or popcorn according to a variable-interval (VI) 60 second schedule in one component and a VI 240 second schedule in the other. Following baseline, resistance to change was assessed by presenting a television program (i.e., Music Television [MTV]) as a disrupter across both components of the multiple schedule. Results showed that when the disruptor was presented, silverware sorting persisted to a greater extent in the component associated with the higher rate of reinforcement.

In Part 2 of the experiment, Mace et al. (1990) replicated Nevin et al.'s (1990) Experiment 1, which we described earlier. In one component of the multiple schedule, reinforcers were delivered for utensil sorting according to a VI 60 second schedule. In the other component, however, participants received reinforcers both dependent on and independent of utensil sorting according to VI 60 second and variable-time (VT) 30 second schedules, respectively. Then, as in Part 1 of the experiment, a television disruptor was presented to assess resistance to change of participants' utensil sorting. Responding was more persistent in the component of the multiple schedule that was associated with higher overall rates of reinforcement (i.e., the condition associated with both sorting-dependent and sorting-independent reinforcement). These findings were an important translational extension of those that had been observed previously in the basic laboratory. They demonstrated that, under multiple-schedule arrangements, higher rates of reinforcement engender greater resistance to change of human behavior, regardless of whether those reinforcers are delivered contingently on the behavior in question.

In addition to rate of reinforcement, McComas et al. (2008) demonstrated that reinforcer magnitude can also influence resistance to change of human behavior under multiple-schedule arrangements. Four graduate students participated and were required to play a simple computer game by clicking on colored shapes to produce points as reinforcers. These points were exchangeable for actual money (i.e., $0.10 or $0.05 per point) after participation. A two-component multiple schedule was arranged. In both components, two squares (one on the left and one on the right of the computer screen) were presented, and the components were signaled by the color of the squares (i.e., yellow or green). Responding to the left and right squares produced different magnitudes of reinforcement both within and across components; that is, in the yellow component, right clicks resulted in 1 point and left clicks resulted in 8 points according to a VI 30 second schedule. In the green component, right clicks resulted in 1 point and left clicks resulted in 2 points, again according to a VI 30 second schedule. After responding had stabilized, resistance to change of square clicking was assessed by suspending point delivery. During this extinction test, three of the four participants most frequently clicked on the left square, which was associated with larger magnitudes of reinforcement, in both of the components. Of those three participants, two of them showed greater resistance to change in the yellow component, which was associated with the larger reinforcer magnitude. These findings suggest that, like Nevin's (1974) pigeons, resistance to change of human behavior may be affected by dimensions of reinforcement beyond simply the rate of its delivery.

In addition, as the study of resistance to change approached the "bed" side of the bench-to-bedside continuum, researchers began to consider additional variables that often are used in real-world settings and that may affect resistance to change. For example, Vargo and Ringdahl (2015) compared the effects of conditioned versus unconditioned reinforcers on the resistance to change with which preschoolers performed various tasks (i.e., number tracing, letter tracing, stringing beads). Unconditioned reinforcers were food items, and conditioned reinforcers were tokens exchangeable for food items. Preliminary assessments showed that both consequences served as reinforcers for task completion and were equally preferred by participants. Next, Vargo and Ringdahl arranged a two-component multiple schedule, wherein the components were signaled by the color of the task materials. During baseline conditions, task completion produced unconditioned reinforcers in one component according to a VI 30 second schedule and conditioned reinforcers in the other according to a VI 30 second schedule. Following baseline conditions, task completion was disrupted in three different ways: extinction, presession exposure to reinforcers, and distraction by presenting access to preferred movies. Results of this study varied depending on the disruptor that was used to challenge task completion, but Vargo and Ringdahl reported systematic outcomes across participants for each disruptor. Specifically, conditioned reinforcers produced greater resistance to change relative to unconditioned reinforcers when task completion was disrupted with either extinction or distraction. When task completion was challenged by presession exposure to reinforcers, however, unconditioned reinforcers produced greater resistance to change relative to conditioned reinforcers.

Leon et al. (2016) also evaluated differences between the effects of conditioned and unconditioned reinforcers on resistance to change. Specifically, they studied the task completion of children with intellectual and developmental disabilities (IDD) when completion produced either food (unconditioned reinforcers) or tokens later exchangeable for food (conditioned reinforcers). Resistance to change of task completion was assessed by progressively increasing the delay between reinforced responses and the delivery of the conditioned or unconditioned reinforcers. Results indicated that unconditioned reinforcers produced greater resistance to change in the face of reinforcer delays than conditioned reinforcers. Unlike Vargo and Ringdahl (2015), Leon et al. (2016) did not assess participants' preferences for unconditioned versus conditioned reinforcers. Therefore, it is possible that participants' preferences may have differentially affected resistance to change; that is, participants may have preferred food reinforcers over token reinforcers, and this difference in reinforcer quality may have been responsible for the differential outcomes obtained. This interpretation aligns with research reported by Mace et al. (1997) that demonstrated higher-quality reinforcers produced greater resistance to change of compliance with demands than did lower-quality reinforcers in children with IDD.

Collectively, the studies reported here show that many of the same variables Nevin (1974) found to impact resistance to change in basic studies conducted with nonhuman subjects impact the behavior of human participants in a similar manner. Given that the goals of many behavioral interventions include (1) quickly reducing problem behavior and (2) developing or supporting appropriate alternative responses, understanding the variables that affect resistance to change continues to be an important focus of basic and translational research. Broadening our understanding of these variables may allow applied researchers to determine whether those same variables impact resistance to change of socially relevant, clinically important behavior. Furthermore, this information provides practitioners with a toolkit of treatment manipulations that may support the resistance to change of socially appropriate behavior and deter the resistance to change of socially inappropriate behavior.

Compared to basic and translational analyses, applied analyses of resistance to chance are less numerous. A growing number of studies, however, have been conducted in the context of treatments for problem behavior in individuals diagnosed with IDD. We next turn to this literature, as it provides an important initial demonstration of the utility of the basic and translational research on resistance to chance so far evaluated.

Extensions to Treatments for Problem Behavior

Mace et al. (2010) conducted a groundbreaking study that provided an example of how not only basic and translational research on resistance to change can meaningfully inform treatments for problem behavior but also how translational research methods can be leveraged to overcome barriers to treatment. For our present purposes, we describe outcomes from their Experiment 1, which offered a point of contact between basic research and clinical work. We discuss in a later section outcomes from their Experiments 2 and 3, which demonstrate the utility of translational research as a means to solve real-world problems.

In their Experiment 1, Mace et al. (2010) examined resistance to change during clinical treatment of problem behavior (e.g., aggression, self-injurious behavior [SIB], food stealing) for three children diagnosed with IDD. Following a baseline condition in which a target problem behavior was reinforced, each child was exposed to two different conditions in a counterbalanced sequence. In one condition, the arranged treatment was differential reinforcement of alternative behavior (DRA) in which problem behavior continued to produce reinforcement as in baseline, but engaging in an alternative behavior (e.g., appropriate toy play, appropriate requests for food) provided a better condition of reinforcement. For example, one participant (Tom) gained access to preferred snack foods contingent on food stealing (target behavior) during baseline. When the DRA treatment was implemented, food stealing continued to be reinforced, but appropriate requests also produced access to preferred snacks and therapist praise. Then, to examine resistance to change, all responses were placed on extinction. In the second condition that followed baseline, participants' problem behavior was placed on extinction immediately, without intervening exposure to the DRA-based treatment.

For two of the three participants, problem behavior was suppressed when it was exposed to the DRA treatment. Interestingly, however, all three participants' problem behavior was more persistent during extinction that followed DRA compared to extinction that followed baseline. One may be tempted to come to the conclusion, then, that DRA-based interventions increase the future resistance to change of the behavior they are arranged to treat. It is important to remember, however, that Mace et al. (2010) continued to reinforce problem behavior during the DRA treatment and they provided comparatively high-quality reinforcers for the alternative behavior. Thus, it may not be the case that DRA per se results in increased resistance to change of problem behavior.

Instead, and consistently with previous research from the laboratory (Nevin et al., 1990, Experiment 2) the *subjectively better conditions of reinforcement* arranged during the DRA treatment may have been the causal variable that increased resistance to extinction.

Wacker et al. (2011) also illustrated the clinical implications of the previously reviewed basic- and translational-research findings by evaluating the resistance to change of both problem behavior (SIB, aggression, property destruction) and adaptive behavior (task completion, communication) within the context of clinical treatment. To do so, the authors repeatedly challenged treatment in a number of ways over the course of several months. Eight children diagnosed with IDD who engaged in problem behavior participated. All experimental procedures took place in the participants' homes, with their parents serving as treatment agents.

The study was comprised of four phases (Wacker et al., 2011). In the first phase, a functional analysis (Iwata et al., 1982, 1994) was conducted to determine the consequences that reinforced and maintained participants' problem behavior. The results from this phase indicated that each participant's problem behavior was maintained, at least in part, by escaping demands. This function subsequently was targeted for treatment. In the second phase of the study, a series of initial extinction sessions was arranged to evaluate the occurrence of problem behavior and adaptive behavior in the absence of reinforcement. The majority of participants displayed elevated levels of problem behavior similar to those observed during the functional analysis. Thus, problem behavior was initially highly resistant to change in the face of extinction. Next, in the third phase, Wacker et al. conducted functional communication training (FCT; Carr & Durand, 1985) while problem behavior was placed on extinction. To facilitate completion of work during the course of treatment, Wacker et al. provided functional reinforcement (escape from demands) for engaging in a communication response (in this case, depressing a microswitch) only after participants met individualized work criteria. Throughout the FCT phase, extinction probes were conducted periodically to evaluate the relative resistance to change of problem and adaptive behavior over the long-term course of treatment. This phase continued until, during probe sessions, adaptive behavior (i.e., compliance and functional communication) persisted and problem behavior did not recur to baseline levels. In the final phase of their study, Wacker et al. arranged four unique challenges to treatment: (1) extended extinction sessions, (2) introduction of new demand materials, (3) removal of communication devices, and (4) a mixed schedule of reinforcement wherein adaptive and problem behavior produced reinforcement.

Wacker et al. (2011) found that FCT produced rapid suppression of problem behavior and increases in adaptive behavior. During the extinction probes, however, problem behavior was likely to recur. Over repeated exposures to extinction, the effects of treatment eventually persisted; that is, participants became more likely to continue to engage in compliance and communication and less likely to engage in problem behavior across probes. Strikingly, the remaining challenges to treatment that were arranged in the final phase of the experiment produced only mild disruptions in behavior, suggesting that the enhanced resistance to change of treatment effects that Wacker et al. observed across probe sessions generalized to other situations that might act to disrupt those effects. Overall, these findings translate and extend those from the laboratory by demonstrating that behavior that has been reinforced in the past is likely to demonstrate resistance to change, and the extent to which behavior persists may be a function of an organism's recent experiences (see Craig et al., 2015); that is, as the duration of an individual's history of reinforcement for engaging in a behavior increases, resistance to change of that behavior may increase. Conversely, as an individual's history of extinction for engaging in a behavior increases, resistance to change of that behavior may decrease. It is important to note, however, that the jury is still out on the robustness of these functional relations, as the outcome from a growing number of basic-research studies have demonstrated weak or null effects of treatment duration on resistance to change (e.g., Nall et al., 2017; Shahan et al., 2020).

Several additional studies have demonstrated the influence of reinforcement-schedule variables on socially important and/or clinically relevant appropriate behavior. For example, Romani et al. (2016) evaluated how reinforcement rate impacted the resistance to change of problem behavior displayed by three children. Participants' problem behavior had been demonstrated to be sensitive to negative reinforcement in the form of escape from demands. During intervention, the researchers arranged a two-component multiple schedule, in which both of the components were associated with different reinforcement rates. Compliance produced reinforcement in both components according to the same VI schedule (the mean inter-reinforcer interval of which differed between participants), but the rate of reinforcement was increased in one of the components by delivering additional reinforcers according to fixed-time (FT) schedules (the mean inter-reinforcer interval of which also differed between participants). After compliance stabilized in both components, reinforcement was discontinued. Results demonstrated that compliance in the schedule component with the higher reinforcement rate (i.e., VI plus FT) was more resistant to change than compliance exhibited during the schedule component with the lower reinforcement rate (i.e., VI only).

In addition to reinforcement variables related to *treatment*, at least two published studies have evaluated how reinforcement rate during *assessment* impacts subsequent resistance to change during extinction. Lerman et al. (1996) compared rates of problem behavior during extinction following exposure to continuous-reinforcement (CRF) schedules and intermittent schedules during baseline. Specifically, the problem behavior of three adults diagnosed with IDD first was maintained during baseline by delivering reinforcers identified during functional analyses according to a CRF schedule. Behavior then was placed on extinction. Next, problem behavior was reestablished under an intermittent reinforcement schedule, followed again by extinction. When extinction patterns were compared across applications for an individual, results indicated that behavior persisted to a greater degree following the CRF baseline than following the intermittent-reinforcement baseline for two of the three participants when expressed as proportion-of-baseline responding.[1] For the third participant, proportion-of-baseline responding during the initial extinction sessions was greater following CRF than following intermittent reinforcement. Subsequently, however, proportion of baseline dropped to near-zero rates more quickly in extinction following CRF than in extinction following the intermittent reinforcement schedule. Given that the CRF baseline produced a higher rate of reinforcement than the intermittent-schedule baseline, these findings are in line with findings from the basic literature regarding the relation between reinforcement history and resistance to change.

MacDonald et al. (2013) replicated the findings from Lerman et al. (1996) by comparing responding during extinction that followed either CRF or intermittent reinforcement

---

[1] The *proportion-of-baseline response rate* is a measure of resistance to change that is helpful when comparing resistance produced by different conditions of reinforcement. Frequently, different conditions of reinforcement produce differences in response rate during baseline. Proportion of baseline allows one to visualize between-condition differences in the slope of resistance-to-change functions independently of differences in the functions' intercepts.

schedules during functional analyses of problem behavior exhibited by four children diagnosed with IDD. The CRF schedules produced higher reinforcement rates compared to the intermittent reinforcement schedules. Subsequent responding during extinction persisted to a greater extent following CRF than following intermittent reinforcement. Again, these results align with findings from the basic literature (e.g., Nevin, 1974), in that responding preceded by higher reinforcement rates was more resistant to change than responding preceded by lower reinforcement rates.

In addition to these published studies, a series of unpublished datasets from Ringdahl's laboratory at the University of Georgia shows a similar phenomenon. Specifically, we evaluated the data from three individuals whose clinical cases met the following criteria: (1) a functional analysis of problem behavior identified two social functions (i.e., escape from demands, accesses to tangible items, and/or access to adult attention), and (2) DRA-based interventions for both functions were conducted separately. For all three cases, we determined that the obtained rates of reinforcement differed across the relevant social-function conditions of the functional analysis, with one condition producing a greater rate of reinforcement than the other (see Figure 18.1 for outcomes of functional analysis). For two of the three cases, as shown in Figure 18.2, greater resistance to

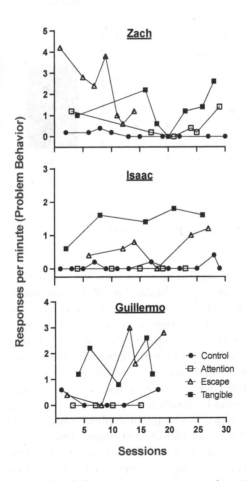

FIGURE 18.1. Instances of problem behavior per minute across functional analysis sessions.

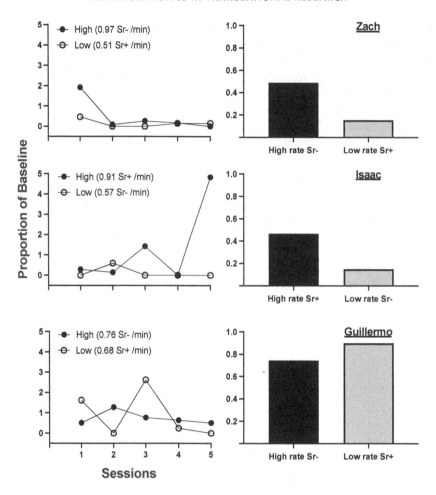

FIGURE 18.2. Proportion of baseline rates of problem behavior across sessions of DRA treatment (left panels) and averaged across sessions of treatment (right panels).

change of problem behavior was noted in the intervention associated with the functional-analysis condition that produced the higher rate of reinforcement. These data again align with findings from basic and translational evaluations of resistance to change in that higher-rate reinforcement tended to produce more persistent behavior than did lower-rate reinforcement. From a practical standpoint, these data also suggest that preintervention assessments that include delivery of reinforcement for problem behavior can impact the initial treatment success of DRA-based interventions.

The studies and clinical demonstrations described in this section highlight the impact that parameters within an individual's reinforcement history, such as reinforcer rate and magnitude, have on resistance to change in applied contexts. Yet these variables do not comprise a comprehensive list of factors that impact resistance to change. For example, the response selected as the alternative behavior has been demonstrated to impact resistance to change. When given the opportunity to earn reinforcement by engaging in different behaviors, individuals often demonstrate preference for one response over another independently of the programmed reinforcement contingencies for those responses. Ringdahl et al. (2016) for example, intervened on the problem behavior of 18 individuals diagnosed with IDD using FCT. During treatment, participants were trained to emit two communication responses (e.g., activating a microswitch and manually signing) to produce functional reinforcers. When participants subsequently were given the opportunity to perform either response for reinforcement under a concurrent fixed-ratio (FR) 1/FR 1 schedule, each participant demonstrated a preference for one response over the other; that is, despite the fact that both responses produced the same consequence according to the same reinforcement schedules, participants chose to emit one response more frequently than the other. This finding replicated earlier studies by Winborn et al. (2009) and Falcomata et al. (2010) showing that not only could FCT be effective across multiple communication topographies, but also that individuals often demonstrate a preference for which topography to use when both produce equal reinforcement.

In an extension of this line of research, Ringdahl et al. (2018) evaluated whether demonstrated preference for communication topography impacted resistance to change. Similar to Falcomata et al. (2009), Ringdahl et al. (2016), and Winborn et al (2009), participants in the Ringdahl et al. (2018) study were individuals diagnosed with IDD whose problem behavior was treated using FCT. Moreover, the FCT treatment incorporated two different communicative responses. These responses were reinforced in the context of a two-component multiple schedule. The components were signaled by differently colored poster boards. One component was associated with reinforcement for one form of communication, and the other component was associated with reinforcement for the other form of communication. Once the responses had been established in the participants' repertoires, a concurrent-schedule evaluation was conducted to identify which response was preferred. All eight participants demonstrated a preference for one of the two communicative responses. The multiple schedule was then reintroduced until rates of communication in the two components were stable, after which resistance to change of communication was assessed by introducing extinction for communication in both components. For seven of eight participants, the preferred communication response during the concurrent-schedule assessment was also the response that demonstrated the most resistance to change during the extinction assessment.

Ringdahl et al.'s (2018) findings are noteworthy, as they provided an illustration that dimensions of the *response* can play a role in determining resistance to change, whereas previous studies have, for the most part, focused exclusively on the role that dimensions of reinforcement play in determining resistance to change. One could reasonably argue, however, that response-related variables that contribute to preference do so because, much like reinforcers that are arranged purposely by experimenters or clinicians, those variables might have reinforcing properties in and of themselves. For example, pushing a microswitch may produce pleasurable sensory consequences (e.g., a satisfying "click" or other tactile stimulation) that are not produced by touching a card. Even if those sensory consequences are insufficiently reinforcing to motivate behavior in the absence of any additional, experimentally arranged reinforcement contingencies, it is conceivable that they might contribute to the value of a response. Other variables may differ between topographically different responses that may further contribute to differences in the subjective value of those responses (e.g., differences in extraexperimental reinforcement histories, response efforts). Consistent with the broader literatures on choice and resistance to change, then, one would expect the more valued response to be preferred over and more persistent than the less valued response (Grace & Nevin, 1997).

A Conceptual Analysis: Behavioral Momentum Theory

In the preceding sections, we have described a handful of variables that reliably impact resistance to change of operant behavior, including, but not limited to, reinforcer rate, magnitude, immediacy, and quality. Moreover, we have reviewed studies that evaluated the effects of these variables across diverse species and populations engaging in myriad different behaviors of focus. Time and time again, the data have suggested that more valuable sources of reinforcement produce behavior that is more persistent than less valuable sources of reinforcement. When a general relation between an independent and dependent variable is identified, a natural next step in the scientific process is to ask, "Why are these variables related?" Nevin et al. (1983) developed "behavioral momentum theory" as a means of answering exactly this question as it relates to reinforcement effects on resistance to change.

Behavioral momentum theory (BMT) draws parallels between the way that an operant behavior resists changes in its rate when that behavior is faced with disruption and the way that a moving object resists changes in its velocity when a force that opposes motion acts on that object. Imagine gently rolling a ping-pong ball across a dinner table toward a desk fan. The breeze from the fan will oppose the ping-pong ball's motion. After a few seconds, and before it reaches the fan, the ping-pong ball will likely stop rolling and probably start rolling back toward you. Try recreating that situation with a bowling ball, and you are likely to need a new desk fan![2] That is, the bowling ball may slow down slightly as it rolls across the table, but the breeze generated by the desk fan is likely to be insufficient to stop the ball's motion before it collides with the fan. As this example illustrates, the larger an object's mass, the more it resists changes in its velocity. Nevin et al. (1983) argued that delivering reinforcers in the presence of a discriminative stimulus produces a Pavlovian (stimulus–stimulus) association between the reinforcers and the stimulus in the presence of which they are delivered. According to BMT, this Pavlovian stimulus–reinforcer relation imparts a mass-like quality to behavior that causes it to persist when disrupted. Reinforcers of higher value produce stronger Pavlovian relations than do reinforcers of lower value, thereby producing more "behavioral mass" and greater resistance to change. Recall the Nevin et al. (1990) and Mace et al. (1990) findings described earlier. These studies have been used as principal support for the notion that *Pavlovian* contingencies instead of *operant* contingencies govern resistance to change.

Since its development 40 years ago, BMT has shaped the way behavior analysts think about resistance to change as we have defined it for the purpose of this chapter (resistance to change in the face of extinction, reinforcer satiation, distraction, etc.). It has strongly influenced research on other topics, too, including relapse (see, e.g., Saini et al., Chapter 19, this volume), attentional (e.g., Nevin et al., 2005; Podlesnik, Thrailkill, et al., 2012), and memorial processes (e.g., Nevin et al., 2003, 2008; Odum et al., 2005). Importantly, for our present purposes, BMT has served as a catalyst for myriad translational and applied work aimed at increasing the efficiency and long-term efficacy of behavioral interventions. By way of example, recall the Mace et al. (2010) findings described earlier: Participants' problem behavior tended to be more resistant to change following relatively high-quality DRA reinforcement than following relatively low-quality reinforcement for problem behavior. From the perspective of BMT, this outcome was observed because DRA reinforcers contributed to the Pavlovian stimulus–reinforcer relation in the

---

[2] Readers, do not try this thought experiment at home. The authors of this chapter take no responsibility for incidents involving desk fans or bowling balls that may ensue.

treatment situation, thus enhancing the behavioral mass and resistance to change of the participants' problem behavior *even though those reinforcers were delivered contingently on a different behavior* (for further discussion, see Craig & Shahan, 2016a; Nevin et al., 2017; Nevin & Shahan, 2011; Shahan & Sweeney, 2011).

Armed with the insights from BMT about *why* DRA might have increased resistance to extinction of participants' problem behavior, Mace et al. (2010) set out to develop a solution to this problem in the basic laboratory (their Experiment 2) and evaluated the viability of this solution in the context of clinically significant problem behavior (their Experiment 3). These experiments were complicated, but their rationale was simple: If an alternative response is established and frequently reinforced in a stimulus context that is different from the context previously associated with reinforcement for problem behavior, those reinforcers should not contribute to the mass, or increase resistance to change, of problem behavior. The procedures used in these experiments were very similar, so we focus specifically on the outcomes from their Experiment 3. Participants were two males who engaged in severe problem behavior. During baseline, three different conditions were arranged across sessions, each of which was associated with different discriminative stimuli (i.e., rooms, therapists' gown colors). In Condition 1, therapists delivered a relatively low rate of reinforcement (48 reinforcers per hour) for problem behavior. In Condition 2, problem behavior produced the same low rate of reinforcement as it had in Condition 1, but an additional 180 reinforcers per hour were available for appropriate requests. Finally, in Condition 3, appropriate requests produced as many as 180 reinforcers per hour, but problem behavior was placed on extinction.

Mace et al. (2010) assessed how the different reinforcement conditions just described affected resistance to change of problem behavior in a follow-up extinction test. Here, participants experienced extinction for problem behavior and appropriate communication in three stimulus situations: The situation previously associated with Condition 1 (reinforcement for problem behavior only during baseline), the situation previously associated with Condition 2 (reinforcement for problem behavior and appropriate requests at the same time during baseline), and a new situation that included a combination of stimuli from Conditions 1 (reinforcement for problem behavior only during baseline) and 3 (reinforcement for appropriate requests only during baseline). They found that participants' problem behavior persisted to the greatest degree in the stimulus situation associated with concurrent reinforcement of problem and alternative behavior during baseline (i.e., Condition 2). Moreover, resistance to change of problem behavior was relatively low and about the same in the tests that included only Condition-1 stimuli and Condition-1 + Condition-3 stimuli. Thus, consistent with the predictions of BMT and the authors' hypothesis, delivering reinforcers for alternative behavior in a stimulus context that was separate from the context in which problem behavior previously was reinforced appeared to prevent those reinforcers from contributing to the resistance to change of problem behavior (for similar findings, see Craig et al., 2018; Podlesnik, Bai, et al., 2012). These findings underscore not only the utility of BMT (and other quantitative theories of behavior) for practice but also, as we alluded to previously, the utility of translational research methods for overcoming barriers to treatment in real-world situations.

In addition to the Mace et al. (2010) findings, there are many other examples of translational applications of BMT to inform clinical interventions. Providing a review, or even a semiexhaustive bibliography, of this work is outside the scope of this chapter (for interested readers, see Fisher et al., 2019; Mace & Nevin, 2017; Podlesnik & DeLeon, 2015). Nevertheless, and despite the wealth of data that provide support for BMT and its implications for research and practice, it is by no means without its limitations. The shortcomings of the theory have been exhaustively reviewed by others (e.g., Craig et al., 2014; Nevin et al., 2017; Shahan & Craig, 2017). We provide a brief overview of two of these problems, however, because they call into question the basic arguments that BMT puts forward. Moreover, when evaluating a way of thinking about a behavior process, it is important to critically analyze all dimensions of the argument put forward: the good, the bad, and the ugly.

As we described earlier when reviewing Nevin (1974), when extinction is applied as a disruptor, higher rates of reinforcement produce greater resistance to change than do lower rates when the different reinforcement conditions are arranged within the components of a multiple schedule. When different reinforcement rates are arranged in single schedules of reinforcement, higher rates tend to produce behavior that is *less* resistant to extinction than lower rates (see Craig & Shahan, 2016a, 2016b, 2018; Shull & Grimes, 2006). Cohen (1998), for example, evaluated the effects of reinforcer rates on resistance to extinction of rats' lever pressing in a series of conditions. In the "Multiple" condition, rats experienced both high- (VI 30 second) and low-rate (VI 120 second) reinforcement for lever pressing within sessions in the components of a multiple schedule. The components of the multiple schedule were signaled by presentation of a steady or blinking house light inside the operant chamber. In the "Alternating" condition, the rate of reinforcement for lever pressing alternated between high and low across successive sessions, and the "Successive" condition arranged protracted phases in which rats experienced only high or low reinforcer rates. In these two conditions, the different reinforcer rates were correlated with either a steady or flashing house light as in the Multiple condition. Thus, the only difference between these three conditions was how often the high- and low-rate reinforcement schedules (and their correlated stimuli) alternated. Resistance to change of lever pressing in the face of extinction was assessed in the Multiple and Alternating conditions by continuing the conditions without reinforcement. In the Successive condition, individual extinction tests followed each reinforcer-rate phase.

As one would predict based on BMT, Cohen (1998) found that lever pressing was more resistant to change in the stimulus situation that was associated with the high rate of reinforcement than in the situation associated with the low rate of reinforcement in the Multiple and Alternating conditions. This prediction did not, however, bear out in the Successive condition. Here, lever pressing was *less* resistant to extinction in the high-rate than in the low-rate stimulus situation. It is unclear why reinforcer rates and the stimulus–reinforcer relations they produce would affect extinction performance differently in these conditions (i.e., enhancing resistance to change in multiple schedules and deterring resistance in single schedules). Thus, these and other, similar findings call into question the generality of the description of resistance to change offered by BMT.[3]

A second complication for BMT relates to the assertion of the theory that response rates and resistance to change are governed by different contingencies (operant response–reinforcer and Pavlovian stimulus–reinforcer contingencies, respectively). If this were

---

[3] Others (e.g., Nevin & Grace, 2005; Shull & Grimes, 2006) have presented methods for using the quantitative framework offered by BMT to account for differences in reinforcer–rate effects on resistance to change during extinction between single and multiple schedules. It is important to note, however, that these approaches entail large and otherwise unexplained variation in model parameters between single and multiple schedules (for discussion, see Craig & Shahan, 2016b). Inasmuch, these approaches offer up as many questions about BMT's description of extinction performance as they claim to solve.

true, the rate at which behavior occurs before it is disrupted should have no impact on how resistant to change it is during disruption. This basic assertion of BMT is not always supported.

Nevin et al. (2001, Experiment 1), for example, trained pigeons to peck keys for food reinforcers in a two-component multiple schedule. One component arranged reinforcement for pecking according to a variable-ratio (VR) 60 schedule, and the other arranged reinforcement according to a VI schedule. The mean value of the VI was titrated across sessions for each pigeon until the rates of reinforcement delivered by the VR and VI schedules were equivalent. Consistent with previous reports (Baum, 1993; Zuriff, 1970), the VR schedule produced higher rates of key pecking than did the VI schedule. When pecking subsequently was disrupted by either extinction of partial reinforcer satiation, responding in the VI component tended to be more resistant to change than responding in the VR component. All else being equal, behavior that occurs at a low rate predisruption tends to persist to a greater degree than behavior that occurs at a high rate predisruption. Moreover, this finding appears to be robust and has been demonstrated when response–rate differentials are produced by different reinforcement schedules (e.g., Nevin et al., 2001), pacing schedules (Lattal, 1989), or even naturally occurring variability in response rate (Kuroda et al., 2018).

These and other complications for BMT have led some, including ourselves, to argue that the underlying processes evoked by BMT need no longer be considered serious candidate processes to explain resistance to change (see Bell & Baum, 2021; Craig, in press; Nevin et al., 2017; Shahan & Craig, 2017). Nevertheless, it is important to acknowledge that the predictions of BMT, though sometimes imprecise or even flat-out contradicted by empirical outcomes, are often supported. Thus, BMT may, at the least, provide a useful heuristic for identifying experimental and treatment variables that may affect resistance to change.

Clinical Implications of Basic, Translational, Applied, and Conceptual Analyses of Resistance to Change

Research related to resistance to change and the relevant variables impacting it began in basic investigations (e.g., Nevin, 1974) and progressed to translational demonstrations (e.g., Mace, 1990; McComas, 2008) and application (e.g., Ringdahl et al., 2018; Wacker et al., 2011). Currently, much of the research on the topic occurs in the context of assessment and intervention related to socially significant clinical concerns such as communication delays and severe problem behavior. For example, both the Ringdahl et al. (2018) and Wacker et al. (2011) studies evaluated resistance to change in the context of intervention for severe problem behavior exhibited by individuals with IDD in which appropriate, alternative responses (i.e., communication) were reinforced, while problem behavior was placed on extinction. Prevalence estimates of severe problem behavior range from 10 to 15% in the population of individuals with IDD (Emerson et al., 2001), and problem behaviors within this population often are communicative in nature (Beavers et al., 2013). Thus, demonstrating how the resistance to change of communicative behavior (Wacker et al., 2011) changes over time and evaluating variables that impact resistance to change of communicative behavior (Ringdahl et al., 2018) represent examples of research that is designed to translate what has been shown in the basic behavioral literature toward the improvement and refinement of interventions conducted in applied contexts.

The current trend of research related to the resistance to change of socially significant behavior highlights the utility of understanding the relations between reinforcement history and resistance to change when developing impactful interventions. Ultimately, any behavior change program has the goal of being durable and affecting lasting behavior change that does not wane immediately upon discontinuation of supporting contingencies. The existing applied literature demonstrates that what is done prior to and during intervention alters resistance to change.

Specifically, the findings of Lerman et al. (1996), MacDonald et al. (2013), and the unpublished clinical data from the University of Georgia reviewed earlier demonstrate that practitioners should be aware of the relative frequency of reinforcement before intervention is implemented, so that they can prepare care providers regarding the likely course of treatment. For example, if problem behavior resulted in a relatively high rate of reinforcement, caregivers could be counseled that intervention may be slow to have the desired impact given the relation between high rates of reinforcement and increased resistance to change. Similarly, these findings suggest that programming relatively lean reinforcement schedules during preintervention baselines may enhance initial intervention effects. Collectively, these demonstrations highlight the potential importance of considering reinforcement history prior to implementing intervention and how reinforcers are programmed during intervention to support alternative, appropriate behavior.

The findings reported by Romani et al. (2016) suggest that reinforcement history during intervention impacts the resistance to change of appropriate, alternative behavior reinforced to replace problem behavior. Specifically, higher rates of reinforcement received during intervention may result in enhanced resistance to change of the replacement behavior. These treatment variables may allow treatment effects to be resilient in the face of challenges such as brief exposures to extinction that might happen when someone unfamiliar with a behavior plan is providing care to the individual.

Finally, data reported by Ringdahl et al. (2018) demonstrated that, in addition to reinforcement variables such as rate, magnitude, quality, or immediacy, response-specific variables may play a role in determining resistance to change. Specifically, to increase the resistance to change of appropriate behavior introduced into a repertoire, practitioners may want to take the additional step of determining whether a preference exists among candidate alternative responses. As currently implemented, many DRA- and FCT-based interventions include selection of alternative responses based on practical or experiential variables. For example, use of a tablet-based augmentative and alternative communication system may be pursued in the context of FCT, because a classroom teacher has access to tablets and the school district owns a subscription to the communication system. In another instance, picture exchange may be selected as the alternative response, because the individual has had previous experience with this communication system and the implementer is familiar with its procedures based on their experience with other students or clients. While these variables may be important to consider, they have not been demonstrated to impact resistance to change, and future research on this topic is warranted.

The conceptual analysis of resistance to change offered by BMT provides additional insights into resistance to change that may be practically useful. Behavioral theories in general are helpful for a number of reasons: (1) They help us to organize the way that we think about behavioral outcomes and functional relations, (2) they allow us to make sense of broad and often complicated bodies of literature using a few key assumptions, and (3) they enable researchers and practitioners to make precise predictions about the effects of an independent variable on a dependent variable. To these ends, we introduced

BMT in the preceding section for several reasons. First, it has played an important role in guiding basic, translational, and applied research on resistance to change. Second, it offers a reasonably straightforward metaphor for understanding why and how variables such as reinforcer rate, magnitude, quality, and immediacy impact resistance to change. We should also note that various quantitative models of resistance to change have been based on the argument put forward by BMT (see Nevin et al., 2017; Nevin & Grace, 2000; Nevin & Shahan, 2011). If practitioners know the specific parameters of reinforcement they plan to arrange during a treatment evaluation, they may use these models to generate predicted behavior during treatment on a session-by-session basis.

We have provided an overview of some of the challenges to the BMT because, just as it is important to understand the potential utility of behavioral theories for practice, it is important to appreciate that BMT is wrong. Earlier, we provided some examples of why BMT is wrong (e.g., the relation between preextinction reinforcer rates and resistance to extinction in single schedules of reinforcement opposes BMT's predictions, response rate and resistance to change appear to be related when the theory suggests that no such relation should exist), but these are not the only reasons to question the theory's assertions (see Craig et al., in press; Nevin et al., 2017). In saying that the theory is wrong, however, we do not mean that it is not useful. To demonstrate this point by way of analogy, consider for a moment the classical mechanics on which BMT is based. Despite its shortcomings, classical mechanics played a critical role in establishing our current understanding of how the physical world works. Only by identifying shortcomings of these basic tenets were researchers and theoreticians able to develop more general physical principles such as quantum mechanics. Likewise, BMT has played a critical role in leading researchers to discover variables that affect resistance to change of operant behavior. Identifying higher-order dependent variables that affect resistance to change could continue to shape our understanding of resistance-to-change mechanisms and operant behavior more generally.

Conclusions

Resistance to change is an important dimension of operant behavior that is directly relevant to clinical applications of behavior analysis. Basic, translational, and conceptual analyses of resistance to change point toward simple manipulations that are likely to make behavior more or less persistent. On the one hand, resistance to change of desirable behavior may be promoted by arranging higher rate, larger magnitude, better quality, or more immediate reinforcers. On the other hand, resistance to change of undesirable behavior may be deterred by arranging lower rate, smaller magnitude, worse quality, or more delayed reinforcers. Many of these functional relations have borne out in real-world situations with clinical populations and socially relevant behaviors.

Moreover, the study of resistance to change highlights the utility of bidirectional translational research in behavior analysis. In the traditional progression of translational research, findings from the bench are translated to the bedside; that is, basic research leads to the discovery of principles and development of technologies that are helpful when translated into application. As we have demonstrated in this chapter, some resistance-to-change research has followed this progression. It has also, however, placed emphasis on reverse translation: moving the analysis of real-world problems into the basic and translational laboratories (e.g., Craig et al., 2018; Mace et al., 2010; Nevin et al., 2016; Sweeney et al., 2014). As this literature demonstrates, the process of cyclical learning (Kasichay-anula & Vankatakrishnan, 2018), of moving from bench to bedside and back again, can help us understand why barriers to treatment exist and how we can overcome them. We encourage readers to embrace this approach to behavior-analytic research.

REFERENCES

Bai, J. Y. H., & Podlesnik, C. A. (2017). No impact of repeated extinction exposures on operant responding maintained by different reinforcement rates. *Behavioural Processes, 138,* 29–33.

Baum, W. M. (1974). On two types of deviation from the matching law: Bias and undermatching. *Journal of the Experimental Analysis of Behavior, 22,* 231–242.

Baum, W. M. (1993). Performances on ratio and interval schedules of reinforcement: Data and theory. *Journal of the Experimental Analysis of Behavior, 59,* 245–264.

Baum, W. M., & Rachlin, H. C. (1969). Choice as time allocation. *Journal of the Experimental Analysis of Behavior, 12,* 861–874.

Beavers, G. A., Iwata, B. A., & Lerman, D. C. (2013). Thirty years of research on the functional analysis of problem behavior. *Journal of Applied Behavior Analysis, 46,* 1–21.

Bell, M. C. (1999). Pavlovian contingencies and resistance to change in a multiple schedule. *Journal of the Experimental Analysis of Behavior, 72,* 81–96.

Bell, M. C., & Baum, W. M. (2021). Resistance to extinction versus extinction as discrimination. *Journal of the Experimental Analysis of Behavior, 115,* 702–716.

Blackman, D. E. (1968). Response rate, reinforcement frequency, and conditioned suppression. *Journal of the Experimental Analysis of Behavior, 11,* 503–516.

Carr, E. G., & Durand, V. M. (1985). Reducing behavior problems through functional communication training. *Journal of Applied Behavior Analysis, 18*(2), 111–126.

Cohen, S. L. (1998). Behavioral momentum: The effects of the temporal separation of rates of reinforcement. *Journal of the Experimental Analysis of Behavior, 69,* 29–47.

Cohen, S. L., Riley, D. S., & Weigle, P. A. (1993). Tests of behavioral momentum in simple and multiple schedules with rats and pigeons. *Journal of the Experimental Analysis of Behavior, 60,* 255–291.

Craig, A. R. (in press). Resistance to change of behavior and theory. *Journal of the Experimental Analysis of Behavior.* [Epub ahead of print]

Craig, A. R., Cunningham, P. J., & Shahan, T. A. (2015). Behavioral momentum and accumulation of bass in multiple schedules. *Journal of the Experimental Analysis of Behavior, 103,* 437–449.

Craig, A. R., Cunningham, P. J., Sweeney, M. M., Shahan, T. A., & Nevin, J. A. (2018). Delivering alternative reinforcement in a distinct context reduces its counter-therapeutic effects on relapse. *Journal of the Experimental Analysis of Behavior, 109,* 492–505.

Craig, A. R., Nevin, J. A., & Odum, A. L. (2014). Behavioral momentum and resistance to change. In F. K. McSweeney & E. S. Murphy (Eds.), *The Wiley Blackwell handbook of operant and classical conditioning* (pp. 249–274). Wiley Blackwell.

Craig, A. R., & Shahan, T. A. (2016a). Behavioral momentum theory fails to account for the effects of reinforcement rate on resurgence. *Journal of the Experimental Analysis of Behavior, 105,* 375–392.

Craig, A. R., & Shahan, T. A. (2016b). Experience with dynamic reinforcement rates decreases resistance to extinction. *Journal of the Experimental Analysis of Behavior, 105,* 291–306.

Craig, A. R., & Shahan, T. A. (2018). Multiple schedules, off-baseline reinforcement shifts, and resistance to extinction. *Journal of the Experimental Analysis of Behavior, 109,* 148–163.

Craig, A. R., & Shahan, T. A. (2022). Non-drug reinforcers contingent on alternative behavior or abstinence increase resistance to extinction and reinstatement of ethanol-maintained behavior. *Journal of the Experimental Analysis of Behavior, 118,* 353–375.

Craig, A. R., Sweeney, M. M., & Shahan, T. A. (2019). Behavioral momentum and resistance to extinction across repeated extinction tests.

Journal of the Experimental Analysis of Behavior, 112, 290–309.

Emerson, E., Kiernan, C., Alborz, A., Reeves, D., Mason, H., Swarbrick, R., . . . Hatton, C. (2001). The prevalence of challenging behaviors: A total population study. *Research in Developmental Disabilities, 22,* 77–93.

Falcomata, T. S., Ringdahl, J. E., Christensen, T. J., & Boelter, E. W. (2010). An evaluation of prompt schedules and mand preference during functional communication training. *The Behavior Analyst Today, 11,* 77–84.

Fisher, W. W., Greer, B. D., Craig, A. R., Retzlaff, B. J., Fuhrman, A. M., & Lichtblau, K. R. (2019). On the predictive validity of behavioral momentum theory for mitigating resurgence of problem behavior. *Journal of the Experimental Analysis of Behavior, 109,* 281–290.

Fleming, A. (1929). On the antibacterial action of cultures of a Penicillium, with special reference to their use in the isolation of B. influenzae. *British Journal of Experimental Pathology, 10,* 226–236.

Gallistel, C. R. (2012). Extinction from a rationalist perspective. *Behavioral Processes, 90,* 66–80.

Grace, R. C., & Nevin, J. A. (1997). On the relation between preference and resistance to change. *Journal of the Experimental Analysis of Behavior, 67,* 43–65.

Grimes, J. A., & Shull, R. L. (2001). Response-independent milk delivery enhances persistence of pellet-reinforced lever pressing by rats. *Journal of the Experimental Analysis of Behavior, 76,* 179–194.

Harper, D. N., & McLean, A. P. (1992). Resistance to change and the law of effect. *Journal of the Experimental Analysis of Behavior, 57,* 317–337.

Herrnstein, R. J. (1961). Relative and absolute strength of response as a function of frequency of reinforcement. *Journal of the Experimental Analysis of Behavior, 4,* 267–272.

Herrnstein, R. J. (1970). On the law of effect. *Journal of the Experimental Analysis of Behavior, 13,* 243–266.

Igaki, T., & Sakagami, T. (2004). Resistance to change in goldfish. *Behavioural Processes, 66,* 139–152.

Iwata, B. A., Dorsey, M. F., Slifer, K. J., Bauman, K. E., & Richman, G. S. (1994). Toward a functional analysis of self-injury. *Journal of Applied Behavior Analysis, 27,* 197–209.

Kasichayanula, S., & Venkatakrishnan, K. (2018). Reverse translation: The art of cyclical learning. *Clinical Pharmacology and Therapeutics, 103,* 152–159.

Kuroda, T., Cook, J. E., & Lattal, K. A. (2018). Baseline response rates affect resistance to change. *Journal of the Experimental Analysis of Behavior, 109,* 164–175.

Lattal, K. A. (1989). Contingencies on response rate and resistance to change. *Learning and Motivation, 20,* 191–203.

Lerman, D. C., Iwata, B. A., Shore, B. A., & Kahng, S. (1996). Responding maintained by intermittent reinforcement: Implications for the use of extinction with problem behavior in clinical settings. *Journal of Applied Behavior Analysis, 29,* 153–171.

Leon, Y., Borrero, J. C., & DeLeon, I. G. (2016). Parametric analysis of delayed primary and conditioned reinforcers. *Journal of Applied Behavior Analysis, 49,* 639–655.

MacDonald, J. M., Ahearn, W. H., Parry-Cruwys, D., & Bancroft, S. (2013). Persistence during extinction: Examining the effects of continuous and intermittent reinforcement on problem behavior. *Journal of Applied Behavior Analysis, 46,* 333–338.

Mace, F. C., & Critchfield, T. S. (2010). Translational research in behavior analysis: Historical traditions and imperative for the future. *Journal of the Experimental Analysis of Behavior, 93,* 293–312.

Mace, F. C., Lalli, J. S., Shea, M. C., Lalli, E. P., West, B. J., Roberts, M., & Nevin, J. A. (1990). The momentum of human behavior in a natural setting. *Journal of the Experimental Analysis of Behavior, 54,* 163–172.

Mace, F. C., Mauro, B. C., Boyajian, A. E., & Eckert, T. L. (1997). Effects of reinforcer quality on behavioral momentum: Coordinated applied and basic research. *Journal of Applied Behavior Analysis, 30,* 1–20.

Mace, F. C., McComas, J. J., Mauro, B. C., Progar, P. R., Taylor, B., Ervin, R., & Zangrillo, A. N. (2010). Differential reinforcement of alternative behavior increases resistance to extinction: Clinical demonstration, animal modeling, and clinical test of one solution. *Journal of the Experimental Analysis of Behavior, 93,* 349–367.

Mace, F. C., & Nevin, J. A. (2017). Maintenance, generalization, and treatment relapse: A behavioral momentum analysis. *Education and Treatment of Children, 40,* 27–42.

McComas, J. J., Hartman, E. C., & Jimenez, A. (2008). Some effects of magnitude of reinforcement on persistence of responding. *The Psychological Record, 58*(4), 517–528.

McIlvane, W. J. (2009). Translational behavior analysis: From laboratory science in stimulus control to intervention with persons with neurodevelopmental disabilities. *Behavior Analyst, 32,* 273–280.

Nall, R. W., Craig, A. R., Browning, K. O., & Shahan, T. A. (2018). Longer treatment with alternative non-drug reinforcement fails to reduce resurgence of cocaine or alcohol seeking in rats. *Behavioral Brain Research, 341,* 54–62.

Nevin, J. A. (1974). Response strength in multiple schedules. *Journal of the Experimental Analysis of Behavior, 21,* 389–408.

Nevin, J. A. (1992). An integrative model for the study of behavioral momentum. *Journal of the Experimental Analysis of Behavior, 57,* 301–316.

Nevin, J. A., Craig, A. R., Cunningham, P. J., Podlesnik, C. A., Shahan, T. A., & Sweeney, M. M. (2017). Quantitative models of persistence and relapse from the perspective of behavioral momentum theory: Fits and misfits. *Behavioural Processes, 141,* 92–99.

Nevin, J. A., Davison, M., & Shahan, T. A. (2005). A theory of attending and reinforcement in conditional discriminations. *Journal of the Experimental Analysis of Behavior, 84,* 281–303.

Nevin, J. A., & Grace, R. C. (2000). Behavioral momentum and the Law of Effect. *Behavioral and Brain Sciences, 23*(1), 73–130.

Nevin, J. A., & Grace, R. C. (2005). Resistance to extinction in the steady state and in transition. *Journal of Experimental Psychology: Animal Behavior Processes, 31,* 199–212.

Nevin, J. A., Grace, R. C., Holland, S., & McLean, A. P. (2001). Variable-ratio versus variable-interval schedules: Response rate, resistance to change, and preference. *Journal of the Experimental Analysis of Behavior, 76,* 43–74.

Nevin, J. A., Mace, F. C., DeLeon, I. G., Shahan, T. A., Shamlian, K. D., Lit, K., ... Craig, A. R. (2016). Effects of signaled and unsignaled alternative reinforcement on persistence and relapse in children and pigeons. *Journal of the Experimental Analysis of Behavior, 106,* 34–57.

Nevin, J. A., Mandell, C., & Atak, J. R. (1983). The analysis of behavioral momentum. *Journal of the Experimental Analysis of Behavior, 39,* 49–59.

Nevin, J. A., Milo, J., Odum, A. L., & Shahan, T. A. (2003). Accuracy of discrimination, rate of responding, and resistance to change. *Journal of the Experimental Analysis of Behavior, 79,* 307–321.

Nevin, J. A., & Shahan, T. A. (2011). Behavioral momentum theory: Equations and applications. *Journal of Applied Behavior Analysis, 44,* 877–895.

Nevin, J. A., Shahan, T. A., & Odum, A. L. (2008). Contrast effects in response rate and accuracy of delayed matching to sample. *Quarterly Journal of Experimental Psychology, 61,* 1400–1409.

Nevin, J. A., Tota, M. E., Torquato, R. D., & Shull, R. L. (1990). Alternative reinforcement increases resistance to change: Pavlovian or operant contingencies? *Journal of the Experimental Analysis of Behavior, 53,* 359–379.

Odum, A. L., Shahan, T. A., & Nevin, J. A. (2005). Resistance to change of forgetting functions and response rates. *Journal of the Experimental Analysis of Behavior, 84,* 65–75.

Podlesnik, C. A., Bai, J. Y. H., & Elliffe, D. (2012). Resistance to extinction and relapse in combined stimulus contexts. *Journal of the Experimental Analysis of Behavior, 98,* 169–189.

Podlesnik, C. A., & Deleon, I. G. (2015). Behavioral momentum theory: Understanding persistence and improving treatment. In F. D. D. Reed & D. D. Reed (Eds.), *Autism and child psychopathology series. Autism service delivery: Bridging the gap between science and practice* (pp. 327–351). Springer Science + Business Media.

Podlesnik, C. A., Jimenez-Gomez, C., Ward, R. D., & Shahan, T. A. (2006). Resistance to change of responding maintained by unsignaled delays to reinforcement: A response-bout analysis. *Journal of the Experimental Analysis of Behavior, 85,* 329–347.

Podlesnik, C. A., & Shahan, T. A. (2009). Behavioral momentum and relapse of extinguished operant responding. *Learning and Behavior, 37,* 357–364.

Podlesnik, C. A., Thrailkill, E., & Shahan, T. A. (2012). Differential reinforcement and resistance to change of divided-attention performance. *Learning and Behavior, 40,* 158–169.

Pyszczynski, A. D., & Shahan, T. A. (2011). Behavioral momentum and relapse of ethanol seeking: Nondrug reinforcement in a context increases relative reinstatement. *Behavioural Pharmacology, 22,* 81–86.

Rau, J. C., Pickering, L. D., & McLean, A. P. (1996). Resistance to change as a function of concurrent reinforcer magnitude. *Behavioural Processes, 38,* 253–264.

Ringdahl, J. E., Berg, W. K., Wacker, D. P., Ryan, S., Ryan, A., Crook, K., & Molony, M. (2016). Further demonstrations of individual preference among mand modalities during functional communication training. *Journal of Developmental and Physical Disabilities, 28,* 905–917.

Ringdahl, J. E., Crook, K., Molony, M. A., Zabala, K., Taylor, C. J., Berg, W. K., . . . Neurnberger, J. E. (2018). Effects of response preference on resistance to change. *Journal of the Experimental Analysis of Behavior, 109,* 265–280.

Romani, P. W., Ringdahl, J. E., Wacker, D. P., Lustig, N. H., Vinquist, K. M., Northup, J., . . . Carrion, D. P. (2016). Relations between rate of negative reinforcement and the persistence of task completion. *Journal of Applied Behavior Analysis, 49,* 122–137.

Shahan, T. A., Browning, K. O., & Nall, R. W. (2020). Resurgence as choice in context: Treatment duration and on/off alternative reinforcement. *Journal of the Experimental Analysis of Behavior, 113,* 57–76.

Shahan, T. A., & Burke, K. A. (2004). Ethanol-maintained responding of rats is more resistant to change in a context with added non-drug reinforcement. *Behavioural Pharmacology, 15,* 279–285.

Shahan, T. A., & Craig, A. R. (2017). Resurgence as choice. *Behavioural Processes, 141,* 100–127.

Shahan, T. A., & Sweeney, M. M. (2011). A model of resurgence based on behavioral momentum theory. *Journal of the Experimental Analysis of Behavior, 95,* 91–108.

Shull, R. L., & Grimes, J. A. (2006). Resistance to extinction following variable-interval reinforcement: Reinforcer rate and amount. *Journal of the Experimental Analysis of Behavior, 85,* 23–39.

Skinner, B. F. (1956). A case history in scientific method. In B. F. Skinner (Ed.), *Cumulative record* (pp. 76–100). Appleton-Century-Crofts.

Skinner, B. F. (1979). *The shaping of a behaviorist: Part two of an autobiography.* Knopf.

Sweeney, M. M., Moore, K., Shahan, T. A., Ahearn, W. H., Dube, W. V., & Nevin, J. A. (2014). Modeling the effects of sensory reinforcers on behavioral persistence with alternative reinforcement. *Journal of the Experimental Analysis of Behavior, 102,* 252–266.

Tan, S. Y., & Tatsumura, Y. (2015). Alexander Fleming (1881–1955): Discoverer of penicillin. *Singapore Medical Journal, 56,* 366–367.

Vargo, K. K., & Ringdahl, J. E. (2015). An evaluation of resistance to change with unconditioned and conditioned reinforcers. *Journal of Applied Behavior Analysis, 48*(3), 643–662.

Wainwright, M., & Swan, H. T. (1986). C. G. Paine and the earliest surviving clinical records of penicillin therapy. *Medical History, 30,* 42–56.

Wacker, D. P., Harding, J. W., Berg, W. K., Lee, J. F., Schieltz, K. M., Padilla, Y. C., . . . Shahan, T. A. (2011). An evaluation of persistence of treatment effects during long-term treatment of destructive behavior. *Journal of the Experimental Analysis of Behavior, 96,* 261–282.

Winborn-Kemmerer, L., Ringdahl, J. E., Wacker, D. P., & Kitsukawa, K. (2009). A demonstration of individual preference for novel mands during functional communication training. *Journal of Applied Behavior Analysis, 42,* 185–189.

Zuriff, G. E. (1970). A comparison of variable-ratio and variable-interval schedules of reinforcement. *Journal of the Experimental Analysis of Behavior, 13,* 369–374.

CHAPTER 19

An Introduction to Laboratory Models of Relapse for Applied Behavior Analysis Therapists and Researchers

Valdeep Saini
Carolyn M. Ritchey
Christopher A. Podlesnik

Behavioral interventions designed to reduce or eliminate challenging behavior often result in near-zero levels of challenging behavior when an intervention is in place. However, the effects of such treatments are not always permanent. *Relapse* refers to the recurrence of a previously eliminated challenging behavior when treatment conditions change and reflects the failure of treatment gains to maintain over time, across settings, or with different individuals (Mace & Nevin, 2017; Podlesnik et al., 2017; Podlesnik & Kelley, 2015; Wathen & Podlesnik, 2018; Pritchard et al., 2014). Relapse following successful intervention can be detrimental to an individual's ability to find or maintain employment, have a meaningful family or social life, and be a productive member of society (DeJong, 1994). Relapse of challenging behavior can take many forms, including alcohol abuse (Vuchinich & Tucker, 1996), gambling addiction (Ledgerwood & Petry, 2006), overeating (Gomez-Rubalcava et al., 2018), fear and avoidance (Smith et al., 2020), and the reemergence of severe challenging behavior exhibited by individuals with intellectual or developmental disabilities (IDDs; Radhakrishnan et al., 2020). Despite being associated with challenging behavior, behavioral principles underlying relapse are also relevant to understanding the reemergence of adaptive forms of behavior (e.g., Garner et al., 2018; Williams & St. Peter, 2020). Our purpose in this chapter is to describe basic research on relapse and its relevance to understanding and mitigating relapse in clinical and natural settings, with a focus on the treatment of severe challenging behavior exhibited by individuals with IDDs.

There have been numerous demonstrations of relapse in clinical and natural settings following treatment of behavior disorders using interventions based on technologies derived from applied behavior analysis (Briggs et al., 2018; Falligant et al., 2021; Muething et al., 2020, 2021; Suess et al., 2020). Historically, relapse following successful behavioral intervention has been viewed as a "generalization failure" due to insufficient training or teaching during the intervention period (Stokes & Baer, 1977). For example, one type of generalization failure may be explained by an oversight to include natural behavior-change agents (e.g., family or friends) during intervention planning (commonly referred to as "incorporating common mediators"). However, viewing relapse through this lens simply describes the result of a behavioral effect, but does not identify or target the specific variables that increase the probability of relapse. Without first grounding the broad spectrum of environmental events that lead to relapse in conceptually systematic experimental frameworks, developing strategies to reduce or eliminate relapse may prove to be difficult (Podlesnik & Kelley, 2017).

Translational research in the area of relapse aims to bridge the gap between basic behavioral research and applied behavioral research on relapse of socially significant challenging behavior. Knowledge derived from basic research is geared toward understanding fundamental *behavioral processes* (or mechanisms) contributing to relapse and developing behavioral technologies needed to better address clinical relapse. As identifying and targeting neurobiological processes can point toward more plausible routes to effective pharmacological interventions, identifying and targeting behavioral processes underlying relapse can offer principled approaches to combating relapse through more effective behavioral interventions. In contrast, applied research can not only directly build on treatment failures to inform, refine, and improve on existing practice, but it can also build on those processes identified in basic research on relapse. This give-and-take between basic and applied research has been referred to as *bidirectional translational research* (Dube, 2013; Mace & Critchfield, 2010). The goal of this research ultimately is to inform novel treatment approaches that are better suited to inhibit the likelihood of relapse occurring in clinical contexts (Podlesnik & Kelley, 2015). Translational research provides the opportunity to study variables that lead to relapse across the continuum of basic and applied research while drawing parallels between the experimental laboratory and natural situations in which relapse is likely to occur.

Models of Relapse

Laboratory models of relapse have been designed to mimic variables occurring in applied situations as a method for systematically investigating the factors contributing to relapse (Wathen & Podlesnik, 2018). Furthermore, these models can serve as a proving ground for testing various methods to mitigate relapse when challenges to behavioral treatments occur. Greater appreciation and understanding of findings from basic research and the fundamental behavioral processes underlying relapse could increase the effectiveness of applied research and treatment approaches to behavior disorders.

There are several advantages and reasons for using laboratory models to study relapse that occurs in clinical settings. First, basing applied research and practice in methods derived from basic behavior analysis is firmly rooted in behavior-analytic tradition and is consistent with the foundation of behavioral science (Baer et al., 1968); that is, the empirical tools of basic behavior analysis apply equally to applied behavior analysis. From this point of view, the procedures used in applied behavior analysis can be seen as a logical extension of laboratory principles (Critchfield & Reed, 2009). Second, using non-human animals as subjects allows researchers to better control environmental and subject factors that may otherwise obscure the variables contributing to relapse (e.g., ontogeny, motivation). Natural settings typically include a complex array of variables influencing treatment effects. In contrast, laboratory models allow researchers to examine these variables systematically in isolation or in combination in ways typically not possible in natural settings. Third, systematically examining even a small subset of variables influencing relapse in clinical situations can be impractical, because studying relapse requires manipulation of a range of variables that could disrupt ongoing intervention.

One of the most common interventions for treating a wide variety of behavioral challenges is differential reinforcement of alternative behavior (DRA; Petscher et al., 2009) in combination with extinction (cf. Brown et al., 2020; Vollmer et al., 2020). This intervention involves withholding reinforcement contingent upon the undesirable response and delivering reinforcement contingent upon a socially appropriate alternative response. This approach to treating behavioral problems has been considerably successful in controlled clinical contexts; however, applied research and clinical case studies rarely demonstrate long-term maintenance of intervention effectiveness (Ghaemmaghami et al., 2021; Neely et al., 2018). For example, Durand and Carr (1991) described a communication-based intervention (e.g., "Help me") in the treatment of escape-maintained challenging behavior in children diagnosed with IDDs in a school setting. Although the initial intervention was effective in the original classroom, challenging behaviors for one individual in particular increased when transitioning to a novel classroom in which a novel teacher made treatment-integrity errors. It is likely that multiple events contributed to the return of challenging behavior, and we address below some environmental events that can contribute to relapse when encountered in isolation or in combination. It is difficult, however, to isolate or systematically examine how different variables contributed to relapse in Durand and Carr's study, as is the case in most other clinical environments. In contrast, laboratory studies of relapse provide a set of well-controlled methods for systematically examining relevant variables in isolation and in combination that contribute to relapse in clinical contexts.

A wide variety of relapse models have assisted both basic and applied researchers to better understand the different processes contributing to relapse, as well as better identify functional relations of practical importance. Each of these models is supported by both basic and applied research, and reveals how laboratory studies can advance clinical assessment and treatment. Furthermore, the parallels between models of relapse in basic studies and clinical relapse in applied settings have led to specific treatment recommendations and provided practitioners with strategies for mitigating future recurrence of challenging behavior (e.g., Fisher et al., 2018; Fisher et al., 2020; Shvarts et al., 2020).

It is worth noting that *models of relapse* can refer both to the procedures used to observe relapse and the effects of those procedures. This distinction is identical to the term *extinction,* referring both to a procedure eliminating a response–reinforcer contingency and the effect of that contingency. In other words, one can define extinction by both the procedural manipulation ("introduce extinction") and the decrease in responding resulting from the procedural manipulation ("extinction of the response"). The procedure does not necessarily lead to the effect. Therefore, each of the models of relapse discussed herein describe both the procedures used to observe relapse and the underlying principle of relapse being studied.

In an individual's typical environment, some challenging behavior contacts reinforcement and is established through a learning history. For example, attention is provided by others when an individual engages in aggression, which serves to reinforce aggression. Next, the challenging behavior is reduced through treatment (e.g., DRA plus extinction).

Finally, it is possible for a variety of environmental changes to disrupt or "challenge" the treatment, which could lead to relapse (Nevin & Wacker, 2013). Common examples we discuss below are failure to reinforce the alternative response or inadvertently reinforcing aggression.

Given the natural trajectory of the development and occurrence of relapse in typical settings described in the preceding paragraph, relapse in the laboratory is often examined in a three-phase procedure. In the first phase, a target response simulating a challenging behavior is learned or acquired and maintained through some individual history of reinforcement. In the second phase, the target response is eliminated by simulating behavioral interventions based on differential reinforcement, extinction, punishment, stimulus control procedures, or some combination thereof. In the third phase, the treatment is challenged by a disruptive environmental event that results in the reemergence of the target response, or relapse. As in the earlier Durand and Carr (1991) example, it is because of the parallel between each of these three phases and examples of clinical relapse (i.e., the initial presence of challenging behavior, implementation of treatment, and subsequent relapse) that both basic and applied research on relapse typically use some variation of this procedure to evaluate the variables affecting relapse. Based on the fact that DRA-based interventions are susceptible to relapse while representing the most common strategy for the treatment of behavior problems, we largely focus our discussion of three-phase relapse procedures in the context of DRA treatments.

Resurgence

Resurgence is a procedure primarily designed to model relapse of a challenging behavior previously eliminated by DRA plus extinction (cf. Bouton et al., 2017; Rey et al., 2020). Resurgence occurs when the alternative behavior itself contacts extinction through omitting the delivery of alternative reinforcers or when deliberately thinning the alternative reinforcement rate to make DRA procedures more manageable (Kestner & Peterson, 2017; Wathen & Podlesnik, 2018; Ringdahl & St. Peter, 2017). Therefore, resurgence as a procedure generally represents the worsening of alternative reinforcement conditions that challenge DRA-treatment effectiveness (Lattal et al., 2017; Shahan & Craig, 2017).

Identifying resurgence due to worsening of alternative reinforcement conditions can provide some clarity about variables contributing to relapse during clinical interventions. In the Durand and Carr (1991) example described earlier, relapse of challenging behavior accompanied changes in both teacher and environmental setting, as well as the introduction of treatment-integrity errors. Resurgence specifically would be any return in challenging behavior as a result of treatment-integrity errors that result in failures to reinforce instances of the alternative communication response. Other models described below address additional environmental changes contributing to relapse. Experimental research using resurgence models can identify variables most likely to contribute to or mitigate resurgence under laboratory conditions—information that can be used for improving the long-term effectiveness of DRA treatments.

Resurgence in Basic Research

Table 19.1 (top panel) displays the basic three-phase procedure examining resurgence and Figure 19.1 shows hypothetical data demonstrating general patterns of responding. In Phase 1 (i.e., baseline), the target response is reinforced and therefore increases

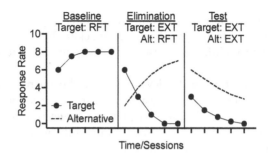

FIGURE 19.1. General patterns of responding observed during resurgence. RFT, reinforcement; EXT, extinction; Alt, alternative.

over time or sessions. This phase simulates the acquisition of challenging behavior in the typical environment through contact with a reinforcement contingency. In Phase 2, the target response is placed on extinction and an alternative behavior is also reinforced. Target responding decreases and alternative responding increases. Phase 2 simulates the behavioral intervention or treatment, wherein DRA plus extinction decrease the challenging behavior. In Phase 3, the alternative response is placed on extinction or exposed to leaner schedules of reinforcement. Target responding increases transiently, while alternative responding decreases across time or sessions. Phase 3 simulates the challenge to the behavioral treatment, which can lead to resurgence. Resurgence typically is said to occur if the target response increases relative to target-response levels toward the end of Phase 2 (i.e., DRA treatment), as shown during the test in the figure. Note that some laboratory studies include other criteria to define a resurgence effect, including target response rates exceeding inactive control responses (e.g., Cox et al., 2019; see Lattal & Oliver, 2020, for discussion).

Basic research has demonstrated the generality of resurgence across a range of species, including fish, mice, rats, hens, pigeons, monkeys, and humans ranging in age both with and without IDDs (Wathen & Podlesnik, 2018). In a number of laboratory experiments with rats, both eliminating and thinning alternative reinforcement rates produced a resurgence of target response rates (e.g., Ho et al., 2018; Schepers & Bouton, 2015; Sweeney & Shahan, 2013; Winterbauer & Bouton, 2012). During Phase 1, Winterbauer and Bouton reinforced target lever presses with food deliveries on average once every 30 seconds in three groups. During Phase 2, they introduced extinction for target responding, and alternative lever pressing received different contingencies among the three groups. One group received a typical-resurgence procedure, with alternative lever pressing reinforced across sessions once every 20 seconds on average. Another group received thinning by initially reinforcing alternative lever pressing once every 20 seconds on average, but the rate of reinforcement was halved in the middle of most Phase-2 sessions (a reinforcer was available, on average, every 20 seconds, then 40 seconds, then 80 seconds, etc.). The third, a control group, experienced only extinction of alternative lever pressing. In Phase 3, all groups experienced extinction of both target and alternative lever pressing to assess whether target lever pressing returned.

In Phase 3 of Winterbauer and Bouton (2012), target lever pressing was greater for the two groups experiencing removal of alternative reinforcement during Phase 2 compared with the control group that did not. For the typical-resurgence group, target lever pressing only increased during Phase 3 when introducing extinction of alternative lever pressing (resembling data in Figure 19.1). While target response rates remained at low levels in Phase 2 for the typical-resurgence and control groups, the group experiencing thinning of alternative reinforcement rates during Phase 2 showed increases in target lever pressing as the rate of alternative reinforcement decreased within and across sessions. Similarly, other studies with rats found that decreasing the number or duration of food deliveries *per alternative reinforcer* during Phase 3 also produced a resurgence of target lever pressing (Craig et al., 2018; Oliver et al., 2018). Moreover, Oliver et al. showed that increasing the amount of alternative reinforcement did not produce resurgence. Therefore, basic research on resurgence revealed that resurgence is a result of a worsening of alternative reinforcement conditions rather than simply a change in reinforcement conditions (see Lattal et al., 2017, for a review). These findings from basic research demonstrate specific functional relations producing resurgence, allowing for further examination of both the behavioral processes involved in resurgence and factors influencing and mitigating resurgence in clinical situations.

Resurgence in Applied Research

Behavior analysts in practice do not often treat discrete forms of challenging behavior, and it may appear as though the simple responses studied in basic research cannot sufficiently represent phenomena that occur in natural settings. Consistent with the numerous studies from basic research, however, a number of applied studies have demonstrated that resurgence is a robust phenomenon that occurs in complex and severe challenging behavior (Briggs et al., 2018; Muething et al., 2020). Furthermore, the resurgence of complex behavior patterns including chains of responding and response-class hierarchies is common, and has implications for studying resurgence with socially significant behavior (e.g., childhood tantrums that consist of different topographies of challenging behavior; St. Peter, 2015).

As described earlier, the experimental procedures used to study resurgence are very similar to the types of treatment procedures used by clinicians. For example, in the treatment of severe challenging behavior demonstrated by individuals with IDDs, the clinician first collects data on baseline levels of the challenging behavior, wherein the response typically contacts some schedule of reinforcement (e.g., aggression contacts continuous reinforcement in the form of access to attention). Next, the clinician may introduce a DRA-based procedure such as functional communication training (FCT) to reduce the challenging behavior and teach an appropriate communicative alternative (e.g., aggression contacts extinction and saying "Look at me!" is reinforced with attention). The clinician may then introduce reinforcement-schedule thinning, in which the alternative response is not reinforced on every occasion to make the intervention more manageable. Because schedule thinning exposes the alternative behavior to brief periods of extinction and reduces the overall density of reinforcement, this clinical procedure challenges the DRA treatment and resembles the worsening conditions described earlier in basic laboratory research (Winterbauer & Bouton, 2012). Under these circumstances, resurgence of the challenging behavior and degradation of the appropriate behavior may occur (e.g., aggression reemerges and communication decreases; Volkert et al., 2009; Briggs et al., 2018; Muething et al., 2021).

Another potential challenge to treatment occurs when natural behavior-change agents (e.g., caregivers of young children with disabilities) implement treatment

TABLE 19.1. Basic and Applied Demonstrations of Resurgence

	Baseline/acquisition	Elimination/treatment	Relapse test
Basic	Reinforce target response	Extinguish target response	Extinguish target response
		Reinforce alternative response	Extinguish alternative response
Applied	Reinforce tantrums with iPad	Tantrums placed on extinction	Tantrums continue to undergo extinction
		Reinforce communication with iPad	Communication is placed on extinction or reinforcement schedule thinned

procedures inconsistently or with omission errors (i.e., failing to provide a reinforcer at a prescribed time). Table 19.1 (bottom panel) displays how resurgence of tantrums could occur when a caregiver fails to implement FCT as prescribed, which inadvertently places the communication response on extinction. In this situation, a child is taught that (1) to gain access to their iPad they must vocally ask for it, and (2) engaging in tantrums will not lead to obtaining the iPad. In natural settings, numerous situations could arise to prevent the caregiver from reinforcing communication responses, such as cooking dinner, speaking on the phone, attending to a sick sibling, and so forth. These situations represent a "worsening condition," because the appropriate response contacts extinction. Such situations resemble those from Durand and Carr (1991) when novel teachers failed to reinforce instances of the newly trained communication response and challenging behavior returned. Therefore, resurgence of the challenging behavior can occur when errors of omission occur and ultimately threaten the integrity of the intervention (Marsteller & St. Peter, 2012).

Reinstatement

Reinstatement is a procedure designed to model relapse of a challenging behavior due to encountering the reinforcer that previously maintained the challenging behavior (e.g., Bouton, 2019; Burokas et al., 2018). Reinstatement has been demonstrated when the target behavior, eliminated by extinction, reemerges when the original reinforcer is presented either response independently or response dependently (e.g., Podlesnik & Shahan, 2009) or when stimuli/cues previously paired with target reinforcement are presented without target reinforcement (e.g., Floresco et al., 2008).[1] One way offered to conceptualize all these methods of producing reinstatement is that re-presenting the cue or reinforcer serves as a discriminative stimulus for the original contingency between target behavior and reinforcement (e.g., Bouton et al., 2012). In other words, whether the event is a cue or primary reinforcer, contingent or noncontingent, re-presentation of the event signals that the original contingency between target behavior and reinforcement might again be present and active, thereby reinstating target responding (i.e., a stimulus–response

---

[1]It is worth noting there is one other common method for producing reinstatement (see Mantsch et al., 2016, for a review), which is exposing organisms to stressful experiences during reinstatement testing after extinction (e.g., shock, forced swimming) but stress-induced reinstatement likely is more appropriately described as another type of model, renewal (see Bouton, 2019; Schepers & Bouton, 2019).

relation). Alternatively, reinstatement with response-dependent events might reflect only the reintroduction of the reinforcement contingency (i.e., a response–stimulus relation). We further address these issues below in the context of basic research on reinstatement.

In the context of DRA plus extinction, reinstatement of a challenging behavior could occur when a reinforcer previously unavailable during DRA is again made available either noncontingently or contingent upon challenging behavior. For example, reprimands maintaining challenging behavior through attention before DRA treatment could reinstate challenging behavior after effective DRA treatment. Reinstatement is relevant to the example from Durand and Carr (1991) described earlier, in which a child's escape-maintained challenging behavior relapsed when moving to a new classroom. It is possible that the teacher provided unrequested breaks or breaks contingent upon problem behavior (i.e., a treatment-integrity error) that contributed to relapse by reinstating challenging behavior. As with resurgence, basic research using reinstatement models can identify variables most likely to contribute to or mitigate reinstatement under laboratory conditions—information that can be used for improving the long-term effectiveness of DRA treatments.

Reinstatement in Basic Research

Table 19.2 (top panel) displays the basic three-phase procedure of an experimental study of reinstatement, and Figure 19.2 shows hypothetical data demonstrating general patterns of responding. In Phase 1 (i.e., baseline), reinforcement increases the target response, and this phase simulates the acquisition of challenging behavior in the typical environment through contact with a reinforcement contingency. In Phase 2, the target response decreases when placed on extinction. Phase 2 provides a general simulation of a behavioral intervention or treatment, although laboratory models of reinstatement typically do not include a DRA component. In Phase 3, the reinforcer originally maintaining the target response in Phase 1 is re-presented, simulating the availability of the reinforcer directly evoking an increase in challenging behavior (see Figure 19.2). In some cases, only a small number of reinforcer deliveries are presented (one to three; e.g., Liggett et al., 2018; Ostlund & Balleine, 2007; Podlesnik & Shahan, 2009, 2010) whereas in other cases, reinforcers have been delivered continually according to an ongoing fixed- or variable-time-based schedule (e.g., Doughty et al., 2004; Rescorla & Skucy, 1969). In a few cases, reinforcers have been delivered contingently on the target response leading

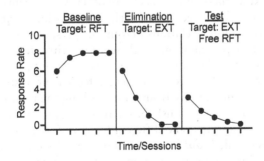

FIGURE 19.2. General patterns of responding observed during reinstatement. RFT, reinforcement; EXT, extinction.

to a reinstatement effect (e.g., Acosta et al., 2008; Podlesnik & Shahan, 2009). As with resurgence, reinstatement typically is said to occur if the target response increases relative to target-response levels toward the end of Phase 2, but target response rates exceeding inactive control responses also are reported frequently (e.g., Panlilio et al., 2003).

Basic research has demonstrated the generality of reinstatement across a range of species and experimental conditions (see Wathen & Podlesnik, 2018). In one example, Ostlund and Balleine (2007) reinforced one lever press with food pellets and another lever press with a sucrose solution in alternating sessions during Phase 1 in two groups of rats. In Phase 2, both levers were available concurrently, but extinction was in place for 15 minutes. Within the extinction session, Phase 3 began when 5 seconds passed without a response, and then a single delivery of either a food pellet or sucrose solution (counter-balanced across rats) served to test for reinstatement. Only the lever previously produc-ing the reinforcer type (food or sucrose) presented during testing increased reliably (for related findings, see Colwill, 1994; Delamater et al., 2003; Leri & Stewart, 2001). The 5-second omission criterion before delivering the reinforcer in Phase 3 guarded against interpretations based on adventitious reinforcement (i.e., superstitious behavior; Skin-ner, 1948). Instead, the findings of Ostlund and Balleine (2007) and others are consis-tent with an interpretation that reinforcers reinstate operant behavior as discriminative stimuli for specific operant responses.

There are considerations briefly mentioned earlier that are relevant to understanding the methods used to examine reinstatement. Researchers have arranged both response-independent and -dependent deliveries of reinforcers to examine reinstatement of target responding. Response-independent and -dependent methods of presenting the reinstating reinforcers have been distinguished empirically. In the only direct comparison to our knowledge, greater overall levels of reinstatement were found with response-dependent than -independent methods of reinforcer delivery with pigeons, but patterns of respond-ing did not differ (Podlesnik & Shahan, 2009). The question is whether the causes of the increases in target responding with the different contingencies are fundamentally differ-ent. As there are no data resolving this question, we present some potential interpreta-tions of the different reinstatement methods.

One interpretation is that response-independent and -dependent reinforcer deliveries reinstate behavior in fundamentally the same way (Bouton et al., 2012). When presented response independently, a number of studies examining reinstatement lend support to the interpretation that reinforcer deliveries reinstate extinguished responding by setting the occasion for target responding (e.g., Baker et al., 2001; Franks & Lattal, 1976; Miranda-Dukoski et al., 2016; Rescorla & Skucy, 1969). In other words, deliveries of the reinforcer following extinction serve as antecedent discriminative stimuli for emitting the target response (i.e., stimulus–response relations). From this perspective, response-independent and -dependent reinforcer presentations both serve to reinstate behavior through ante-cedent/discriminative control (i.e., stimulus–response relations).

Another interpretation of the reinstatement effects from response-dependent rein-forcer deliveries is they result entirely from reestablishing the reinforcement contingency itself (i.e., response–stimulus relations). From this interpretation, reinstatement from response-dependent presentations is no different from increases in extinguished respond-ing from what has been called *rapid reacquisition* (e.g., Bouton et al., 2012). Studies of rapid reacquisition extinguish a target response before re-introducing the reinforcement contingency during testing. With rapid reacquisition, reinforcement contingencies reintro-duced following extinction produce faster acquisition than the first phase of acquisition, demonstrating the influence of prior learning. These studies typically compare conditions that might facilitate or impede reacquisition of the target response to levels observed before extinction (e.g., Willcocks & McNally, 2011). From this perspective, reinstatement from response-dependent reinforcer presentations simply reflects the influence of a reinforcement contingency. Therefore, response-independent deliveries set the occasion for target responding, while response-dependent deliveries and the rapid-reacquisition model explicitly reinforce target responding.

A final interpretation is that response-dependent deliveries increase target behavior by a combination of events. Antecedent–discriminative control (i.e., stimulus–response relations) contributes in the same way it did with response-independent presentations in combination with the reinforcement contingency itself (i.e., response–stimulus relations). Regardless of what interpretation ultimately contributes to reinstatement, both methods serve to model relapse by producing increases in target responding through re-presenting the target reinforcer. In this way, the reinstatement and reacquisition models can be generally contrasted with the resurgence model, which typically involves the removal or reduction of alternative reinforcement.

Reinstatement in Applied Research

Laboratory studies of reinstatement and rapid reacquisition have direct relevance to clinical relapse given that these models are principally concerned with relapse due to the delivery of reinforcers previously maintaining operant behavior, as with errors of commission (i.e., providing a reinforcer at a nonprescribed time; St. Peter Pipkin et al., 2010) in clinical contexts. Such events pose significant challenges to the treatment of challenging behavior because errors of commission can occur during and following treatment (Brand et al., 2019). These relapse phenomena have been observed to occur in nonhuman and human models of drug addiction (Shaham et al., 2003), obesity (Bodnar et al., 2020; Burokas et al., 2018), and severe challenging behavior (Falcomata et al., 2013). For example, DeLeon et al. (2005) treated attention-maintained aggression in one adult with extinction. Following reduction of aggression, the experimenters continued to implement extinction but also provided response-independent attention (e.g., FT 60 seconds schedule). During this phase, they observed the reinstatement of aggression consistent with laboratory models.

TABLE 19.2. Basic and Applied Demonstrations of Reinstatement

	Baseline/acquisition	Elimination/treatment	Relapse test
Basic	Reinforce target response	Extinguish target response	Extinguish target response
			Response-independent reinforcer presentations
Applied	Reinforce aggression with attention	Reinforce communication for attention	Reinforce communication for attention
	Reinforce self-injury with tangible items	Reinforce communication for tangible items	Free access to attention
			Reinforce communication for tangible items
			Free access to tangible items

Table 19.2 (bottom panel) illustrates how reinstatement can occur for multiple topographies of challenging behavior maintained by different social reinforcers (Beavers & Iwata, 2011) in an example resembling the experimental study presented earlier (Ostlund & Balleine, 2007). A child might engage in aggression to obtain attention from others and in self-injury to obtain tangible items (e.g., toys). Following independent FCT interventions, the presentation of one of those reinforcers alone may facilitate the relapse of a specific topography of challenging behavior. For instance, the free delivery of a tangible item (e.g., teacher provides toys independent of a communication response) could reinstate self-injury, whereas the free delivery of attention (e.g., classmate provides attention independent of a communication response) could reinstate aggression. Presentation of one of the reinforcers could produce reinstatement potentially by setting the occasion for the specific challenging behavior functionally related to the reinforcer presented, similar to Ostlund and Balleine (2007).

Both reinstatement and rapid reacquisition are clinically relevant for similar reasons and are believed to promote clinical relapse due to the same or similar underlying mechanisms, as reinforcer deliveries can signal the returned availability of reinforcement for challenging behavior (Wathen & Podlesnik, 2018). As described earlier, *rapid reacquisition* is a model of relapse similar to reinstatement and occurs when a reinforcer is delivered contingent upon a challenging behavior (i.e., an error of commission). Clinically, commission errors occasionally occur such that the reinforcer is presented immediately following the target challenging behavior, on a response-contingent basis (as opposed to time). In the typical environment, after the successful reduction of challenging behavior following treatment, a caregiver might inadvertently deliver a functional reinforcer for challenging behavior for one of many reasons. For example, the challenging behavior may begin occurring at a level of severity that is unmanageable, and the caregiver delivers the reinforcer in order to prevent further escalation. Alternatively, the intervention may include many components that require the caregiver's attention. In this case, the effort involved in implementing the intervention may lead to an integrity error in which the caregiver provides the functional reinforcer freely (i.e., in the absence of an appropriate alternative response).

The findings across laboratory and applied studies of reinstatement and reacquisition indicate that errors of commission should be minimized during and following treatment to prevent reinstatement of the challenging behavior that might hinder treatment progress. Function-based treatments for challenging behavior involve the presentation of a putative reinforcer that maintained challenging behavior. However, it is important to recognize that the reinforcers used during treatment, even when functionally the same, are not always exactly like those that maintained challenging behavior. For an example with attention, a child's tantrums might be maintained by caregiver reprimands (e.g., the caregiver scolding the child for tantrums) but the function-based intervention might involve the caregiver providing approval for an alternative appropriate behavior (e.g., smiling and hugging the child when they request their caregiver's attention vocally). This difference in the qualitative aspects of reinforcement delivered during treatment and nontreatment conditions is one potential reason why reinstatement effects might not be observed during function-based treatments implemented with high integrity. When implemented with less integrity, functional reinforcers could reinstate challenging behavior.

The ease with which commission errors (or response-dependent reinforcement for challenging behavior) can be minimized does depend, in part, on the challenging behavior being treated and the environment in which treatment is delivered. For example, avoiding errors of commission might be easier in the treatment of attention-maintained tantrums when trained therapists are implementing the intervention versus when a class-room teacher is implementing the intervention. Ultimately, clinicians should consider specific strategies designed to reduce the probability of relapse if such an error does occur by programming relapse-mitigation strategies during the course of intervention. Basic and applied research on resurgence and reinstatement in isolation imply that interventions implemented with perfect integrity would eliminate any concerns about relapse. How-ever, the next laboratory model of relapse we discuss should undermine this impression.

Renewal

Thus far, we have discussed the relevance of laboratory models for understanding relapse due to errors of omission (e.g., resurgence) and commission (e.g., reinstatement, rapid reacquisition). In such cases, relapse occurs as a result of reinforcement contingencies. However, relapse can occur independently from changes in the contingencies and could occur as a function of antecedents in the form of changes in contextual variables. Spe-cifically, *renewal* is a procedure used to assess relapse due to changes in environmental context (Bouton, 2019; Podlesnik et al., 2017). Renewal of the target behavior occurs when transitioning to an environmental context after eliminating the target behavior in the presence of a different environmental context. To return to the example of Durand and Carr (1991), the transition itself to a novel classroom with a new teacher might have been sufficient to produce some level of increase in challenging behavior independent of any breakdowns in treatment integrity. Such effects with FCT would be consistent with the type of relapse observed during laboratory studies of renewal.

Behavioral interventions for severe challenging behavior are often conducted in a setting different from one's typical environment, such as receiving treatment for chal-lenging behavior in a clinic rather than in the home. Moreover, treatments are often implemented by trained therapists as opposed to natural behavior-change agents (e.g., caregivers). Within clinical settings, interventions are usually quite effective (Petscher et al., 2009). However, treatment gains established in one setting do not always maintain in other settings, and relapse of challenging behavior may occur when clients transition to natural or novel environments (e.g., home, new school; Podlesnik et al., 2017). Relapse may also occur when treatments are transitioned to novel therapists or natural behavior-change agents as part of a generalization strategy. The relapse of undesirable behavior as a result of changing stimulus contexts, including to new individuals, is termed a *renewal* effect. This relapse phenomenon describes the recurrence of challenging behavior as a function of the interaction between learning processes related to contingencies and the contexts in which learning occurs (Bouton & Todd, 2014; Podlesnik et al., 2017; Saini & Mitteer, 2020).

Renewal in Basic Research

Table 19.3 (top panel) and the two panels of Figure 19.3 display the basic three-phase procedures of experimental studies of renewal. In the first phase, the target response is reinforced in a distinctive stimulus context, typically referred to as Context A. This phase simulates the acquisition of reinforced challenging behavior in a specific setting, which oftentimes will be a child's challenging behavior occurring at home. In the second phase, the target response is eliminated in a novel context, typically referred to as Context B.

In experimental research, responding in Phase 2 usually is eliminated through simple extinction of a target response, but clinical evaluations of renewal have also arranged DRA treatments (e.g., Falligant et al., 2021; Muething et al., 2020; Kelley et al., 2018; Saini et al., 2018). Experimentally, this phase simulates treatment delivered in a setting different from the setting in which the behavior usually occurs, such as an inpatient behavioral therapy program in a hospital setting. In the final phase, the original context (A), or a novel context (C), is introduced with the treatment contingency (e.g., extinction or DRA plus extinction) still in place. Phase 3 simulates the transfer of the treatment to the natural environment, such as transitioning back home (A) or to a new school (C) from the hospital following intervention. The relapse of challenging behavior when the initial context, or a novel context, is introduced despite ongoing treatment is termed the *renewal effect* (Nakajima et al., 2000).

Like resurgence and reinstatement, the renewal of operant behavior has been demonstrated under a range of experimental conditions, using a number of different species, and in different populations (for reviews, see Podlesnik et al., 2017; Saini & Mitteer, 2020; Wathen & Podlesnik, 2018). The word *context* has been used to refer to a range of different types of events (for discussion, see Bouton et al., 2021; Podlesnik & Kelley, 2015, Podlesnik et al., 2017). Contextual stimuli in laboratory research, for example, have included various visual, tactile, and olfactory stimuli embedded in the operant chamber (Todd et al., 2014), another laboratory animal (Browning & Shahan, 2018; Nieto et al., 2017), motivational state (Schepers & Bouton, 2017), drug effects (Bouton et al., 1990), and presence–absence of stressors (Schepers & Bouton, 2019), among others. Thus, context appears to refer broadly to a range of changes to environmental stimuli that affect behavior. In a fairly typical example, Bouton et al. (2011) reinforced rats' lever pressing with food pellets every 30 seconds on average during Phase 1 in the presence of Context A. Contexts were defined by various visual, tactile, and olfactory stimuli embedded in the

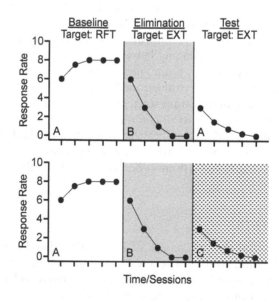

FIGURE 19.3. General patterns of responding observed during ABA (top panel) and ABC (bottom panel) renewal. RFT, reinforcement; EXT, extinction.

operant chamber. During Phase 2, the constellation of stimuli changed to comprise Context B, in which extinction of responding was introduced. Finally, returning to Context A or transitioning to yet another novel context (C) produced an increase in responding—the renewal effect. These two renewal effects are referred to as ABA and ABC renewal, respectively.

Another form of renewal (called AAB renewal) occurs when acquisition and extinction across Phases 1 and 2, respectively, occur in the same context (A) while testing occurs in a novel context (B). For example, Cohenour et al. (2018) extinguished a lever pull by children diagnosed with autism spectrum disorder. They suggested that presenting either a novel light or buzzer during extinction served as a novel Context B and produced AAB renewal. As with ABC renewal, these findings indicate that renewal results from transitioning out of the context in which target behavior was eliminated (see Bouton, 2019). In addition, the presentation of a discrete stimulus to comprise a context is indicative, as suggested earlier, of the broad use of the word *context* to refer to a range of different types of changes to environmental stimuli that affect behavior (see Podlesnik et al., 2017, for a discussion). As such, it is likely that AAB renewal is related to another relapse model called *disinhibition*. Disinhibition involves introducing novel stimuli into a context following extinction, in which those stimuli serve to increase responding (Brimer, 1970). A clinical example might be having a fire alarm (i.e., novel stimulus) suddenly go off at a behavior therapy clinic (i.e., context) that evokes challenging behavior in a child with IDD after a DRA treatment has successfully been implemented. The alarm sounding serves as a novel stimulus that has been introduced into a context with which the child is already familiar (i.e., a context with an existing conditioning history). Nevertheless, these three forms of renewal (ABA, ABC, AAB) demonstrate that operant behavior will return when transitioning out of the context in which behavior was extinguished.

Laboratory demonstration of ABC and AAB renewal indicate that relapse due to contextual changes is not simply a function of returning to the original context in which initial learning occurred. Instead, renewal is a more general result in which the original learning appears to generalize well beyond the original training context, even after being eliminated within or outside that original training context (for reviews, see Bouton, 2019; Bouton et al., 2012). Therefore, basic research on renewal demonstrates the susceptibility of operant behavior to relapse any time that aspects of the environmental context change from those arranged during treatment.

Renewal in Applied Research

The relapse of challenging behavior as a function of contextual variables, like those described in experimental models of renewal, may be of particular importance in clinical applications of behavior analysis. Their relevance stems primarily from interventions for behavior disorders often being conducted in settings outside of the individual's typical environment, and are usually first introduced by clinicians or therapists as opposed to natural behavior-change agents (Saini & Mitteer, 2020); that is, behavioral interventions often require the transfer of an intervention across settings and among individuals.

Models of renewal suggest that a change in the stimulus conditions or context is sufficient to produce clinical relapse of previously eliminated challenging behavior. The implication for behavioral treatments is that undesirable behavior learned in one context (e.g., child aggression toward caregivers at home) and treated in a different context (e.g., trained therapists implement extinction for aggression in a classroom), could relapse

TABLE 19.3. Basic and Applied Demonstrations of Renewal

	Baseline/acquisition	Elimination/treatment	Relapse test
Basic	Context A:	Context B:	Context A or C:
	Reinforce target response	Extinguish target response	Extinguish target response
Applied	Context A:	Context B:	Context A or C:
	Aggression reinforced with attention by caregiver at home	Aggression is placed on extinction by therapist in clinic	Aggression is placed on extinction by caregiver at home or playground
		Communication is reinforced with attention by therapist in clinic	Communication is reinforced with attention by caregiver at home or playground

when the intervention is transferred to the original context (i.e., home with therapists), a novel context (e.g., grocery store with therapists), or a combination of these (e.g., home or grocery store with caregivers). Table 19.3 (bottom panel) draws a direct parallel to laboratory studies of renewal and describes how treatment of attention-maintained aggression occurring in a home setting might renew when a DRA-based intervention is implemented in a clinic setting and then transferred to the child's home (i.e., the original setting) or to the child's school (i.e., a novel setting).

Although renewal is typically studied in laboratory settings using extinction, and extinction-induced renewal has been observed in clinical settings (Ibañez et al., 2019), interventions to treat complex challenging behavior are more likely to rely on DRA-based interventions, such as FCT, in combination with extinction. Clinical investigations of relapse have demonstrated that the renewal effect is observed when a behavioral intervention based on differential reinforcement is transferred from a treatment setting to the natural environment (Pritchard et al., 2016; Saini et al., 2018) and contexts within a treatment setting (Kelley et al., 2018). Therefore, renewal is not an extinction-specific effect and can occur with a variety of intervention procedures.

Findings from clinical investigations of relapse further validate the notion that the same types of contextual variables studied in laboratory experiments of relapse also contribute to clinical relapse in applied settings in the form of renewal. The collective findings across basic and applied studies suggest that if relapse of challenging behavior depends in part on the reinforcement history established in a given context, the generality and maintenance of behavioral interventions might also depend on contextual variables.

Considerations for Practice

Laboratory models of relapse have implications for behavior analysts in practice who routinely work with individuals who engage in challenging or harmful behavior (e.g., drug addiction, self-harm). The results of experiments based on these models provide specific guidelines for strategies to improve treatment generality and reduce the likelihood of relapse occurring in clinical situations. Given that clinically oriented behavior-analytic research of relapse is only just emerging, these recommendations should be considered preliminary in nature. Nonetheless, reducing or eliminating relapse should be on the forefront of all behavioral interventions given the deleterious outcomes associated with recidivism of challenging behavior.

Interactions among Relapse Models

Laboratory models are useful for identifying the specific environmental variables that contribute to relapse, and these models have produced a rich and robust literature base from which to study relapse through a behavior-analytic lens. Although models of different relapse phenomena are often studied and described individually, relapse in natural or clinical environments is likely due to the interaction of variables described in each model; that is, in applied and clinical contexts, the variables described by these models likely interact and cannot be easily isolated. For example, a child who engages in disruptive behavior at home may be prescribed FCT as an intervention by a behavior analyst in a clinic setting. If FCT is successful in reducing disruptions at the clinic, the behavior analyst may then transfer the intervention to the home setting with caregivers. This scenario resembles the renewal procedure described in the clinical example in Table 19.3. However, other complications can often arise during clinical interventions. When FCT is first introduced, the caregiver may inadvertently reinforce disruptions or fail to reinforce communication. This arrangement, which is common in the treatment of challenging behavior, consists of contextual changes that could precipitate renewal (i.e., transferring treatment from a clinic setting to a home setting), as well as errors of omission and commission, which could precipitate resurgence and reinstatement, respectively (see Mitteer et al., 2018).

Translational research on relapse has begun exploring the degree to which relapse of challenging behavior might be amplified when multiple variables affecting relapse are present simultaneously. In other words, combinations of variables known to produce relapse result in greater relapse than any in isolation. Such combinations have been examined in at least four ways, and each of these combinations shows how standard models of relapse might interact in applied settings.

First, laboratory research with nonhuman animals and humans with and without IDDs diagnoses demonstrated such effects with resurgence and renewal (Podlesnik et al., 2019; for related findings, see also Kincaid et al., 2015; Nakajima et al., 2002; Nighbor et al., 2018; Trask & Bouton, 2016). After reinforcing an operant response within Context A and arranging DRA during Context B, removing alternative reinforcers produced greater resurgence when returning to Context A than when remaining in Context B. These findings demonstrate the confluence of omission errors (resurgence) and a context change (renewal). The collective findings suggest that relapse in clinical situations may be exacerbated when omission errors and context changes occur together.

Second, Todd et al. (2014) demonstrated faster reacquisition of reinforced lever pressing in rats when returning to the training context (ABA renewal) or transitioning to a novel context (AAC renewal) than when remaining in the context in which extinction occurred (see also Willcocks & McNally, 2011). These findings demonstrate the confluence of commission errors (reacquisition/reinstatement) and a context change (renewal), and suggest that relapse in clinical situations may be exacerbated when commission errors and context changes occur together.

Third, Liggett et al. (2018) simulated omission and commission errors in isolation or in combination in a laboratory study with children diagnosed with autism spectrum disorder. The combination of errors produced greater relapse than either in isolation, indicating the confluence of resurgence and reinstatement effects. The clinical implication of this finding is that relapse may be exacerbated when omission errors and commission errors co-occur (e.g., following intervention, a caregiver fails to reinforcer an appropriate communication response and accidentally reinforces a challenging behavior).

Finally, *spontaneous recovery* describes the extent to which responding recurs when there has been some absence or break from the context in which extinction was arranged. Spontaneous recovery can occur clinically after suspension of treatment implementation, such as following a long weekend or holiday. Gámez and Bernal-Gamboa (2019) found in a game-like laboratory task with university students that extinguished responses recurred to a greater extent when testing after a 48-hour delay compared with no delay. Moreover, renewal by changing the onscreen context was increased when testing after a 48-hour delay compared with no delay. These findings demonstrate the confluence of a break from treatment (spontaneous recovery) and a context change (renewal), and suggest that relapse in clinical settings can be exacerbated when a context change occurs following some absence in treatment (e.g., an intervention is temporarily suspended and restarted in a new clinic).

The range of findings presented here clearly demonstrate that multiple environmental variables that contribute individually to relapse can combine to exacerbate relapse effects. Furthermore, it is important to take into account the fact that some forms of relapse can initiate others. For example, a change in context or failure to reinforce the alternative response could result in an increase in challenging behavior through renewal or resurgence, respectively. With the challenging behavior returning to greater frequency, the likelihood increases that someone with insufficient training will reinforce instances of challenging behavior, resulting in further increases through reinstatement or rapid reacquisition. Therefore, developing strategies to minimize the likelihood of relapse is important for the long-term maintenance of behavioral treatments.

Translational Research on Mitigation Strategies and Implications for Practice

An additional benefit of laboratory research, beyond identifying and understanding how environmental variables influence relapse, is the capability to evaluate specific approaches to reducing the likelihood of relapse. A number of approaches exist and show promise for mitigating specific forms of relapse described earlier, while others could be more general and effectively reduce relapse resulting from a number of sources. We briefly review these approaches, but other sources are available for additional information (see Podlesnik et al., 2017; Wathen & Podlesnik, 2018). It is important to state that these approaches are unlikely to eliminate entirely all relapse, especially in isolation. As combinations of variables contribute to exacerbating relapse, combinations of strategies likely will prove to mitigate relapse more effectively than any in isolation (see also Falcomata & Wacker, 2013).

Incorporating Treatment-Correlated Cues

Increasing generalization between treatment and nontreatment conditions can make treatments more durable and has been an important component of improving the effectiveness of DRA treatments for decades (Stokes & Baer, 1977). One approach examined in laboratory research has been to present discrete stimuli during simulated treatment in

Phase 2 and continue presenting those stimuli during relapse testing in Phase 3. These have variously been referred to as *extinction cues, treatment cues,* and *retrieval cues.*

Originally developed to mitigate renewal in studies of respondent conditioning (e.g., Brooks & Bouton, 1993, 1994), these findings have been extended to operant behavior both in studies of renewal (Gámez & Bernal-Gamboa, 2019; Nieto et al., 2017, 2020) and resurgence (Craig et al., 2018; Shvarts et al., 2020; Trask, 2019). In the studies of renewal, stimuli presented response independently in Context B during simulated treatment in Phase 2 reduce renewal when those stimuli are maintained during testing upon returning to Context A in Phase 3. With some individuals and populations, appropriate instructions might serve this purpose (see Mystkowski et al., 2006, for relevant findings).

In the studies of resurgence, brief stimuli have been paired with delivery of alternative reinforcers during DRA in Phase 2 (Craig et al., 2018; Shvarts et al., 2020; Trask, 2019). Such stimuli might be conceptualized as conditioned reinforcers, but there is some evidence against this interpretation (Shvarts et al., 2020). When removing the alternative reinforcer during testing in Phase 3, maintaining the delivery of the brief stimuli contingent on alternative responses decreases resurgence of target responding relative to removing the brief stimuli as well.

The implication of treatment-related cues as a strategy to mitigate relapse for applied practice is that associating unique stimuli with an intervention could mitigate renewal or resurgence of challenging behavior given that a unique learning history of reinforcement for appropriate behavior is established in the presence of that stimulus. In other words, this strategy is used to establish discriminative control over appropriate and inappropriate behaviors, and reduce the likelihood of relapse whenever discriminative stimuli are present (for examples of this strategy used in practice, see Fisher et al., 2020; Greer et al., 2019).

Conducting Multiple-Context Training

Another procedure directly relevant to enhancing generalization aims to establish treatment effects across a range of contexts (e.g., various clinical and/or community settings) before introducing the treatment into a clinically relevant context (e.g., home, school). Also established originally with respondent behavior (Gunther et al., 1998), laboratory studies with rats and university students have shown that ABA and ABC renewal can be mitigated when extinguishing operant behavior across multiple contexts compared with extinguishing responding in only a single context (Bernal-Gamboa et al., 2017, 2020).

The implication of multiple-context training in applied settings is that one strategy for mitigating relapse due to contextual factors, such as in renewal, is to introduce the treatment successively in multiple contexts prior to the target context. For example, Busch et al. (2018) described using a DRA procedure to reduce the pica of one man with IDDs by first implementing the intervention on a secure hospital unit, then transferring the treatment across subsequent contexts before implementing DRA in the community (e.g., secure hospital unit, lunchroom, hospital grounds, community).

Conducting Separate-Context Training

An approach related to both arranging treatment cues and multiple-context training is born out of research on behavioral momentum theory (Nevin & Grace, 2000). This approach arranges reinforcement of an alternative response in a context separate (when clinically possible) from contexts in which the challenging behavior occurs (see Mace et al., 2010). Once the alternative response is trained, features of the alternative context can be combined with features of the target context. A number of studies with rats, pigeons, and children have demonstrated that target responding within the combined context is less resistant to extinction and less likely to result in resurgence and reinstatement than when target and alternative responding are trained and reinforced within the same context (Craig et al., 2018; Dube et al., 2017; Mace et al., 2010; Podlesnik et al., 2012, 2016, 2017).

The implication of this strategy for practice settings is that it may be beneficial to introduce DRA-based treatments in settings different than the one in which the challenging behavior occurs. For example, it may be therapeutically beneficial to assess and treat behavior disorders in clinical settings (e.g., outpatient or day program) when they occur in typical settings (e.g., school or home). Similar to the strategy of treatment cues, it is likely that establishing discriminative control over appropriate and inappropriate behaviors in different contexts prior to introducing treatment in the target context reduces the likelihood of relapse (e.g., Suess et al., 2020).

Training Multiple Alternative Responses

Some laboratory research suggests that the availability of multiple alternative responses within an individual's repertoire could be effective for mitigating resurgence relative to the availability of only a single alternative response (Diaz-Salvat et al., 2020; Lambert et al., 2015). Lambert et al. arranged arbitrary switch responses for adults diagnosed with developmental disabilities to examine an analogue DRA treatment. They arranged two conditions that alternated successively as a multielement (or alternating-treatments) design. In the control condition, DRA consisted of a single reinforced response with target responding contacting extinction. In the experimental condition, Lambert et al. reinforced and then extinguished three successively available alternative responses. They found the successively trained alternative responses mitigated resurgence relative to the single alternative. However, Diaz-Salvat et al. (2020) replicated and extended these findings with university students and revealed that the effectiveness in mitigating resurgence was likely a result of multiple responses being available rather than successively reinforcing alternative responses per se.

The clinical implication of using this strategy to mitigate relapse is that reinforcing multiple topographies of appropriate behavior during the course of intervention may increase the probability that appropriate behaviors persist when treatment challenges are presented (e.g., error of omission during resurgence). Although this strategy has not yet been conclusively demonstrated in applied settings (Lambert et al., 2017), it may be a method to improve DRA-based interventions when combined with methods that promote behavioral variability (see Falcomata et al., 2018, for a demonstration of how this might be accomplished). Establishing a repertoire of appropriate behavior beyond a single response may also be warranted in clinical contexts given that relapse of multiple topographies of challenging behavior can be common (Sullivan et al., 2020). A larger repertoire of appropriate behavior could increase the possibility that appropriate behaviors emerge (as opposed to challenging responses) when treatments are challenged. Finally, training a larger repertoire of appropriate behavior would contribute to meeting the general treatment goal of increasing communication and independence of clients.

Extending DRA Treatment

One fairly straightforward approach that could potentially increase the long-term effectiveness of DRA treatments is to ensure that individuals are provided with sufficiently extensive exposure to the treatment (see Wacker et al., 2011). Several laboratory studies with rats provide empirical support for this approach (Leitenberg et al., 1975; Shahan et al., 2020) but other studies found no reduction in resurgence with longer DRA treatments (Nall et al., 2018; Trask et al., 2018; Winterbauer et al., 2013). Therefore, some, but not all, evidence suggests that relatively longer exposures to DRA treatment could mitigate relapse upon exposure to treatment challenges, such as omission errors or thinning of alternative reinforcement.

In applied settings, the magnitude of certain relapse effects (e.g., resurgence) could be reduced when the duration of the intervention period is extended. For example, Wacker et al. (2011) found that resurgence occurred at smaller magnitudes when exposure to FCT was extended. It is important to note that Wacker et al. also exposed challenging behavior to relapse probes during the course of extended FCT, which suggests that exposure to relapse challenges could also have a reductive effect on later relapse (see also Shahan et al., 2020). Nonetheless, Greer et al. (2020) suggested that the extent to which this strategy is effective might depend on the level of discriminability between treatment and nontreatment conditions; that is, even during situations in which DRA treatments are extended, the degree to which contextual variables come to establish discriminative control over appropriate and inappropriate behaviors may play an important role in mitigating relapse. Ultimately, it may behoove practitioners to increase the duration for which interventions are in place prior to beginning schedule thinning or transferring to other contexts.

Introducing Punishment

It is well known that punishment contingencies can be effective in decreasing challenging behavior when in place, but a concern is that responding will return when punishment contingencies are removed (i.e., recovery from punishment; Estes, 1944; Lerman & Iwata, 1996). Recent laboratory research on relapse suggests these concerns are warranted, as punished target responses can renew upon changing contexts (e.g., Kuroda et al., 2020; Bouton & Schepers, 2015; Pelloux et al., 2018), be reinstated by reexposure to the functional reinforcer (e.g., Panlilio et al., 2003, 2005), and resurge when removing both alternative-reinforcement and punishment contingencies (e.g., Bolívar & Dallery, 2020; Kestner et al., 2015, 2018; Kuroda et al., 2020). The evidence on whether punishment contingencies present during DRA mitigate resurgence is mixed. Studies with laboratory animals showed that including a punisher during DRA decreased resurgence compared with a typical resurgence procedure arranging no punisher during DRA (Kestner et al., 2015; Kuroda et al., 2020). However, examining the effects of response cost as punishers with point reinforcers with humans revealed no effect of including a punishment contingency on resurgence (Bolívar & Dallery, 2020; Kestner et al., 2018). Moreover, Kuroda et al. (2020) found that including a punisher during extinction of target responding *increased* ABA renewal relative to arranging no punishment during extinction, perhaps by enhancing the difference of Context B relative to Context A (see Todd et al., 2014, for related findings). Overall, there is some indication that punishment contingencies could reduce the likelihood of relapse, but further study of these conditions is needed, especially as they relate to clinical applications of behavioral interventions.

Combining Multiple Approaches

As any medical treatment often takes multiple approaches to be effective, no one mitigation approach is going to be a panacea for relapse of challenging behavior. Furthermore, basic research with respondent conditioning suggests that renewal is more effectively decreased when combining multiple-context training with more extensive exposure to extinction (Laborda & Miller, 2013; Thomas et al., 2009). Therefore, research programs are needed to identify mitigation approaches effective in isolation and combination under laboratory conditions, with translational and applied research identifying best practices for clinical settings. It is important to reiterate that the development of mitigation strategies in structured and systematic laboratory research is the route to conceptually systematic approaches to treatment (Baer et al., 1968; see also Podlesnik et al., 2017).

In practice, clinicians might consider implementing multiple mitigation strategies simultaneously to reduce the overall or global probability of relapse (Podlesnik et al., 2017; Wathen & Podlesnik, 2018). Doing so could simultaneously address several of the environmental events that contribute to relapse, such as omission errors and context changes. Nevertheless, it should be noted that the effectiveness of any of these mitigation strategies will interact with the historical and current conditions contributing to challenging behavior. For example, more extensive reinforcement histories will likely enhance the probability that challenging behavior will relapse. The implication for practice is that clinicians should minimize exposure to baseline contingencies whenever possible while increasing dosage and methods of intervention (Fisher et al., 2018, 2019).

Conclusion

The relapse of challenging behavior poses a serious challenge to the longevity of behavioral interventions, as evidenced by recent research demonstrating the prevalence of relapse across a variety of contexts, populations, and interventions (Briggs et al., 2018; Falligant et al., 2021; Muething et al., 2020, 2021; Radhakrishnan et al., 2020; Saini & Mitteer, 2020). Determining the variables responsible for relapse in clinical contexts can be labor-intensive, unethical, and in some cases even impossible. Fortunately, laboratory models of relapse do not as readily suffer from these problems. Compared with clinical research, laboratory models have the advantage of establishing greater control over both environmental variables present during experimentation and subject ontogeny and phylogeny when employing nonhuman laboratory animals. These methods can be used to arrange specific conditions to measure behavioral patterns respectively analogous to human health behaviors. These models can then serve as the foundation from which basic principles and processes upon which relapse in applied contexts can be understood.

The robust literature base on relapse and maintenance of behavioral interventions suggests that understanding how to promote durable treatment effects is best achieved through a bidirectional process in which applied technology is enhanced by advances in basic research and experimental studies can be leveraged to investigate the mechanisms involved in complex clinical problems (Dube, 2013; Mace & Critchfield, 2010). Although we introduced the most basic models of relapse in accordance with this bidirectional process, a number of additional variables not discussed herein can influence the size and pattern of the effects described (see Wathen & Podlesnik, 2018, for a description of these and other variables). Furthermore, healthy debate exists over the learning and behavioral processes underlying relapse effects, and these accounts may further illuminate the variables and functional relations related to treatment maintenance (for conceptual and theoretical accounts of relapse, see Bouton, 2019; Greer & Shahan, 2019; Nevin et al., 2017).

Although clinical translations of relapse effects are still in their infancy, and the models of relapse described herein require replications and extension to a broader array of behavioral health problems and treatment contexts, it is clear that experimental analysis of behavior and applied behavior analysis are intimately interconnected. We affirm that the relapse of challenging behavior is best understood within a unified field of behavior analysis that bridges basic and applied investigations of behavior through translational research.

REFERENCES

Acosta, J. I., Thiel, K. J., Sanabria, F., Browning, J. R., & Neisewander, J. L. (2008). Effect of schedule of reinforcement on cue-elicited reinstatement of cocaine-seeking behavior. *Behavioural Pharmacology, 19*, 129–136.

Baer, D. M., Wolf, M. M., & Risley, T. R. (1968). Some current dimensions of applied behavior analysis. *Journal of Applied Behavior Analysis, 1*(1), 91–97.

Baker, D., Tran-Nguyen, L., Fuchs, R., & Neisewander, J. L. (2001). Influence of individual differences and chronic fluoxetine treatment on cocaine-seeking behavior in rats. *Psychopharmacology, 155*, 18–26.

Beavers, G. A., & Iwata, B. A. (2011). Prevalence of multiply controlled problem behavior. *Journal of Applied Behavior Analysis, 44*(3), 593–597.

Bernal-Gamboa, R., Nieto, J., & Gámez, A. M. (2020). Conducting extinction in multiple contexts attenuates relapse of operant behavior in humans. *Behavioural Processes, 181*, Article 104261.

Bernal-Gamboa, R., Nieto, J., & Uengoer, M. (2017). Effects of extinction in multiple contexts on renewal of instrumental responses. *Behavioural Processes, 142*, 64–69.

Bodnar, H., Denyko, B., Waenke, P., & Ball, K. T. (2020). Vulnerability to diet-induced obesity is associated with greater food priming-induced reinstatement of palatable food seeking. *Physiology and Behavior, 213*, Article 112730.

Bolívar, H. A., & Dallery, J. (2020). Effects of response cost magnitude on resurgence of human operant behavior. *Behavioural Processes, 178*, Article 104187.

Bouton, M. E. (2019). Extinction of instrumental (operant) learning: Interference, varieties of context, and mechanisms of contextual control. *Psychopharmacology, 236*, 7–19.

Bouton, M. E., Kenney, F. A., & Rosengard, C. (1990). State-dependent fear extinction with two benzodiazepine tranquilizers. *Behavioral Neuroscience, 104*, 44–55.

Bouton, M. E., Maren, S., & McNally, G. P. (2021). Behavioral and neurobiological mechanisms of Pavlovian and instrumental extinction learning. *Physiological Reviews, 101*(2), 611–681.

Bouton, M. E., & Schepers, S. T. (2015). Renewal after the punishment of free operant behavior. *Journal of Experimental Psychology: Animal Learning and Cognition, 41*, 81–90.

Bouton, M. E., Thrailkill, E. A., Bergeria, C. L., & Davis, D. R. (2017). Preventing relapse after incentivized choice treatment: A laboratory model. *Behavioural Processes, 141*, 11–18.

Bouton, M. E., & Todd, T. P. (2014). A fundamental role for context in instrumental learning and extinction. *Behavioural Processes, 104*, 13–19.

Bouton, M. E., Todd, T. P., Vurbic, D., & Winterbauer, N. E. (2011). Renewal after the extinction of free operant behavior. *Learning and Behavior, 39*, 57–67.

Bouton, M. E., Winterbauer, N. E., & Todd, T. P. (2012). Relapse processes after the extinction of instrumental learning: Renewal, resurgence, and reacquisition. *Behavioural Processes, 90*, 130–141.

Brand, D., Henley, A. J., Reed, F. D. D., Gray, E., & Crabbs, B. (2019). A review of published studies involving parametric manipulations of treatment integrity. *Journal of Behavioral Education, 28*(1), 1–26.

Briggs, A. M., Fisher, W. W., Greer, B. D., & Kimball, R. T. (2018). Prevalence of resurgence of destructive behavior when thinning reinforcement schedules during functional communication training. *Journal of Applied Behavior Analysis, 51*(3), 620–633.

Brimer, C. J. (1970). Disinhibition of an operant response. *Learning and Motivation, 1,* 346–371.

Brooks, D. C., & Bouton, M. E. (1993). A retrieval cue for extinction attenuates spontaneous recovery. *Journal of Experimental Psychology: Animal Behavior Processes, 19,* 77–89.

Brooks, D. C., & Bouton, M. E. (1994). A retrieval cue for extinction attenuates response recovery (renewal) caused by a return to the conditioning context. *Journal of Experimental Psychology: Animal Behavior Processes, 20,* 366–379.

Brown, K. R., Greer, B. D., Craig, A. R., Sullivan, W. E., Fisher, W. W., & Roane, H. S. (2020). Resurgence following differential reinforcement of alternative behavior implemented with and without extinction. *Journal of the Experimental Analysis of Behavior, 113*(2), 449–467.

Browning, K. O., & Shahan, T. A. (2018). Renewal of extinguished operant behavior following changes in social context. *Journal of the Experimental Analysis of Behavior, 110,* 430–439.

Burokas, A., Martín-García, E., Espinosa-Carrasco, J., Erb, I., McDonald, J., Notredame, C., . . . Maldonado, R. (2018). Extinction and reinstatement of an operant responding maintained by food in different models of obesity. *Addiction Biology, 23*(2), 544–555.

Busch, L. P. A., Saini, V., Zorzos, C., & Duyile, L. (2018). Treatment of life-threatening pica with 5-year follow-up. *Advances in Neurodevelopmental Disorders, 2,* 335–343.

Cohenour, J. M., Volkert, V. M., & Allen, K. D. (2018). An experimental demonstration of AAB renewal in children with autism spectrum disorder. *Journal of the Experimental Analysis of Behavior, 110,* 63–73.

Colwill, R. M. (1994). Associative representations of instrumental contingencies. In D. L. Medin (Ed.), *The psychology of learning and motivation* (Vol. 31, pp. 1–72). Academic Press.

Cox, D. J., Bolívar, H. A., & Barlow, M. A. (2019). Multiple control responses and resurgence of human behavior. *Behavioural Processes, 159,* 93–99.

Craig, A. R., Cunningham, P. J., Sweeney, M. M., Shahan, T. A., & Nevin, J. A. (2018). Delivering alternative reinforcement in a distinct context reduces its counter-therapeutic effects on relapse. *Journal of the Experimental Analysis of Behavior, 109,* 492–505.

Critchfield, T. S., & Reed, D. D. (2009). What are we doing when we translate from quantitative models? *Behavior Analyst, 32*(2), 339–362.

DeJong, W. (1994). Relapse prevention: An emerging technology for promoting long-term drug abstinence. *International Journal of the Addictions, 29*(6), 681–705.

Delamater, A. R., LoLordo, V. M., & Sosa, W. (2003). Outcome-specific conditioned inhibition in Pavlovian backward conditioning. *Learning and Behavior, 31,* 393–402.

DeLeon, I., Williams, D. C., Gregory, M. K., & Hagopian, L. (2005). Unexamined potential effects of the noncontingent delivery of reinforcers. *European Journal of Behavior Analysis, 6,* 57–69.

Diaz-Salvat, C. C., St. Peter, C., & Shuler, N. J. (2020). Increased number of responses may account for reduced resurgence following serial training. *Journal of Applied Behavior Analysis, 53,* 1552–1558.

Doughty, A. H., Reed, P., & Lattal, K. A. (2004). Differential reinstatement predicted by preextinction response rate. *Psychonomic Bulletin and Review, 11,* 1118–1123.

Dube, W. V. (2013). Translational research in behavior analysis. In G. J. Madden (Ed.) & W. V. Dube, T. D. Hackenberg, G. P. Hanley, & K. A. Lattal (Assoc. Eds.), *APA handbook of behavior analysis: Vol. 1. Methods and principles* (pp. 65–78). American Psychological Association.

Dube, W. V., Thompson, B., Silveira, M. V., & Nevin, J. A. (2017). The role of contingencies and stimuli in a human laboratory model of treatment of problem behavior. *Psychological Record, 67,* 463–471.

Durand, V. M., & Carr, E. G. (1991). Functional communication training to reduce challenging behavior: Maintenance and application in new settings. *Journal of Applied Behavior Analysis, 24,* 251–264.

Estes, W. K. (1944). An experimental study of punishment. *Psychological Monographs, 57,* i–40.

Falcomata, T. S., Hoffman, K. J., Gainey, S., Muething, C. S., & Fienup, D. M. (2013). A preliminary evaluation of reinstatement of destructive behavior displayed by individuals with autism. *Psychological Record, 63*, 453–466.

Falcomata, T. S., Muething, C. S., Silbaugh, B. C., Adami, S., Hoffman, K., Shpall, C., & Ringdahl, J. E. (2018). Lag schedules and functional communication training: Persistence of mands and relapse of problem behavior. *Behavior Modification, 42*(3), 314–334.

Falcomata, T. S., & Wacker, D. P. (2013). On the use of strategies for programming generalization during functional communication training: A review of the literature. *Journal of Developmental and Physical Disabilities, 25*, 5–15.

Falligant, J. M., Kranak, M. P., McNulty, M. K., Schmidt, J. D., Hausman, N. L., & Rooker, G. W. (2021). Prevalence of renewal of problem behavior: Replication and extension to an inpatient setting. *Journal of Applied Behavior Analysis, 54*, 367–373.

Fisher, W. W., Fuhrman, A. M., Greer, B. D., Mitteer, D. R., & Piazza, C. C. (2020). Mitigating resurgence of destructive behavior using the discriminative stimuli of a multiple schedule. *Journal of the Experimental Analysis of Behavior, 113*(1), 263–277.

Fisher, W. W., Greer, B. D., Fuhrman, A. M., Saini, V., & Simmons, C. A. (2018). Minimizing resurgence of destructive behavior using behavioral momentum theory. *Journal of Applied Behavior Analysis, 51*(4), 831–853.

Fisher, W. W., Saini, V., Greer, B. D., Sullivan, W. E., Roane, H. S., Fuhrman, A. M., . . . Kimball, R. T. (2019). Baseline reinforcement rate and resurgence of destructive behavior. *Journal of the Experimental Analysis of Behavior, 111*(1), 75–93.

Floresco, S. B., McLaughlin, R. J., & Haluk, D. M. (2008). Opposing roles for the nucleus accumbens core and shell in cue-induced reinstatement of food-seeking behavior. *Neuroscience, 154*(3), 877–884.

Franks, G. J., & Lattal, K. A. (1976). Antecedent reinforcement schedule training and operant response reinstatement in rats. *Animal Learning and Behavior, 4*, 374–378.

Gámez, A. M., & Bernal-Gamboa, R. (2019). The reoccurrence of voluntary behavior in humans is reduced by retrieval cues from extinction. *Acta Psychologica, 200*, Article 102945.

Garner, J., Neef, N. A., & Gardner, R. (2018). Recurrence of phonetic responding. *Journal of Applied Behavior Analysis, 51*(3), 596–602.

Ghaemmaghami, M., Hanley, G. P., & Jessel, J. (2021). Functional communication training: From efficacy to effectiveness. *Journal of Applied Behavior Analysis, 54*(1), 122–143.

Gomez-Rubalcava, S., Stabbert, K., & Phelan, S. (2018). Behavioral treatment of obesity. In T. A. Wadden & G. A. Bray (Eds.), *Handbook of obesity treatment* (2nd ed., pp. 336–348). Guilford Press.

Greer, B. D., Fisher, W. W., Briggs, A. M., Lichtblau, K. R., Phillips, L. A., & Mitteer, D. R. (2019). Using schedule-correlated stimuli during functional communication training to promote the rapid transfer of treatment effects. *Behavioral Development, 24*(2), 100–119.

Greer, B. D., Fisher, W. W., Retzlaff, B. J., & Fuhrman, A. M. (2020). A preliminary evaluation of treatment duration on the resurgence of destructive behavior. *Journal of the Experimental Analysis of Behavior, 113*, 251–262.

Greer, B. D., & Shahan, T. A. (2019). Resurgence as choice: Implications for promoting durable behavior change. *Journal of Applied Behavior Analysis, 52*, 816–846.

Gunther, L. M., Denniston, J. C., & Miller, R. R. (1998). Conducting exposure treatment in multiple contexts can prevent relapse. *Behaviour Research and Therapy, 36*, 75–91.

Ho, T., Bai, J. Y. H., Keevy, M., & Podlesnik, C. A. (2018). Resurgence when challenging alternative behavior with progressive ratios in children and pigeons. *Journal of the Experimental Analysis of Behavior, 110*, 474–499.

Ibañez, V. F., Piazza, C. C., & Peterson, K. M. (2019). A translational evaluation of renewal of inappropriate mealtime behavior. *Journal of Applied Behavior Analysis, 52*(4), 1005–1020.

Kelley, M. E., Jimenez-Gomez, C., Podlesnik, C. A., & Morgan, A. (2018). Evaluation of renewal mitigation of negatively reinforced socially significant operant behavior. *Learning and Motivation, 63*, 133–141.

Kestner, K. M., & Peterson, S. M. (2017). A review of resurgence literature with human participants. *Behavior Analysis: Research and Practice, 17*(1), 1–17.

Kestner, K., Redner, R., Watkins, E. E., & Poling, A. (2015). The effects of punishment on resurgence in laboratory rats. *Psychological Record, 65*, 315–321.

Kestner, K. M., Romano, L. M., St. Peter, C. C., & Mesches, G. A. (2018). Resurgence following response cost in a human-operant procedure. *Psychological Record, 68*, 81–87.

Kincaid, S. L., Lattal, K. A., & Spence, J. (2015). Super-resurgence: ABA renewal increases resurgence. *Behavioural Processes, 115*, 70–73.

Kuroda, T., Gilroy, S. P., Cançado, C. R. X., & Podlesnik, C. A. (2020). Effects of punishing target response during extinction on resurgence and renewal in zebrafish (Danio rerio). *Behavioural Processes, 178*, Article 104191.

Laborda, M. A., & Miller, R. R. (2013). Preventing return of fear in an animal model of anxiety: Additive effects of massive extinction and extinction in multiple contexts. *Behavior Therapy, 44*, 249–261.

Lambert, J. M., Bloom, S. E., Samaha, A. L., & Dayton, E. (2017). Serial functional communication training: Extending serial DRA to mands and problem behavior. *Behavioral Interventions, 32*, 311–325.

Lambert, J. M., Bloom, S. E., Samaha, A. L., Dayton, E., & Rodewald, A. M. (2015). Serial alternative response training as intervention for target response resurgence. *Journal of Applied Behavior Analysis, 48*, 765–780.

Lattal, K. A., Cançado, C. R. X., Cook, J. E., Kincaid, S. L., Nighbor, T. D., & Oliver, A. C. (2017). On defining resurgence. *Behavioural Processes, 141*, 85–91.

Lattal, K. A., & Oliver, A. C. (2020). The control response in assessing resurgence: Useful or compromised tool? *Journal of the Experimental Analysis of Behavior, 113*(1), 77–86.

Ledgerwood, D. M., & Petry, N. M. (2006). What do we know about relapse in pathological gambling? *Clinical Psychology Review, 26*(2), 216–228.

Leitenberg, H., Rawson, R. A., & Mulick, J. A. (1975). Extinction and reinforcement of alternative behavior. *Journal of Comparative and Physiological Psychology, 88*(2), 640–652.

Leri, F., & Stewart, J. (2001). Drug-induced reinstatement to heroin and cocaine seeking: A rodent model of relapse in polydrug use. *Experimental and Clinical Psychopharmacology, 9*, 297–306.

Lerman, D. C., & Iwata, B. A. (1996). Developing a technology for the use of operant extinction in clinical settings: An examination of basic and applied research. *Journal of Applied Behavior Analysis, 29*, 345–382.

Liggett, A. P., Nastri, R., & Podlesnik, C. A. (2018). Assessing the combined effects of resurgence and reinstatement in children diagnosed with autism spectrum disorder. *Journal of the Experimental Analysis of Behavior, 109*(2), 408–421.

Mace, F. C., & Critchfield, T. S. (2010). Translational research in behavior analysis: Historical traditions and imperative for the future. *Journal of the Experimental Analysis of Behavior, 93*(3), 293–312.

Mace, F. C., McComas, J. J., Mauro, B. C., Progar, P. R., Taylor, B., Ervin, R., & Zangrillo, A. N. (2010). Differential reinforcement of alternative behavior increases resistance to extinction: Clinical demonstration, animal modeling, and clinical test of one solution. *Journal of the Experimental Analysis of Behavior, 93*, 349–367.

Mace, F. C., & Nevin, J. A. (2017). Maintenance, generalization, and treatment relapse: A behavioral momentum analysis. *Education and Treatment of Children, 40*(1), 27–42.

Mantsch, J. R., Baker, D. A., Funk, D., Lê, A. D., & Shaham, Y. (2016). Stress-induced reinstatement of drug seeking: 20 years of progress. *Neuropsychopharmacology, 41*(1), 335–356.

Marsteller, T. M., & Peter, C. C. S. (2012). Resurgence during treatment challenges. *Mexican Journal of Behavior Analysis, 38*(1), 7–23.

Miranda-Dukoski, L., Bensemann, J., & Podlesnik, C. A. (2016). Training reinforcement rates, resistance to extinction, and the role of context in reinstatement. *Learning and Behavior, 44*, 29–48.

Mitteer, D. R., Greer, B. D., Fisher, W. W., Briggs, A. M., & Wacker, D. P. (2018). A laboratory model for evaluating relapse of undesirable caregiver behavior. *Journal of the Experimental Analysis of Behavior, 110*, 252–266.

Muething, C., Call, N., Pavlov, A., Ringdahl, J., Gillespie, S., Clark, S., & Mevers, J. L. (2020). Prevalence of renewal of problem behavior during context changes. *Journal of Applied Behavior Analysis, 53*(3), 1485–1493.

Muething, C., Pavlov, A., Call, N., Ringdahl, J., & Gillespie, S. (2021). Prevalence of resurgence during thinning of multiple schedules of reinforcement following functional communication training. *Journal of Applied Behavior Analysis, 54*, 813–823.

Mystkowski, J. L., Craske, M. G., Echiverri, A. M., & Labus, J. S. (2006). Mental reinstatement of context and return of fear in spider-fearful participants. *Behavior Therapy, 37*, 49–60.

Nakajima, S., Tanaka, S., Urushihara, K., & Imada, H. (2000). Renewal of extinguished lever-press responses upon return to the training context. *Learning and Motivation, 31,* 416–431.

Nakajima, S., Urushihara, K., & Masaki, T. (2002). Renewal of operant performance formerly eliminated by omission or noncontingency training upon return to the acquisition context. *Learning and Motivation, 33,* 510–525.

Nall, R. W., Craig, A. R., Browning, K. O., & Shahan, T. A. (2018). Longer treatment with alternative non-drug reinforcement fails to reduce resurgence of cocaine or alcohol seeking in rats. *Behavioural Brain Research, 341,* 54–62.

Neely, L., Garcia, E., Bankston, B., & Green, A. (2018). Generalization and maintenance of functional communication training for individuals with developmental disabilities: A systematic and quality review. *Research in Developmental Disabilities, 79,* 116–129.

Nevin, J. A., Craig, A. R., Cunningham, P. J., Podlesnik, C. A., Shahan, T. A., & Sweeney, M. M. (2017). Quantitative models of persistence and relapse from the perspective of behavioral momentum theory: Fits and misfits. *Behavioural Processes, 141,* 92–99.

Nevin, J. A., & Grace, R. C. (2000). Behavioral momentum and the Law of Effect. *Behavioral and Brain Sciences, 23,* 73–130.

Nevin, J. A., & Wacker, D. P. (2013). Response strength and persistence. In G. J. Madden, W. V. Dube, T. D. Hackenberg, G. P. Hanley, & K. A. Lattal (Eds.), *APA handbook of behavior analysis: Vol. 2. Translating principles into practice* (pp. 109–128). American Psychological Association.

Nieto, J., Mason, T. A., Bernal-Gamboa, R., & Uengoer, M. (2020). The impacts of acquisition and extinction cues on ABC renewal of voluntary behaviors. *Learning and Memory, 27,* 114–118.

Nieto, J., Uengoer, M., & Bernal-Gamboa, R. (2017). A reminder of extinction reduces relapse in an animal model of voluntary behavior. *Learning and Memory, 24,* 76–80.

Nighbor, T. D., Kincaid, S. L., O'Hearn, C. M., & Lattal, K. A. (2018). Stimulus contributions to operant resurgence. *Journal of the Experimental Analysis of Behavior, 110,* 243–251.

Oliver, A. C., Nighbor, T. D., & Lattal, K. A. (2018). Reinforcer magnitude and resurgence. *Journal of the Experimental Analysis of Behavior, 110,* 440–450.

Ostlund, S. B., & Balleine, B. W. (2007). Selective reinstatement of instrumental performance depends on the discriminative stimulus properties of the mediating outcome. *Learning and Behavior, 35,* 43–52.

Panlilio, L. V., Thorndike, E. B., & Schindler, C. W. (2003). Reinstatement of punishment-suppressed opioid self-administration in rats: An alternative model of relapse to drug abuse. *Psychopharmacology, 168,* 229–235.

Panlilio, L. V., Thorndike, E. B., & Schindler, C. W. (2005). Lorazepam reinstates punishment-suppressed remifentanil self-administration in rats. *Psychopharmacology, 179,* 374–382.

Pelloux, Y., Hoots, J. K., Cifani, C., Adhikary, S., Martin, J., Minier-Toribio, A., . . . Shaham, Y. (2018). Context-induced relapse to cocaine seeking after punishment-imposed abstinence is associated with activation of cortical and subcortical brain regions. *Addiction Biology, 23,* 699–712.

Petscher, E. S., Rey, C., & Bailey, J. S. (2009). A review of empirical support for differential reinforcement of alternative behavior. *Research in Developmental Disabilities, 30*(3), 409–425.

Podlesnik, C. A., Bai, J. Y., & Elliffe, D. (2012). Resistance to extinction and relapse in combined stimulus contexts. *Journal of the Experimental Analysis of Behavior, 98,* 169–189.

Podlesnik, C. A., Bai, J. Y. H., & Skinner, K. A. (2016). Assessing the role of alternative response rates and reinforcer rates in resistance to extinction of target responding when combining stimuli. *Journal of the Experimental Analysis of Behavior, 105,* 427–444.

Podlesnik, C. A., & Kelley, M. E. (2015). Translational research on the relapse of operant behavior. *Mexican Journal of Behavior Analysis, 41*(2), 226–251.

Podlesnik, C. A., & Kelley, M. E. (2017). Beyond intervention: Shaping policy for addressing persistence and relapse of severe problem behavior. *Policy Insights from the Behavioral and Brain Sciences, 4,* 17–24.

Podlesnik, C. A., Kelley, M. E., Jimenez-Gomez, C., & Bouton, M. E. (2017). Renewed behavior produced by context change and its implications for treatment maintenance: A review. *Journal of Applied Behavior Analysis, 50*(3), 675–697.

Podlesnik, C. A., Kuroda, T., Jimenez-Gomez, C., Abreu-Rodrigues, J., Cançado, C., Blackman, A. L., . . . Teixeira, I. (2019). Resurgence is greater following a return to the training context than remaining in the extinction context. *Journal of the Experimental Analysis of Behavior, 111*, 416–435.

Podlesnik, C. A., & Shahan, T. A. (2009). Behavioral momentum and relapse of extinguished operant responding. *Learning and Behavior, 37*(4), 357–364.

Podlesnik, C. A., & Shahan, T. A. (2010). Extinction, relapse, and behavioral momentum. *Behavioural Processes, 84*, 400–411.

Pritchard, D., Hoerger, M., & Mace, F. C. (2014). Treatment relapse and behavioral momentum theory. *Journal of Applied Behavior Analysis, 47*(4), 814–833.

Pritchard, D., Hoerger, M., Mace, F. C., Penney, H., Harris, B., & Eiri, L. (2016). Clinical translation of the ABA renewal model of treatment relapse. *European Journal of Behavior Analysis, 17*(2), 182–191.

Radhakrishnan, S., Gerow, S., & Weston, R. (2020). Resurgence of challenging behavior following functional communication training for children with disabilities: A literature review. *Journal of Developmental and Physical Disabilities, 32*(2), 213–239.

Rescorla, R. A., & Skucy, J. C. (1969). Effect of response-independent reinforcers during extinction. *Journal of Comparative and Physiological Psychology, 67*, 381–389.

Rey, C. N., Thrailkill, E. A., Goldberg, K. L., & Bouton, M. E. (2020). Relapse of operant behavior after response elimination with an extinction or an omission contingency. *Journal of the Experimental Analysis of Behavior, 113*, 124–140.

Ringdahl, J. E., & St. Peter, C. (2017). Resurgence: The unintended maintenance of problem behavior. *Education and Treatment of Children, 40*(1), 7–26.

Saini, V., & Mitteer, D. R. (2020). A review of investigations of operant renewal with human participants: Implications for theory and practice. *Journal of the Experimental Analysis of Behavior, 113*(1), 105–123.

Saini, V., Sullivan, W. E., Baxter, E. L., DeRosa, N. M., & Roane, H. S. (2018). Renewal during functional communication training. *Journal of Applied Behavior Analysis, 51*(3), 603–619.

Schepers, S. T., & Bouton, M. E. (2015). Effects of reinforcer distribution during response elimination on resurgence of an instrumental behavior. *Journal of Experimental Psychology: Animal Learning and Cognition, 41*, 179–192.

Schepers, S. T., & Bouton, M. E. (2017). Hunger as a context: Food seeking that is inhibited during hunger can renew in the context of satiety. *Psychological Science, 28*, 1640–1648.

Schepers, S. T., & Bouton, M. E. (2019). Stress as a context: Stress causes relapse of inhibited food seeking if it has been associated with prior food seeking. *Appetite, 132*, 131–138.

Shaham, Y., Shalev, U., Lu, L., De Wit, H., & Stewart, J. (2003). The reinstatement model of drug relapse: History, methodology and major findings. *Psychopharmacology, 168*(1–2), 3–20.

Shahan, T. A., Browning, K. O., & Nall, R. W. (2020). Resurgence as choice in context: Treatment duration and on/off alternative reinforcement *Journal of the Experimental Analysis of Behavior, 113*, 57–76.

Shahan, T. A., & Craig, A. R. (2017). Resurgence as choice. *Behavioural Processes, 141*, 100–127.

Shvarts, S., Jimenez-Gomez, C., Bai, J. Y., Thomas, R. R., Oskam, J. J., & Podlesnik, C. A. (2020). Examining stimuli paired with alternative reinforcement to mitigate resurgence in children diagnosed with autism spectrum disorder and pigeons. *Journal of the Experimental Analysis of Behavior, 113*(1), 214–231.

Skinner, B. F. (1948). "Superstition" in the pigeon. *Journal of Experimental Psychology, 38*, 168–172.

Smith, B. M., Smith, G. S., & Dymond, S. (2020). Relapse of anxiety-related fear and avoidance: Conceptual analysis of treatment with acceptance and commitment therapy. *Journal of the Experimental Analysis of Behavior, 113*(1), 87–104.

St. Peter, C. C. (2015). Six reasons why applied behavior analysts should know about resurgence. *Mexican Journal of Behavior Analysis, 41*, 252–268.

St. Peter Pipkin, C. C., Vollmer, T. R., & Sloman, K. N. (2010). Effects of treatment integrity failures during differential reinforcement of alternative behavior: A translational model. *Journal of Applied Behavior Analysis, 43*(1), 47–70.

Stokes, T. F., & Baer, D. M. (1977). An implicit technology of generalization. *Journal of Applied Behavior Analysis, 10*, 349–367.

Suess, A. N., Schieltz, K. M., Wacker, D. P., Detrick, J., & Podlesnik, C. A. (2020). An evaluation of resurgence following functional communication training conducted in alternative antecedent contexts via telehealth. *Journal of the Experimental Analysis of Behavior, 113*(1), 278–301.

Sullivan, W. E., Saini, V., DeRosa, N. M., Craig, A. R., Ringdahl, J. E., & Roane, H. S. (2020). Measurement of nontargeted problem behavior during investigations of resurgence. *Journal of Applied Behavior Analysis, 53*, 249–264.

Sweeney, M. M., & Shahan, T. A. (2013). Effects of high, low, and thinning rates of alternative reinforcement on response elimination and resurgence. *Journal of the Experimental Analysis of Behavior, 100*, 102–116.

Thomas, B. L., Vurbic, D., & Novak, C. (2009). Extensive extinction in multiple contexts eliminates the renewal of conditioned fear in rats. *Learning and Motivation, 40*, 147–159.

Todd, T. P., Vurbic, D., & Bouton, M. E. (2014). Mechanisms of renewal after the extinction of discriminated operant behavior. *Journal of Experimental Psychology: Animal Learning and Cognition, 40*, 355–368.

Trask, S. (2019). Cues associated with alternative reinforcement during extinction can attenuate resurgence of an extinguished instrumental response. *Learning and Behavior, 47*, 66–79.

Trask, S., & Bouton, M. E. (2016). Discriminative properties of the reinforcer can be used to attenuate the renewal of extinguished operant behavior. *Learning and Behavior, 44*, 151–161.

Trask, S., Keim, C. L., & Bouton, M. E. (2018). Factors that encourage generalization from extinction to test reduce resurgence of an extinguished operant response. *Journal of the Experimental Analysis of Behavior, 110*, 11–23.

Volkert, V. M., Lerman, D. C., Call, N. A., & Trosclair-Lasserre, N. (2009). An evaluation of resurgence during treatment with functional communication training. *Journal of Applied Behavior Analysis, 42*(1), 145–160.

Vollmer, T. R., Peters, K. P., Kronfli, F. R., Lloveras, L. A., & Ibañez, V. F. (2020). On the definition of differential reinforcement of alternative behavior. *Journal of Applied Behavior Analysis, 53*(3), 1299–1303.

Vuchinich, R. E., & Tucker, J. A. (1996). Alcoholic relapse, life events, and behavioral theories of choice: A prospective analysis. *Experimental and Clinical Psychopharmacology, 4*(1), 19–28.

Wacker, D. P., Harding, J. W., Berg, W. K., Lee, J. F., Schieltz, K. M., Padilla, Y. C., . . . Shahan, T. A. (2011). An evaluation of persistence of treatment effects during long-term treatment of destructive behavior. *Journal of the Experimental Analysis of Behavior, 96*(2), 261–282.

Wathen, S. N., & Podlesnik, C. A. (2018). Laboratory models of treatment relapse and mitigation techniques. *Behavior Analysis: Research and Practice, 18*(4), 362–387.

Willcocks, A. L., & McNally, G. P. (2011). The role of context in re-acquisition of extinguished alcoholic beer-seeking. *Behavioral Neuroscience, 125*, 541–550.

Williams, C. L., & St. Peter, C. C. (2020). Resurgence of previously taught academic responses. *Journal of the Experimental Analysis of Behavior, 113*(1), 232–250.

Winterbauer, N. E., & Bouton, M. E. (2012). Effects of thinning the rate at which the alternative behavior is reinforced on resurgence of an extinguished instrumental response. *Journal of Experimental Psychology: Animal Behavior Processes, 38*, 279–291.

Winterbauer, N. E., Lucke, S., & Bouton, M. E. (2013). Some factors modulating the strength of resurgence after extinction of an instrumental behavior. *Learning and Motivation, 44*, 60–71.

CHAPTER 20

Operant Variability

Terry S. Falcomata
Allen Neuringer

The variability of operant behavior is directly affected by reinforcement contingencies. Research shows that when reinforcement is contingent on high (or low) variability, then high (or low) variability is generated and maintained (e.g., Arantes et al., 2012; Doughty & Lattal, 2001; Page & Neuringer, 1985). The study of the *operant nature of variability*, or *operant variability*, as well as potential applications to clinically relevant populations and socially important behaviors, has been a focus of researchers in the experimental analysis of behavior (EAB) and applied behavior analysis (ABA). In this chapter, we discuss (1) basic research on operant variability and (2) applied research focusing on clinical applications, with a particular focus on autism spectrum disorder (ASD). The operant nature of variability has robust support in both the basic and applied literatures. Furthermore, procedures based on the reinforcement of variability can assist in the promotion of positive behavior change, across a variety of skills and behaviors of excess, in individuals with ASD diagnoses.

Basic/EAB Research on Operant Variability

Variability Is an Operant Dimension

Page and Neuringer (1985) asked, "Is response variability controlled by contingent reinforcers, as are other behavioral dimensions, such as response rate, location, duration, force, and topography?" (p. 429). Earlier studies had reported inconsistent results. Several indicated that highly variable responding was maintained by reinforcers contingent upon it (e.g., Blough, 1966; Bryant & Church, 1974; Pryor et al., 1969), but others (i.e., Schwartz, 1980, 1982) reported failures to reinforce variability. Subsequently, Page and Neuringer (1985) performed a series of six experiments in which pigeons were reinforced for pecking two keys under lag schedules similar to Schwartz (1980) with one exception. In Page and Neuringer (1985), a sequence of eight L(efts) and R(ights) responses constituted a "trial," and reinforcement depended on the current L and R pattern differing from the just-prior trial (Lag 1), or, under different conditions, each of the previous five trials (Lag 5). Schwartz (1980, 1982), too, employed lag schedules but with an additional constraint. Under Schwartz's Lag 1, reinforcement was provided if the current sequence differed from the just prior sequence *and if the trial contained exactly four L's and four R's*. Page and Neuringer (1985; Experiments 1 and 2) showed that the four L and four R constraint was responsible for Schwartz's failure to reinforce variability. Subsequently (i.e., Experiment 3), Page and Neuringer found that response variability increased as the schedule demands became more stringent. For example, under Lag 50, more than two-thirds of the birds' sequences differed from each of the preceding 50 sequences. Page and Neuringer went on to show (Experiment 5) that variability was, in fact, controlled by reinforcement and was not a respondent (or induced) effect. To do so, responding during a Lag-50 schedule was compared to responding under a schedule that was yoked to the Lag 50 (i.e., pigeons were provided with the same frequencies of reinforcement that had occurred during previous Lag-50 sessions but independently of variability). The results confirmed that variability was controlled by the Lag-50 reinforcement contingencies (i.e., variability was significantly higher during the lag condition than under the yoked schedule). Last, Page and Neuringer (Experiment 6; see also Denney & Neuringer, 1998) demonstrated stimulus control: Pigeons exhibited high variability in the presence of one discriminative stimulus (i.e., red lights) and repeated a single sequence in the presence of a different stimulus (i.e., blue lights). Taken together, the results demonstrated the operant nature of variability by (1) clarifying inconsistencies in previous studies (i.e., Schwartz (1980, 1982a); (2) showing that variability was maintained at high levels under schedule arrangements that based reinforcement on those levels; (3) demonstrating that variable responding increased as the schedule requirements of the lag increased; (4) showing that the variability depended on its reinforcement rather than being an elicited or respondent effect; and (5) showing that discriminative stimuli controlled the variable responding.

The Page and Neuringer (1985) procedures have been replicated and the results confirmed in numerous subsequent studies, both basic and applied. More specifically, the three defining characteristics of operant behavior are demonstrated when variability is reinforced: (1) sensitivity of variability to contingencies of reinforcement, (2) allocation (choice) of levels of variability as a function of the relative values of available reinforcers (Neuringer, 1992), and (3) control by discriminative stimuli. Furthermore, the operant nature of variability has been demonstrated across a variety of procedures including *recency-based methods, frequency-based methods*, and *statistical feedback methods,* with consistent and robust results (for reviews of the literature, see Neuringer, 2002, 2004; Neuringer & Jensen, 2012; Silbaugh, Murray, et al., 2020; for additional discussion of methods, see Neuringer & Jensen, 2013; and for alternative views, see Barba, 2012; Nergaard & Holth, 2020). Below, we describe some of these methods and studies that have utilized them.

Recency-Based Methods

The lag schedule used by Page and Neuringer (1985) provides an example of a *recency-based schedule* . Under such schedules, for reinforcement, a particular response cannot have been emitted for a predetermined number of recent responses. Lag schedules, for example, require a response or response pattern to have differed from a given number (the lag value) of previously exhibited responses or patterns. Recency-based methods have been used regularly in both basic and applied research (e.g., Galizio et al., 2020; Abreu-Rodrigues et al., 2005). As we discuss later in this chapter, recency-based methods are predominant in the applications of reinforcement-of-variability procedures to individuals with ASD.

Frequency-Based Methods

Frequency-based methods entail the reinforcement of responses that have occurred *less frequently*—relative to other available responses—than some predetermined level (Denney & Neuringer, 1998; Machado, 1989). Denney and Neuringer (1998), for example, reinforced rats for emitting relatively infrequent response sequences across two levers. They calculated the frequencies of each of 16 possible sequences on a trial-by-trial basis. A particular sequence was reinforced only if its relative frequency fell below a designated threshold value. Their results showed that, as with lag schedules, frequency threshold procedures resulted in highly variable responding that was maintained across many sessions. The Denney and Neuringer experiment also supported the claim that variability is an operant dimension by showing discriminative control. Specifically, a schedule that reinforced variability was cued by specific stimuli (i.e., light on/tone off), while a yoked control condition was cued by other stimuli (i.e., light off/tone on). Under the yoked control, response sequences were reinforced at exactly the same frequency as under the variability stimulus but independently of response variations. The results showed that stimulus control was established, with variable responding significantly higher under the stimulus for variability than under the yoke stimulus. Additional demonstrations of stimulus control have reported variable responding in the presence of one stimulus and a fixed pattern (e.g., Right Right Left Left [RRLL]), in the presence of an alternative stimulus (e.g., Odum et al., 2006).

Percentile-Reinforcement Schedules

Percentile schedules, which provide a form of automatic shaping of performance, have been shown to increase or maintain high levels of response variability. A fictional example will illustrate the basic procedure. John wants to increase the number of push-up exercises that he performs in a period. He keeps track of that number each day. He then establishes the following percentile-reinforcement schedule for himself. If his number of push-ups today is greater than the median number over the last 10 days, then he rewards himself with the opportunity to watch his favorite online program. Note that the median may change across weeks or months, but it will always be based on John's own performance and will always be "pushing" him to be better than his prior average. Percentile schedules have been used regularly in basic research on operant variability including (but not limited to) persistence of variability (e.g., Arantes et al., 2012; Doughty & Lattal, 2001), the effects on variability of reinforcement delays (Wagner & Neuringer, 2006) and of reinforcement magnitude (Doughty et al., 2013).

Statistical Feedback Methods

Recency- and frequency-based schedules are useful when the focus is on nonrepetitive or variable responding, but if the goal is to test whether humans can respond "randomly" (or, more precisely, in random-like ways), recency and frequency methods are limited (see Neuringer & Jensen, 2013 for a discussion). To test whether human participants could generate random-like sequences, feedback was provided from as many as 10 different statistical tests (Neuringer, 1986; Neuringer & Jensen, 2013, p. 517). Participants were initially directed to respond as randomly as possible during a baseline phase in which no feedback was provided. Baseline responses were found to differ significantly from what would be expected from a random generator (i.e., from a computer-based random number generator). Next was a feedback condition in which, following each trial (100 responses), the participants saw the results of one statistical test (computer's random generator vs. the participant's responses), then two tests, then three, and so on. Eventually, participants learned to generate sequences that were indistinguishable, according to as many as 10 statistics, from the computer's random sequences. Said another way, participants learned to emit random-like responses. The demonstration that statistical feedback results in acquisition of random-like behavior provides further evidence that variability—in this case, to the highest degree—can be acquired and maintained as an operant. Additional evidence for random-like operant responding was reported in Page and Neuringer (1985).

Operant Variability and Learning

The training of operant responses depends on baseline levels of variability (Mazur, 1998; Skinner, 1984). Response variability is necessary when reinforcement is based on successive approximations of target behaviors. Several studies have demonstrated that explicit reinforcement of such variability facilitates the learning of new responses in both nonhuman animals (e.g., Grunow & Neuringer, 2002; Neuringer, 1993; Neuringer et al., 2000) and in humans (e.g., Hansson & Neuringer, 2018). For example, Neuringer et al. (2000) showed that speed of learning of target responses (for high-value reinforcers) was facilitated by concurrent reinforcement of variable responding (for lower-value reinforcers). Specifically, a group of rats that was exposed to variability-based contingencies learned to emit target sequences more quickly than a control group that had not been exposed. Grunow and Neuringer (2002; Experiment 2) examined the effects of different levels of baseline variability. Specifically, they first trained four groups of rats to respond at different levels of variability. Next, they exposed the four groups to conditions in which reinforcement was concurrently contingent on both variable response sequences and repetitions of an easy-to-learn sequence, and found that all four groups learned to repeat equally well. However, when repetitions of a difficult-to-learn sequence was required, speed of acquisition and levels of success were a function of the concurrently reinforced levels of variability. The rats reinforced for highest variability acquired the difficult target most rapidly and to the highest level. Thus, levels of variability were critical to the learning of target responses in terms of both speed of acquisition and terminal performance.

Although robust findings with pigeons and rats have demonstrated that learning is facilitated by reinforcement of variable responding, findings with human participants have been less consistent (e.g., Doolan & Bizo, 2013; Maes & van der Goot, 2006). The most recent human study indicated reasons for the disconnect. Hansson and Neuringer (2018) modified the procedures used in the previous human studies to enhance engagement with the task and increase reinforcing qualities of target sequences. Specifically, (1) to increase engagement in the task, participants "played" a computer-based soccer game by controlling a virtual soccer player's L and R moves toward a goal; (2) points earned in the soccer game were used to win real money via a virtual slot machine; (3) effort was increased by separating the location of L and R responses; and (4) the value of emitting the target sequence (12 points) was greater than that earned from response variations (3 points). The participants, 37 college students, were randomly assigned to three groups (i.e., VAR, YOKE, CON). All three groups received high-value, 12-point reinforcers for emission of either of two difficult target response sequences (e.g., LLRLR). Concurrently, VAR participants received low-value reinforcers (i.e., three tokens) contingent on variable responses that met a threshold-variability requirement. YOKE participants, in addition to high-value reinforcement for the target sequences, received low-value reinforcement at the same rate as participants in the VAR group but independently of their sequence variability. CON participants were reinforced (12 points) only for the target sequences (i.e., no concurrent low-value reinforcers were administered). The VAR participants learned to emit difficult target sequences at significantly higher frequencies than YOKE and CON participants, thus replicating with humans the findings from nonhuman animal studies (Grunow & Neuringer, 2002; Neuringer, 1993; Neuringer et al., 2000).

Translational Research

Several translational studies bridge the gap between the previously described basic research and applied work (e.g., Galizio et al., 2020; Miller & Neuringer, 2000; Murray & Healy, 2013). Importantly, these translational studies examined operant variability with clinically relevant populations (e.g., individuals with ASD diagnoses). The studies by Miller and Neuringer (2000) and Murray and Healy (2013) were directed at basic research with clinically relevant human populations. They helped to define behavioral mechanisms associated with operant variability while at the same time demonstrating relevance to individuals with ASD. Such transitional studies allow for the circumspect investigation, with clinically relevant populations, of mechanisms and associated procedures before applying them to socially important dependent variables (e.g., communication; problem behavior; feeding; social skills; play behaviors). For example, Miller and Neuringer (2000) demonstrated reinforcement-of-variability effects with individuals with autism diagnoses. Three groups (adolescents diagnosed with autism, a control group of college-age adults with no diagnoses, and a second control group of typically developing children) were exposed to a series of conditions in which they played a computer-based game requiring sets of four L and R responses, each set constituting a "trial." In one condition, reinforcement was provided independent of the variability of the response patterns via a random ratio schedule (reinforcement was provided following 50% of trials). In a second condition, a percentile reinforcement schedule was applied in which reinforcement was provided contingent on variable patterns (i.e., relative frequency [RF] values were calculated on a trial-by-trial basis and reinforcement was provided contingent on patterns with RF values that were less than the 11th lowest in the 20 most recent trials). The results showed that, for all three groups, variable patterns of response increased relative to the random ratio schedule when the percentile schedule was applied. Levels of variation were lowest throughout in the ASD group, but importantly, their variability was controlled by the variability contingencies in a manner similar to the control groups. Furthermore, when the random ratio schedule was reimplemented following the percentile schedule, all three groups persisted in their emissions of variable response sequences despite the fact that reinforcement was no longer contingent on variability. The results of Miller and Neuringer were noteworthy because they demonstrated that previous findings from basic studies on operant variability translated to an autism population. The results were also noteworthy in that they demonstrated persistence of variable responding after contingencies for variability were removed. Last, the results provided an antecedent for evaluations of potential applications further "downstream" along the basic–translational–applied continuum (Hake, 1982).

Applications of Operant Variability Procedures

A robust literature focusing on applications of reinforcement-of-variability contingencies has emerged over the last two decades. Reinforcement of variability has been applied to a variety of socially relevant dependent variables (e.g., interview skills; O'Neill & Rehfeldt, 2017; O'Neill et al., 2015), and application to ASD is particularly important. This is because one of the core features of ASD is excessive engagement in restricted and repetitive patterns of responding, sometimes conceptualized as a deficit in behavioral variability (see Rodriguez & Thompson, 2015, for a discussion). We next review applications of operant variability to individuals with ASD.

Responding to Social Questions

Subsequent to Miller and Neuringer (2000), Lee et al. (2002) provided an initial, "downstream" demonstration of the applied benefit of reinforcing variability with individuals with ASD diagnoses. Specifically, Lee et al. evaluated the effects of a lag schedule of reinforcement on variable appropriate verbal responding exhibited by three individuals with ASD. The participants were first exposed to a condition in which differential reinforcement of appropriate behaviors (DRA) was implemented such that, regardless of variability, appropriate responses to social questions were reinforced. Next, a Lag-1 schedule was implemented in which reinforcement was provided only for appropriate responses that differed from the previously emitted response. The results showed that when the Lag-1 schedule was applied, variable responding clearly increased for all three participants. Lee et al. also implemented reversals between the DRA and lag conditions with two participants and found that variable responding persisted during DRA, despite the removal of variability-based contingencies, before eventually decreasing to zero levels. This result was similar to the Miller and Neuringer (2000) finding of persistence of variable responding. The findings of Lee et al. (2002) provided a significant contribution to the research stream pertaining to operant variability, because (1) they, along with Miller and Neuringer (2000), showed that invariant responding by individuals with ASD diagnoses could be impacted by variability-reinforcing contingencies and (2) the Lee et al. (2002) study demonstrated these effects with a socially relevant behavior (i.e., appropriate responses to social questions). Furthermore, Lee et al.'s focus on variability *and* language/communication skills allowed the researchers to evaluate two distinct core characteristics of ASD (i.e., deficits in communication and stereotypies). The Lee et al. findings have been replicated consistently in subsequent studies focusing on appropriate responding to social questions (e.g., Lee & Sturmey, 2014; Olin et al., 2020; Radley, Dart, Moore, Lum, et al., 2017; Radley et al., 2019; Susa & Schlinger, 2012). Lee et al. (2002) also provided the first clinical application of recency-based methods (lag schedules in this case) to produce variable responding that had, to that point, been utilized only in basic EAB arrangements.

Other Language/Communication-Based Skills and ASD

Subsequent to Lee et al. (2002), numerous studies on ASD and other developmental disability have successfully reinforced linguistic variability: in tacts (Heldt & Schlinger, 2012), mands (e.g., Silbaugh, Swinnea, et al., 2020; Silbaugh, Falcomata, et al., 2018; Silbaugh & Falcomata, 2019), intraverbals (e.g., Contreras & Betz, 2016), naming within categories (e.g., Wiskow et al., 2018; Wiskow & Donaldson, 2016), vocal responding (Esch et al., 2009), and phonemic variability (Koehler-Platten et al., 2013). As with Lee et al. (2002), these studies focused on two distinct core characteristics of ASD: deficits in variability and language/communication. For example, Silbaugh, Falcomata, et al. (2018) examined the utility of lag schedules with embedded progressive time delays (TDs) to increase and maintain manding with two individuals with ASD. Progressive TD involves providing a prompt after a predetermined interval in which the individual had not responded (e.g., 2 seconds). Silbaugh et al. initially implemented a Lag-0 schedule in which all mands, regardless of variability, were reinforced. Next, the authors implemented a Lag 1 plus TD in which they prompted variable mands if the participant did not respond within 2 seconds of the presentation of the establishing operation and reinforced all mands that differed from the immediately preceding mand. In addition to demonstrating higher variability in manding during Lag-1 plus TD, both individuals also demonstrated novel mands (i.e., those not previously emitted).

Lepper et al. (2017) provided an example of the positive effects of reinforcement of variable verbal behavior on perseverative speech exhibited by two individuals with ASD. The participants, both of whom had histories of perseveration on limited interests during conversations, were exposed to three conditions in which conversation partners reinforced conversational behavior (1) regardless of variability (i.e., Lag 0), (2) contingent on the participants' engaging in conversation on topics that differed from the previous topic (i.e., Lag 1), and (3) contingent on the participants' engaging in conversation on topics that differed from the previous two topic (i.e., Lag 2). The results showed that, during the lag conditions, both participants engaged in conversational topics that differed from their perseverative circumscribed interests. For one participant, the Lag-1 schedule increased engagement in nonperseverative topics, while engagement in perseverative topics continued at levels similar to baseline. During the Lag-2 condition, the participant's engagement in nonperseverative topics further increased, while engagement in perseverative topics decreased. The second participant exhibited increases in nonperseverative topics during the Lag-1 condition, with similar levels exhibited during Lag 2. The second participant also exhibited decreases in perseverative topics during the Lag-1 condition, with similar levels exhibited during Lag 2. The results of Lepper et al. are consistent with a growing number of studies that have demonstrated positive effects of reinforcing variability of other types of previously repetitive behaviors (e.g., play skills; Lang et al., 2014, 2020).

Social Skills

Based on current classification systems, individuals with ASD demonstrate marked impairments in social interaction. Therefore, social skills training is often a primary component of educational programming with such individuals. Researchers have recently combined social skills training with reinforcement of variability (e.g., Radley, Moore, et al., 2019; Radley et al., 2018; Radley, Dart, Moore, Battaglia, et al., 2017). Social skills training involves teaching individuals a variety of skills that produce positive social interactions (Gresham & Elliott, 1987; Gresham, 1986). Social skills are needed for successful interactions with others that are consistent with social conventions (e.g., eye contact, maintaining conversation, asking questions; responding to questions). Radley, Dart, Moore, Battaglia, et al. (2017) combined multiple exemplar training with lag schedules to promote the acquisition and variable emission of four social skills (i.e., responding to questions; maintaining a conversation; expressing wants and needs; participating) with four individuals with ASD. The program was implemented in a university-based clinic twice per week during 2-hour sessions. The authors first implemented social skills training using multiple response exemplars and reinforced accurate responses via a fixed-ratio (FR) 1 schedule; thus, accurate responses were reinforced regardless of variability. Radley et al.'s multiple response exemplar training consisted of modeling and teaching three responses (e.g., "May I have that dinosaur?"; "Can I play with the puzzle?"; p. 91) to specific skill prompts (e.g., "Go ask [name] for a toy"; p. 91). The combination of multiple exemplar training and the FR 1 schedule resulted in emergence and maintenance of accurate responding; however, invariant responding was also observed. The authors subsequently modified the schedule of reinforcement to Lag 2 and then Lag 4 while continuing multiple exemplar training. The combination of multiple exemplar training and lag schedules produced the emergence and maintenance of variable and accurate responding. Radley et al. (2018) replicated and extended Radley, Dart, Moore, Battaglia, et al. (2017) with three additional individuals with ASD by (1) demonstrating the positive effects of the multiple exemplar training with lag schedules combination in a natural setting (i.e., school setting) and (2) implementing the procedures in a brief format (i.e., training occurred once per week over 8 weeks). Subsequently, Radley, Moore, et al. (2019) further replicated and extended their previous studies by applying the same procedure in participants with more severe ASD diagnoses and assessing parent perceptions posttraining (with positive findings regarding parent perceptions). Overall, Radley and colleagues' findings support application of reinforcement-of-variability contingencies to the social interaction core characteristic of ASD.

Play

Similar to other target behaviors often associated with ASD (e.g., language/communication; perseverative speech; social skills), the issue of restricted, or invariant play/leisure activities also lends itself to possible benefit from reinforcement of variability. Several studies have demonstrated positive effects of reinforcing variable play by individuals with ASD (e.g., Baruni et al., 2014; Lang et al., 2014, 2020; Napolitano et al., 2010). For example, Lang et al. (2014) evaluated generalization and maintenance of acquired play skills following lag reinforcement of variable play. The authors initially taught play skills to three children with ASD in an early childhood special education setting. Although all three participants demonstrated stimulus generalization (i.e., the acquired play skills generalized across settings), two of the participants did not demonstrate response generalization of the acquired play skills (i.e., play skills did not generalize across toys). The authors subsequently applied a lag schedule with the two participants, and both subsequently demonstrated response generalization of the play skills. Lang et al. also found that in addition to increasing generalization and maintenance of acquired play skills, decreases in stereotypy were observed even though no contingencies were directly applied to the

behavior (i.e., reinforcement was contingent on play skills and no programmed consequences were provided for stereotypy). Lang et al. (2020) extended their previous results
to a distinct setting (playground with typical playground equipment) with different-age
participants and showed that reinforcing variable play behavior during skills training (1)
increased appropriate play, (2) increased the variety of play-based items with which the
participants interacted, and (3) decreased stereotypies. Lang et al. (2014, p. 870) hypothesized that reinforcing play behavior, including variable responding, may have promoted
contact of novel, functional behaviors, with "new communities of reinforcement, potentially displacing stereotypy."

Feeding

Individuals with ASD often exhibit feeding problems including food selectivity (e.g., Curtin et al., 2015; Badalyan & Schwartz, 2012). In fact, ASD's core symptoms may interact with food selectivity and mealtime problem behavior (i.e., repetitive and restrictive
behavior patterns; deficits in social and communication skills; Curtin et al., 2015). The
restricted and repetitive nature of food selectivity exhibited by such individuals with ASD
suggests possible benefits of reinforcing food-selection variability. Several studies (i.e.,
Silbaugh & Falcomata, 2017; Silbaugh et al., 2017; Silbaugh, Swinnea, et al., 2018) have
tested this hypothesis. Silbaugh and Falcomata (2017) evaluated the effects of a Lag-1
schedule on food selectivity exhibited by a 4-year-old boy diagnosed with ASD and a
history of consuming a limited variety of foods. First implemented was a Lag-0 condition
in which reinforcement in the form of access to preferred nonfood items was provided
contingent on bites consumed among any of five foods presented in an array. After the
participant demonstrated invariant food choices, a Lag-1 schedule was implemented in
which reinforcement was made contingent on variability of foods independently eaten
(i.e., reinforcement was contingent on independent bites of foods that differed from the
immediately preceding independent bite). The Lag-1 schedule resulted in both increases
in variable consumption of foods and the total number of different foods consumed.
When lag schedules alone do not produce variability, subsequent studies have combined
such schedules with other behavioral procedures (e.g., response blocking: Silbaugh et al.,
2017; physical guidance: Silbaugh, Swinnea, et al., 2018) and have shown the combination to be effective at increasing variable food selectivity.

Problem Behavior

Many individuals with ASD exhibit problem behaviors such as aggression, self-injury,
disruptions, inappropriate vocalizations, and tantrums. Such problem behaviors are
often interpreted as negatively reinforced (e.g., escape from nonpreferred activities), or
positively reinforced (access to attention and/or preferred activities). Functional communication training (FCT; Carr & Durand, 1985) is a common treatment that involves
training and reinforcement of appropriate communicative responses (mands) to enable
the individual to access reinforcers that previously maintained problem behavior. In this
way, mands come to replace problem behavior in the individual's repertoire as a way
to produce functional reinforcers. Despite numerous demonstrations of its effectiveness,
FCT sometimes results in relapse in the form of resurgence (e.g., Volkert et al., 2009;
Wacker et al., 2011; see Saini et al., Chapter 19, this volume). Resurgence is the recurrence
of previously reinforced behaviors when a second, subsequently reinforced behavior, is

undergoing extinction (Epstein, 1983). It has been described as the "transient recurrence, with consideration of the stimulus context, of some dimension of previously established but not currently occurring activity when reinforcement conditions of current behavior are worsened" (Lattal et al., 2017, p. 90). Resurgence of problem behavior is observed when challenges occur during treatment (Wacker et al., 2011), such as lapses in treatment integrity (i.e., failure to reinforce appropriate communication; reinforcement of problem behavior), as well as disruptions prior to treatment (e.g., accidental misplacement of communication materials; battery shortage on iPad-based communication system). The training of multiple modalities of communication (e.g., communication card, manual sign, iPad-based communication system, voice-output device) during FCT is one strategy for inoculating against resurgence, in that the use of alternative mands is promoted when a preferred mand goes unreinforced (e.g., Lambert et al., 2015).

Reinforcement of mand variability across multiple modalities of communication via lag schedules is another strategy that may be helpful in the prevention of resurgence. Previous basic studies (e.g., Arantes et al., 2012; Doughty & Lattal, 2001) demonstrated that when reinforcement was omitted during an extinction phase operant variability persisted (i.e., responding continued despite contacting extinction) longer than operant repetition (however, see Neuringer et al., 2001). Thus, there is support for the notion that persistence of multiple mands when they go unreinforced may be augmented via reinforcement of variability. Following this logic, Adami et al. (2017) and Falcomata et al. (2018) evaluated the effects of embedding lag schedules within FCT procedures. Specifically, Adami et al. (2017) studied the effects of lag schedules and FCT on (1) variable responding across multiple mand topographies and (2) persistence of multiple mands when invariant mands were not reinforced (i.e., invariant mands did not meet the lag requirements) leading possibly to resurgence of problem behavior. Adami et al. first conducted a functional analysis and identified the function(s) of problem behavior exhibited by three individuals with ASD. Next, they used a reversal design to compare the effects of FCT with a Lag 1 to FCT with a Lag 0 in terms of their effects on mand variability and problem behavior. With all three participants, variable manding during the FCT with Lag 1 was considerably higher than during the FCT with Lag 0. Both treatment arrangements were effective at reducing problem behavior. Falcomata et al. (2018) extended the work of Adami et al. (2017) by increasing the value of the lag schedule during FCT from Lag 0 to Lag 5 with two individuals with ASD and histories of problem behavior. With both participants, mand variability increased as the value of the lag schedule increased from Lag 0 to Lag 4; however, no differences in variability were observed between the Lag-4 and Lag-5 conditions, similar to findings from the basic research literature (Page & Neuringer, 1985). Problem behavior remained low relative to baseline at each lag value, including the Lag 5. Thus, despite the similarity between clinical conditions that evoke resurgence and FCT with lag schedules (i.e., both entail the nonreinforcement of mands after problem behavior has been extinguished via extinction), problem behavior did not recur in either Adami et al. (2017) or Falcomata et al. (2018) when mands went unreinforced within the lag. Their results suggest possible utility of lag schedules during FCT to mitigate or prevent resurgence. Said another way, it is possible that the reinforcement of variability during FCT via lag promoted persistence of functional mands and prevented recurrence of problem behaviors. In summary, the results of Adami et al. (2017) and Falcomata et al. (2018) showed that reinforcement of mand variability during FCT (1) can increase variable manding and promote use of multiple modalities of communication and (2) may have utility in the mitigation of resurgence of problem behavior.

Conclusion

Variability was critically important to both Charles Darwin and B. F. Skinner. Darwin is of particular importance because Skinner related the shaping of operant behaviors to Darwinian theory-based variation and selection. Darwin spent many years analyzing the data from his 5-year journey on the *Beagle,* a 90-foot sailboat, trying to explain how species came to be (Darwin, 1859; Darwin, 2001). His insight, seminal to this day, was that environmental and social conditions selected for adaptive phenotypes, but that idea not only solved a problem, it created one. If a particular environment selects particular individuals (i.e., those having adaptive attributes or phenotypes) and the selection process is replicated across generations, then over time, shouldn't species become increasingly stereotyped or homogeneous? What, then, maintains the variability necessary for the evolution of species? Darwin's answer, long in its gestation, was that the environment selects for variability within and across species. Selection of individual phenotypes and selection of phenotype variability work together, each depending on the other.

At the beginning of his professional career, B. F. Skinner was attracted to Pavlovian reflex psychology. However, in studying eating behaviors in rats, Skinner observed high levels of variability (i.e., how rats pressed levers to produce food pellets) that could not be explained by Pavlovian principles. The variations appeared to be controlled by the same reinforcing event, the food pellets, causing Skinner to posit the operant as a "generic response class" that comprised individual actions, each of which led to a reinforcing event (Skinner, 1938). At least initially, the different actions emerged unpredictably. Skinner and many researchers who followed him, showed that, after a response had been acquired, variability tended to decrease under conditions of continued reinforcement (e.g., Antonitis, 1951; Iversen, 2002; Stebbins & Lanson, 1962). For new behaviors to be shaped, however, variability must be present. As in the Darwinian case, a question confronted researchers: What generated and maintained that variability? One answer was that variability was always present, at least at some levels; another was that withholding reinforcers (extinction) increased variability. A third contributor parallels Darwinian selection: Behavioral variability is itself selected by consequences; that is, variability can be shaped, controlled, and maintained by contingent reinforcers.

We conclude by noting the importance of cross talk between laboratory-based, basic research on variability and applications to clinically relevant populations. Laboratory research with both nonhuman animals and human populations has documented precise control by reinforcement contingencies and discriminative stimuli over levels of variability. These studies have led to clinically relevant applications (e.g., successful reinforcement of variable behaviors in individuals diagnosed with ASD). Thus, clinicians have profited from basic research and have successfully applied the same reinforcement-of-variability contingencies studied in basic-science laboratories. Basic researchers, on their part, have profited from the extensions by clinicians to new methods of reinforcement, to different classes of behaviors, and to demonstrations of generalization of effects.

REFERENCES

Abreu-Rodrigues, J., Lattal, K. A., Dos Santos, C. V., & Matos, R. A. (2005). Variation, repetition, and choice. *Journal of the Experimental Analysis of Behavior, 83,* 147–168.

Adami, S., Falcomata, T. S., Muething, C. S., & Hoffman, K. (2017). An evaluation of lag schedules of reinforcement during functional communication training: Effects on varied mand responding and challenging behavior. *Behavior Analysis in Practice, 10*, 209–213.

Antonitis, J. J. (1951). Response variability in the white rat during conditioning, extinction, and reconditioning. *Journal of Experimental Psychology, 42*, 273–281.

Arantes, J., Berg, M. E., Le, D., & Grace, R. C. (2012). Resistance to change and preference for variable versus fixed response sequences. *Journal of the Experimental Analysis of Behavior, 98*, 1–21.

Badalyan, V., & Schwartz, R. H. (2012). Mealtime feeding behaviors and gastrointestinal dysfunction in children with classic autism compared with normal sibling controls. *Journal of Pediatrics, 2*, 150–160.

Barba, L. S. (2012). Operant variability: A conceptual analysis. *Behavior Analyst, 35*, 213–227.

Baruni, R. R., Rapp, J. T., Lipe, S. L., & Novotny, M. A. (2014). Using lag schedules to increase toy play variability for children with intellectual disabilities. *Behavioral Interventions, 29*, 21–35.

Blough, D. S. (1966). The reinforcement of least-frequent interresponse times. *Journal of the Experimental Analysis of Behavior, 9*, 581–591.

Bryant, D., & Church, R. M. (1974). The determinants of random choice. *Animal Learning and Behavior, 2*, 245–248.

Carr, E., & Durand, V. (1985). Reducing behavior problems through Functional Communication Training. *Journal of Applied Behavior Analysis, 18*, 111–126.

Contreras, B. P., & Betz, A. M. (2016). Using lag schedules to strengthen the intraverbal repertoires of children with autism. *Journal of Applied Behavior Analysis, 49*, 3–16.

Curtin, C., Hubbard, K., Anderson, S. E., Mick, E., Must, A., & Bandini, L. G. (2015). Food selectivity, mealtime behavior problems, spousal stress, and family food choices in children with and without autism spectrum disorder. *Journal of Autism and Developmental Disorders, 45*, 3308–3315.

Darwin, C. (1859). *The origin of species by means of natural selection*. John Murray.

Darwin, C. (2001). *Charles Darwin's beagle diary*. Cambridge University Press.

Denney, J., & Neuringer, A. (1998). Behavioral variability is controlled by discriminative stimuli. *Animal Learning and Behavior, 26*, 154–162.

Doolan, K. E., & Bizo, L. A. (2013). Reinforced behavioral variability in humans. *Psychological Record, 63*(4), 725–734.

Doughty, A. H., Giorno, K. G., & Miller, H. L. (2013). Effects of reinforcer magnitude on reinforced behavioral variability. *Journal of the Experimental Analysis of Behavior, 100*, 355–369.

Doughty, A. H., & Lattal, K. A. (2001). Resistance to change of operant variation and repetition. *Journal of the Experimental Analysis of Behavior, 76*, 195–215.

Epstein, R. (1983). Resurgence of previously reinforced behavior during extinction. *Behaviour Analysis Letters, 3*, 391–397.

Esch, J. W., & Esch, B. E. (2009). Increasing vocal variability in children with autism using a lag schedule of reinforcement. *The Analysis of Verbal Behavior, 25*, 73–78.

Falcomata, T. S., Muething, C. S., Silbaugh, B. C., Adami, S., Hoffman, K., Shpall, C., & Ringdahl, J. E. (2018). Lag schedules and functional communication training: Persistence of mands and relapse of problem behavior. *Behavior Modification, 42*, 314–334.

Galizio, A., Friedel, J. E., & Odum, A. L. (2020). An investigation of resurgence of reinforced behavioral variability in humans. *Journal of the Experimental Analysis of Behavior, 114*, 381–393.

Galizio, A., Higbee, T. S., & Odum, A. L. (2020). Choice for reinforced behavioral variability in children with autism spectrum disorder. *Journal of the Experimental Analysis of Behavior, 113*, 495–514.

Gresham, F. M. (1986). Conceptual and definitional issues in the assessment of children's social skills: Implications for classifications and training. *Journal of Clinical Child Psychology, 15*(1), 3–15.

Gresham, F. M., & Elliott, S. N. (1987). The relationship between adaptive behavior and social skills: Issues in definition and assessment. *Journal of Special Education, 21*(1), 167–181.

Grunow, A., & Neuringer, A. (2002). Learning to vary and varying to learn. *Psychonomic Bulletin and Review, 9*, 250–258.

Hake, D. F. (1982). The basic–applied continuum and the possible evolution of human operant social and verbal research. *The Behavior Analyst, 5*, 21–28.

Hansson, J., & Neuringer, A. (2018). Reinforcement of variability facilitates learning in humans. *Journal of the Experimental Analysis of Behavior, 110*, 380–393.

Heldt, J., & Schlinger, H. D. (2012). Increased

variability in tacting under a lag 3 schedule of reinforcement. *The Analysis of Verbal Behavior, 28,* 131–136.

Iversen, I. H. (2002). Response-initiated imaging of operant behavior using a digital camera. *Journal of the Experimental Analysis of Behavior, 77,* 283–300.

Koehler-Platten, K., Grow, L. L., Schulze, K. A., & Bertone, T. (2013). Using a lag reinforcement schedule to increase phonemic variability in children with autism spectrum disorders. *The Analysis of Verbal Behavior, 29,* 71–83.

Lambert, J. M., Bloom, S. E., Samaha, A. L., Dayton, E., & Rodewald, A. M. (2015). Serial alternative response training as intervention for target response resurgence. *Journal of Applied Behavior Analysis, 48,* 765–780.

Lang, R., Machalicek, W., Rispoli, M., O'Reilly, M., Sigafoos, J., Lancioni, G., . . . Didden, R. (2014). Play skills taught via behavioral intervention generalize, maintain, and persist in the absence of socially mediated reinforcement in children with autism. *Research in Autism Spectrum Disorders, 8,* 860–872.

Lang, R., Muharib, R., Lessner, P., Davenport, K., Ledbetter-Cho, K., & Rispoli, M. (2020). Increasing play and decreasing stereotypy for children with autism on a playground. *Advances in Neurodevelopmental Disorders, 4,* 146–154.

Lattal, K. A., Cançado, C. R., Cook, J. E., Kincaid, S. L., Nighbor, T. D., & Oliver, A. C. (2017). On defining resurgence. *Behavioural Processes, 141,* 85–91.

Lee, R., McComas, J. J., & Jawor, J. (2002). The effects of differential and lag reinforcement schedules on varied verbal responding by individuals with autism. *Journal of Applied Behavior Analysis, 35,* 391–402.

Lee, R., & Sturmey, P. (2014). The effects of script-fading and a Lag-1 schedule on varied social responding in children with autism. *Research in Autism Spectrum Disorders, 8,* 440–448.

Lepper, T. L., Devine, B., & Petursdottir, A. I. (2017). Application of a lag contingency to reduce perseveration on circumscribed interests. *Developmental Neurorehabilitation, 20,* 313–316.

Machado, A. (1989). Operant conditioning of behavioral variability using a percentile reinforcement schedule. *Journal of the Experimental Analysis of Behavior, 52,* 155–166.

Maes, J. H. R., & van der Goot, M. (2006). Human operant learning under concurrent reinforcement of response variability . *Learning and Motivation, 37*(1), 79–92.

Mazur, J. E. (1998). *Learning and behavior* (4th ed.). Prentice Hall.

Miller, N., & Neuringer, A. (2000). Reinforcing variability in adolescents with autism. *Journal of Applied Behavior Analysis, 33,* 151–165.

Murray, C., & Healy, O. (2013). Increasing response variability in children with autism spectrum disorder using lag schedules of reinforcement. *Research in Autism Spectrum Disorders, 7,* 1481–1488.

Napolitano, D. A., Smith, T., Zarcone, J. R., Goodkin, K., & McAdam, D. B. (2010). Increasing response diversity in children with autism. *Journal of Applied Behavior Analysis, 43,* 265–271.

Nergaard, S. K., & Holth, P. (2020). A critical review of the support for variability as an operant dimension . *Perspectives on Behavior Science, 43,* 579–603.

Neuringer, A. (1986). Can people behave "randomly?": The role of feedback. *Journal of Experimental Psychology: General, 115,* 62–75.

Neuringer, A. (1992). Choosing to vary and repeat. *Psychological Science, 3,* 246–251.

Neuringer, A. (1993). Reinforced variation and selection. *Animal Learning and Behavior, 21,* 83–91.

Neuringer, A. (2002). Operant variability: Evidence, functions, and theory. *Psychonomic Bulletin and Review, 9,* 672–705.

Neuringer, A. (2004). Reinforced variability in animals and people: Implications for adaptive action. *American Psychologist, 59,* 891–906.

Neuringer, A., Deiss, C., & Olson, G. (2000). Reinforced variability and operant learning. *Journal of Experimental Psychology: Animal Behavior Processes, 26,* 98–111.

Neuringer, A., & Jensen, G. (2012). The predictably unpredictable operant. Comparative *Cognition and Behavior Reviews, 7,* 55–84.

Neuringer, A., & Jensen, G. (2013). Operant variability. In G. J. Madden, W. V. Dube, T. D. Hackenberg, G. P. Hanley, & K. A. Lattal (Eds.), *APA handbook of behavior analysis: Vol. 1. Methods and principles* (pp. 513–546). American Psychological Association.

Neuringer, A., Kornell, N., & Olufs, M. (2001). Stability and variability in extinction. *Journal of Experimental Psychology: Animal Behavior Processes, 27,* 79–94.

Odum, A. L., Ward, R. D., Barnes, C. A., &

Burke, K. A. (2006). The effects of delayed reinforcement on variability and repetition of response sequences. *Journal of the Experimental Analysis of Behavior, 86,* 159–179.

Olin, J., Sonsky, A., & Howard, M. (2020). Using a lag schedule of reinforcement to increase response variability in children with autism spectrum disorders. *The Analysis of Verbal Behavior, 36,* 169–179.

O'Neill, J., Blowers, A. P., Henson, L., & Rehfeldt, R. A. (2015). Further analysis of selection-based instruction, lag reinforcement schedules, and the emergence of topography-based responses to interview questions. *The Analysis of Verbal Behavior, 31,* 126–136.

O'Neill, J., & Rehfeldt, R. A. (2017). Computerized behavioral skills training with selection-based instruction and lag reinforcement schedules for responses to interview questions. *Behavior Analysis: Research and Practice, 17,* 42–54.

Page, S., & Neuringer, A. (1985). Variability is an operant. *Journal of Experimental Psychology, 11,* 429–452.

Pryor, K. W., Haag, R., & O'Reilly, J. (1969). The creative porpoise: Training for novel behavior. *Journal of the Experimental Analysis of Behavior, 12,* 653–661.

Radley, K. C., Battaglia, A. A., Dadakhodjaeva, K., Ford, W. B., & Robbins, K. (2018). Increasing behavioral variability and social skill accuracy in children with autism spectrum disorder. *Journal of Behavioral Education, 27*(3), 395–418.

Radley, K. C., Dart, E. H., Helbig, K. A., Schrieber, S. R., & Ware, M. E. (2019). An evaluation of the additive effects of lag schedules of reinforcement. *Developmental Neurorehabilitation, 22,* 180–191.

Radley, K. C., Dart, E. H., Moore, J. W., Battaglia, A. A., & LaBrot, Z. C. (2017). Promoting accurate variability of social skills in children with autism spectrum disorder. *Behavior Modification, 41*(1), 84–112.

Radley, K. C., Dart, E. H., Moore, J. W., Lum, J. D. K., & Pasqua, J. (2017). Enhancing appropriate and variable responding in young children with autism spectrum disorder. *Developmental Neurorehabilitation, 20*(8), 538–548.

Radley, K. C., Moore, J. W., Dart, E. H., Ford, W. B., & Helbig, K. A. (2019). The effects of lag schedules of reinforcement on social skill accuracy and variability. *Focus on Autism and Other Developmental Disabilities, 34,* 67–80.

Rodriguez, N. M., & Thompson, R. H. (2015). Behavioral variability and autism spectrum disorder. *Journal of Applied Behavior Analysis, 48,* 167–187.

Schwartz, B. (1980). Development of complex, stereotyped behavior in pigeons. *Journal of the Experimental Analysis of Behavior, 33,* 153–166.

Schwartz, B. (1982). Reinforcement-induced behavioral stereotypy: How not to teach people to discover rules. *Journal of Experimental Psychology: General, 111,* 23–59.

Silbaugh, B. C., & Falcomata, T. S. (2017). Translational evaluation of a lag schedule and variability in food consumed by a boy with autism and food selectivity. *Developmental Neurorehabilitation, 20,* 309–312.

Silbaugh, B. C., & Falcomata, T. S. (2019). Effects of a lag schedule with progressive time delay on sign mand variability in a boy with autism. *Behavior Analysis in Practice, 12,* 124–132.

Silbaugh, B. C., Falcomata, T. S., & Ferguson, R. H. (2018). Effects of a lag schedule of reinforcement with progressive time delay on topographical mand variability in children with autism. *Developmental Neurorehabilitation, 21,* 166–177.

Silbaugh, B. C., Murray, C., Kelly, M. P., & Healy, O. (2020). A systematic synthesis of lag schedule research in individuals with autism and other populations. *Review Journal of Autism and Developmental Disorders, 8,* 92–107.

Silbaugh, B. C., Swinnea, S., & Falcomata, T. S. (2018). Clinical evaluation of physical guidance procedures in the treatment of food selectivity . *Behavioral Interventions, 33,* 403–413.

Silbaugh, B. C., Swinnea, S., & Falcomata, T. S. (2020). Replication and extension of the effects of lag schedules on mand variability and challenging behavior during functional communication training. *The Analysis of Verbal Behavior, 36,* 49–73.

Silbaugh, B. C., Wingate, H. V., & Falcomata, T. S. (2017). Effects of lag schedules and response blocking on variant food consumption by a girl with autism. *Behavioral Interventions, 32,* 21–34.

Skinner, B. F. (1938). *The behavior of organisms: An experimental analysis* . Appleton-Century.

Skinner, B. F. (1984). Selection by consequences. *Behavioral and Brain Sciences, 7,* 477–510.

Stebbins, W. C., & Lanson, R. N. (1962). Response latency as a function of reinforcement schedule. *Journal of the Experimental Analysis of Behavior, 5*(3), 299–304.

Susa, C., & Schlinger, H. D. (2012). Using a lag schedule to increase variability of verbal responding in an individual with autism. *The Analysis of Verbal Behavior, 28*, 125–130.

Volkert, V. M., Lerman, D. C., Call, N. A., & Trosclaire-Lasserre, N. (2009). An evaluation of resurgence during treatment with functional communication training. *Journal of Applied Behavior Analysis, 42*, 145–160.

Wacker, D. P., Harding, J. W., Berg, W. K., Lee, J. F., Schieltz, K. M., Padilla, Y. C., . . . Shahan, T. A. (2011). An evaluation of persistence of treatment effects during long-term treatment of destructive behavior. *Journal of the Experimental Analysis of Behavior, 96*, 261–282.

Wagner, K., & Neuringer, A. (2006). Operant variability when reinforcement is delayed. *Learning and Behavior, 34*, 111–123.

Wiskow, K. M., & Donaldson, J. M. (2016). Evaluation of a lag schedule of reinforcement in a group contingency to promote varied naming of categories items with children. *Journal of Applied Behavior Analysis, 49*(3), 472–484.

Wiskow, K. M., Matter, A. L., & Donaldson, J. M. (2018). An evaluation of lag schedules and prompting methods to increase variability of naming category items in children with autism spectrum disorder. *The Analysis of Verbal Behavior, 36*, 251–272.

CHAPTER 21

Behavioral Economics for Applied Behavior Analysts

Gregory J. Madden
Derek D. Reed
Dorothea C. Lerman

Many readers have heard of *behavioral economics*, likely through Kahneman and Tversky's influential theories (Kahneman & Tversky, 2013), popular books such as *Nudge* (Thaler & Sunstein, 2009), or the *Freakonomics Radio* podcast. What readers may not know is that there are two categories of behavioral economics. The famous category is the one focused on the "predictable irrationality" of human behavior, that is, the many ways in which humans defy the "laws" of economics (Ariely et al., 2009; Thaler, 1981). This form of behavioral economics has produced important discoveries that have led to practical applications (e.g., Thaler & Benartzi, 2004), but this category of behavioral economics is not the primary focus of this chapter—sorry to disappoint.

Instead, the category of behavior economics we focus on is that which explores the relevance of microeconomic principles to the behavior of individuals, the latter being the traditional focus of behavior analysis. These microeconomic principles are myriad—consumer demand and indifference curves, income and price constraints, the continuum from substitutes to complements—and most have only begun to be explored empirically in applied behavior-analytic research. Thus, this chapter is partially empirical and partially aspirational. Our intent is to give the reader a different prism through which to view a behavior-change challenge. The design of the prism stands things on their head a bit. Doing so may be initially disorienting, but the momentary discomfort could be rewarded with new insights, new problems never noticed, new solutions within reach.

The chapter begins with a brief primer on the economics of supply and demand. Thereafter, we focus on two broad categories of behavior of interest to applied behavior analysts: appropriate behavior and problem behavior. Appropriate behavior includes academic, independent living, and social behaviors, to name just a few. In applied settings, these appropriate behaviors are maintained with therapeutic reinforcers, which we abbreviate throughout this chapter as R_T. Because these behaviors are appropriate, the goal is to increase their frequency to a level that would be suitable in the current environment. At the same time, constantly providing R_T's is often impractical; therefore, intermittent reinforcement is important; maintaining appropriate behavior with fewer R_T's enhances the probability that interventions will be continued and that behavior can be maintained in less supportive environments. Later, the chapter integrates into the discussion those interventions designed to reduce problem behavior. These unwanted behaviors are maintained by reinforcing consequences (abbreviated R_P) that are often outside the control of the applied practitioner. Therefore, the therapeutic approach is often to arrange a choice between R_P and a newly arranged R_T. We view this choice context through the prism of behavioral economics, conceptualizing the context as a marketplace in which commodities (R_T and R_P) interact and compete for the limited resources of the consumer. But for now, let's talk about the basics.

A Primer on Supply and Demand

How many appropriate responses will my client make to earn one reinforcer?
How many tokens should I require before a backup reinforcer is provided?
Why isn't this therapeutic reinforcer competing effectively with problem behavior?

If you've ever asked questions like these, then you have recognized that economic factors play a role in your behavior-change plan. In many of our behavioral interventions, client behavior is exchanged for a reinforcer, just like the way consumers spend their limited resources of time, effort, and money to acquire products and services. When we arrange reinforcement contingencies—setting and manipulating the amount of the clients' behavioral resources that must be expended to acquire reinforcers with a type/size/quality that we determine—we are manipulating economic variables, whether we know it or not. Economic research has uncovered principles that govern how these variables should be changed when the goal is (as it is in behavior-analytic practice) to encourage spending (client responding for R_T's) while also keeping the supplier of the product afloat (developing a behavior plan that may be practically implemented).

Economics may be broadly defined as the study of supply and demand (Robbins, 1932). *Supply* refers to the scarcity or abundance of goods/services in the marketplace, while *demand* refers to the operant goods/services-seeking behaviors of consumers. In the economic marketplace, suppliers set prices and they use consumer demand (spending) to guide this activity. If demand is low, prices must be decreased and profits will suffer; if demand is high, prices will be increased and profits will soar. Suppliers also consider the prices of other goods; it is important not to price your product out of contention with its competitors.

Practicing behavior analysts operate in a behavioral-economic marketplace (Reed et al., 2013). The behavior analyst, like the supplier, determines the price of their R_T (again, "R_T" is the therapeutic reinforcer used to maintain appropriate behavior). Before we consider how these pricing decisions might be made, we should define what we mean by the "price" of a reinforcer. *Price* refers to a cost–benefit ratio, which aligns nicely with the response–reinforcer contingency about which readers of this chapter already know. In the behavioral economist's price ratio, *cost* refers to the resources the consumer must sacrifice to acquire the reinforcer. For example, clients expend time and effort to acquire our R_T's; these resources could be withheld or allocated elsewhere. The *benefit* part of the price ratio refers to the characteristics of the reinforcer itself: its type, size, quality, and so forth. Thus, price changes can be implemented by manipulating costs (e.g., asking for more correct responses per R_T) or by changing the benefits (e.g., increasing the size of R_T).

One of those economic principles that we alluded to earlier—principles that should be understood by those who manipulate prices (or reinforcement contingencies)—is that price has an orderly effect on consumers' consumption of a product. All else being equal, when a product is available at a low price, it will be consumed more than when it is available at a high price. This price effect on consumption is illustrated in Figure 21.1. This effect has been verified by behavioral economists with so many products, in so many consumers, and with so many species that it is referred to as the "demand law" (Hursh, 1980, 1984; Hursh et al., 2013; Hursh & Roma, 2016; Koffarnus et al., 2015; Winkler, 1971). Beyond this simple prediction that price increases decrease consumption (which has a "duh" quality to it) the *shape* of the curve—the "demand curve"—shown in Figure 21.1—enjoys substantial empirical support[1] (Gilroy et al., 2021; Hursh & Silberberg, 2008; Koffarnus et al., 2015).

The three things to notice quickly about the demand curve in Figure 21.1 are as follows. First, consumption of the product is completely unconstrained at price zero. This is akin to a daylong session in which the R_T is available for free throughout. In a session like this, the client's consumption will peak at a level reflecting their "intensity" of demand. When unconstrained by price, consumption is limited only by factors such as reinforcer satiety, habituation, or the costs of acquiring surpluses of the reinforcer (McSweeney & Roll, 1998). Second, as the price of the reinforcer increases from left to right along the horizontal axis of Figure 21.1, consumption decreases along an exponentially declining demand curve that, again, enjoys substantial empirical support (Hursh & Silberberg, 2008; Johnson & Bickel, 2006; Madden et al., 2007; Murphy et al., 2011; Oleson & Roberts, 2009). Third, eventually, a high enough price is reached that the consumer is no longer consuming, nor working to acquire, the reinforcer.

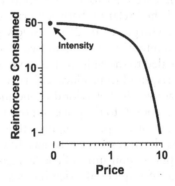

FIGURE 21.1. A demand curve illustrating the effects of price changes on the number of reinforcers consumed per day. Note that the graph's axes are logarithmically scaled.

---

[1]Demand curves are depicted on logarithmic axes to facilitate evaluating the *relative* magnitude of changes in reinforcers consumed and price manipulations (see Gilroy et al., 2020).

Pricing R_T and Its Effects on Appropriate Behavior

Given the orderliness of price effects on consumption of reinforcers, it should be clear that setting the price of R_T is critical in applied behavior analysis. The client, like the consumer, will choose whether to pay the price we have set to acquire our R_T. If the practitioner has set the price too high, appropriate behavior will not occur, and it will appear that the reinforcer is ineffective. If the price of R_T is set too low, then many reinforcers will be consumed, but the client engages in very little appropriate behavior—the intervention is inefficient; more client behavior could be maintained with fewer reinforcers by increasing the price of R_T.

So, how does one find the "just-right" price for R_T? Not much guidance on this is provided in our behavior-analytic textbooks. We are frequently encouraged to increase R_T prices by thinning the schedule of reinforcement from continuous to intermittent. This price change is often implemented so the appropriate behavior may be maintained with fewer artificial reinforcers, and a variety of intermittent schedules of reinforcement are discussed. But elsewhere, we are told that a different type of price increase—increasing the effort needed to acquire R_P—will decrease (problem) behavior. While there are kernels of wisdom in these pieces of advice, they are seemingly at odds with one another (i.e., increasing the price of R_T is supposed to maintain behavior, while increasing the price of R_P is expected to decrease behavior). What is needed is a roadmap that would be useful in predicting the effects of price increases on behavior, something that would do more than warn us about the impending, and dimly lit cliff of "ratio stain." Behavioral economics can further illuminate these warnings with a roadmap to the edge; the road is not straight, but it is predictable.

If the demand curve in Figure 21.1 illustrates the orderly, empirically supported relation between price and consumption, then the amount of responding to acquire those reinforcers must also be orderly.[2] In an applied setting, if the focus of our intervention is on maintaining more instances of appropriate behavior—more academic, independent living, and appropriate social behavior—then this orderly relation between R_T price and response output is critically important.

Figure 21.2 illustrates what we refer to as the "behavioral-economic roadmap"; the predictable, empirically established relation between price changes and response output (e.g., Johnson & Bickel, 2006; Murphy et al., 2011). At low prices, consumption approximates the previously discussed intensity of demand (see "Demand Curve" in figure), but response output (gray curve scaled to the right vertical axis, the "Work Curve") is low. At this price, very little effort is required to produce satiety, or other consumption-limiting states. As R_T price increases across the behavioral-economic roadmap, so does response output as the client/consumer responds to the price-imposed constraint on their consumption. Minimizing reductions in consumption requires that the client/consumer increase response output. Readers who have responded to gasoline price increases by spending more (increased response output) to consume a little less gas per month can empathize.

In Figure 21.2, the range of sequential price increases that decrease consumption but continuously increase response output is referred to as the "inelastic" portion of the roadmap (Gilroy et al., 2020; Hursh, 1980). As prices further increase, a price (P_{max}) is eventually reached at which peak response output (O_{max}) occurs; if price is increased

---

[2] This statement assumes there is a direct relation between how many responses are made and how many reinforcers are earned, as is true of all ratio schedules of reinforcement.

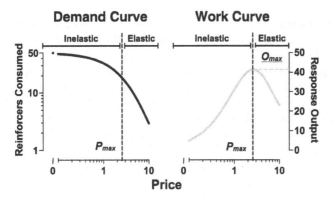

FIGURE 21.2. A prototypical pair of demand (reinforcers consumed) and work (response output) curves, plotted as a function of reinforcer price. Also depicted are the ranges of inelastic and elastic demand, P_{max}, and O_{max} (see text for details).

further still, response output will decrease (Madden et al., 2005, 2007; Murphy et al., 2011). The range of price increases across which consumption and response output both decrease is referred to as the "elastic" portion of the curve. Because considerable empirical evidence supports the demand law and the shape of the curves in Figures 21.1 and 21.2, the behavioral-economic roadmap has predictive utility. This is a set of predictions that the applied behavior analyst may use to foresee the likely effects of changing the price of R_T on appropriate-response output.

At this point, it is worth noting that to many readers, the expected effects of a price increase will not match up with the behavioral-economic roadmap. Price increases, such as increasing the amount of effort required to complete a response and obtain a reinforcer, are expected to decrease response output, not increase it. Indeed, reviews of the response-effort literature mostly attest to the response-suppressing effects of increasing effort requirements (e.g., Friman & Poling, 1995; Wilder et al., 2021). However, this response-suppressing effect of increased effort requirements is difficult to square with our daily experiences. Do we universally respond to a price increase by exerting less effort, or by giving up? Anyone who has exerted more effort when a jar was unusually difficult to open will say "no." Similarly, when the reader has shifted a client's behavior from reinforcement to extinction (the ultimate price increase) or, less drastically, just asked for one more response per reinforcer, has the universal outcome been an immediate reduction in responding? No.

We suggest that at least three factors underlie the apparent discrepancy between the behavioral-economic roadmap and the response-effort literature. First, in some of the studies examining the effects of effort on behavior, the dependent measure is a *consumption* measure—reinforcers obtained—not a response-output measure; that is, these studies report that making a problem behavior more effortful has the beneficial effect of decreasing the number of $R_{p}s$ obtained (Wilder et al., 2021). Such reductions in R_P *consumption* are consistent with the demand law—price increases decrease consumption. What often goes unmeasured, however, is response output (i.e., client efforts, successful or not, in acquiring R_P). If response output was measured and reported, it would be expected to conform to the behavioral-economic roadmap in Figure 21.2, as it does when measured in the lab (see Lamb et al., 2016; Pinkston & Libman, 2017).

Second, price increases will decrease response output if demand for the reinforcer at the higher price is assessed in the elastic portion of the demand curve (see Figure 21.2). This is more likely to occur when responding is assessed at only two prices, which is a common practice in the response-effort literature (e.g., Buckley & Newchok, 2005). Third, and as discussed later in the chapter, price increases can decrease response output if a lower priced substitute reinforcer is concurrently available for a different response (e.g., Cagliani et al., 2019; Shore et al., 1997). All else being equal, behavior is allocated to the lowest-price reinforcer (Herrnstein & Loveland, 1975; Shabani et al., 2009). Therefore, if a cheaper, substitute reinforcer is available, small price increases will have a disproportionate effect on response output. Again, we will discuss this substitute effect in greater detail later in the chapter, when the focus shifts to using R_Ts as alternative reinforcers designed to reduce demand for R_P. For now, we return to the discussion of the potential utility of the roadmap.

As previously mentioned, the behavioral-economic roadmap is useful in applied settings when attempting to predict the effects of R_T price changes on response output. But a second factor that affects the decision to implement a price change is supplier costs; that is, suppliers of products must consider how costly it is to produce the product; they must set the price of the product at a level that allows them to recover their costs. Analogously, the applied behavior analyst will consider the costs of bringing R_T to the client. These costs comprise primarily the labor involved in monitoring the desired response and delivering R_T when the price contingency is met. If therapists, parents, and so forth, do not have the capacity to reinforce the desired behavior every time it occurs, then the price of R_T must be increased, lest the return on investment not justify the expense of supplying R_T. The twofold good news provided by the behavioral-economic roadmap is that (1) price increases will decrease consumption of R_T (increasing the practicality of the intervention for therapists, parents, etc.) and (2), as long as the higher price is at or below P_{max}, the behavioral-economic roadmap predicts an increase in the output of client appropriate behavior. Thus, when the goal is to increase appropriate behavior, it would be useful to know the R_T price corresponding to P_{max}. Not only is this the price at which R_T is most efficiently arranged, but it is also the "just right" price at which peak response output (O_{max}) is observed.

Finding P_{max}

Although the inverted U-shape of the behavioral-economic roadmap is lawful and predictable, its height (rising to the point of O_{max}) and span from zero to P_{max} is not; that is, one cannot easily predict how sensitive the behavior of an individual client will be to R_T price increases. For suppliers of products in the natural marketplace in which we all shop, consumers' willingness to pay can be surveyed by asking them how much of the product they would purchase under hypothetically different prices. Behavioral economists studying substance-use disorders have used this validated survey method to quantify demand for drugs, the likely impact of contemplated price changes, and the predictive relation between demand and treatment outcomes (Amlung et al., 2012; Mackillop et al., 2016; Reed et al., 2020; Zvorsky et al., 2019). To our knowledge, this "purchase task" methodology has not been explored in applied behavior-analytic settings with clients who have the verbal skills needed to make prospective decisions about how much of a reinforcer they would consume at a range of hypothetical prices. Given the need to know the height and span parameters of the behavioral-economic roadmap, both for therapeutic reinforcers and, as discussed later in the chapter, the reinforcers that maintain problem behavior, this may be a fruitful area of future inquiry.

A second approach to identifying the height (O_{max}) and span (zero to P_{max}) of the behavioral-economic roadmap is to actually increase the price of R_T and measure the effects on response output. This was the approach taken by Delmendo et al. (2009) in their study of demand for edibles reinforcers among typically developing 3- to 6-year-olds. As illustrated in the top panels of Figure 21.3, when price was increased from two to four responses per reinforcer, Elijah and Anna defended their reinforcer consumption by increasing their response output (inelastic demand), but further price increases decreased response output (elastic demand). These data suggest that the location of P_{max} was somewhere in the shaded area of the graph; further data at additional prices could more precisely identify P_{max}, if that were important to treatment efficacy/efficiency.

For the remaining participants, Keelan and Elizabeth, demand for the reinforcer was elastic throughout the price range explored (i.e., each price hike decreased response output and consumption, which is not shown). The shaded zone in which P_{max} might be located for these participants is speculative; fixed-ratio (FR) 2 might prove to be the P_{max} for these individuals with these edible reinforcers, but without additional data, one cannot be certain. Presumably the inverted-U-shaped behavioral economic roadmap would have been observed had lower prices been explored; for example, if the cost–benefit ratio was one response for five edibles (price = 0.2), then it is likely that response output would decline below the peaks seen in Figure 21.3.

The inverted U-shape of the behavioral-economic roadmap illustrates the importance of at least approximately knowing the price at which demand will shift from

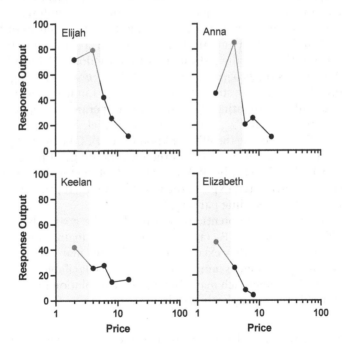

FIGURE 21.3. Response output of four children as a function of edible reinforcer prices. Data replotted based on Delmendo et al. (2009).

inelastic to elastic (P_{max}). If the edible reinforcers in Figure 21.3 had been R_T's used in a behavioral intervention (which they were not), then it would be important to know that for Elijah and Anna, more appropriate behavior could be maintained as R_T prices increased from 0 to P_{max}, which was approximately four responses per edible. This "just-right" price of R_T allows us to maximize appropriate responding while delivering fewer reinforcers than at lower prices, thereby enhancing the efficiency and practicality of the intervention.

An important detail when determining demand curves is that consumption cannot be artificially capped by the experimenter (e.g., by ending the session after 5 minutes or 20 reinforcers, whichever comes first). Finding P_{max} requires that the only constraint on consumption be a price constraint, not an experimenter-imposed constraint. Thus, the best method is to set the price and leave it in place for an entire day, leaving it to the client to decide how often they will emit the appropriate response and "consume" R_T at that price. As prices are gradually increased, the experimenter monitors response output, looking for progressively smaller increases in response output with successive price increases. As the response output curve begins to flatten, we know we are approaching P_{max} and nearing peak response output (O_{max}). At that point, there may be little reason to attempt further price increases. We are sensitive to the criticism that this assessment method may be impractical, but we will also attempt to plant a seed: If we expect our interventions to work throughout the day, then perhaps we should evaluate reinforcer efficacy at a comparable timescale.

Having said this, a third, more practical strategy is to arrange a progressive-ratio (PR) schedule (Roane, 2008). This strategy can aid in approximately locating P_{max}, but without obtaining a complete response-output curve. To implement the PR schedule, R_T is first arranged at a very low price (typically FR 1). After each reinforcer is obtained, the ratio requirement is progressively increased (e.g., FR 1, 2, 4, 8, and so on[3]). The assessment concludes when the participant fails to respond for a specified duration (Jarmolowicz & Lattal, 2010) or they verbally indicate that they are done (Delmendo et al., 2009). The outcome of interest is the *progressive-ratio* (PR) *breakpoint*—the highest ratio value completed before the individual stops working for R_T. Limited evidence suggests PR breakpoints are useful in estimating P_{max}. In human operant and applied settings, PR breakpoints are correlated with P_{max} (e.g., Johnson & Bickel, 2006; Reed et al., 2009) but they do not *specify* P_{max}. Because the PR breakpoint specifies the highest price completed before giving up, it is a price likely to fall in the inelastic range of prices in Figure 21.2; P_{max} is presumably higher than the breakpoint. Those looking for P_{max} might set the price at the breakpoint and, thereafter, explore the effects of gradual price changes, in accord with the guidelines of the preceding paragraph.

This third strategy is also potentially useful when the goal is behavior reduction. Identifying the PR breakpoint for R_P (again, the reinforcer maintaining problem behavior) and then arranging prices that exceed that breakpoint may redirect behavior away from R_P and toward R_T seeking, assuming the latter is (1) available at a lower price and (2) substitutes for R_P. This approach may offer a practical solution in cases when caregivers are unable or unlikely to completely withhold R_P.

---

[3]A variety of strategies have been used to increase the response requirement in a PR schedule. The progression provided here is informed by Weber's law. In a nutshell, the difference between FR 1 and FR 2 is far more discriminable than the difference between FR 100 and FR 101 (despite an identical change in the amount of the response requirement). Therefore, the change should be proportional throughout.

One caveat to this third strategy, when applied to the pricing of problem behavior, comes from the learned-industriousness literature (Eisenberger, 1992). A large number of studies with human and nonhuman subjects reveals that systematic experience with progressively increasing effort requirements can increase "willingness" to work to obtain a reinforcer (Eisenberger et al., 1979; Eisenberger & Adornetto, 1986; Peck & Madden, 2021). Thus, when assessing the PR breakpoint for R_P, we suggest doing so only once or twice—further exposure to the progressively increasing prices that comprise the PR may inadvertently provide participants with industriousness training. Similarly, after determining the PR breakpoint for R_P, it may be important to abruptly set its price above that breakpoint; that is, do not gradually increase the price of R_P. A drastic price increase may decrease the probability that R_P will be acquired, and industrious R_P seeking reinforced.

DeLeon et al. (2000) provides a positive example of this strategy. They found the breakpoint-exceeding price for R_P was 20 aggressive responses. At this R_P price, the client reallocated their efforts to appropriate behavior (mands), which produced the same reinforcer at a lower price (FR 1). At lower R_P prices (i.e., FR 2, FR 5, FR 10), aggression was the more prevalent response. A subsequent evaluation confirmed that treatment with functional communication training (FCT) was effective when the price of R_P was FR 20, but not when it was FR 2. Identifying the PR breakpoint for R_P also may be useful for determining whether a planned intervention is likely to be effective within the context of naturally occurring schedules of reinforcement for problem behavior.

Preference Assessments and P_{max}

In applied cases in which it would be helpful to know the height (O_{max}) and span (zero to P_{max}) of the behavioral-economic roadmap, the methods discussed thus far may be impractical, taking time away from the core mission of positively influencing client behavior (Poling, 2010). Practicality is important in applied settings and, perhaps for this reason, when applied behavior analysts evaluate the likelihood that a stimulus will maintain appropriate behavior, they use a stimulus preference assessment (DeLeon & Iwata, 1996; Fisher et al., 1992; Pace et al., 1985). A variety of procedures are available, as are excellent reviews on the relative merits of these methods (Haddock & Hagopian, 2020; Kang et al., 2013). In most preference assessments, the individual makes a simple response (FR 1) to choose their preferred item among several goods/activities (i.e., potential reinforcers). The items reliably chosen first are identified as high-preferred (HP) stimuli, while those reliably foregone are classified as low-preferred (LP) stimuli. In between are the stimuli filling the LP to HP continuum (i.e., the rank-ordered list, or "preference hierarchy").[4]

Is a stimulus's position within this preference hierarchy useful in predicting which stimulus will maintain a higher peak response-output (O_{max}) or a wider span of R_T prices across which demand will prove inelastic? Can we use the preference assessment to set the "just-right" price (P_{max}) of R_T, so as to maximize therapeutic behavior while increasing the practicality of the intervention? To our knowledge, no studies have evaluated the ability of a preference assessment to predict P_{max}; indeed, it is difficult to imagine how a

---

[4]It is worth noting that the results of a preference assessment make no predictions about which stimulus will be consumed in the greatest quantity, when little or no constraints are placed on consumption (demand intensity; see Figure 21.1). Because rapid satiety will make R_T less useful in many applied settings, this is a limitation on the utility of the results of a stimulus preference assessment.

preference assessment could do more than rank-order predicted P_{max} values among the stimuli. Considerable research, however, has evaluated the predictive validity of the preference assessment in maintaining operant behavior, sometimes at escalating prices. We turn our attention to those findings next.

Three preparations are most commonly used when evaluating the predictive validity of a stimulus preference assessment: (1) single-operant experiments with R_T available at a low-price, (2) single-operant PR experiments, or (3) choice preparations with escalating prices. Figure 21.4 shows the first of these. Specifically, the x-axis shows the percent preference for each stimulus, as assessed in the stimulus preference assessment, and the y-axis shows response-output in a single-operant preparation that puts minimal constraint on access to the stimuli (e.g., FR 1; Higbee et al., 1999; Horrocks & Higbee, 2008; Lee et al., 2010; Mangum et al., 2012; Nix, 2016; Paramore & Higbee, 2005).[5] Each panel shows data from all participants in the study (each with a unique symbol) and all sessions. Across these studies, the relation between preference and subsequent

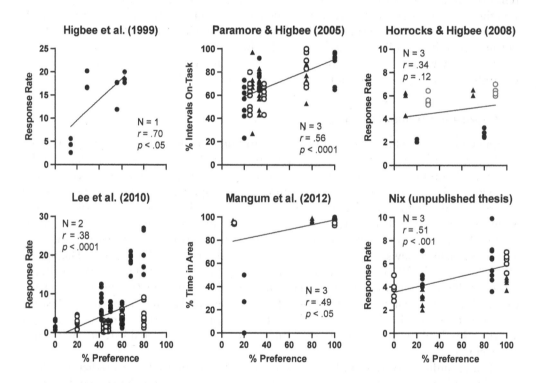

FIGURE 21.4. Response rate or time spent in a reinforcement area, plotted as a function of percent preference as assessed by a stimulus preference assessment. Spearman correlation coefficients based on all participants' data (different symbols denote different individuals) in all sessions reported.

---

[5] Two frequently cited studies are omitted from Figure 21.4 (Francisco et al., 2008; Roscoe et al., 1999). In both studies, only the low-preference (LP) stimulus is evaluated in a single-operant arrangement. Prior papers citing these studies have compared those single-operant LP response rates with concurrent-operant high-preference (HP) rates, which is an inappropriate comparison given that the latter rates will be influenced by responding allocated to the LP alternative.

responding is positive (Spearman's *r*), although in Horrocks and Higbee (2008), one of the three participants' data rendered the correlation nonsignificant at the group level. In Mangum et al. (2012), the opposite is true—the correlation is significant, but this is due to one out of three participants.

These positive relations make it clear that there is predictive utility in conducting a preference assessment, provided that our goal is to maintain appropriate behavior at a very low price. Sometimes this is all that is needed, and if this is the case, then the preference assessment can be an evidence-based practice (DeLeon & Iwata, 1996; Fisher et al., 1992). But what is the relation between single-operant response rates under an FR 1 and response persistence at higher prices (i.e., the height and span of the roadmap)? As noted some time ago by Tustin (1994) and Hursh (1980), the picture here is mixed. In many cases, responding at a low price is a poor predictor of continued responding at higher prices. This was illustrated in a study in which rats worked in a single-operant context for either grain-based pellets or, in a different phase, a fat solution (Madden et al., 2007). All six rats responded at higher rates for the fat solution when it was available on an FR 1, but as prices increased, all of the rats worked harder for high-priced food than for high-priced fat. Indeed, at some prices in the upper range, pellets maintained considerable responding, whereas fat maintained none at all.

Lest the reader wonder if these findings are unique to rats, fats, or studies conducted in one of our labs, this same outcome was reported with cigarette smokers by Johnson and Bickel (2006). At the lowest price (one puff per response or, in a different phase, $0.08 per response) all five participants responded at higher rates for money than for puffs. However, as price increased, all five smokers reached a price at which they continued to make hundreds of responses for puffs but, in separate sessions, none at all for money. In summary, preference assessment outcomes are often valid in predicting response rates at low prices, but those rates may be a poor predictor of response persistence at higher prices (for additional supporting evidence, see Bickel & Madden, 1999; Elsmore et al., 1980; Foster et al., 2009; Hursh, 1984; Jacobs & Bickel, 1999; Johnson & Bickel, 2006; Shahan et al., 1999; Tan & Hackenberg, 2015; Tustin, 1994).

Which takes us to the second dependent measure used to evaluate the predictive validity of stimulus preference assessments—the previously defined PR breakpoint. Is a stimulus's position within the preference hierarchy predictive of its PR breakpoint? Figure 21.5 shows the results of 12 studies that have evaluated this question; the outcomes are mixed. Glover et al. (2008) reported a strong-positive correlation between relative preferences (*x*-axis) and PR breakpoints (*y*-axis), but for two of their three participants, the LP stimulus was almost never selected in the stimulus-preference assessment. It is unsurprising then that the HP stimulus (selected 100% of the time in the preference assessment) had a higher breakpoint than a strongly unpreferred stimulus (for similar outcomes, see Fiske et al., 2014; Jerome & Sturmey, 2008). The remaining panels better fill in the continuum of the preference hierarchy between LP and HP stimuli (Call et al., 2012; DeLeon et al., 2009; Hoffmann et al., 2017; Kenzer et al., 2013; Linn, 2016; Nix, 2016; Penrod et al., 2008; Reed et al., 2009; Trosclair-Lasserre et al., 2008) and the relation is less uniformly positive. That three datasets in Figure 21.5 showing no relation between preferences-assessment outcomes and PR breakpoints were unpublished (separate theses by Linn and Nix) raises the possibility of a file-drawer problem; that is, other datasets with nonsignificant correlations exist but remain unpublished.

In other published studies using PR schedules, stimuli that were equally preferred in the preference assessment later proved to have very different PR breakpoints (Roane et al.,

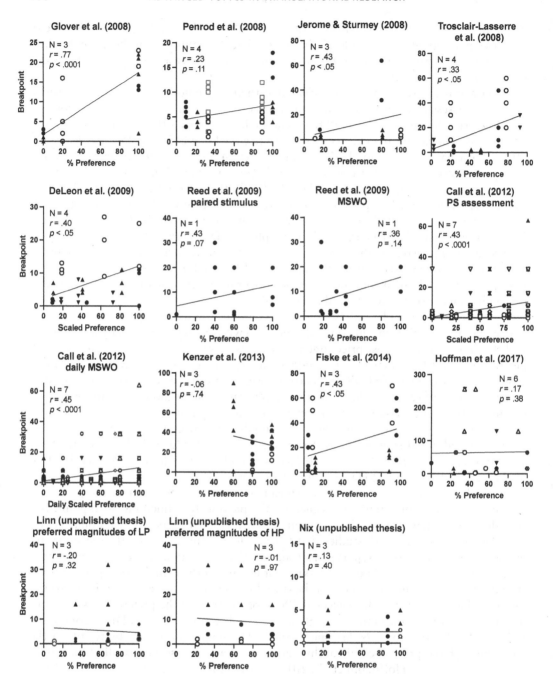

FIGURE 21.5. Progressive-ratio breakpoints plotted as a function of percent preference, as assessed by a stimulus preference assessment. Spearman correlation coefficients based on all participants' data (different symbols denote different individuals) in all sessions reported.

2001; Trosclair-Lasserre et al., 2008; data not shown in Figure 21.5); that is, preference was a poor predictor of which reinforcer would be reliably purchased at a higher price. Of applied importance, in Roane et al. (2001), the more inelastic reinforcer proved more effective in reducing problem behavior in a subsequent intervention. In summary, the results of a stimulus-preference assessment may have limited utility as a predictor of the ability of a reinforcer to maintain single-operant behavior when the R_T price increases; that is, the preference assessment tells us very little about the height (O_{max}) and span (zero to P_{max}) of the behavioral-economic roadmap.

And this takes us to the third dependent measure commonly used in evaluating the predictive validity of the stimulus preference assessment—choice. Two studies that we are aware of have evaluated choice between LP and HP stimuli under concurrent FR-1 schedules (Francisco et al., 2008; Roscoe et al., 1999). To our reading, these tests have limited utility given their close resemblance to the preference assessment itself; that is, in both phases, the participant is choosing between reinforcers available at minimal cost. Further limiting utility, an R_T will not be asked to compete with an LP stimulus. Instead, it must compete against an R_P that is effective enough to warrant an intervention.

A more useful test of the predictive validity of the preference assessment is the concurrent PR schedule arrangement. Here, the prices of both concurrently available stimuli start low (e.g., FR 1) and independently escalate (FR 2, 4, 8, etc.) after a reinforcer is obtained. In each session, two breakpoints are obtained; therefore, from a practical perspective, the concurrent PR arrangement is a tool for quickly identifying the most price inelastic of two potentially effective R_T's.

To date, only three studies have used concurrent PR schedules to evaluate the predictive validity of the stimulus preference assessment (left three panels of Figure 21.6). In two studies, stronger preferences were predictive of higher breakpoints (Francisco et al., 2008; Glover et al., 2008), but as was the case before, the continuum between LP and HP stimuli was not examined in those studies. In Kenzer et al. (2013), which compared familiar and unfamiliar HP stimuli, preference was not predictive of concurrent PR breakpoints. More research is clearly needed in which the LP to HP continuum is evaluated under the concurrent PR procedure.

The fourth panel in Figure 21.6 shows the results of the oft-cited Tustin (1994) study. Here a single participant (S3) chose between two different computer-generated stimuli, access to both on an FR 1. Because this approximates a preference assessment, this participant's preferences for these stimuli are shown on the x-axis (e.g., 41.9% preference for the LP stimulus). Thereafter, the prices of the two concurrently available stimuli increased in unison (not independently) between sessions (FR 2–20). The y-axis shows the total responses made to obtain these stimuli at these higher prices. This quasi-preference assessment was not predictive of responding at any of the higher prices (see DeLeon et al., 1997, for similar outcomes with edible reinforcers).

To summarize, the empirical evidence reviewed here suggests that preference assessments can be useful when the task is to identify a reinforcer that will maintain behavior at low prices (Figure 21.4). They can also help to rule out LP stimuli that are unlikely to maintain much behavior when R_T prices increase (Figure 21.5). But if the goal is to discriminate among several non-LP stimuli, to find the R_T that will maintain the most behavior as its price increases (i.e., the zero to P_{max} span of the roadmap), then the record is mixed at best (Reed et al., 2015). We can see this at a glance by holding a hand over the left halves of the graphs in Figures 21.5 and 21.6. When we exclude the LP stimuli, the

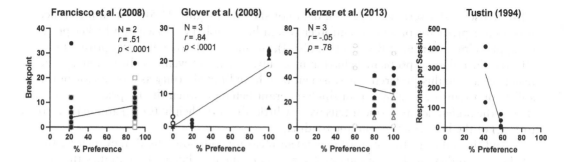

FIGURE 21.6. Left three panels show concurrent progressive-ratio breakpoints plotted as a function of the results of a preference assessment; details as in Figures 21.4 and 21.5. The right panel (Tustin, 1994) shows the inverse relation between stimulus preference at concurrent FR 1 and response output in subsequent sessions when the prices of the two stimuli were simultaneously increased.

relation between preference (x-axis) and the highest price that will be paid for R_T (y-axis) is not at all clear.

If preference assessments are not predictive of a client's response to increases in the price of R_T, can behavioral economics address this shortcoming? If addressing it means supplying a rapid test allowing the applied behavior analyst to accurately predict which contingent consequence will best maintain behavior when prices are inevitably increased, then no, it cannot. What it offers instead is the orderliness of the behavioral-economic roadmap—R_T price increases from zero throughout a range of positive values will increase response output until it peaks at P_{max}; thereafter, additional price increases will decrease responding for R_T. As previously discussed in the section "Finding P_{max}," the most efficient method for estimating the approximate location of P_{max} has yet to be identified and empirically evaluated. This may prove to be an important area of research in applied behavior analysis, one designed to address the shortcomings of the preference assessment.

The Marketplace in Which R_T and R_P Compete

To this point in the chapter, the focus has been on the effects of price changes on single-operant behavior. How much behavior will a reinforcer maintain when its price increases; at what price does response output peak; what is the "just-right" price of an R_T? However, these questions ignore a reality of the applied setting—therapeutic behavior maintained by R_T often occurs in a context of choice in which undesirable, problem behavior is maintained by R_P. Such choice contexts resemble the economic marketplace in which products/services compete for the limited resources of the consumer. In this marketplace, consumers compare the relative prices of products/services (i.e., their costs and benefits) and, *all else being equal,* they choose the cheaper product/service (lower costs and/or greater benefits). Behavior analysts are well aware of this relative pricing effect; it is built into their quantitative model of choice, the matching law (Herrnstein, 1970).

But as noted by behavioral economists (e.g., Green & Freed, 1993; Green & Rachlin, 1991; Hursh, 1980; Tustin, 1994), the "all else being equal" clause of the sentence above is not always true; indeed, outside the lab, it is rarely true. The rats and pigeons in the experiments summarized by Herrnstein (1970) chose between two identical reinforcers—food and food—so "all else being equal" was true and they preferred the supplier offering food at a lower price. But in applied settings, our clients are often choosing between two nonidentical reinforcers; for example, when the reinforcer maintaining problem behavior can't be identified or controlled. If the "all else being equal" clause is violated, then introducing an R_T to compete with R_P may fail to work as expected. Such outcomes may lead us to conclude that R_T is an ineffective reinforcer, but an alternative conclusion is possible—R_T does not *substitute* for R_P.

In behavioral economics, reinforcers are known to interact in a variety of ways, and one of those ways is as a *substitute*. These reinforcer interactions are considered "cross-price" effects, meaning we can determine the kind of interaction between reinforcers by examining what happens when the price of Commodity A increases while Commodity B remains fixed. There are two separate stimulus relations that can be identified in cross-price analyses: *substitutes* and *complements*. Substitutes and complements both exist within continuums ranging from independent to fully substitutable or complementary, with partial interactions in between (interested readers can learn more about these relations and how to quantify them by reading Imam, 1993). Understanding the potential interactions of R_T and R_P within these stimulus classes can help inform how the behavioral-economic roadmap can be used in a context of choice.

When reinforcers are in all ways identical, they are perfect substitutes: They are functionally identical; they serve the same "purpose"; they are readily traded for one another; they address the same establishing operation (EO), just as the food and food reinforcers in experiments summarized by Herrnstein (1970) identically addressed the animals' hunger. When R_T perfectly substitutes for R_P, the matching law makes accurate predictions; all else is equal, so behavior is differentially allocated to the lower priced alternative.[6] This prediction is illustrated in the form of the behavioral-economic roadmap in Figure 21.7. Here the behavioral output of interest is problem behavior maintained by R_P. At baseline (dashed curve), when R_T is unavailable, the height (O_{max}) and span (zero to P_{max}) of the roadmap indicate demand for R_P is strong (strong enough to warrant a behavioral intervention). If the R_T used in therapy perfectly substitutes for R_P, then the height and the span of the roadmap will both decrease, shifting the curve down and to the left. The extent to which this happens depends on the relative price of R_T. Relatively lower priced R_Ts are frequently arranged in applied settings by putting minimal constraint on the acquisition of R_T (e.g., FR 1) and increasing the price of R_P; the latter is often accomplished by increasing the effort required to obtain R_P (Wilder et al., 2021) or by imperfectly implementing an extinction contingency (DeLeon et al., 2000; Worsdell et al., 2000). When the R_T perfectly substitutes for R_P, problem behavior becomes more sensitive to R_P price increases because, for all intents and purposes, the exact same reinforcer (i.e., a perfect substitute) may be obtained at a lower price. Such differential

---

[6]It is interesting that in the previously discussed DeLeon et al. (2000) case study that R_T and R_P were identical (1-minute access to toys) but aggressive behavior predominated unless the price of aggression-produced toy access was increased to FR 20. This might be due to differences in the duration of history of reinforcement. Because of the extended history of reinforced problem behavior, it may have become habitual (i.e., shifted from consequence control to antecedent stimulus control of "automatic" responding). The habit-formation literature may have important implications for applied behavior analysis (Gardner, 2015).

reinforcement strategies have proven effective in applied settings for decades (Bonner & Borrero, 2018; Chowdhury & Benson, 2011; Petscher et al., 2009).

But what happens when "all else" is not equal, when R_T does not perfectly substitute for R_P? Well, it depends on the interaction between R_T and R_P. If R_T *partially substitutes* for R_P, then the shift illustrated in Figure 21.7 will be diminished. An everyday example may help us to see why. Imagine that you are cooking a new recipe and it calls for fresh peppermint (R_P). You go to the fresh herbs market to buy some but find the price of peppermint is a bit more than you hoped to pay. So, you do a quick Google search asking, "What substitutes for peppermint?" The answer, tarragon (R_T), is available at a much lower price. You find it hard to believe that tarragon would perfectly match the taste of peppermint (if it did, it would function as a perfect substitute and you would buy no peppermint at all), so you buy the amount of herbs needed for the recipe but substitute R_T for half of the R_P that you originally planned to buy.

Two applied implications of partial substitute relations between R_P and R_T are worth considering. First, if our therapeutic R_T only partially substitutes for R_P, then in order for it to attract client behavior, it will have to be the much less expensive reinforcer; the less it functions as a perfect substitute, the lower its price will need to be relative to R_P. Second, if R_T is only partially substituting for R_P, then some consideration should be given to why it is not a perfect substitute for R_P. What functional characteristic is it missing? If that characteristic can be identified and ameliorated, it may allow the applied behavior analyst to increase the price of R_T and, thereby, maintain more appropriate behavior than before.

The Shore et al. (1997) study provides a possible example of this partial substitute relation. In their study, continuous, free access to preferred leisure materials nearly eliminated stereotypical self-injurious behavior (SIB) in three adults with developmental disabilities. The R_T for object manipulation may have partially substituted for the R_P for SIB. This treatment effect vanished, however, when the experimenters increased the price of R_T (e.g., by increasing the physical effort necessary to engage in object manipulation). Again, the less fully R_T substitutes for R_P, the more it must enjoy a large price advantage to be competitive in the reinforcer marketplace.

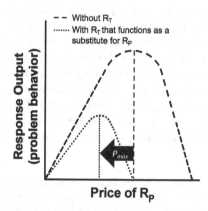

FIGURE 21.7. An illustration of the behavioral-economic roadmap applied to problem behavior maintained by R_P. When a therapeutic reinforcer (R_T) that substitutes for R_P is made contingent upon appropriate behavior, the roadmap (and P_{max}) shifts downward and to the left.

Continuing our journey through the categories of reinforcer interactions, we leave the zone of partial substitutes and enter the *independents* zone. These reinforcers do not interact; that is, if problem behavior is maintained by R_P and the R_T is an independent, it will have no effect whatsoever on demand for R_P. To revisit the grocery store analogy, if R_P is a bunch of peppermint, then an *independent* R_T is a toothbrush. In this instance, R_T in no way addresses the EO that sent us to the grocery store. Regardless of the price of the independent R_T, the height and span of the behavioral-economic roadmap for R_P will be unchanged. In an applied setting, an HP stimulus identified within a stimulus-preference assessment will have no impact on problem behavior if that R_T is in an *independent* relation with R_P; that is, demand for R_P will not be more (or less) elastic when R_T is concurrently available, regardless of its price.

The final category of reinforcer interactions is, perhaps, the one least considered in applied settings—*complements*. By definition, a *complementary relation* exists between reinforcers when the price of one reinforcer (e.g., cigarettes) increases and consumption of that reinforcer *and* its complement (e.g., alcohol) decreases, despite the price of the complement being unchanged (Hursh et al., 2013). But from an applied perspective, a different framing of complements is in order. Complements are goods that are consumed together, preferably in a constant ratio (e.g., two parts cereal to one part milk). Having the complementary good on hand (cereal) increases the essential value of the other good (milk). If the price of milk increases, then (1) consumption of milk will decrease, (2) consumption of cereal will decrease, and (3) responding is reallocated to the *more* expensive reinforcer (milk). Note that effect (3) is the opposite of what would occur if milk was a substitute for cereal.

Chips and salsa are in a similar complementary relation. They are consumed together, and if the price of chips increases, then (1) consumption of chips will decrease, (2) consumption of salsa will decrease, and (3) responding will be reallocated to chip-seeking behavior. Conversely, if the price of chips decreases (e.g., the waiter brings a basket of chips but no salsa), then the value of salsa increases and, so do salsa-seeking behaviors that were absent moments earlier (e.g., flagging down another waiter, entering the kitchen to ask for help).

As illustrated in Figure 21.8, if R_T is in a complementary relation with R_P, then the availability of R_T will have an unintended effect—it will increase demand for R_P; shifting P_{max} to the right and increasing peak response output for R_P. This outcome was illustrated in an experiment conducted by Spiga et al. (2005; data presented in Hursh et al., 2013). In their experiment, human smokers could work for cigarette puffs (R_P) across a range of prices. In one condition, cigarettes alone were available. In a second condition, alcoholic beverages (R_T, if you will) were available for purchase. Because cigarettes and alcohol are consumed together, one enhancing the value of the other, the availability of R_T increased R_P consumption and, as illustrated in Figure 21.8, increased R_P-seeking behavior throughout the range of cigarette prices explored (for replications with these and other reinforcers, see Green & Rachlin, 1991; Hursh, 1978; Rachlin et al., 1976; Spiga et al., 2005). Obviously, an applied behavior analyst would never seek to reduce cigarette smoking by opening a bottle of scotch. The point is that if, unbeknownst to the therapist, R_T is in a complementary relation with R_P, then the well-meaning introduction of R_T to the therapeutic setting could have the unintended effect of increasing problem behavior. Such a relation may have been demonstrated by Van Camp et al. (2000), who found that providing access to certain types of toys or to social interaction increased levels of two children's problem behavior that was maintained by automatic reinforcement.

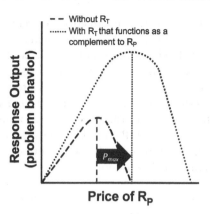

FIGURE 21.8. An illustration of the behavioral-economic roadmap applied to problem behavior maintained by RP. When a therapeutic reinforcer (RT) that complements RP is made contingent upon appropriate behavior, the roadmap (and Pmax) is expected to shift upward and to the right.

Figure 21.8 might be interpreted as suggesting that complements should be avoided in therapeutic settings. However, we think applied behavior analysts could use them skillfully. Specifically, once an R_T that substitutes for R_P has been identified, the practitioner should consider things that might be in a complementary relation with R_T: Is there something with which R_T is typically consumed? If complements enhance the reinforcing efficacy of the commodity with which they are usually consumed (like salsa does for chips), then finding a complement to R_T could enhance the efficacy of that therapeutic reinforcer. For example, points within a video game are "consumed" along with the game narrative (e.g., the hero's journey). The contingent delivery of points within this narrative enhances the fun of the game (e.g., when points are used to purchase new and better equipment that aids in the hero's quest and, complementarily, enhances the value of points. This complementary relation between a game narrative and point reinforcers has been used to increase children's healthy eating and exercise in schools (Jones et al., 2014; Joyner et al., 2017, 2019; Wengreen et al., 2021).

How does one identify complementary reinforcers? The advice given by economists is highly technical but it can be oversimplified by suggesting one *look for goods and services that, when access to them is unconstrained, are consumed together, often in a constant ratio.* To stay within the realm of gaming, some games are played alone (solitaire) where other games are played socially (Words with Friends). In the latter, the game and online social contact are in a complementary relation. Imposing a monetary cost on playing Words with Friends will decrease time spent playing the game *and* online social contact. From an applied perspective, if access to an iPad game like Risk is the R_T, then the value of that R_T might be increased by making a human opponent available (a social-contact *complement*) instead of playing the game against the less challenging artificial intelligence. In therapeutic settings, measuring simultaneous consumption of putative R_Ts and R_Ps in a free-operant arrangement (Roane et al., 1998) might be an efficient way to identify potential complementary reinforcers. Suppose, for example, that a child rarely plays with a toy kitchen in the absence of engaging with a doll as a pretend "chef," or vice versa. Such information might be useful for enhancing the reinforcing value of either R_T by ensuring that its complement is available. We recognize the challenge of identifying complements to R_Ts, and hope this chapter functions as an EO that generates new research that seeks more systematic means of identifying complements to our therapeutic R_Ts.

Open and Closed Economies

Readers may be familiar with the behavioral-economic concept of open and closed economies (Hursh, 1980). The distilled-down version is that demand for R_T is diminished in an open economy, when free or low-cost access to the R_T is provided elsewhere, relative to a closed economy, when the only way to acquire R_T is to satisfy the contingency of reinforcement.[7] Connecting this to a previous section of this chapter, free or low-cost access to R_T outside of therapy has the effect of decreasing effort expended during therapy, because the extramural R_T perfectly substitutes for the therapist-provided R_T. In an applied evaluation of this prediction, Roane et al. (2005) found that individuals with developmental disabilities engaged in more task responding under PR schedules when R_T could only be earned during work sessions (closed economy) than when unearned R_Ts were available after the completion of the work session (open economy). Effort was impacted during therapeutic sessions even when extramural R_T was not available until 4 hours later. The implication of open and closed economies is clear—applied behavior analysts should create a monopoly on the client's access to R_T.

But this advice is qualified in important ways by the prior discussion of substitutes and complements. Perhaps the behavior analyst has cornered the market on R_T, but a free or low-cost nonidentical reinforcer available elsewhere partially substitutes for R_T. If so, then, despite our best efforts to create a monopoly, this substitute good will decrease demand for R_T (see Figure 21.7). Kodak et al. (2007) evaluated this phenomenon within the context of choice for concurrently available food items. Children with developmental disabilities completed more academic tasks to earn a less preferred but (apparently) substitutable reinforcer when the therapist increased the price of the more preferred reinforcer. However, they were less willing to expend effort to receive the costlier (more preferred) reinforcer when the substitutable reinforcer was available for free after the session. Therefore, the best R_Ts are those for which there are few substitutes; the ubiquitous use of access to the iPad may be an example of an R_T with few nonidentical substitutes.

But if the free reinforcer is an independent, then it will have no effect at all on the ability of R_T to maintain the desired behavior. Most interestingly, making a complementary reinforcer available will, at least theoretically, have the *desired effect* of enhancing the efficacy of R_T. We are aware of no empirical tests of this theoretical proposition but, once again, hope this chapter serves as an EO to inspire such investigations. In summary, it may not be as simple as open-economy bad, closed-economy good—it depends on how the other reinforcer interacts with R_T.

---

[7] The concept of open and closed economies is more complicated than this distilled version. Interested readers are encouraged to read (Hursh, 1980).

Summary and Conclusions

Reinforcement is an essential component of therapeutic interventions in applied behavior analysis. Knowledge drawn from behavioral economics indicates that the efficacy of therapeutic reinforcement contingencies to promote optimal clinical outcomes depends on the complex interplay between demand for R_T and R_P, relative pricing of those reinforcers, and potential interactions between those and other reinforcers available in the "marketplace." Familiarity with these findings may better prepare applied behavior analysts to answer questions like the following:

> *What reinforcement schedule for appropriate behavior will be both effective and practical for caregivers to implement?*
> *How can I arrange reinforcers for appropriate behavior so that they will compete with those maintaining problem behavior?*

Applied behavior analysts are well trained in behavior-change methodology, but existing methods make it difficult to accurately predict reinforcer efficacy when schedules must inevitably be leaned out. Decades of basic, translational, and applied studies have informed the behavioral-economic roadmap shown in Figure 21.2. The general shape of the roadmap may help practicing behavior analysts navigate the future of an intervention, finding the "just right" price at which optimal levels of appropriate behavior (response output) may be efficiently maintained. These roadmaps may help identify reinforcer interactions in substitute or complementary relations (Figures 21.7 and 21.8). We have discussed some ways in which identifying these interactions may help to amplify behavior-change plans, to understand why some plans are ineffective, and to suggest novel plans in need of clinical evaluation.

For now, clinicians must draw inspiration from the findings of basic and translational research on behavioral-economic principles, because applied research on these relations remains in its infancy. We hope this chapter provides guidance/inspiration for those engaged in clinical practice and those planning the next stages of their clinical research.

ACKNOWLEDGMENT

We wish to thank Joseph Lambert of Vanderbilt University for helpful comments on a draft of this chapter.

REFERENCES

Amlung, M. T., Acker, J., Stojek, M. K., Murphy, J. G., & MacKillop, J. (2012). Is talk "cheap"?: An initial investigation of the equivalence of alcohol purchase task performance for hypothetical and actual rewards. *Alcoholism: Clinical and Experimental Research, 36*(4), 716–724.

Ariely, D., Gneezy, U., Loewenstein, G., & Ma-zar, N. (2009). Large stakes and big mistakes. *Review of Economic Studies, 76*(2), 451–469.

Bickel, W. K., & Madden, G. J. (1999). A comparison of measures of relative reinforcing efficacy and behavioral economics: Cigarettes and money in smokers. *Behavioural Pharmacology, 10*(6–7), 627–637.

Bonner, A. C., & Borrero, J. C. (2018). Differential reinforcement of low rate schedules reduce severe problem behavior. *Behavior Modification, 42*(5), 747–764.

Buckley, S. D., & Newchok, D. K. (2005). Differential impact of response effort within a response chain on use of mands in a student with autism. *Research in Developmental Disabilities, 26*(1), 77–85.

Cagliani, R. R., Ayres, K. M., Ringdahl, J. E., & Whiteside, E. (2019). The effect of delay to reinforcement and response effort on response variability for individuals with autism spectrum disorder. *Journal of Developmental and Physical Disabilities, 31*(1), 55–71.

Call, N. A., Trosclair-Lasserre, N. M., Findley, A. J., Reavis, A. R., & Shillingsburg, M. A. (2012). Correspondence between single versus daily preference assessment outcomes and reinforcer efficacy under progressive-ratio schedules. *Journal of Applied Behavior Analysis, 45*(4), 763–777.

Chowdhury, M., & Benson, B. A. (2011). Use of differential reinforcement to reduce behavior problems in adults with intellectual disabilities: A methodological review. *Research in Developmental Disabilities, 32*(2), 383–394.

DeLeon, I. G., Fisher, W. W., Herman, K. M., & Crosland, K. C. (2000). Assessment of a response bias for aggression over functionally equivalent appropriate behavior. *Journal of Applied Behavior Analysis, 33*(1), 73–77.

DeLeon, I. G., Frank, M. A., Gregory, M. K., & Allman, M. J. (2009). On the correspondence between preference assessment outcomes and progressive-ratio schedule assessments of stimulus value. *Journal of Applied Behavior Analysis, 42*(3), 729–733.

DeLeon, I. G., & Iwata, B. A. (1996). Evaluation of a multiple-stimulus presentation format for assessing reinforcer preferences. *Journal of Applied Behavior Analysis, 29*(4), 519–533.

DeLeon, I. G., Iwata, B. A., Goh, H. L., & Worsdell, A. S. (1997). Emergence of reinforcer preference as a function of schedule requirement and stimulus similarity. *Journal of Applied Behavior Analysis, 30*(3), 439–449.

Delmendo, X., Borrero, J. C., Beauchamp, K. L., & Francisco, M. T. (2009). Consumption and response output as a function of price: Manipulation of cost and benefit components. *Journal of Applied Behavior Analysis, 42*(3), 609–625.

Eisenberger, R. (1992). Learned industriousness. *Psychological Review, 99*(2), 248–267.

Eisenberger, R., & Adornetto, M. (1986). Generalized self-control of delay and effort. *Journal of Personality and Social Psychology, 51*(5), 1020–1031.

Eisenberger, R., Carlson, J., Guile, M., & Shapiro, N. (1979). Transfer of effort across behaviors. *Learning and Motivation, 10*(2), 178–197.

Elsmore, T. F., Fletcher, G. V., Conrad, D. G., & Sodetz, F. J. (1980). Reduction of heroin intake in baboons by an economic constraint. *Pharmacology Biochemistry and Behavior, 13*(5), 729–731.

Fisher, W. W., Piazza, C. C., Bowman, L. G., Hagopian, L. P., Owens, J. C., & Slevin, I. (1992). A comparison of two approaches for identifying reinforcers for persons with severe and profound disabilities. *Journal of Applied Behavior Analysis, 25*(2), 491–498.

Fiske, K. E., Cohen, A. P., Bamond, M. J., Delmolino, L., LaRue, R. H., & Sloman, K. N. (2014). The effects of magnitude-based differential reinforcement on the skill acquisition of children with autism. *Journal of Behavioral Education, 23*(4), 470–487.

Foster, T. M., Sumpter, C. E., Temple, W., Flevill, A., & Poling, A. (2009). Demand equations for qualitatively different foods under fixed-ratio schedules: A comparison of three conversions. *Journal of the Experimental Analysis of Behavior, 92*(3), 305–326.

Francisco, M. T., Borrero, J. C., & Sy, J. R. (2008). Evaluation of absolute and relative reinforcer value using progressive-ratio schedules. *Journal of Applied Behavior Analysis, 41*(2), 189–202.

Friman, P. C., & Poling, A. (1995). Making life easier with effort: Basic findings and applied research on response effort. *Journal of Applied Behavior Analysis, 28*(4), 583–590.

Gardner, B. (2015). A review and analysis of the us of "habit" in understanding, predicting and influencing health-related behaviour. *Health Psychology Review, 9*(3), 277–295.

Gilroy, S. P., Kaplan, B. A., & Reed, D. D. (2020). Interpretation(s) of elasticity in operant demand. *Journal of the Experimental Analysis of Behavior, 114*(1), 106–115.

Gilroy, S. P., Kaplan, B. A., Schwartz, L. P., Reed, D. D., & Hursh, S. R. (2021). A zero-bounded model of operant demand. *Journal of the Experimental Analysis of Behavior, 115*(3), 729–746.

Glover, A. C., Roane, H. S., Kadey, H. J., &

Grow, L. L. (2008). Preference for reinforcers under progressive- and fixed-ratio schedules: A comparison of single and concurrent arrangements. *Journal of Applied Behavior Analysis, 41*(2), 163–176.

Green, L., & Freed, D. E. (1993). The substitutability of reinforcers. *Journal of the Experimental Analysis of Behavior, 60*(1), 141–158.

Green, L., & Rachlin, H. (1991). Economic substitutability of electrical brain stimulation, food, and water. *Journal of the Experimental Analysis of Behavior, 55*(2), 133–143.

Haddock, J. N., & Hagopian, L. P. (2020). Competing stimulus assessments: A systematic review. *Journal of Applied Behavior Analysis, 53*(4), 1982–2001.

Herrnstein, R. J. (1970). On the law of effect. *Journal of the Experimental Analysis of Behavior, 13*(2), 243–266.

Herrnstein, R. J., & Loveland, D. H. (1975). Maximizing and matching on concurrent ratio schedules. *Journal of the Experimental Analysis of Behavior, 24*(1), 107–116.

Higbee, T. S., Carr, J. E., & Harrison, C. D. (1999). The effects of pictorial versus tangible stimuli in stimulus-preference assessments. *Research in Developmental Disabilities, 20*(1), 63–72.

Hoffmann, A. N., Samaha, A. L., Bloom, S. E., & Boyle, M. A. (2017). Preference and reinforcer efficacy of high- and low-tech items: A comparison of item type and duration of access. *Journal of Applied Behavior Analysis, 50*(2), 222–237.

Horrocks, E., & Higbee, T. S. (2008). An evaluation of a stimulus preference assessment of auditory stimuli for adolescents with developmental disabilities. *Research in Developmental Disabilities, 29*(1), 11–20.

Hursh, S. R. (1978). The economics of daily consumption controlling food- and water-reinforced responding. *Journal of the Experimental Analysis of Behavior, 29*(3), 475–491.

Hursh, S. R. (1980). Economic concepts for the analysis of behavior. *Journal of the Experimental Analysis of Behavior, 34*(2), 219–238.

Hursh, S. R. (1984). Behavioral economics. *Journal of the Experimental Analysis of Behavior, 42*(3), 435–452.

Hursh, S. R., Madden, G. J., Spiga, R., DeLeon, I. G., & Francisco, M. T. (2013). The translational utility of behavioral economics: The experimental analysis of consumption and choice. In G. J. Madden, W. V. Dube, T. D.

Hackenberg, G. P. Hanley, & K. A. Lattal (Eds.), *APA handbook of behavior analysis: Vol. 2. Translating principles into practice* (pp. 191–224). American Psychological Association.

Hursh, S. R., & Roma, P. G. (2016). Behavioral economics and the analysis of consumption and choice. *Managerial and Decision Economics, 37*(4–5), 224–238.

Hursh, S. R., & Silberberg, A. (2008). Economic demand and essential value. *Psychological Review, 115*(1), 186–198.

Imam, A. A. (1993). Response-reinforcer independence and the economic continuum: A preliminary analysis. *Journal of the Experimental Analysis of Behavior, 59*(1), 231–243.

Jacobs, E. A., & Bickel, W. K. (1999). Modeling drug consumption in the clinic using simulation procedures: Demand for heroin and cigarettes in opioid-dependent outpatients. *Experimental and Clinical Psychopharmacology, 7*(4), 412–426.

Jarmolowicz, D. P., & Lattal, K. A. (2010). On distinguishing progressively increasing response requirements for reinforcement. *Behavior Analyst, 33*(1), 119–125.

Jerome, J., & Sturmey, P. (2008). Reinforcing efficacy of interactions with preferred and nonpreferred staff under progressive-ratio schedules. *Journal of Applied Behavior Analysis, 41*(2), 221–225.

Johnson, M. W., & Bickel, W. K. (2006). Replacing relative reinforcing efficacy with. behavioral economic demand curves. *Journal of the Experimental Analysis of Behavior, 85*(1), 73–93.

Jones, B. A., Madden, G. J., Wengreen, H. J., Aguilar, S. S., & Desjardins, E. A. (2014). Gamification of dietary decision-making in an elementary-school cafeteria. *PLOS One, 9*(4), Article e93872.

Joyner, D., Wengreen, H., Aguilar, S., & Madden, G. J. (2019). Effects of the FIT game on physical activity in sixth graders: A pilot reversal design intervention study. *JMIR Serious Games, 7*(2), Article e13051.

Joyner, D., Wengreen, H. J., Aguilar, S. S., Spruance, L. A., Morrill, B. A., & Madden, G. J. (2017). The FIT Game III: Reducing the operating expenses of a game-based approach to increasing healthy eating in elementary schools. *Games for Health Journal, 6*(2), 111–118.

Kahneman, D., & Tversky, A. (2013). Choices, values, and frames. In L. C. MacLean & W. T.

Ziemba (Eds.), *Handbook of the fundamentals of financial decision making* (pp. 269–278). World Scientific.

Kang, S., O'Reilly, M., Lancioni, G., Falcomata, T. S., Sigafoos, J., & Xu, Z. (2013). Comparison of the predictive validity and consistency among preference assessment procedures: A review of the literature. *Research in Developmental Disabilities, 34*(4), 1125–1133.

Kenzer, A. L., Bishop, M. R., Wilke, A. E., & Tarbox, J. R. (2013). Including unfamiliar stimuli in preference assessments for young children with autism. *Journal of Applied Behavior Analysis, 46*(3), 689–694.

Kodak, T., Lerman, D. C., & Call, N. (2007). Evaluating the influence of postsession reinforcement on choice of reinforcers. *Journal of Applied Behavior Analysis, 40*(3), 515–527.

Koffarnus, M. N., Franck, C. T., Stein, J. S., & Bickel, W. K. (2015). A modified exponential behavioral economic demand model to better describe consumption data. *Experimental and Clinical Psychopharmacology, 23*(6), 504–512.

Lamb, R. J., Schindler, C. W., & Pinkston, J. W. (2016). Conditioned stimuli's role in relapse: Preclinical research on Pavlovian instrumental transfer. *Psychopharmacology, 233*(10), 1933–1944.

Lee, M. S. H., Yu, C. T., Martin, T. L., & Martin, G. L. (2010). On the relation between reinforcer efficacy and preference. *Journal of Applied Behavior Analysis, 43*(1), 95–100.

Linn, T. L. (2016). *Consideration of reinforcer magnitude with respect to preference and reinforcer assessment outcomes* (*Culminating Projects in Community Psychology, Counseling and Family Therapy*, Vol. 16). Master's thesis, St. Cloud State University, St. Cloud, MN. Retrieved from *https://repository. stcloudstate.edu/cpcf_etds/16.*

Mackillop, J., Murphy, C. M., Martin, R. A., Stojek, M., Tidey, J. W., Colby, S. M., & Rohsenow, D. J. (2016). Predictive validity of a cigarette purchase task in a randomized controlled trial of contingent vouchers for smoking in individuals with substance use disorders. *Nicotine and Tobacco Research, 18*(5), 531–537.

Madden, G. J., Dake, J. M., Mauel, E. C., & Rowe, R. R. (2005). Labor supply and consumption of food in a closed economy under a range of fixed- and random-ratio schedules: Tests of unit price. *Journal of the Experimental Analysis of Behavior, 83*(2), 99–118.

Madden, G. J., Smethells, J. R., Ewan, E. E., & Hursh, S. R. (2007). Tests of behavioral-economic assessments of relative reinforcer efficacy: Economic substitutes. *Journal of the Experimental Analysis of Behavior, 87*(2), 219–240.

Mangum, A., Fredrick, L., Pabico, R., & Roane, H. (2012). The role of context in the evaluation of reinforcer efficacy: Implications for the preference assessment outcomes. *Research in Autism Spectrum Disorders, 6*(1), 158–167.

McSweeney, F. K., & Roll, J. M. (1998). Do animals satiate or habituate to repeatedly presented reinforcers? *Psychonomic Bulletin and Review, 5*(3), 428–442.

Murphy, J. G., Mackillop, J., Tidey, J. W., Brazil, L. A., & Colby, S. M. (2011). Validity of a demand curve measure of nicotine reinforcement with adolescent smokers. *Drug and Alcohol Dependence, 113*(2–3), 207–214.

Nix, L. D. (2016). *An evaluation of a stimulus preference assessment of iPad applications for young children with autism.* Master's thesis, Utah State University, Logan, UT. Retrieved from *https://digitalcommons.usu.edu/cgi/ viewcontent.cgi?article=5911&context=etd.*

Oleson, E. B., & Roberts, D. C. (2009). Behavioral economic assessment of price and cocaine consumption following self-administration histories that produce escalation of either final ratios or intake. *Neuropsychopharmacology, 34*, 796–804.

Pace, G. M., Ivancic, M. T., Edwards, G. L., Iwata, B. A., & Page, T. J. (1985). Assessment of stimulus preference and reinforcer value with profoundly retarded individuals. *Journal of Applied Behavior Analysis, 18*(3), 249–255.

Paramore, N. W., & Higbee, T. S. (2005). An evaluation of a brief multiple-stimulus preference assessment with adolescents with emotional disorders in an educational setting. *Journal of Applied Behavior Analysis, 38*(3), 399–403.

Peck, S., & Madden, G. J. (2021). Effects of effort training on effort-based impulsive choice. *Behavioural Processes, 189*, Article 104441.

Penrod, B., Wallace, M. D., & Dyer, E. J. (2008). Assessing potency of high- and low-preference reinforcers with respect to response rate and response patterns. *Journal of Applied Behavior Analysis, 41*(2), 177–188.

Petscher, E. S., Rey, C., & Bailey, J. S. (2009). A review of empirical support for differential reinforcement of alternative behavior. *Research in Developmental Disabilities, 30*(3), 409–425.

Pinkston, J. W., & Libman, B. M. (2017). Aversive functions of response effort: Fact or artifact? *Journal of the Experimental Analysis of Behavior, 108*(1), 73–96.

Poling, A. (2010). Looking to the future: Will behavior analysis survive and proper? *The Behavior Analyst, 33*(1), 7–17.

Rachlin, H., Green, L., Kagel, J. H., & Battalio, R. C. (1976). Economic demand theory and psychological studies of choice. *Psychology of Learning and Motivation: Advances in Research and Theory, 10*, 129–154.

Reed, D. D., Kaplan, B. A., & Becirevic, A. (2015). Basic research on the behavioral economics of reinforcer value. In F. D. Digennaro Reed & D. D. Reed (Eds.), *Autism service delivery: Bridging the gap between science and practice* (pp. 279–306). Springer.

Reed, D. D., Luiselli, J. K., Magnuson, J. D., Fillers, S., Vieira, S., & Rue, H. C. (2009). A comparison between traditional economical and demand curve analyses of relative reinforcer efficacy in the validation of preference assessment predictions. *Developmental Neurorehabilitation, 12*(3), 164–169.

Reed, D. D., Naudé, G. P., Salzer, A. R., Peper, M., Monroe-Gulick, A. L., Gelino, B. W., . . . Higgins, S. T. (2020). Behavioral economic measurement of cigarette demand: A descriptive review of published approaches to the cigarette purchase task. *Experimental and Clinical Psychopharmacology, 28*(6), 688–705.

Reed, D. D., Niileksela, C. R., & Kaplan, B. A. (2013). Behavioral economics: A tutorial for behavior analysis in practice. *Behavior Analysis in Practice, 6*(1), 34–54.

Roane, H. S. (2008). On the applied use of progressive-ratio schedules of reinforcement. *Journal of Applied Behavior Analysis, 41*(2), 155–161.

Roane, H. S., Call, N. A., & Falcomata, T. S. (2005). A preliminary analysis of adaptive responding under open and closed economies. *Journal of Applied Behavior Analysis, 38*(3), 335–348.

Roane, H. S., Lerman, D. C., & Vorndran, C. M. (2001). Assessing reinforcers under progressive schedule requirements. *Journal of Applied Behavior Analysis, 34*(2), 145–166.

Roane, H. S., Vollmer, T. R., Ringdahl, J. E., & Marcus, B. A. (1998). Evaluation of a brief stimulus preference assessment. *Journal of Applied Behavior Analysis, 31*(4), 605–620.

Robbins, L. (1932). *An essay on the nature and significance of economic science.* Macmillan.

Roscoe, E. M., Iwata, B. A., & Kahng, S. (1999). Relative versus absolute reinforcement effects: Implications for preference assessments. *Journal of Applied Behavior Analysis, 32*(4), 479–493.

Shabani, D. B., Carr, J. E., & Petursdottir, A. I. (2009). A laboratory model for studying response-class hierarchies. *Journal of Applied Behavior Analysis, 42*(1), 105–121.

Shahan, T. A., Bickel, W. K., Madden, G. J., & Badger, G. J. (1999). Comparing the reinforcing efficacy of nicotine containing and denicotinized cigarettes: A behavioral economic analysis. *Psychopharmacology, 147*(2), 210–216.

Shore, B. A., Iwata, B. A., DeLeon, I. G., Kahng, S., & Smith, R. G. (1997). An analysis of reinforcer substitutability using object manipulation and self-injury as competing responses. *Journal of Applied Behavior Analysis, 30*(1), 21–41.

Spiga, R., Martinetti, M. P., Meisch, R. A., Cowan, K., & Hursh, S. (2005). Methadone and nicotine self-administration in humans: A behavioral economic analysis. *Psychopharmacology, 178*(2–3), 223–231.

Tan, L., & Hackenberg, T. D. (2015). Pigeons' demand and preference for specific and generalized conditioned reinforcers in a token economy. *Journal of the Experimental Analysis of Behavior, 104*(3), 296–314.

Thaler, R. H. (1981). Some empirical evidence on dynamic inconsistency. *Economics Letters, 8*(3), 201–207.

Thaler, R. H., & Benartzi, S. (2004). Save More Tomorrow™: Using behavioral economics to increase employee saving. *Journal of Political Economy, 112*(Suppl. 1), S164–S187.

Thaler, R. H., & Sunstein, C. R. (2009). *Nudge: Improving decisions about health, wealth, and happiness.* Penguin.

Troslair-Lasserre, N. M., Lerman, D. C., Call, N. A., Addison, L. R., & Kodak, T. (2008). Reinforcement magnitude: An evaluation of preference and reinforcer efficacy. *Journal of Applied Behavior Analysis, 41*(2), 203–220.

Tustin, R. D. (1994). Preference for reinforcers under varying schedule arrangements: A behavioral economic analysis. *Journal of Applied Behavior Analysis, 27*(4), 597–606.

Van Camp, C. M., Lerman, D. C., Kelley, M. E., Roane, H. S., Contrucci, S. A., & Vorndran, C. M. (2000). Further analysis of idiosyncratic antecedent influences during the assessment and treatment of problem behavior. *Journal of Applied Behavior Analysis, 33*(2), 207–221.

Wengreen, H. J., Joyner, D., Kimball, S. S., Schwartz, S., & Madden, G. J. (2021). A randomized controlled trial evaluating the FIT game's efficacy in increasing fruit and vegetable consumption. *Nutrients, 13*(8), Article 2646.

Wilder, D. A., Ertel, H. M., & Cymbal, D. J. (2021). A review of recent research on the manipulation of response effort in applied behavior analysis. *Behavior Modification, 45*, 740–768.

Winkler, R. C. (1971). The relevance of economic theory and technology to token reinforcement systems. *Behaviour Research and Therapy, 9*(2), 81–88.

Worsdell, A. S., Iwata, B. A., Hanley, G. P., Thompson, R. H., & Kahng, S. (2000). Effects of continuous and intermittent reinforcement for problem behavior during functional communication training. *Journal of Applied Behavior Analysis, 33*(2), 167–179.

Zvorsky, I., Nighbor, T. D., Kurti, A. N., DeSarno, M., Naudé, G., Reed, D. D., & Higgins, S. T. (2019). Sensitivity of hypothetical purchase task indices when studying substance use: A systematic literature review. *Preventive Medicine, 128*, Article 105789.

CHAPTER 22

Translating Impulsivity

David P. Jarmolowicz
Robert S. LeComte

Impulsivity. It is one of those words that we hear a lot. Teachers complain about the challenges associated with working with impulsive students. Exasperated parents blame their ever-growing frustration on their children's impulsivity. Your doctor hints that it's your impulsivity that stands between you and the beach body that the media suggests is so important. We read stories of impulsive adolescents experimenting with drugs and spreading sexually transmitted infections (STIs). Substance abuse and other behavioral disorders are talked about in terms of difficulties with impulse control.

Despite its ubiquity, it can be somewhat difficult to come up with a solid operational definition of impulsivity. We can catalogue examples of impulsive behavior, yet the topographies differ widely. For example, blurting out answers in class looks very different from choosing to consume the chocolate cake you know will go straight to your hips. As such, topographical definitions, like those favored in applied behavior analysis (ABA), may be preempted. This is perhaps unsurprising given that we are probably talking about a behavioral process rather than discrete instances of aberrant behavior.

The sorts of functional definitions used in the experimental analysis of behavior (EAB) provide a different approach. Specifically, rather than building a definition that captures the entire range of topographies referred to as *impulsive,* behaviors can be grouped by similar impacts on the environment (i.e., function). In doing so, the behaviors are said to share an operant class. This is not unlike the approach taken in foundational behavioral research dating back to the 1930s (Skinner, 1938). For example, when foundational behavioral researchers report the number of lever presses made by a rat per session, the number includes lever presses made by any part of the animal's body such as its right paw, its left paw, both paws, or its nose. In fact, "lever press" represents the number of times that the lever was moved from its starting position, such that a sensor picks up its movement, not a specific topography of behavior. While this approach may seem foreign to many working in ABA, it has dominated EAB since its inception.

Unfortunately, the issues entailed in defining impulsivity are not entirely resolved via the use of functional definitions. For example, many instances of "impulsive behavior" entail premature responses, such as students blurting out the answers to questions prior to being called upon. The topography of these premature responses may vary widely (e.g., vocalizing "blue," "red," saying "chili dog") but their impact on the environment remains the same—interruption of ongoing instruction. This sort of premature responding is seen in many populations and settings, which can vary across a vast array of topographies. In fact, many instances that we call *impulsive* may fit under this umbrella. Others, however, do not. For example, impulsive spending often entails choosing to spend money on small yet immediately available trinkets rather than saving for long-term goals (e.g., retirement, larger and cooler trinkets). The environmental impact of these choices is access to the immediate consumption of the small reward at the expense of larger yet delayed rewards. Although this type of present-focused choice occurs across a wide range of persons, places, and things, it differs from the premature responding described earlier.

Thus, impulsivity can—at best—be thought of as a series of interlinked operant responses. For a behavior analyst, however, this can be somewhat discomforting. Specifically, this is only a small step away from viewing "impulsivity" as a thing that is manifest through these linked operant classes. This position risks attributing the cause of the observed behavior to "impulsivity," a calling card for the sort of surplus meaning seen with hypothetical constructs. As behavior analysts, we have been trained to eschew explanations that rely on *hypothetical constructs* (i.e., statement to unobserved entities that are not wholly reducible to groupings of empirically demonstrable events; MacCorquodale & Meehl, 1948) for good reason—they move the cause of the behavior into the organism. This slippery slope can lead one to posit that "little Jonny blurts out the answers because of his impulsivity"—a behavioral situation that is nearly untreatable.

Being small steps away from a hypothetical construct, however, does not make something a hypothetical construct. Taking a small step in the other direction, these linked operant classes can be conceptualized with "impulsivity" as an *intervening variable* (i.e., a grouping of observable and empirically demonstrable events (MacCorquodale & Meehl, 1948). In doing so, the term *impulsivity* simply serves as a placeholder summarizing the observed relations. In doing so, it does not become a causal entity for the observed behavior—it is the behavior. This approach would be typified by the statement "because little Johnny blurts out the answers, they say he is impulsive." Although this change in stance may seem small, the entity causing the participant's behavior is not placed inside of the organism. As a result, control of such behavior remains in the environment, a much easier treatment situation. To quote one of the first author's graduate school instructors, "Inside bad, outside good" (Michael Perone, personal communication of his mentor's [Alan Baron] maxim).

Defining Impulsivity

The previously mentioned challenges notwithstanding, a definition of impulsivity is needed. This dilemma is not new. Researchers across a wide range of disciplines/orientations have struggled to define impulsivity. Famously, in the special issue of *Psychopharmacology* on impulsivity, Evenden (1999) catalogued 21 distinct types of impulsivities. These varieties of impulsivity are pulled from conceptualizations of impulsivity dominant at the time during which Evenden was writing. These range from Dickman's (1993) "reflection impulsivity" and "disinhibition," to Buss and Plomin's (1975) "inhibitory control," "decision time," "lack of persistence," and "boredom/sensation seeking," to trait-based conceptualizations such as "motor," cognitive," and "nonplanning" impulsivity of the Barratt Impulsiveness Scale (BIS-11; Patton et al., 1995).

Our goal in this chapter is not to repeat the struggles of other well-intentioned researchers. As such, we do not provide "the" account of impulsivity, settling instead for "an" account of impulsivity that we hope is defensible. In doing so, we adopt an account of impulsivity found useful in prior work (Bickel, Jarmolowicz, Mueller, Gatchalian, et al., 2012). As such, our overall definition for impulsivity is pulled from Durana and Barnes's (1993) book-length treatment of the topic. Namely, we note that "the behavioral universe thought to reflect impulsivity encompasses actions that appear poorly conceived, prematurely expressed, unduly risky, or inappropriate to the situation and that often result in undesirable consequences" (p. 23). From a behavioral perspective, several features of this definition are somewhat appealing. First and foremost, the definition implies no internal mechanism, instead placing the focus on observable aspects of behavior. While clear operational definitions of "appear poorly conceived, prematurely expressed, unduly risky, or inappropriate to the situation" are not provided, they are definable. Second, consistent with the research traditions of EAB, the definition includes a functional consequence of the behavior (i.e., "often result in undesirable consequences"). While this component of the definition is also left underdefined it can—in principle—be defined.

An astute reader will note that the definition of impulsivity provided here is quite vague. The blanket definition provided can more accurately be thought of as setting the context within which more detailed descriptions can reside—with each of these subtypes of impulsivity being fully nested within the overall definition. Consistent with Bickel, Jarmolowicz, Mueller, Gatchalian, et al. (2012), impulsivity can be divided into several subtypes.

Trait Impulsivities

A considerable body of impulsivity literature has been conducted within the framework of personality traits. While traditional behavior analysts have spent little to no time talking about trait variables, this need not be the case. Simply put, a "trait variable is a relatively stable pre-existing characteristic an individual brings to a situation" (Odum, 2011, p. 1). Hence, traits can be conceptualized as stable patterns of behavior that individuals exhibit across a range of contexts—not unlike many of the other response patterns behavior analysts are called upon to change.

In the context of impulsivity, there are many traits to consider. The widely used BIS-11 (Patton et al., 1995) asks 30 questions, the answers to which are thought to give information of participant's persistent patterns of inattention, motor impulsivity, and failures to appropriately plan responses before making them. Although inattention has no direct link to our overall definition, motor impulsivity results in behavior that appears to be "prematurely expressed" and failures to plan make behavior appear "poorly conceived." Thus, with two of the three response patterns identified being directly related to our overall definition, responding on the BIS-11 will remain part of our framework.

Behavioral Disinhibition

Once a response has been initiated, it is often difficult to stop. For example, it can be challenging to stop yourself from eating potato chips once the package has been opened and you have begun to bring the chips to your mouth. As is the case with each of the subtypes of impulsivity that we discuss, most people experience these challenges with disinhibition problems being an issue of degree. *Behavioral disinhibition* refers to a relative lack of ability to suppress a prepotent response (Dalley et al., 2011). This covers a wide range of situations, from the student who blurts out the answer to questions before she can be called upon to writing the wrong year on checks every January. Behavioral disinhibition is typically measured via neurocognitive tests that prompt the initiation of a response, quickly followed by a prompt to cancel the response (i.e., stop-signal reaction-time task: Logan & Cowan, 1984; go/no-go tasks: Drewe, 1975). In general, these behaviors appear "prematurely expressed," providing a clear linkage to our overall definition of impulsivity.

Attention-Deficit Impulsivity

Attention deficits are often thought of when we speak of impulsivity. For example, the prototype childhood impulse control disorder is attention-deficit/hyperactivity disorder (ADHD). Associated with various types of impulsivity (e.g., trouble paying attention, controlling impulsive behaviors, or overactivity; Centers for Disease Control and Prevention, 2021) a defining feature of ADHD is difficulty with sustained attention. As such, we define *attention-deficit impulsivity* as a diminished ability to sustain engagement with relevant stimuli while in the presence of additional irrelevant stimuli. The focus in assessing attention-deficit impulsivity is on the individual's ability to respond to the appropriate stimuli (i.e., responses to other stimuli are implied rather than assessed). Thus, neurocognitive tasks that assess attention-deficit impulsivity require that participants monitor for and report the presence of briefly presented stimuli. For example, the computerized Conners Continuous Performance Task (Conners, 1992) has participants watch closely and press the spacebar whenever any letter other than X appears on the screen.

Reflection Impulsivity

Even the best of us can fail to think things through before acting. We may drive to the store to find out it's already closed. We may arrive at the DMV to find out that we don't have all the documentation we need. Or we may come to class without all of the materials so clearly described in the syllabus. Common to all of these lapses is a failure to gather important information before acting. Thus, we define *reflection impulsivity* as a deficit in gathering and evaluating available information prior to acting/decision making (Clark et al., 2009). This potential deficit is assessed via tasks such as the matching familiar figures task, wherein the participant views a sample stimulus (e.g., butterfly) followed by five to six comparison stimuli, each of which differ from each other by a single attribute. One of the comparison stimuli matches the sample stimulus, and the participant's job is to identify that stimulus. A tendency to act before gathering all information, however, often leads to errors on this widely used task.

Impulsive Choice

In behavioral science, a considerable body of literature has accumulated surrounding impulsive choice. Often discussed within the conceptualization of behavioral economics, impulsive choice tasks often entail trade-offs between one reward attribute and another. Strictly speaking, impulsive choice tasks examine trade-offs between reward magnitude and immediacy—but in this section, we consider another reward trade-off (i.e., magnitude vs. certainty). Although there are important differences between these tasks, we discuss them together to draw attention to their commonalities.

Delay Discounting

Over the past few decades, a considerable literature has accumulated examining individuals' choices between rewards that differ in both their size and immediacy. *Delay discounting* describes how individuals' subjective value of a given reward decreases as the delay to that reward increases (Green & Myerson, 2004). A conceptual descendant of Mischel and Ebbesen's (1970) famous marshmallow test, delay discounting tasks often require that participants make choices between amounts of immediate versus delayed hypothetical money. For example, a participant may be required to report whether she would prefer $500 now, or $1,000 tomorrow. If the participant chooses to wait for the larger reward, larger immediate amounts (e.g., $750 today vs. $1,000 tomorrow) are offered on future trials, until a point at which the participant is indifferent between the immediate and delayed reward, with the amount of immediately offered money at that point being called the *indifference point*. Similarly, if the participant chooses the immediate reward, amounts of that immediate reward will systematically decrease (e.g., $250 today vs. $1,000 tomorrow) across future trials, until the indifference point is identified. This process is used to determine indifference points across a range of delays (e.g., 1 day, 1 week, 1 month, 3 months, 6 months, 1 year, and 5 years), and nonlinear regression (Subjective value = Amount/[1 + Delay * k]; Mazur, 1987) is used to quantify the entire parametric function. In doing so, k represents the discounting rate and provides a single number that represents the shape of the entire parametric function. Higher k values correspond to a steeper curve, indicating higher rates of delay discounting—a response pattern said to represent impulsivity/impulsive choice.

An interesting wrinkle to delay discounting assessment is that discounting rates can differ based on the commodity examined. While monetary rewards may be the standard, understanding individuals' valuation of disorder-specific rewards can be highly illuminating. For example, for individuals who are concerned with their overeating, examining their delay discounting of food may be particularly relevant (Hendrickson & Rasmussen, 2017). Similarly, for those suffering from substance abuse disorder, their discounting of delayed drugs may provide novel information (Madden et al., 1997). This process is relatively straightforward once the commodity of interest is translated to monetary terms. For example, Madden et. al. asked heroin users how much heroin would be worth $1,000 to them. By doing so, they were able to use the same sort of process to determine indifference points for delayed money and delayed heroin. Unsurprisingly, heroin users discounted delayed heroin much more rapidly than they discounted delayed money. This general finding has been widely replicated, including in individuals who abuse alcohol (Lemley et al., 2016; Petry, 2001a), use cannabis (Jarmolowicz et al., 2020), and smoke cigarettes (Odum & Baumann, 2007).

Probability Discounting

While delay discounting may cover a wide range of impulsive choices, we sometimes think of needlessly risky choices as impulsive (Green & Myerson, 2013). This is reflected in our overall definition of impulsivity, which includes behavior that is "unduly risky." In behavioral economics, these sorts of risky choices are often investigated via probability discounting. Most simply put, *probability discounting* represents the rate at which individuals devalue rewards as they become increasingly unlikely. Measured and quantified in ways that are similar to those used to measure delay discounting (i.e., with the exception that the choices are between certain rewards and probabilistic rewards; e.g., $500 for sure or a 95% chance of $1,000), nonlinear regression (Subjective value = Amount/ [1 + Odds against receiving the reward * h]; Rachlin et al., 1991) yields an h value, said to represent probability discounting rate. Unlike delay discounting, however, lower h values—indicative of very little devaluation of rewards as they become improbable—is indicative of risky choice.

Impulsivity as a Participant Characteristic

Behavior-analytic discomfort with impulsivity research may stem from the tendency of researchers to describe impulsivity as a participant characteristic that explains other portions of their behavioral repertoires (Bickel et al., 2012; Green & Myerson, 2013). This concern is fair. Many researchers working in impulsivity come from theoretical orientations that are more comfortable with hypothetical constructs than most behavior analysts. As such, their descriptions and conceptual schemes often differ markedly from those put forth by Skinner and our other pioneers. Despite these theoretical differences, these are often well-conducted experiments that yield interesting data. As behavior analysts, we must remember "the scientific truism that good data are notoriously fickle. They change their allegiance from theory to theory, and even maintain their importance in the presence of no theory at all" (Sidman, 1960, pp. 6–7).

A different conceptualization is that these behavioral patterns we label impulsivity reflect an interplay between participants' genetic makeup/capacity and behavioral history that influences the way they respond across a wide range of circumstances. From that viewpoint, there is value in assessing these repertoires, because they could predict participants' behavior across a range of contexts. Researchers working from a behavior-analytic and/or neurocognitive perspective have spent considerable time cataloguing populations associated with these aberrant repertoires, which we review below.

Trait Impulsivities

Measures such as the BIS-11 (Patton et al., 1995) and the Sensation Seeking Scale–V (SSS-V; Zuckerman et al., 1978), have been used to identify differences in trait impulsivity among groups. Moreno et al. (2012), for example, noted significantly higher scores on the BIS-11 and SSS-V among recreational cannabis users and binge drinkers compared to non-drug-using controls. Similarly, higher levels of trait impulsivities have been observed among both recreational and dependent cocaine users compared to healthy, cocaine-naive controls (Vonmoos et al., 2013). Outside of substance-abuse populations, Bénard et al. (2017) found that individuals with higher scores on the BIS-11 were more likely to be obese compared to individuals with lower levels of trait impulsivities.

Behavioral Disinhibition

Numerous studies have identified deficits in the ability to withhold an already initiated response among several populations of substance abusers. Comparing performance on a response inhibition task (stop-signal reaction-time test) between healthy controls and alcohol-dependent individuals, for example, Lawrence et al. (2009) noted significantly slower reaction times to a stop signal among those in the alcohol-dependent group. Slower stop-signal reaction times (SSRTs) were further correlated with the severity of alcohol-use disorder among the sample. Similar deficits in response inhibition have been shown among other substance-using populations, including cocaine (Kaufman et al., 2003), methamphetamine (Monterosso et al., 2005), and nicotine users (Mashoon et al., 2018). Outside of substance-abusing populations, response inhibition deficits have also been observed in samples of pathological gamblers (Billieux et al., 2012) and among obese individuals when responding in the presence of food-related stimuli (Gerdan & Kurt, 2020). Research also suggests that behavioral disinhibition is a component of sexual risk behavior (e.g., multiple sexual partners, sex under the influence of drugs) among adolescents (Epstein et al., 2014).

Attention-Deficit Impulsivity

Perhaps unsurprisingly, persistent deficits in the ability to attend to relevant versus irrelevant environmental stimuli are a characteristic of mental health disorders such as attention-deficit disorder and ADHD (National Institutes of Health, 2011). Interestingly, however, attention-deficit impulsivity has also been identified in various populations struggling with addiction. Salgado et al. (2009), for example, observed poorer performance in attention tasks among alcohol-dependent individuals compared to healthy controls during a continuous performance task (CPT). Similarly, Moeller et al. (2005) found decreased brain activity in areas associated with attention among cocaine-dependent individuals as compared to nondependent controls.

Reflection Impulsivity

A tendency to inadequately collect information prior to making decisions has been identified among several groups, notably in populations of younger adult substance abusers. Banca et al. (2016), for example, noted that young binge drinkers compiled less evidence before making decisions in a sorting task compared to healthy, non-binge-drinking controls. Furthermore, Townshend et al. (2014), found significant correlations between low performance on a reflection impulsivity task (Information Sampling Task [IST]; Cambridge Cognition Ltd., Bottisham, Cambridge, UK) and greater numbers of unplanned sexual encounters among a sample of high binge-drinking college students. Similar findings have been observed in populations of current opioid and amphetamine users (Clark et al., 2006), 3,4-methylenedioxymethamphetamine (MDMA; "ecstasy") users (Quednow et al., 2007), and adolescent cannabis users (Solowij et al., 2012). Outside of substance abuse disorders, planning deficits have also been observed in samples of individuals diagnosed with ADHD (Jepsen et al., 2018). Additionally, research has also identified impairments in reflection impulsivity among obese children (Breat et al., 2007).

Impulsive Choice

Notably, patterns of impulsive choice are often associated with several problematic behaviors (e.g., substance abuse, overeating, gambling).

Delay Discounting

The rate at which reinforcers are devalued as a function of the delay to their receipt has shown to differ widely among groups. Individuals who use opioids (Madden et al., 1997), use stimulants (Coffey et al., 2003; Monterosso et al., 2007), smoke cigarettes (Bickel, Jarmolowicz, Mueller, Franck, et al., 2012; Bickel et al., 1999; Jarmolowicz et al., 2012), and/or drink heavily (Bickel, Jarmolowicz, Mueller, Franck, et al., 2012; Petry, 2001a; Vuchinich & Simpson, 1998) all tend to discount delayed rewards at higher rates than healthy controls, prompting the supposition that excessive discounting of delayed rewards may be a trans-disease process (Bickel, Jarmolowicz, Mueller, Koffarnus, et al., 2012; Bickel & Mueller, 2009) that undergirds a wide range of behaviors. Among non-substance-abusing populations, evidence suggests significant differences in delay discounting among obese and healthier weight individuals for monetary (Bickel et al., 2014; Jarmolowicz et al., 2014; Rasmussen et al., 2010; Weller et al., 2008) and food rewards (Epstein et al., 2010; Rasmussen et al., 2010). Research on pathological gamblers has also revealed significant differences in rates of delay discounting compared to healthy controls (Dixon et al., 2003; Petry, 2001b).

Probability Discounting

Based on previous discussions of impulsivity, we may view substance abusers as engaging in or demonstrating a preference for risk taking even when the likelihood for reinforcement is low. Research on the rate at which probabilistic rewards are discounted in these groups, however, reveals some interesting effects. Studies of cigarette smokers, for example, have shown significantly higher rates of discounting for probabilistic rewards (i.e., were more risk-averse) compared to nonsmokers (Reynolds et al., 2004; Yi et al., 2007). Similarly, Garami and Moustafa (2019) found greater rates of probability discounting among opioid-dependent individuals compared to non-using controls. Such contradictory findings may suggest the presence of different mechanisms or processes involved in choice behavior for delayed and probabilistic rewards (McKerchar & Renda, 2012).

Impulsivity and Context

Like all patterns of behavior, impulsive behavior may be expressed differently depending on environmental and physiological contexts. These context-based differences can result from stimulus control, differences in motivational states, or other setting events. The nature of this research, however, is more focused on demonstrating environmental/context control over impulsive response patterns than on determining the precise behavioral influences that drive them. As such, we have a cataloguing of behavioral effects—with a less precise accounting of their etiology. While this status is not satisfactory, it represents an important starting point for future research.

Behavioral Disinhibition

Acute exposure to several classes of drugs has been shown to affect the ability to withhold responding. Among other things (e.g., changes in motivational variables, stimulus discriminability, and/or physical capacities), consuming psychoactive substances changes the context under which responding occurs—as evidenced by the widely acknowledged phenomenon of "state-dependent learning"/dissociation (i.e., skills learned in one context [e.g., while on drug] are not available in another context [i.e., when not on drug]; Radu-lovic et al., 2017).

In the case of alcohol use, acute consumption was shown to significantly impact inhibition responding during a go/no-go task and a simulated driving procedure. More specifically, results showed a dose-dependent relationship between alcohol and increases in stopping failures and lane line crossing (Fillmore et al., 2008). Even without physical consumption, alcohol-related cues have been shown to affect behavioral inhibition performance among sober drinkers (Weafer & Fillmore, 2015).

Attention-Deficit Impulsivity

Effects of acute drug administration on attention-deficit impulsivity have also been noted in the literature. Dougherty et al. (2000), for example, examined the effects of low (0.5 gram/kilogram of body weight) and high doses (1.0 gram/kilogram of body weight) of alcohol on participants' attentional performance in a version of the CPT. High doses of alcohol were shown to decrease the percentage of correctly identified stimuli, increase errors of commission, and decrease participants' ability to discriminate between stimuli during the task. Similarly, Kuypers et al. (2007) noted decreased performance during a divided attention task under acute doses of MDMA (ecstasy).

Interestingly, in addition to acute drug exposure affecting attention, individuals with higher baseline attention deficits may not be able to accurately perceive drug effects themselves. McCloskey et al. (2010), for example, found that participants who demonstrated lower performance on attention and reaction-time tasks prior to drug administration did not show expected increases in reports of drug-liking and euphoria under various doses of D-amphetamine compared to participants with higher preadministration performance. Such findings may indicate that individuals with higher attention-deficit impulsivity are less sensitive to overall drug effects and may consume more drugs as a result.

Reflection Impulsivity

A tendency to prematurely express behavior prior to sufficiently gathering information is also shown to be exacerbated by acute drug administration. Voon et al. (2016), for example, found that participants made more premature decisions during a sorting task (beads task; Phillips and Edwards, 1966) under acute doses of methylphenidate compared to baseline conditions. Similarly, van Wel et al. (2012) found that acute doses of MDMA increased participants' reaction time during a reflection impulsivity task (Matching Familiar Figures Task; Cairns & Cammock, 1978), making them more prone to committing errors.

Interestingly, the expectation of cognitive and behavioral impairments from substance use can affect reflection impulsivity. Specifically, Caswell et al. (2013) found that participants who indicated greater expected impairment from alcohol showed reduced performance on a reflection impulsivity task prior to drug administration. Outside of substance-related research, partial sleep deprivation is also shown to affect reflection impulsivity (Salfi et al., 2020).

Impulsive Choice

Individuals make impulsive choices in a range of contexts, and those contexts consistently impact impulsive choice.

Delay Discounting

As observed with other subtypes of impulsivity, delay discounting can also be differentially expressed by the context in which it is measured. Dixon et al. (2006) demonstrated such effects on discounting in a sample of pathological gamblers. One group of participants completed a monetary discounting task in a gambling-related context, which included a betting facility containing two bars and multiple TVs showing horse races. Another group of participants completed the same discounting task in a nongambling context, including restaurants, coffee shops, and other common public settings. Significantly higher rates of discounting (i.e., greater preference for immediate rewards) were observed for participants in the gambling-related context compared to those in the nongambling setting. In the physiological sense, research also points to the context-altering effects of acute substance administration on subjective reward valuation. Johnson et al. (2017), for example, noted significantly higher rates of discounting for sex and condom use under acute cocaine administration compared to placebo. Effects were also dose-dependent, such that greater rates of discounting were observed following high doses of cocaine versus low doses. Such findings relate to those observed by Reynolds et al. (2006), wherein preference for immediate rewards was increased under high doses of alcohol during an experiential discounting task.

Another context-altering setting event is the experience of withdrawal in addicted individuals. Specifically, while withdrawal may be a powerful motivating variable for acquiring drug, it also impacts a wide range of correlated non-drug-related behavior. Subjectively, withdrawal is a highly discriminable context—thus, its ability to exert contextual control cannot be ignored. Field et al. (2006), for example, found that discounting rates for monetary and cigarette rewards were significantly higher during conditions of nicotine deprivation compared to postsmoking satiation. Similar increases in delay discounting were noted during food deprivation when participants considered both future food and non-food-related rewards (Skrynka & Vincent, 2019). These findings are highly consistent with those of Giordano et al. (2002), who found that individuals with their opioid addictions managed via medication discounted at higher rates before receiving their daily dose (i.e., when in mild withdrawal) than after receiving their daily dose.

Probability Discounting

Conditions of acute drug administration and deprivation also affect the subjective valuation of uncertain rewards. Johnson et al. (2016), for example, observed significantly greater probability discounting of monetary rewards under acute doses of alcohol compared to placebo conditions. Furthermore, during the alcohol condition, participants indicated a greater likelihood of engaging in unprotected sex despite a high hypothetical risk of contracting an STI, as measured in a sexual probability discounting task. Similarly, Johnson et al. (2017) found that both low and high doses of cocaine increased sexual probability discounting, such that participants were more likely to have unprotected sex despite high odds of STI contraction.

Impulsivity as a Treatment Target

As behavior analysts, we are often deeply concerned with improving the sort of behavioral excesses and/or deficits we classify as impulsivity. To some, the cataloguing of deficits we have undertaken thus far in this chapter may not seem particularly impactful. This may be part of the reason why behavior analysts are not currently the dominant force in this research area. For those who have ventured into this area, however, their impact is perceivable and the tide is turning.

Changing impulsive patterns of behavior is becoming an active research area—with many noteworthy contributions from behavior analysts. While much of the work—to date—has emphasized changing rates of delay discounting (Bickel et al., 2015; Koffarnus et al., 2013), other repertoires are also viable targets that will surely receive considerable attention as evidence accumulates. In covering these changes, we cast a wide net—covering treatments with varying degrees of connection to Skinner's science of behavior. Behavior analysts do not have the market on effective treatments cornered, and understanding a range of variables that control behavior can only serve to improve our understanding of how behavior works.

Altering these patterns of impulsive behavior has the potential to spur robust and lasting changes with considerable generality. Although we divide impulsivity into discrete subtypes, these subtypes are not based on topography. Instead, the subtypes represent distinct response classes. Said another way, each of our impulsivities are functionally rather than topographically defined. As a result, interventions that decrease impulsivity alter that entire impulsive response class rather than a specific topography. For example, if one changes delay discounting, one expects the participant to be better able to choose delayed yet beneficial rewards across a range of contexts.

While the potential to create robust and lasting change by decreasing impulsivity is substantial, the case can be oversold. For example, the delay discounting framework is often evoked to explain why some may eat too much, in lieu of the long-term benefits of exercise. While a stunted ability to value delayed rewards certainly contributes to overeating, the reality is more complex. As Skinner noted, most behaviors are caused/maintained by multiple interacting influences—a concept generally called *multiple causation* (Skinner, 1957). As for overeating at any given meal, impulsivity is certainly part of the equation, but so are an inability to discriminate portion sizes, environments designed to facilitate eating, and a host of biological factors, such as differences in one's feeling of fullness. This is not to diminish the role of impulsivity, which is part of the equation across a host of maladaptive behaviors, but rather to point out that while impulsivity is a behavioral influence across a range of situations, it is seldom the only influence on behavior.

Impulsive Choice

One robust area of research has been development of techniques that decrease impulsive choice—specifically, delay discounting. While few of these techniques are ready for immediate application, this research represents an important new frontier, as evidenced by the relatively recent special issue of the *Journal of the Experimental Analysis of Behavior* on the topic. It is our hope that translations of these efforts for use in practice are forthcoming.

Based on the observation that those who discount delayed rewards at lower rates tend to do better in substance abuse treatment than their more impulsive counterparts (Stanger et al., 2012), many addiction researchers have turned their focus to decreasing delay discounting rates. One of the earliest bits of progress on this front came from one of the most unexpected places. Specifically, based on the observation that the same brain areas are used to choose delayed rewards and to remember things for a short period of time, Bickel et al. (2011) tested whether having individuals who rapidly discount delayed rewards engage in working memory exercises would decrease their discounting rates. Specifically, 14 stimulant (i.e., cocaine and/or methamphetamine) users came to the lab three times a week (up to 15 sessions) to undergo a series of computerized working memory exercises. Participants were compensated for attending sessions and if their performance improved relative to their previous session. Thirteen additional stimulant users participated in a control group, wherein they completed the same memory exercises but with the answers provided. Their compensation was also tied to that of one of the participants in the treatment group. Delay discounting rates, which were measured at the beginning and end of the experiment, decreased in the patients who underwent working memory training, but not those from the control group. Simply put, working memory training decreased delay discounting in a clinically relevant sample.

Another successful approach for decreasing delay discounting rates entails getting individuals to think about the future. Episodic future thinking (EFT), or the self-projection and preexperience of future goals and/or circumstances (Atance & O'Neill, 2001), has been adapted as an approach to reducing rates of impulsive choice in clinical populations. In a study of cigarette smokers, for example, Stein et al. (2016) asked participants to consider three positive life events, unrelated to smoking, that were likely to occur following delays of 1 day, 1 week, 1 month, 3 months, and 1 year. Participants were then asked to rate these future life events based on vividness, excitement, enjoyment, and importance. Conversely, participants assigned to a control group were asked to imagine a series of similar events that occurred in the past, referred to as episodic recent thinking (ERT). Next, participants in both EFT and ERT groups wrote and recorded two to three sentences about each future or past event, which would be used as prompts during delay discounting and cigarette self-administration tasks. During the discounting assessment, participants made a series of choices between receiving smaller, immediate or larger, delayed sums of money. Audio and text prompts (related to EFT/ERT) were presented on screen throughout the task. In the cigarette administration phase, participants could earn single puffs by manipulating plungers on a fixed-ratio schedule. Participant-generated cues were also presented throughout this phase. Results showed that participants in the EFT group discounted delayed monetary rewards less steeply (i.e., retained greater subjective value over time) and consumed fewer cigarette puffs when compared to controls in the ERT group.

In addition to changing rates of discounting among cigarette smokers, EFT interventions are also shown to be effective for reducing alcohol demand intensity for individuals with alcohol dependence (Snider et al., 2016) and within at-risk drinking groups, such as college students (Bulley & Gullo, 2017). Further adaptations to EFT procedures have been geared toward reducing food-related discounting among populations with obesity (Stein et al., 2017) and are also demonstrated to reduce food consumption (Dassen et al., 2016; O'Neill et al., 2016).

Exercise also seems to decrease rates of delay discounting in both humans and non-humans. For example, Strickland et al. (2016) housed one group of rats (n = 8) in home cages that contained running wheels and another group of rats in standard cages (i.e., no running wheels; n = 8) for 11 weeks. Delay discounting rates, assessed via a well-validated delay discounting task (Evenden & Ryan, 1996), were lower in the rats that were given access to exercise. Follow-up analyses indicated that exercise impacted rats' sensitivity to both reward magnitude and delay. More directly relevant to ABA, Sofis et al. (2017) conducted a pair of studies wherein sedentary adults were provided access to a free exercise program. Evaluated in a multiple-baseline design (concurrent in Experiment 1, nonconcurrent in Experiment 2), delay discounting rates decreased when participants exercised three times a week with the experimenter. These effects, demonstrated in two separate experiments, lasted for at least 1 month after intervention.

Another promising approach to decreasing delay discounting rates is providing specialized learning histories that are compatible with choosing delayed rewards. These approaches represent a straightforward application of behavior analytic principles, yet they have not been demonstrated in humans, to date. For example, Stein et al. (2013) compared delay discounting rates in rats that had undergone extensive training (i.e., 120 days) with all rewards being delivered after a 17.5-second delay (n = 14) to rats that had received all of their rewards after no delay (n = 14), or after a delay that started at 17.5 seconds but progressively increased throughout training. Delay discounting rates were markedly lower in the rats that had experienced delays during their training. This finding has been replicated several times (Renda & Madden, 2016; Renda et al., 2018; Renda et al., 2021) including in a follow-up study demonstrating that this improved self-control lasts 4+ months after training (Renda & Madden, 2016).

Response Inhibition

Due to its relation to a range of outcomes, researchers have undergone considerable efforts to decrease response disinhibition. In a notable study, Ludyga et al. (2021) evaluated preadolescent's (n = 9) response inhibition (assessed via a go/no-go task) before and after engaging in 3 months of martial arts (i.e., judo). Their responding was compared to that of students in a waitlist control condition (i.e., students who did not receive intervention until after the study; n = 10). Students who underwent judo training had marked improvements in their responding on the go/no-go task, whereas no notable improvement was seen in the control group's responding.

As was seen with delay discounting, developing specific learning histories can also produce improvements in response inhibition. For example, Honma et al. (2021) exposed Parkinson's disease patients to 4 weeks of training to accurately judge the passage of time. This training was compared to training to accurately judge distance. Two groups experienced both training conditions, with a third group of patients receiving no training. Measures of response inhibition were taken after each 4-week training period. Response inhibition (go/no-go and Stroop tasks) only improved after patients were trained to judge the passage of time, suggesting that learning history is important for effective response inhibition.

Reflection Impulsivity

Consistent with our observations from delay discounting and response inhibition, establishing specialized behavioral histories can also improve reflection impulsivity. For example, in a randomized controlled trial, Valls-Serrano et al. (2016) demonstrated that goal management training with a mindfulness meditation program was sufficient to decrease reflection impulsivity in treatment-seeking polysubstance users. Specifically, after being randomized into the treatment group (*n* = 16), patients underwent 8 weeks of training wherein they learned to inhibit automatic behaviors/focus on the present, set/maintain goals, divide tasks into manageable pieces, and reassess/adjust their behavior as needed. These patients' performance was compared to individuals in a treatment-as-usual control group. Performance on the information sampling task (a measure of reflection impulsivity) improved in the goals management training group, but not in the treatment-as-usual group. Thus, establishing targeted learning histories improved reflection impulsivity.

Conclusions and Directions

In this chapter we have presented a brief overview of concepts and findings surrounding impulsivity. While this is not an area that behavior analysts often discuss, it is a huge research area (over 70,000 results for a PubMed search on "impulsivity" [conducted July 22, 2021]). As such, an exhaustive description of this literature is not possible. Instead, the goal has been to introduce this research area. Given that behavior-analytic curricula seldom cover "impulsivity" and that few traditional behavior-analytic researchers are embedded in this research area, an introduction may be enough.

Our hope is that the relevance of these overarching behavioral repertoires will be apparent. These are skills that enter every behavior that individuals emit. As such, they are important targets for behavioral intervention. On the bright side, improving targeted behavioral repertoires is one of our science's biggest strengths. As such, impulsivity represents a golden opportunity for behavior analysts looking to expand our practice beyond the populations and/or treatment modalities seen in most of our work/research. There is nothing about this shift that is non-behavior analytic—but it will certainly entail adjustment. For those who rise to the challenge, there is much work to be done, and our sense is that this hard work will be met with ample reward.

REFERENCES

Atance, C. M., & O'Neill, D. K. (2001). Episodic future thinking. *Trends in Cognitive Sciences, 5*(12), 533–539.

Banca, P., Lange, I., Worbe, Y., Howell, N. A., Irvine, M., Harrison, N. A., . . . Voon, V. (2016). Reflection impulsivity in binge drinking: Behavioural and volumetric correlates. *Addiction Biology, 21*, 504–515.

Bénard, M., Camilleri, G. M., Etilé, F., Mejean, C., Bellisle, F., Reach, G., . . . Péneau, S. (2017). Association between impulsivity and weight status in a general population. *Nutrients, 9*(3), Article 217.

Bickel, W. K., Jarmolowicz, D. P., Mueller, E. T., Franck, C. T., Carrin, C., & Gatchalian, K. M. (2012). Altruism in time: Social temporal discounting differentiates smokers from problem drinkers. *Psychopharmacology, 224*(1), 109–120.

Bickel, W. K., Jarmolowicz, D. P., Mueller, E. T., Gatchalian, K. M., & McClure, S. M. (2012). Are executive function and impulsivity antipodes?: A conceptual reconstruction with special reference to addiction. *Psychopharmacology, 221*(3), 361–387.

Bickel, W. K., Jarmolowicz, D. P., Mueller, E. T., Koffarnus, M. N., & Gatchalian, K. M. (2012). Excessive discounting of delayed reinforcers as a trans-disease process contributing to addiction and other disease-related vulnerabilities: Emerging evidence. *Pharmacology and Therapeutics, 134*(3), 287–297.

Bickel, W. K., MacKillop, J., Madden, G. J., Odum, A. L., & Yi, R. (2015). Experimental manipulations of delay discounting and related processes: An introduction to the special issue. *Journal of the Experimental Analysis of Behavior, 103*, 1–9.

Bickel, W. K., & Mueller, E. T. (2009). Toward the study of trans-disease processes: A novel approach with special reference to the study of co-morbidity. *Journal of Dual Diagnosis, 5*(2), 131–138.

Bickel, W. K., Odum, A. L., & Madden, G. J. (1999). Impulsivity and cigarette smoking: Delay discounting in current, never, and ex-smokers. *Psychopharmacology, 146*(4), 447–454.

Bickel, W. K., Wilson, G. A., Franck, C. T., Mueller, E. T., Jarmolowicz, D. P., Koffarnus, M. N., & Fede, S. J. (2014). Using crowdsourcing to compare temporal, social temporal, and probability discounting among obese and non-obese individuals. *Appetite, 75*, 82–89.

Bickel, W. K., Yi, R., Landes, R. D., Hill, P. F., & Baxter, C. (2011). Remember the future: Working memory training decreases delay discounting among stimulant addicts. *Biological Psychiatry, 69*(3), 260–265.

Billieux, J., Lagrange, G., Van der Linden, M., Lancon, C., Adida, M., & Jeanningros, R. (2012). Investigation of impulsivity in a sample of treatment-seeking pathological gamblers: A multidimensional perspective. *Psychiatry Research, 198*, 291–296.

Breat, C., Claus, L., Verbeken, S., & Van Vlierberghe, L. (2007). Impulsivity in overweight children. *European Journal of Adolescent Psychiatry, 16*, 473–783.

Bulley, A., & Gullo, M. (2017). The influence of episodic foresight on delay discounting and demand for alcohol. *Addictive Behaviors, 66*, 1–6.

Buss, A. H., & Plomin, R. (1975). *A temperament theory of personality development.* Wiley.

Cairns, E., & Cammock, T. (1978). Development of a more reliable version of the Matching Familiar Figures Test. *Developmental Psychology, 14*(5), 555–560.

Caswell, A. J., Morgan, M. J., & Duka, T. (2013). Acute alcohol effects on subtypes of impulsivity and the role of alcohol-outcome expectancies. *Psychopharmacology, 229*(1), 21–30.

Centers for Disease Control and Prevention. (2021). Attention-deficit/hyperactivity disorder (ADHD). Retrieved July 23, 2021, from *www.cdc.gov/ncbddd/adhd/facts.html.*

Clark, L., Robbins, T. W., Ersche, K. D., & Sahakian, B. J. (2006). Reflection impulsivity in current and former substance users. *Biological Psychiatry, 60*(5), 515–522.

Clark, L., Roiser, J. P., Robbins, T. W., & Sahakian, B. J. (2009). Disrupted "reflection" impulsivity in cannabis users but not current or former ecstasy users. *Journal of Psychopharmacology, 23*(1), 14–22.

Coffey, S. F., Gudleski, G. D., Saladin, M. E., & Brady, K. T. (2003). Impulsivity and rapid discounting of delayed hypothetical rewards in cocaine-dependent individuals. *Experimental and Clinical Psychopharmacology, 11*(1), 18–25.

Conners, C. (1992). *Conners Continuous Performance Test.* Multi-Health Systems.

Dalley, J. W., Everitt, B. J., & Robbins, T. W. (2011). Impulsivity, compulsivity, and top-down cognitive control. *Neuron, 69*(4), 680–694.

Dassen, F. C. M., Jansen, A., Nederkoorn, C., & Houben, K. (2016). Focus on the future: Episodic future thinking reduces discount rate and snacking *Appetite, 96*, 327–332.

Dickman, S. J. (1993). Impulsivity and information processing. In W. G. McCown, J. L. Johnson, & M. B. Shure (Eds.), *The impulsive client: Theory, research, and treatment* (pp. 151–184). American Psychological Association.

Dixon, M. R., Jacobs, E. A., & Sanders, S. (2006). Contextual control of delay discounting by pathological gamblers. *Journal of Applied Behavior Analysis, 39*(4), 413–422.

Dixon, M. R., Marley, J., & Jacobs, E. A. (2003). Delay discounting by pathological gamblers. *Journal of Applied Behavior Analysis, 36*(4), 449–458.

Dougherty, D. M., Marsh, D. M., Moeller, F. G., Chokshi, R. V., & Rosen, V. C. (2000). Effects of moderate and high doses of alcohol on attention, impulsivity, discriminability, and response bias in immediate and delayed memory task performance. *Alcoholism: Clinical and Experimental Research, 24*(11), 1702–1711.

Drewe, E. (1975). Go–no go learning after frontal lobe lesions in humans. *Cortex, 11*(1), 8–16.

Durana, J., & Barnes, P. (1993). A neurodevelopmental view of impulsivity and its relationship to the superfactors of personality. In W. McCown, J. Johnson, & M. Shure (Eds.), *The impulsive client: Theory, research and treatment* (pp. 23–37). American Psychological Association.

Epstein, L. H., Salvy, S. J., Carr, K. A., Dearing, K. K., & Bickel, W. K. (2010). Food reinforcement, delay discounting and obesity. *Physiology and Behavior, 100*(5), 438–445.

Epstein, M., Bailey, J. A., Manhart, L. E., Hill, K. G., & Hawkins, J. D. (2014). Sexual risk behavior in young adulthood: Broadening the scope beyond early sexual initiation. *Journal of Sex Research, 51*(7), 721–730.

Evenden, J. L. (1999). Varieties of impulsivity. *Psychopharmacology, 146*(4), 348–361.

Evenden, J. L., & Ryan, C. N. (1996). The pharmacology of impulsive behaviour in rats: The effects of drugs on response choice with varying delays of reinforcement. *Psychopharmacology, 128*(2), 161–170.

Field, M., Santarcangelo, M., Sumnall, H., Goudie, A., & Cole, J. (2006). Delay discounting and the behavioural economics of cigarette purchases in smokers: The effects of nicotine deprivation. *Psychopharmacology, 186*(2), 255–263.

Fillmore, M. T., Blackburn, J. S., & Harrison, E. L. R. (2008). Acute disinhibiting effects of alcohol as a factor in risky driving behavior. *Drug and Alcohol Dependence, 95*, 97–106.

Garami, J., & Moustafa, A. A. (2019). Probability discounting of monetary gains and losses in opioid-dependent adults. *Behavioral Brain Research, 364*, 334–339.

Gerdan, G., & Kurt, M. (2020). Response inhibition according to the stimulus and food type in exogenous obesity. *Appetite, 150*, Article 104651.

Giordano, L., Bickel, W. K., Loewenstein, G., Jacobs, E. A., Marsch, L., & Badger, G. J. (2002). Mild opioid deprivation increases the degree that opioid-dependent outpatients discount delayed heroin and money. *Psychopharmacology, 163*(2), 174–182.

Green, L., & Myerson, J. (2004). A discounting framework for choice with delayed and probabilistic rewards. *Psychological Bulletin, 130*(5), 769–792.

Green, L., & Myerson, J. (2013). How many impulsivities?: A discounting perspective. *Journal of the Experimental Analysis of Behavior, 99*, 3–13.

Hendrickson, K. L., & Rasmussen, E. B. (2017). Mindful eating reduces impulsive food choice in adolescents and adults. *Health Psychology, 36*, 226–235.

Honma, M., Murakami, H., Yabe, Y., Kuroda, T., Akinori, F., Sugimoto, A., . . . Ono, K. (2021). Stopwatch training improves cognitive functions in patients with Parkinson's disease. *Journal of Neuroscience Research, 99*, 1325–1336.

Jarmolowicz, D. P., Bickel, W. K., Carter, A. E., Franck, C. T., & Mueller, E. T. (2012). Using crowdsourcing to examine relations between delay and probability discounting. *Behavioural Processes, 91*(3), 308–312.

Jarmolowicz, D. P., Cherry, J. B., Reed, D. D., Bruce, J. M., Crespi, J. M., Lusk, J. L., & Bruce, A. S. (2014). Robust relation between temporal discounting rates and body mass. *Appetite, 78*, 63–67.

Jarmolowicz, D. P., Reed, D. D., Stancato, S. S., Lemley, S. M., Sofis, M. J., Fox, A. T., & Martin, L. E. (2020). On the discounting of cannabis and money: Sensitivity to magnitude vs. delay. *Drug and Alcohol Dependence, 212*, Article 107996.

Jepsen, J. R. M., Rydkjaer, J., Fagerlund, B., Pagsberg, A. K., Jepersen, R. A. F., Glenthoj, B. Y., & Oranje, B. (2018). Overlapping and disease specific trait, response, and reflection impulsivity in adolescents with first-episode schizophrenia spectrum disorders or attention-deficit/hyperactivity disorder *Psychological Medicine, 48*, 604–616.

Johnson, M. W., Herrmann, E. S., Sweeney, M. M., LeComte, R. S., & Johnson, P. S. (2017). Cocaine administration dose-dependently increases sexual desire and decreases condom use likelihood: The role of delay and probability discounting in connecting cocaine with HIV. *Psychopharmacology, 234*(4), 599–612.

Johnson, P. S., Sweeney, M. M., Herrmann, E. S., & Johnson, M. W. (2016). Alcohol increases delay and probability discounting of condom-protected sex: A novel vector for alcohol-related HIV transmission. *Alcoholism: Clinical and Experimental Research, 40*(6), 1339–1350.

Kaufman, J. N., Ross, T. J., Stein, E. A., & Garavan, H. (2003). Cingulate hypoactivity in cocaine users during a GO–NOGO task as revealed by event-related functional magnetic resonance imaging. *Journal of Neuroscience, 23*(21), 7839–7843.

Koffarnus, M. N., Jarmolowicz, D. P., Mueller, E. T., & Bickel, W. K. (2013). Changing discounting in light of the competing neurobehavioral decision systems theory. *Journal of the Experimental Analysis of Behavior, 99*(1), 32–57.

Kuypers, K. P. C., Wingen, M., Samyn, N., Limbert, N., & Ramaekers, J. G. (2007). Acute effects of nocturnal doses of MDMA on measures of impulsivity and psychomotor performance throughout the night. *Psychopharmacology, 192,* 111–119.

Lawrence, A. J., Luty, J., Bogdan, N. A., Sahakian, B. J., & Clark, L. (2009). Impulsivity and response inhibition in alcohol dependence and problem gambling. *Psychopharmacology, 207*(1), 163–172.

Lemley, S. M., Kaplan, B. A., Reed, D. D., Darden, A. C., & Jarmolowicz, D. P. (2016). Reinforcer pathologies: Predicting alcohol related problems in college drinking men and women. *Drug and Alcohol Dependence, 167,* 57–66.

Logan, G. D., & Cowan, W. B. (1984). On the ability to inhibit thought and action: A theory of an act of control. *Psychological Review, 91*(3), 295–327.

Ludyga, S., Trankner, S., Gerber, M., & Puhse, U. (2021). Effects of judo on neurocognitive indices of response inhibition in preadolescent children: A randomized controlled trial. *Medicine and Science in Sports and Exercise, 53,* 1648–1655.

MacCorquodale, K., & Meehl, P. E. (1948). On a distinction between hypothetical constructs and intervening variables. *Psychological Review, 55,* 95–107.

Madden, G. J., Petry, N. M., Badger, G. J., & Bickel, W. K. (1997). Impulsive and self-control choices in opioid-dependent patients and non-drug-using control participants: Drug and monetary rewards. *Experimental and Clinical Psychopharmacology, 5*(3), 256–262.

Mashoon, Y., Betts, J., Farmer, S. L., & Lukas, S. E. (2018). Early onset tobacco cigarette smokers exhibit deficits in response inhibition and sustained attention *Drug and Alcohol Dependence, 184,* 48–56.

Mazur, J. E. (1987). An adjusting procedure for studying delayed reinforcement. In M. L. Commons, J. E. Mazur, J. A. Nevin, & H. Rachlin (Eds.), *Quantitative analysis of behavior* (Vol. 5, pp. 55–73). Erlbaum.

McCloskey, M., Palmer, A. A., & de Wit, H. (2010). Are attention lapses related to d-amphetamine liking? *Psychopharmacology, 208*(2), 201–209.

McKerchar, T. L., & Renda, C. R. (2012). Delay and probability discounting in humans: An overview. *Psychological Record, 62,* 817–834.

Mischel, W., & Ebbesen, E. B. (1970). Attention in delay of gratification. *Journal of Personality and Social Psychology, 16,* 329–337.

Moeller, F. G., Hasan, K. M., Steinberg, J. L., Kramer, L. A., Dougherty, D. M., Santos, R. M., . . . Narayana, P. A. (2005). Reduced anterior corpus callosum white matter integrity is related to increased impulsivity and reduced discriminability in cocaine-dependent subjects: Diffusion tensor imaging. *Neuropsychopharmacology, 30*(3), 610–617.

Monterosso, J. R., Ainslie, G., Xu, J., Cordova, X., Domier, C. P., & London, E. D. (2007). Frontoparietal cortical activity of methamphetamine-dependent and comparison subjects performing a delay discounting task. *Human Brain Mapping, 28*(5), 383–393.

Monterosso, J. R., Aron, A. R., Cordova, X., Xu, J., & London, E. D. (2005). Deficits in response inhibition associated with chronic methamphetamine abuse. *Drug and Alcohol Dependence, 79*(2), 273–277.

Moreno, M., Estevez, A. F., Zaldivar, F., Montes, J. M. G., Gutiérrez-Ferre, V. E., Esteban, L., . . . Flores, P. (2012). Impulsivity differences in recreational cannabis users and binge drinkers in a university population. *Drug And Alcohol Dependence, 124*(3), 355–362.

National Institute of Mental Health. (2011). Attention deficit hyperactivity disorder (ADHD). Retrieved from *www.nimh.nih.gov/health/topics/attention-deficit-hyperactivity-disorder-adhd*

O'Neill, J., Daniel, T. O., & Epstein, L. H. (2016). Episodic future thinking reduces eating in a food court. *Eating Behaviors, 20,* 9–13.

Odum, A. L. (2011). Delay discounting: Trait variable? *Behavioral Processes, 87,* 1–9.

Odum, A. L., & Baumann, A. A. (2007). Cigarette smokers show steeper discounting of both food and cigarettes than money. *Drug and Alcohol Dependence, 91*(2–3), 293–296.

Patton, J. H., Stanford, M. S., & Barratt, E. S. (1995). Factor structure of the Barratt Impulsiveness Scale. *Journal of Clinical Psychology, 51*(6), 768–774.

Petry, N. M. (2001a). Delay discounting of money and alcohol in actively using alcoholics, currently abstinent alcoholics, and controls. *Psychopharmacology, 154*(3), 243–250.

Petry, N. M. (2001b). Pathological gamblers, with and without substance use disorders, discount delayed rewards at high rates. *Journal of Abnormal Psychology, 110*(3), 482–487.

Phillips, L. D., & Edwards, W. (1966). Conservatism in a simple probability inference task. *Journal of Experimental Psychology, 72*(3), 346–354.

Quednow, B. B., Kuhn, K. U., Hoppe, C., Westheide, J., Maier, W., Daum, I., & Wagner, M. (2007). Elevated impulsivity and impaired decision-making cognition in heavy users of MDMA ("Ecstasy"). *Psychopharmacology, 189*(4), 517–530.

Rachlin, H., Raineri, A., & Cross, D. (1991). Subjective probability and delay. *Journal of the Experimental Analysis of Behavior, 55*(2), 233–244.

Radulovic, J., Jovasevic, V., & Meyer, M. A. A. (2017). Neurobiological mechanisms of state-dependent learning. *Current Opinion in Neurobiology, 45*, 92–98.

Rasmussen, E. B., Lawyer, S. R., & Reilly, W. (2010). Percent body fat is related to delay and probability discounting for food in humans. *Behavioural Processes, 83*(1), 23–30.

Renda, C. R., & Madden, G. J. (2016). Impulsive choice and pre-exposure to delays: III. Four-month test–retest outcomes in male Wistar rats. *Behavioural Processes, 126*, 108–112.

Renda, C. R., Rung, J. M., Hinnenkamp, J. E., Lenzini, S. N., & Madden, G. J. (2018). Impulsive choice and pre-exposure to delays: IV. Effects of delay- and immediacy-exposure training relative to maturational changes in impulsivity. *Journal of the Experimental Analysis of Behavior, 109*(3), 587–599.

Renda, C. R., Rung, J. M., Peck, S., & Madden, G. J. (2021). Reducing impulsive choice: VII. Effects of duration of delay-exposure training. *Animal Cognition, 24*, 11–21.

Reynolds, B., Richards, J. B., & de Wit, H. (2006). Acute-alcohol effects on the Experiential Discounting Task (EDT) and a question-based measure of delay discounting. *Pharmacology Biochemistry and Behavior, 83*(2), 194–202.

Reynolds, B., Richards, J. B., Horn, K., & Karraker, K. (2004). Delay discounting and probability discounting as related to cigarette smoking status in adults. *Behavioral Processes, 30*(65), 35–42.

Salfi, F., D'Atri, A., Tempesta, D., De Gennaro, L. D., & Ferrara, M. (2020). Boosting slow oscillations during sleep to improve memory function in elderly people: A review of the literature. *Brain Science, 10*, Article 300.

Salgado, J. V., Malloy-Diniz, L. F., Campos, V. R., Abrantes, S. S., Fuentes, D., Bechara, A., & Correa, H. (2009). Neuropsychological assessment of impulsive behavior in abstinent alcohol-dependent subjects. *Revista Brasileira de Psiquiatria, 31*(1), 4–9.

Sidman, M. (1960). *Tactics of scientific research: Evaluating experimental data in psychology.* Basic Books.

Skinner, B. F. (1938). *The behavior of organisms.* Appleton-Century-Crofts.

Skinner, B. F. (1957). Multiple causation. In *Verbal behavior* (pp. 227–252). Appleton-Century-Crofts.

Skrynka, J., & Vincent, B. T. (2019). Hunger increases delay discounting of food and nonfood rewards. *Psychological Bulletin and Review, 26*, 1729–1737.

Snider, S. E., LaConte, S. M., & Bickel, W. K. (2016). Episodic future thinking: Expansion of the temporal window in individuals with alcohol dependence. *Alcohol: Clinical and Experimental Research, 40*, 1558–1566.

Sofis, M. J., Carrillo, A., & Jarmolowicz, D. P. (2017). Maintained physical activity induced changes in delay discounting. *Behavior Modification, 41*(4), 499–528.

Solowij, N., Jones, K. A., Rozman, M. E., Davis, S. M., Ciarrochi, J., Heaven, P. C. L., ... Yucel, M. (2012). Reflection impulsivity in adolescent cannabis users: A comparison with alcohol-using and non-substance-using adolescents. *Psychopharmacology, 219*, 575–586.

Stanger, C., Ryan, S. R., Fu, H., Landes, R. D., Jones, B. A., Bickel, W. K., & Budney, A. J. (2012). Delay discounting predicts adolescent substance abuse treatment outcome. *Experimental and Clinical Psychopharmacology, 20*(3), 205–212.

Stein, J. S., Johnson, P. S., Renda, C. R., Smitts, R. R., Liston, K. J., Shahan, T. A., & Madden, G. J. (2013). Early and prolonged exposure to reward delay: Effects on impulsive choice and alcohol self-administration in male rats. *Experimental and Clinical Psychopharmacology, 21*, 172–180.

Stein, J. S., Sze, Y. Y., Athamneh, L., Koffarnus, M. N., Epstein, L. H., & Bickel, W. K. (2017). Think fast: Rapid assessment of the effects of episodic future thinking on delay discounting in overweight/obese participants. *Journal of Behavioral Medicine, 40*(5), 832–838.

Stein, J. S., Wilson, A. G., Koffarnus, M. N., Daniel, T. O., Epstein, L. H., & Bickel, W. K. (2016). Unstuck in time: Episodic future thinking reduces delay discounting and cigarette smoking. *Psychopharmacology, 233,* 3771–3778.

Strickland, J. C., Feinstein, M. A., Lacy, R. T., & Smith, M. A. (2016). The effects of physical activity on impulsive choice: Influence of sensitivity to reinforcement amount and delay. *Behavioural Processes, 126,* 36–45.

Townshend, J. M., Kambouropoulos, N., Griffin, A., Hunt, F. J., & Milani, R. M. (2014). Binge drinking, reflection impulsivity, and unplanned sexual behavior: Impaired decision-making in young social drinkers. *Alcohol: Clinical and Experimental Research, 38,* 1143–1150.

Valls-Serrano, C., Caracuel, A., & Verdejo-Garcia, A. (2016). Goal management training and mindfulness meditation improve executive functions and transfer to ecological tasks of daily life in polysubstance users enrolled in therapeutic community treatment *Drug and Alcohol Dependence, 165,* 9–14.

van Wel, J. H., Kuypers, K. P., Theunissen, E. L., Bosker, W. M., Bakker, K., & Ramaekers, J. G. (2012). Effects of acute MDMA intoxication on mood and impulsivity: Role of the 5-HT2 and 5-HT1 receptors. *PLOS One, 7*(7), Article e40187.

Vonmoos, M., Hulka, L. M., Preller, K. H., Jenni, D., Schulz, C., Baumgartner, M. R., & Quednow, B. B. (2013). Differences in self-reported and behavioral measures of impulsivity in recreational and dependent cocaine users. *Drug and Alcohol Dependence, 133*(1), 61–70.

Voon, V., Chang-Webb, Y. C., Morris, L. S., Cooper, E., Sethi, A., Baek, K., . . . Harrison, N. A. (2016). Waiting impulsivity: The influence of acute methylphenidate and feedback. *International Journal of Neuropsychopharmacology, 19*(1), Article pyv074.

Vuchinich, R. E., & Simpson, C. A. (1998). Hyperbolic temporal discounting in social drinkers and problem drinkers. *Experimental and Clinical Psychopharmacology, 6*(3), 292–305.

Weafer, J., & Fillmore, M. T. (2015). Alcohol-related cues potentiate alcohol impairment of behavioral control in drinkers. *Psychology of Addictive Behavior, 29,* 290–299.

Weller, R. E., Cook, E. W., III, Avsar, K. B., & Cox, J. E. (2008). Obese women show greater delay discounting than healthy-weight women. *Appetite, 51*(3), 563–569.

Yi, R., Chase, W. D., & Bickel, W. K. (2007). Probability discounting among cigarette smokers and nonsmokers: Molecular analysis discerns group differences. *Behavioural Pharmacology, 18*(7), 633–639.

Zuckerman, M., Eysenck, S. B., & Eysenck, H. J. (1978). Sensation seeking in England and America: Cross-cultural, age, and sex comparisons. *Journal of Consulting and Clinical Psychology, 46*(1), 139–149.

CHAPTER 23

Behavioral Pharmacology

Alison D. Cox
Craige Wrenn
Maria G. Valdovinos

Up to 50% of individuals with intellectual and developmental disabilities (IDD) engage in problem behavior (PB; Sheehan et al., 2015). These behaviors often interfere with skills acquisition and service access, and disrupt daily-life activities. Treatment approaches typically include behavioral, psychopharmacological, or combined interventions (i.e., concurrent application of behavioral and psychopharmacological); with psychotropic drug prescriptions being particularly widespread (Lunsky et al., 2018; Scheifes et al., 2013). Using psychotropic drugs to treat PB often means they are being used off-label; that is, the drug is being used in a manner that was not specified in the Food and Drug Administration's approved packaging label. Many individuals receiving psychotropic drugs to treat PB are being prescribed more than one drug concurrently, referred to as *polypharmacy* (Deb et al., 2015). Also, when polypharmacy is observed, individuals are often being prescribed more than one drug from the same drug class (Scheifes et al., 2016).

A focus on specific disorders reveals those diagnosed with autism spectrum disorder (ASD) are generally prescribed more psychotropic drugs, with prevalence rates varying between 2.7% to as high as 80%, and a median reported prevalence of 45.7% (Jobski et al., 2017; Lamy et al., 2020). Other predictors of psychotropic drug use include comorbid diagnoses such as ASD and attention-deficit/hyperactivity disorder (ADHD; Rasmussen et al., 2019), engagement in PB (e.g., Bowring et al., 2017), and age (e.g., Jobski et al., 2017).

A neurological basis of behavior is one argument for using psychotropic drugs to treat PB (Willner, 2015). However, behavior is a complex interaction between environment and biology. Although neurotransmitters such as dopamine, gamma-aminobutyric acid (GABA) and serotonin are implicated in aggression, solely modulating these neurotransmitters is not sufficient to alter behavior.

Given how often psychotropic drugs are used to treat PB in persons with IDD, it is important that behavior analysts working with these individuals understand how psychotropic drugs impact physiology and the mechanisms by which they can exert an effect on behavior. This chapter provides a brief overview of pharmacology, presentation of the effects of commonly prescribed psychotropic drugs, a brief applied behavioral pharmacology literature review, relevant ethical considerations, and a case study illustrating how behavior analysts may approach monitoring drug impact on behavior outcomes.

An Introduction to Pharmacology

Stated simply, *pharmacology* is the study of the alteration of biological processes by chemical agents. The chemical agent can be an endogenous compound (e.g., a neurotransmitter), a toxin (e.g., mustard gas), or a drug (e.g., Prozac). In the case of brain function, the biological processes altered by these chemical agents are primarily the electrical activity of neurons and the chemical communication between neurons. Because behavior is the end product of the electrical and chemical activity of neurons, a chemical agent that alters these processes can lead to profound changes in behavior. The study of how chemical agents, such as drugs, alter behavior is referred to as *behavioral pharmacology.*

An understanding of all areas of pharmacology, including behavioral pharmacology, depends on an understanding of two broad concepts. The first of these is *pharmacodynamics*, which is the name given to a drug's interaction with its target tissues and molecules. A useful colloquialism is that pharmacodynamics is concerned with what the drug does to the body. Of course, a drug's effect on behavior cannot be fully understood by considering only what the chemical agent does to the brain. One must also consider the processes that govern the time course and extent of a drug's arrival and entry into the brain tissue. These processes include absorption into the circulation, distribution from the site of administration, metabolism, and excretion. The study of these processes and their time courses is the second broad concept, known as *pharmacokinetics.* Colloquially, pharmacokinetics is concerned with what the body does to the drug. What follows is a general description of pharmacodynamics and pharmacokinetics in relation to behavioral pharmacology.

Pharmacodynamics

To begin to understand the pharmacodynamics of psychotropic drugs, one should become familiar with their primary cellular target—the synapse (see Figure 23.1). The *synapse* is the gap, or space, that is found between communicating neurons. The usual arrangement is for the *presynaptic neuron* to release a chemical messenger that diffuses across the synapse and ultimately interacts with the *postsynaptic neuron,* altering its function. The chemical messenger is referred to as a *neurotransmitter.* The processes used by the neurotransmitter to alter the function of the postsynaptic neuron are referred to collectively as *synaptic transmission.* It is the facilitation or inhibition of synaptic transmission that forms the pharmacodynamic basis of a drug's impact on behavior.

Synaptic transmission is accomplished through the interaction of neurotransmitter molecules with large proteins found on the surface of the postsynaptic neuron. These proteins are called *postsynaptic receptors* and have highly specific neurotransmitter binding sites. Following release into the synapse, neurotransmitter molecules bind to these receptors, causing the receptor's three-dimensional shape to change. This change in shape triggers a cascade of biochemical reactions inside the postsynaptic neuron. These reactions are the biochemical basis of how neurons alter their function and, in turn, produce behavior. Thus, any drug that can mimic the action of a neurotransmitter at the receptor

Synaptic Transmission

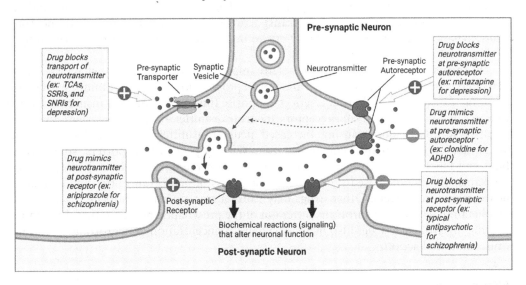

FIGURE 23.1. Illustration of synaptic transmission, with important drug targets. Neurotransmitter (small circles) is stored in vesicles in the presynaptic neuron. Vesicles fuse (represented by diagonal arrow) with the presynaptic membrane and release neurotransmitter into the synapse. Synaptic signaling is accomplished by neurotransmitters binding to postsynaptic receptors, activating biochemical reactions inside the postsynaptic neuron. Postsynaptic receptors are important drug targets for agonists and antagonists. Important drug targets are also present on the presynaptic neuron. Presynaptic transporters regulate synaptic concentration of neurotransmitter by performing reuptake (represented by horizontal arrow). Drugs that block reuptake increase synaptic neurotransmitter and synaptic transmission. When bound by a neurotransmitter, presynaptic autoreceptors regulate synaptic concentration of neurotransmitter by inhibiting release (represented by a dotted arrow). Agonists that mimic the neurotransmitter at autoreceptors decrease synaptic transmission. Antagonists that block autoreceptors increase synaptic transmission. Drug mechanisms that enhance synaptic transmission are indicated by a plus sign. Drug mechanisms that decrease synaptic transmission are indicated by a minus sign. (The figure was prepared using Biorender.)

can produce behaviors similar to those produced by the neurotransmitter. Drugs that mimic the action of neurotransmitters at receptors are referred to as *agonists*. Alternatively, drugs that bind the receptor without producing an effect block signal transduction and prevent stimulation of the receptor by the neurotransmitter. Such drugs are called *antagonists* and may produce behavioral alterations by decreasing the signal transduction of the endogenous neurotransmitter.

On the surface of the presynaptic neuron are important proteins that regulate neurotransmitter action. Two major types of these regulators are the *inhibitory autoreceptors* and the *transporters*. A similarity of these two molecules is that both decrease signal transduction by neurotransmitters. However, they accomplish this function through entirely different mechanisms. In the case of the inhibitory autoreceptors, released neurotransmitters bind to a specific binding site on the autoreceptor, producing a change in the autoreceptor's shape. This results in a biochemical cascade that causes inhibition of further neurotransmitter release. In this way, the autoreceptor is a mechanism of negative feedback that limits postsynaptic neurotransmitter action. Transporters also decrease synaptic transmission by performing *reuptake*. They perform this function by binding the neurotransmitter and physically transporting it back into the presynaptic neuron. Thus, synaptic transmission is reduced due to decreased neurotransmitter concentration in the synapse.

Both autoreceptors and transporters are important drug targets in behavioral pharmacology. Drugs that act as agonists at autoreceptors (neurotransmitter mimics) decrease synaptic transmission and produce effects opposite those of the neurotransmitter. Drugs that act as antagonists at autoreceptors (neurotransmitter blockers) interfere with the negative feedback loop, causing increased neurotransmitter release and effects that are similar to those of the neurotransmitter. With respect to transporters, some drugs bind and block transporters (e.g., selective serotonin reuptake inhibitor [SSRI] antidepressants) causing increased synaptic concentrations of neurotransmitter and enhanced neurotransmitter effects. Other drugs may cause a transporter to work in reverse (e.g., amphetamine), moving neurotransmitter out of the presynaptic neuron rather than transporting inward. Such drugs also increase synaptic concentration of neurotransmitter and cause enhanced action.

Pharmacokinetics

In addition to the pharmacodynamic mechanisms we have described, clinical outcomes with psychotropic drugs are a function of pharmacokinetics. All pharmacokinetic processes (absorption, distribution, metabolism, and excretion) are important, but in the case of psychotropic drugs, the processes that determine clearance of the drug from the body are especially salient. Drug clearance is principally accomplished by the chemical alteration of the compound (metabolism) followed by excretion, usually by the kidney. Metabolism happens primarily (but not exclusively) in the liver.

Phase I metabolism refers to chemical reactions, catalyzed by enzymes found in the liver, that oxidize, reduce, or hydrolyze the drug. In chemical terms, these reactions produce a compound that is more polar. A helpful general rule is that when a compound is made to be more polar, it becomes less able to enter the brain and more able to enter urine for excretion.

Phase II metabolism refers to chemical reactions that conjugate (add) the drug or the drug's metabolite to a molecule, increasing the polarity and often yielding a compound that is ionized at physiological pH. Ionized molecules cannot enter the brain (with a few exceptions), but they readily distribute into urine. Hence, clearance from the body is promoted by Phase II metabolism.

Because drug clearance depends on metabolism by the liver and excretion by the kidney, the function of these organs is critical to the outcome that is seen with a drug. So any condition in which these organs are impaired will result in impaired clearance of the drug from the body. In the case of psychotropic drugs, the impact of liver or kidney dysfunction is often increased toxicity and adverse side effects (ASEs) due to slow clearance and the accumulation of the drug at levels greater than needed for therapy. In some cases, downward dose adjustments can solve this problem and improve clinical outcomes for patients with hepatic or renal dysfunction.

A convenient measure that is commonly employed to quantify the time course of a drug's clearance from the body is *half-life* $(t_{1/2})$. The half-life is defined as the amount of time required for half of the drug to be removed from the blood. Half-life is an important property of a drug, because it determines the dosing interval needed to maintain a drug level at a desired, constant concentration in the blood. For any given dosing interval, a constant blood concentration of the drug is achieved after approximately five half-lives. This constant blood concentration occurs when the rates of absorption and distribution of the drug are equal to the rates of metabolism and excretion. This "sweet spot" of pharmacotherapy is called the *steady state*. Ideally, steady-state blood concentration is at a level that gives the therapeutic effect without producing toxicity or ASE.

Pharmacology of Psychotropic Drug Classes

The mechanism of action, therapeutic effects, and toxicities of psychotropic drugs are all dependent on the pharmacodynamic and pharmacokinetic concepts we have described. Below we identify psychotropic drug classes that are frequently administered to individuals with IDD. For each class, we highlight what is known about how the drugs work in the brain and which concepts and processes are of particular important for understanding each drug class. For fulsome summaries of these drug classes see Brunton et al. (2018), Stahl (2013), and Meyer and Quenzer (2019).

Typical Antipsychotics

The typical antipsychotics are the first generation of drugs discovered to treat the so-called "positive" symptoms of schizophrenia, principally delusions and hallucinations. Their mechanism of action is to act as an antagonist of dopamine receptors in the brain. Dopamine is a neurotransmitter that is critical to a wide variety of behavioral functions including cognition, reward processing, modulation of movement, and endocrine regulation. Most of the desired and undesired effects of the typical antipsychotics can be understood in terms of their ability to block dopamine receptors and reduce dopamine signal transduction in the brain.

The hallucinations and delusions of psychosis are hypothesized to be due to excessive dopamine signal transduction in limbic areas of the brain. Thus, the dopamine antagonists are thought to diminish psychosis by blocking this excessive signaling. Unfortunately, these drugs do not distinguish between limbic dopamine receptors and dopamine receptors in different brain pathways that serve functions unrelated to psychosis.

The blockade of dopamine receptors not involved in psychosis are the mechanism by which the major side effects of the typical antipsychotics arise. Dopamine signaling plays a major role in the modulation of movement through action at receptors in the striatum. The blockade of striatal dopamine receptors can cause tremor, slowed movement, and postural disturbances within about 2 months of starting therapy. In the longer term (after years of use), tardive dyskinesia of the mouth and face manifesting as lip-smacking or other tic-like involuntary movements of mouth, tongue, or eyelids can arise.

Neuroendocrine side effects of the typical antipsychotics are due to the blockade of dopamine receptors in the pituitary. The function of dopamine in the pituitary is to provide inhibition of prolactin release. Without this inhibition, the pituitary performs high intrinsic secretion of prolactin. The consequence of blocking this inhibition by a typical antipsychotic is elevated plasma prolactin (hyperprolactinemia). In women, hyperprolactinemia manifests as breast pain/tenderness, milk discharge unrelated to nursing (galactorrhea), disruption of the menstrual cycle, and infertility. In men, antipsychotic-induced hyperprolactinemia results in development of the breasts (gynecomastia), galactorrhea, erectile dysfunction, and low sperm counts. For both men and women, these endocrine side effects can negatively affect adherence to antipsychotic therapy. In addition to motor and endocrine regulation, dopamine plays a crucial role in the brain's processing of reward. Thus, it is reasonable to hypothesize that antipsychotic drugs alter reward processing, which could impact behavioral therapies relying on operant principles.

Atypical Antipsychotics

The atypical antipsychotics are the second generation of drugs for the treatment of schizophrenia (see Stahl, 2013). Their therapeutic advantage over typical antipsychotics is that they are much less likely to cause dopamine-related motor and endocrine side effects. Furthermore, clozapine is an atypical antipsychotic that is more effective than the typicals at reducing the negative symptoms of schizophrenia such as inappropriate affect, lack of motivation, and social apathy.

The mechanism of action of the atypical antipsychotics is a complex mix of receptor interactions that varies considerably from drug to drug. Despite the complexity, it can be generally stated that all atypical antipsychotics are antagonists at dopamine and serotonin receptors. Compared to typical antipsychotics, atypical antipsychotics have a higher serotonin receptor-to-dopamine receptor binding ratio. This binding ratio is thought to contribute to the lack of dopamine-related side effects (for a thorough discussion, see Stahl, 2013) that make the atypical antipsychotics preferable for most patients.

Although atypical antipsychotics infrequently cause motor and endocrine side effects, they have their own ASE profile that can be problematic for some patients. For example, several have metabolic effects that lead to weight gain, elevated plasma cholesterol, and increased risk of diabetes mellitus. Notably, weight gain is most prominent in adolescents. These metabolic effects are believed to be the consequence of antagonism of histamine and serotonin receptors in brain areas that regulate satiety.

Antidepressants

Antidepressants comprise a wide range of drugs with a variety of mechanisms of action. The three most common drug classes that are prescribed for major depression are the tricyclic antidepressants (TCAs), the SSRIs, and the serotonin–norepinephrine reuptake inhibitors (SNRIs). The rationale for these drugs in treating depression is based on the monoamine hypothesis of depression, a decades-old idea stating that major depression is due to deficient action of monoamine neurotransmitters (chiefly, norepinephrine and serotonin).

Consistent with the monoamine hypothesis, drugs that effectively treat depression increase norepinephrine and/or serotonin signaling in the brain. The TCA's mechanism of action is to block presynaptic norepinephrine and serotonin transporters. Individual agents vary in terms of the relative selectivity, with some favoring to block the norepinephrine transporter (e.g., desipramine) while others equally bind norepinephrine and serotonin transporters (e.g., amitriptyline). It is important to note that TCAs favoring norepinephrine transporter blockade do so only in relative terms. They also block serotonin reuptake, albeit to a lesser extent.

SSRIs are highly selective for the serotonin transporter. At therapeutic doses, these drugs do not appreciably block norepinephrine reuptake. For this reason, SSRIs can be thought of as providing targeted action on increasing serotonin concentrations in brain synapses.

SNRIs are similar mechanistically to the TCAs owing to their ability to block both norepinephrine and serotonin reuptake. SNRIs are categorized separately, because they do not have the tricyclic chemical structure to which the TCAs owe their name.

Choosing a drug to treat depression focuses on ASE profile rather than efficacy. Each of these categories is approximately equivalent in its efficacy to reduce depression symptoms, but their variety in ASEs requires careful consideration of a patient's medical history when choosing an agent. The ASEs of TCAs include sedation and parasympatholytic effects (e.g., blurred vision, dry mouth, constipation, urinary retention, and elevated heart rate). Orthostatic hypotension and effects on the conduction of electrical signals in the heart are also concerns. The cardiac ASEs are particularly troublesome and are life threatening with overdose. The complex ASE profile of the TCAs is directly related to their pharmacology. In addition to blocking monoamine transporters, they are high-affinity antagonists of muscarinic, histaminic, and adrenergic receptors. Thus, TCAs are generally not used as a first-line therapy and are avoided in patients with heart disease.

SSRIs have a *cleaner* pharmacological profile than TCAs. This makes them the first-line therapy for depression treatment. SSRIs do not bind muscarinic, histaminic, or adrenergic receptors, and thus eliminate the concern for sedative, parasympatholytic, and cardiovascular side effects at therapeutic doses. SSRI ASEs are due to elevated signaling of serotonin through various subtypes of serotonin receptors. This signaling may result in insomnia, irritability, and decreased libido. Action in the spinal cord may result in erectile dysfunction and difficulty achieving orgasm. Nausea, diarrhea, and vomiting may occur due to action at serotonin receptors in the central nervous system (CNS) and peripheral sites. SNRIs have a similar ASE profile to that of the SSRIs.

Psychostimulants

Psychostimulants, also known as *psychomotor stimulants*, are drugs that increase alertness, arousal, and behavioral excitement. There is some mechanistic variability among drugs in this class that includes very powerful agents such as amphetamine and cocaine, and milder drug such as nicotine and caffeine. The more powerful agents owe much of their effects to the ability to activate the signaling of the noradrenergic system of the brain. The noradrenergic system is summarily described as a diffusely projecting, activating system. This system originates primarily in the locus coeruleus of the brainstem. The locus coeruleus contains densely packed neurons that send their axonal projections to nearly all parts of the CNS. These neurons use norepinephrine as their neurotransmitter. When released, this norepinephrine has an activating effect on its targets. The activating effect plays an important role in arousal in response to stimuli and in the focusing and orientation of attention.

Amphetamines, which include the chemical forms L-amphetamine, D-amphetamine, and methamphetamine, are a classical example of psychostimulants. Their mechanism of action is multifaceted and includes the blockade of reuptake by presynaptic transporters, the reversal of presynaptic transports, the inhibition of vesicular storage of neurotransmitter, and inhibition of metabolism of neurotransmitter. These mechanisms act in concert to cause a significant increase in synaptic concentrations of neurotransmitters, primarily dopamine and norepinephrine. The increased signaling by norepinephrine is the reason that amphetamines have such a profound effect on alertness, arousal, and behavioral excitement.

Methylphenidate (MPH) is a psychostimulant with a chemical structure distinct from amphetamines. The mechanism of action of MPH is not as multifaceted as that of the amphetamines, as it primarily blocks reuptake by the dopamine and norepinephrine transporters. MPH is frequently prescribed to treat ADHD. Its effectiveness for this condition is a result of increased noradrenergic and dopaminergic signaling in the prefrontal cortex.

ASEs of the amphetamines and MPH can be understood as pathological manifestations of their mechanism of action. Agitated behavior, increased anxiety, and insomnia are examples of adverse, excessive levels of behavioral arousal. In ADHD treatment, current thinking posits that the relationship between stimulant-enhanced neurotransmitter signaling and properly functioning attention is an inverted-U-shaped function (Arnsten, 2009). So, increased norepinephrine and dopamine signaling must be kept in the *just-right* range. Exceeding this range results in distracted and disorganized behavior similar to that seen in the untreated condition.

An important ASE of psychostimulants is the development of psychological dependence and withdrawal symptoms, both of which can drive stimulant abuse disorder. These drugs' ability to increase dopamine signaling in the reward system of the brain is the primary pharmacological reason for the significant abuse potential.

Brief Overview of Behavioral Pharmacology Research

As described earlier, psychotropic drugs affect neurotransmitter availability, which in turn impact behavioral processes. For example, Couppis and Kennedy (2008) demonstrated how dopaminergic activity in the nucleus accumbens can serve as a reinforcer. Specifically, they found that when mice were required to perform an operant task (i.e., nose poke) that produced access to an intruder mouse in which aggression ensued, the mice engaged in high rates of nose poking. However, when a dopamine antagonist was administered, rates of nose poking decreased in a dose-dependent fashion. Notably, movement was not impacted, so decreases in nose poking was not attributed to an inability to engage in the response. This finding suggests that behavior function and psychotropic agent effects on neurotransmitter activity are interrelated.

Typical and Atypical Antipsychotic Drugs

Research has examined how the effects of antipsychotic drugs interact with and impact behavioral processes. For example, Varvel et al. (2002) examined the effects of chronic and acute administration of several antipsychotics (both typical and atypical) at varying doses in rats on multiple fixed-ratio 30 (FR 30) and fixed-interval 60 seconds (FI 60) schedules. Through this work, they found that acute dosing of antipsychotic drugs administered produced dose-dependent decreased responding on the FR and FI components. Except for haloperidol and risperidone, antipsychotic drugs increased response durations, while also significantly decreasing response rates below a minimal threshold. Repeated dosing of the drugs revealed that responding under all of the drugs administered (except for clozapine and thioridazine to a certain extent) showed no tolerance to the drug and continued to show suppressed rates of responding. These results may suggest that the acute dosing of antipsychotics may serve to abolish the magnitude of reinforcer strength as evidenced by the decrease in response rate. More recently, Bédard et al. (2011) documented haloperidol's ability to increase the value of a reinforcer cue when rats were deprived of water and presented with a light-tone stimulus prior to the presentation of water. Their findings suggested that chronic haloperidol use may serve to potentiate the value of reinforcers, as well as strengthen the controlling effects of discriminative stimuli.

Research has also evaluated the effects of antipsychotic drug administration on avoidance responding. Antipsychotic drugs were found to affect avoidance responding at lower doses than necessary to affect escape behavior (Rodriguez, 1992). For example, Arenas et al. (1999) evaluated the effects of haloperidol on avoidance and escape responding in mice using a two-way shuttle box. Illumination of a house light for 5 seconds preceded the presentation of a 10-second foot shock on one side of the box (occupied by the mouse). *Avoidance* was defined as crossing to the opposite side when the light was on, and *escape* was defined as crossing to the opposite side after the onset of the shock. Haloperidol was found to decrease avoidance responding and increase the latencies of escape responses at both doses (0.1, 0.2 milligrams/kilogram body weight). However, increasing nonresponding or decreasing escape response frequency required higher doses. This study also found gender differences in drug response; that is, male mice required less of the drug than female mice to decrease performance on both tasks. Shannon et al. (1999) conducted a separate study evaluating the effects of haloperidol, chlorpromazine, and clozapine on rats on avoidance and escape responding. These authors found that all the antipsychotic drugs evaluated produced dose-dependent decreases in avoidance responding. This suggests they may decrease sensitivity to aversive stimuli, and thus may function as an abolishing operation for negative reinforcers.

The effects of several atypical antipsychotic drugs (i.e., olanzapine, clozapine, risperidone) on responding under punishment paradigms has also been evaluated in pigeons using a multiple FR 30/FR 30 schedule (Benvenga & Leander, 1995). In this series of studies, responding in the presence of white light (on an FR 30 schedule) produced access to food. Alternatively, in the presence of a red light, responding on an FR 30 schedule produced access to food and an electric shock. Each of the drugs was found to differentially affect punished responding. Nonetheless, all atypical antipsychotics drugs were associated with increased responding in the presence of the red light and limited changes in responding in the presence of the white light for at least one dose. These results also support the potential role of antipsychotic drug effects as motivating operations (MOs); that is, their effects served to either decrease the aversiveness of stimuli (e.g., shock delivery) or increase the value of the reinforcer (e.g., food) producing an observed increase in responding during the punishment contingency.

Antidepressants

Research featuring nonhuman animals has also evaluated the potential effects of antidepressants on behavioral processes. Dekeyne and Millan (2003) compared how antidepressants (TCAs and SSRIs) affected performance on differential schedules of reinforcement (i.e., differential reinforcement of low rate [DRL] 72 seconds) when administered to rats. Imipramine produced dose-dependent decreases in response rates and increases in reinforcement rates. However, performance on the SSRIs administered produced mixed results depending on the drug and dosage administered. Generally, it appeared that the SSRI was associated with less efficient responding, suggesting decreased value of the reinforcer; that is, SSRI effects may have served as an abolishing operation. Sokolowski and Seiden (1999) also evaluated the effects of differing doses of SSRIs but found enhanced efficiency in responding.

Additional studies of SSRI antidepressants have used FR schedules to determine drug effects. Ginsburg et al. (2005) evaluated the potential abolishing operation of fluvoxamine using a mixed schedule consisting of three 5-minute FR 5 components. Reinforcement was alternated between food, ethanol, and food across the three components. Dose-dependent decreases were observed in responding across all components of the mixed schedule. Significant decreases were often observed at lower doses of fluvoxamine for ethanol reinforcement compared to food reinforcement. This study suggests that fluvoxamine may differentially alter the reinforcing properties of select stimuli (e.g., ethanol consumption). Collectively, these studies do not clearly indicate whether SSRIs alter reinforcer magnitude of stimuli maintaining behavior.

Joel et al. (2004) evaluated antidepressant effects on extinction and suggested they may impart differential effects. The researchers used an extinction procedure with rats as a paradigm for obsessive–compulsive disorder. They evaluated the effects of several drugs, including two SSRIs (i.e., paroxetine and fluvoxamine) on *compulsive* lever presses. *Compulsive lever presses* were defined as the number of lever presses beyond the first press after which the rat did not insert its head into the food magazine. Paroxetine and fluvoxamine dose-dependently decreased the number of *compulsive* lever presses and the number of lever presses followed by head insertions into the food magazine. Their results suggest that extinction may be facilitated by the featured SSRIs.

Beaufour et al. (1999) investigated the effects of chronic desipramine, imipramine, and fluoxetine administration on punished responding in rats. They alternated reinforcement delivery (food) with periods of random punishment (50% of responses produced foot shock). The researchers established high-response rates when reinforcement was available and suppressed responding during punishment periods. Saline, chronic imipramine, and fluoxetine administration resulted in low-response rates during the punishment periods. However, imipramine also resulted in statistically significant decreases in responding during reinforcement periods. Fluoxetine and saline administration were not associated with differences in responding during reinforcement periods. By contrast, chronic desipramine administration produced statistically significant increases in responding during punishment periods and decreases in responding during reinforcement periods as the study progressed. These data might suggest behavioral interventions that include punishment procedures to reduce behavior may not be as effective combined with desipramine.

Psychostimulants

There are many studies evaluating the impact of psychostimulants on behavioral processes, varying from caffeine to cocaine. Arguably, MPH may be the most clinically relevant in relation to this chapter's content, and therefore is the focus of this section.

Researchers examined MPH effects on the relative value of two reinforcers, sucrose and social stimulation (i.e., access to another rat) using progressive ratio (PR; Martin et al., 2018). Interestingly, during MPH administration, break points were unchanged in the sucrose-alone condition, but break points were lower during the sucrose concurrent with social stimulation condition. These results were interpreted as MPH functioning as a possible abolishing operation for sucrose and establishing operation for social stimulation.

Another paradigm involved the presentation of two levers (Evenden & Ko, 2005). Rats were trained to press the left lever via a fixed consecutive number schedule (i.e., minimum six consecutive times; FCN 6) before pressing the right reinforcement lever once. If the rats pressed the right lever before the required number of responses were made on the left, a time-out was introduced, and the schedule was restarted. Following this, the researchers introduced a new consequence; that is, responses made on the right lever before completing the FCN 6 (on the left) produced food delivery concurrent with a foot shock. Administration of MPH did not impact responding during the original consequence (time-out). However, in the reinforcement concurrent with foot-shock condition, MPH was associated with an increased number of consecutive lever presses; that is, rats were less likely to press the right lever before completing the response requirement on the left. Researchers suggested that MPH may serve to enhance punishment effects.

Psychotropic Drugs as MOs

The aforementioned content clearly indicates that psychotropic drugs affect operant behavior in nonhuman animals. Specifically, they appear to impact stimulus control and may also serve to enhance or alter reinforcers and punishers. Thus, conceptualizing psychotropic drug effects as MOs may be appropriate. An MO is described as an event, operation, or stimulus condition that alters the effectiveness of reinforcers and punishers, and thus alters the frequency of behaviors associated with these consequences (Laraway et al., 2003). Altering stimuli effectiveness can serve to either establish (increase) or abolish (decrease) the effectiveness of a stimulus (Michael, 1982). Regarding establishing operations, psychotropic drug effects may enhance the value of positive and negative reinforcers. For example, thirst establishes liquids as a strong positive reinforcer, which could be enhanced by psychotropic drug effects (e.g., ASE of *dry mouth*). This would make liquids a more powerful reinforcer, resulting in water-seeking behavior that could manifest as a variety of topographies (e.g., aggression, elopement, wandering). Regarding negative reinforcers, light sensitivity establishes escape from bright environments as a stronger negative reinforcer, which could be enhanced by psychotropic drug effects (e.g., ASE of *headache*).

Applied Behavioral Pharmacology

Although relatively limited, behavioral researchers have extended the exploration of drug-behavior phenomena into the applied realm (e.g., individuals with IDD living in group homes; Valdovinos et al., 2009). This work has produced some interesting outcomes.

Functional Analysis and Problem Behavior
Exposed to Psychotropic Drugs

It is widely accepted that behavior function is central to the effects of behavioral treatment (Beavers et al., 2013). Therefore, researchers and clinicians use a functional analysis (FA) to identify the environmental variables maintaining PB. Since the standard protocol was first described by Iwata et al. (1982/1994), researchers have developed many FA variations to refine test and control conditions. This work has resulted in improved accuracy and implementation ease across a range of behaviors, settings, and participants (Beavers et al., 2013). It has also facilitated many empirical inquiries, including how MOs may affect behavior function (e.g., Simó-Pinatella et al., 2013). Given that psychotropic drugs may be functioning as MOs, FA is central in applied behavioral pharmacology research exploring drug–behavior phenomena.

To date, researchers have used FA to assess whether the form and function of PB interact with the effects of stimulant drugs (e.g., Northup et al., 1999; Torelli et al., 2019), opiate agonists (Garcia & Smith, 1999), some atypical antipsychotics (Cox & Virues-Ortega, 2022; Valdovinos et al., 2016), and antidepressants (Valdovinos et al., 2009). For example, Crosland et al. (2003) conducted a double-blind, placebo-controlled study. PB was recorded directly during each FA condition across psychotropic drug phases, as well as indirectly through common self-report questionnaires. The authors observed that risperidone was associated with lower rates of PB in the demand condition for both participants. However, decreases in PB during the access-to-tangible condition were not apparent. They suggested that risperidone may differentially affect escape-maintained PB (also called *function-specific effects*). Northup et al. (1999) also demonstrated function-specific effects by showing that environmental conditions may interact with the presence or absence of MPH.

Zarcone et al. (2004) conducted a study that was similar to that of Crosland et al. (2003). However, some of their results contradicted earlier findings; that is, Zarcone et al. (2004) suggested risperidone was effective in reducing destructive behavior across several FA conditions, including demand, for seven of the 10 responders. Thus, function-specific effects were not consistently observed.

A reanalysis of existing applied behavioral pharmacology literature evaluated the overall effects of psychotropic drugs on PB, and drug-induced changes in behavior function (Cox & Virues-Ortega, 2016). At the time, this systematic literature review revealed only 11 studies with 23 participants, for a total of 37 participant datasets. The psychotropic drugs evaluated in this context included primarily antidepressants, antipsychotics, and stimulants. Out of the 37 datasets reviewed, 17 showed small-to-negligible reductive effects or incremental effects on PB. Sixteen showed moderate reductive effects, and only four showed relatively large reductive effects. Regarding function-specific effects, 73% showed function correspondence, 22% showed function subtraction, 3% showed function addition, and 3% showed a function change. The review highlights the scarcity of research, as well as how few psychotropic drugs have been evaluated to date. Given existing barriers in conducting methodologically rigorous studies on this topic (see Courtemanche et al., 2011; van Haaren & Weeden, 2013), behavior analysts and researchers should endeavor to work with prescribers to create clinical research opportunities to better understand drug–behavior phenomena in applied settings. They may also consider applying creative analyses to conduct retrospective studies using large clinical datasets to inform possible prospective research, or possibly inform next treatment steps (see, e.g., Cox et al., 2022).

Despite the research scarcity, valuable clinical information may still be gleaned. Most importantly, we recommend behavior analysts conduct individualized objective assessments (e.g., repeated functional analysis across psychotropic drug conditions) because (1) it cannot be assumed that psychotropic drugs will have the intended effect (e.g., reduced PB), (2) other nontarget behavior may be differentially affected by the same drug adjustment (e.g., adaptive behavior, secondary PB; Cox & Virues-Ortega, 2022), and (3) drug adjustments could impact behavioral programming (function shift).

Assessing ASEs of Psychotropic Drugs

Many ASE examples were provided earlier (e.g., cardiac events, vomiting, nausea, erectile dysfunction) and are described as "undesirable, unintended, or unwanted reactions because of the known pharmacological effects of a [drug]" (Kalachnik 1999, p. 156). They are an important consideration because persons with IDD are highly likely to experience ASEs associated with psychotropic drugs (Scheifes et al., 2016), and may be less able to accurately report their experiences (Sheehan et al., 2019). Importantly, individuals who engage in more *severe* (or intense) PB may be more likely to experience higher doses of psychotropic drugs (Deb et al. 2015), polypharmacy (Bowring et al., 2017), or both. Furthermore, individuals with severe PB often have a longer history of psychotropic drug use, and prescribers may be less likely to attempt to initiate discontinuation due to a fear of client *destabilization* (de Kuijper & Hoekstra, 2017). These prescribing trends could mean individuals may be more vulnerable to experiencing ASEs more intensely or experiencing a greater ASE profile (Hess et al., 2010; Sommi et al., 1998; Valdovinos, Caruso, et al., 2005). This may also mean an increased likelihood of receiving prescriptions for nonpsychotropic drugs to offset ASEs coinciding with higher doses or polypharmacy (Charlot et al., 2020).

As described earlier in the chapter, psychotropic drug classes are often associated with specific ASE profiles. Alternatively, Valdovinos, Caruso, et al. (2005) described common ASE classes, categorizing them into six groups: (1) gastrointestinal, (2) neurological, (3) mood, (4) speech, (5) sleep, and (6) overall health. Adverse side effects can be tricky to identify, because some can be subtle in presentation. For example, risperidone has been known to produce muscle tension and headaches (Byrne et al., 2010). Subtle ASEs can profoundly affect behavior, and what remains to be determined is how these ASEs may impact the PB that psychotropic drugs are being prescribed to treat.

Even though ASEs are an important consideration, they are seldom adequately assessed (Lunsky et al., 2018; Matson & Hess, 2011). This may be in part because indirect assessment strategies (e.g., rating scales, interviews) are more often applied (Huffman et al., 2011). Select indirect assessment shortcomings include respondents' over- or underestimating ASE presence (Cleary et al., 2012), fair-to-poor convergent validity with direct assessments (e.g., Healy et al., 2013), and primacy and recency effects. Indirect assessments are further limited because they may be inappropriate for use with persons with communication difficulties (Matson & Neal, 2009). This could mean that open-label studies using indirect assessments to capture ASEs may produce unreliable results.

To date, Valdovinos et al. (2017) is the only behavioral study to comprehensively (and directly) assess ASEs. They conceptualized ASEs as MOs, and so developed FA-like conditions to measure the most likely ASEs associated with featured psychotropic drugs. Their results depict response-rate differences across assessment conditions, such that type of drug adjustment appeared to impact ASE-related behavior presentation. They also observed PB increases alongside ASE-related behavior increases, as well as an absence of PB alongside ASE-related behavior increases. More research aimed at directly assessing ASEs is sorely needed, because their impact on PB is not predictable. Despite some considerable study limitations, Valdovinos et al. (2017) takes an important step toward demonstrating viable approaches to directly evaluating ASEs, while also furthering applied behavioral pharmacology inquiry into drug–behavior phenomena.

One final ASE assessment approach may be physical examination (e.g., blood pressure, body weight, blood and urine samples). This would require coordination between the clinical and medical team, and at times adequate client cooperation may be difficult to ensure regular monitoring. Regardless, given the likelihood that persons with IDD will experience ASEs, behavior analysts can help by developing behavioral programming to establish clients' tolerance to undergoing physical examinations for the purpose of ASE evaluation (e.g., Cox et al., 2017). To be effective, behavior analysts must become familiar with the most likely ASEs associated with their clients' psychotropic drugs to work toward accurate direct measurement (Valdovinos, Caruso, et al., 2005; Valdovinos, Roberts, et al., 2005; Valdovinos, 2019). An active working relationship with the medical team may make the previously mentioned tasks more feasible. Furthermore, caregiver feedback and reliable ASE monitoring informed by existing literature may facilitate developing an individualized monitoring system to directly assess ASEs. See the section "Behavioral–Clinical Considerations in Monitoring Psychotropic Drugs Effects."

Assessing Preference in the Context of Psychotropic Drugs

Preference can be defined as the relative strength of behaviors among two or more choice options and is often measured as a choice pattern (Martin et al., 2006). Behavior analysis has a rich history evaluating preference: from developing and validating a range of stimulus preference assessments (Virues-Ortega et al., 2014) to evaluating preference across stimulus classes (i.e., displacement; DeLeon et al., 1997). Recent displacement research by Conine and Vollmer (2019) evaluated stimulus-class displacement in young children with ASD following similar methodology described by earlier work (DeLeon et al., 1997). Out of 26 participants, 17 displaced leisure stimuli with edible stimuli (65%). However, only six of the 17 participants showed total displacement. The authors suggest a few possible explanations for their findings, including psychotropic drug use. They refer to previous studies demonstrating food more often displacing leisure stimuli but note that those studies evaluated preference in adult populations in which the likelihood of psychotropic drug use is greater. Ultimately, Conine and Vollmer (2019) suggest evaluating the effects of psychotropic drugs on displacement. It is surprising that applied behavioral pharmacology research has yet to examine this phenomenon, given that basic behavioral pharmacology literature has described the relationship between psychotropic drugs, neurotransmitter activity, and reinforcing stimuli. Moreover, the theory that psychotropic drugs may act as MOs suggests that it may be reasonable to speculate that psychotropic drugs likely influence individuals' choice patterns (Carlson et al., 2012). That is, preference for foods, toys, items, or activities may shift in accordance with drug adjustments.

Although displacement has not been examined, some earlier applied behavioral pharmacology research suggests preference shifts may be observed in association with stimulant drug adjustments (Northup et al., 1997a, 1997b). Northup et al. (1997) explored the impact of MPH (stimulant) on preference by conducting repeated reinforcer assessments across MPH and placebo conditions. Participants completed math problems (neutral stimuli) in exchange for tokens that could be traded for a variety of reinforcers (e.g., edibles, activities, escape from tasks). The results suggested MPH altered the relative reinforcing effectiveness of some token coupons for various stimuli. This phenomenon may also be explored via FA of PB. For example, Dicesare et al. (2005) replicated and extended earlier work by conducting repeated FA during drugs administration of

MPH and no-MPH. They found MPH administration may be associated with a decrease in responding during the attention condition. They tentatively concluded that MPH may be associated with a decrease in the relative reinforcing effectiveness of attention. Important information may be gleaned via FA. However, conducting preference and reinforcer assessments may garner additional information by providing evidence of controlling contingencies that may not be identified readily through FA.

Apart from stimulants, researchers have yet to explore whether other psychotropic drugs (e.g., atypical antipsychotics, anxiolytics) alter preference (Carlson et al., 2012). Regardless, behavior analysts should monitor preference across drug adjustments for several reasons. First, function-based behavioral interventions rely heavily on whether the behavior analyst has correctly identified clients' preferred stimuli. If a drug adjustment has shifted preference unbeknownst to the behavior analyst, the behavioral intervention may cease to be effective, and the behavior analyst may not realize why. In the context of establishing adaptive skills, drug adjustments could render the consequence (delivery of preferred stimulus for correct, independent responding) less reinforcing, resulting in stalled acquisition. If behavior analysts are not reliably evaluating preference, the stalled progress associated with an adjustment may be incorrectly attributed to an ASE (e.g., impaired cognition).

Augmented by caregiver input, a robust preference and/or reinforcer assessment schedule, as well as direct measurement of ASEs, may help determine how a drug is imparting its affect. This may enable behavior analysts to take appropriate steps to alleviate discomfort, where applicable (e.g., Valdovinos, Roberts, et al., 2005); to adjust the behavioral intervention according to preference shift; or to advocate for expedited medical consultation in response to alarming ASEs that may or may not be physically harmful. Moreover, conducting FA to monitor drug effects on PB (likely the primary purpose for pursuing a prescription) may help determine if a sudden change in behavioral intervention effectiveness may be attributed to a function change associated with drug adjustment. A comprehensive behavioral assessment protocol may also help the team in their cost–benefit considerations; that is, if it appears ASEs are profoundly impacting the client and PB reduction is small to negligible, it may be appropriate to advocate for a substantial drug adjustment (e.g., withdrawal).

Ethics and Psychotropic Drugs in the Treatment of Challenging Behavior

Literature describing decision-making frameworks around treating PB with psychotropic drugs suggest it should be done in the context of a multidisciplinary team, with serious ethical deliberations spearheading decisions to introduce, adjust, and withdraw psychotropic drugs (Sheehan et al., 2018). This topic is ethically complex, with the complexity likely stemming from several issues. First, there is limited evidence supporting psychopharmacology efficacy in treating PB in persons with IDD (Ji & Findling, 2016). This could be the result of many individual drugs being used off-label, with infinite possible combinations of these often used off-label drugs. This makes it difficult empirically to generate compelling conclusions. Second, once a psychotropic drug is prescribed, it is rarely removed (Esbensen et al., 2009). Third, persons with IDD may be more likely to experience ASEs (Sheehan et al., 2017). Fourth, drugs should be considered a last resort, and only after a comprehensive behavioral intervention has been tried (Lloyd et al., 2016). When psychotropic drugs are prescribed, a combined intervention approach may be best (Lloyd et al., 2016). Finally, there appears to be an increasing trend in psychotropic drug use (Song et al., 2020), even though this population is often described as being overmedicated (Branford et al., 2019).

Behavior analysts may look to the Professional and Ethical Compliance Code (Behavior Analyst Certification Board, 2020) for guidance. First, prescribing drugs are beyond their boundaries of competence (1.02). However, behavior analysts should be considered a vital part of the treatment team, because their assessment skills may enable them to generate evidence that can help in advocating on behalf of their client (2.02) for the prudent use of psychotropic drugs. Behavior analysts also have a duty to "review and appraise the effects of *any* treatments about which they are aware that might impact the goals of the behavior-change program" (2.09d; Behavior Analyst Certification Board, 2020, p. 8, emphasis added). It follows that they are responsible for explaining assessment results in a language that is understandable (3.04). This should include disseminating assessment results to the medical treatment team (after obtaining appropriate client consent to do so; 9.03), an activity that could promote data-driven drug adjustments.

Prescribing physicians (e.g., psychiatrist, family physician) operate within the ethical boundaries of their discipline and are offering a treatment within their scope of competence. Psychiatric ethical guidelines mention working within a multidisciplinary team, and respecting carers and guardians on that team (Molina-Ruiz et al., 2017). However, no mention of specific disciplines, apart from *nonpharmacological* ones, are made. It is possible that prescribers may not know about behavior analysis, let alone how it can support their decision-making process. Relatedly, a peer-reviewed commentary mentions using individualized evidence to inform treatment decisions but then refers only to standardized rating scales as a means of information gathering (Sheehan, 2018). This commentary also describes *medication optimization* as an approach that encourages prescribers to consider individual preferences and values alongside the evidence base and clinical judgment to "inform safe, effective, and collaborative management decisions" (Sheehan, 2018, p. 22). Prescribers are urged to operate within this optimization framework whose tenets appear to align with applied behavior-analytic perspectives and approaches on treatment. This shared orientation (i.e., common ground) may provide an opportunity for a behavior analyst to propose augmenting indirect assessment with direct, which could then be incorporated into decision-making processes (Valdovinos, 2019).

Other, related empirical content on physician decision making suggests several specific factors may influence choices around discontinuing psychotropic drugs, including clients' (1) living situation status (appropriate or inappropriate); (2) PB severity; (3) diagnosis status (e.g., ASD); and (4) symptoms of restlessness. Physicians have also reported a fear of client *destabilization* (de Kuijper & Hoekstra, 2017) as a reason for electing not to discontinue psychotropic drugs.

Behavior analysts have an ethical duty to ensure that clients receive the least intrusive, most effective treatment (2.09a), which may be best achieved by fostering a working relationship with prescribers.

Behavioral–Clinical Considerations in Monitoring Psychotropic Drugs Effects

It is well understood that psychopharmacological interventions are commonly prescribed to persons with IDD, despite controversy around efficacy (Ji & Findling, 2016), poorly understood behavioral mechanisms of action (Pitts, 2014) and high risk for ASEs (Scheifes et al., 2016). Taken together, it is imperative that applied behavioral pharmacology research initiatives are pursued. However, this work can be tricky to facilitate, and the publication process is lengthy. In the meantime, behavior analysts are highly likely to be supporting clients taking psychotropic drugs (Li & Poling, 2018). Thus, necessitating a basic understanding of relevant behavioral pharmacology content and psychotropic drug characteristics to develop comprehensive drug monitoring systems to adequately capture relevant drugs effects in applied settings. Recently, Cox et al. (2022) demonstrated how behavior analysts may apply creative analysis strategies to capture separate and combined interventions effects informed by extended clinical data. Their analysis featured four participants for whom systematic data had been collected across many behavioral and psychopharmacological intervention adjustments spanning several years. The authors showed how effect size, confidence intervals, correlation and partial-correlation analyses may reveal subtle trends not easily captured via visual analysis. They also suggest behavior analysts may be able to use outcomes to inform the next treatment steps, showcasing an additional benefit of ongoing, comprehensive drug-monitoring systems.

Ideas for Monitoring Drugs Effects

Creatively analyzing existing clinical data may be an important step in better understanding drug–behavior phenomena. However, for analyses to produce usable results (for research or clinical purpose), a comprehensive behavioral assessment protocol must be established. Otherwise, unreliable data entered into the analysis will produce inaccurate results. Generally, behavior analysts are advised to conduct a battery of direct assessments, including (1) preference and/or reinforcer assessments, (2) FA, and (3) daily data collection to capture both adaptive and PB changes. It will also be important to augment caregiver reports by generating ways to directly assess possible ASEs. Valdovinos (2019) offers a thorough description of drug-monitoring recommendations (Table 23.1 summarizes these recommendations), while Table 23.2 features a step-by-step process on considerations for monitoring behavioral effects of psychotropic drugs.

The following section is *not* meant to be proscriptive. Instead, it serves as one example, of many possible approaches to generating a comprehensive behavioral assessment strategy.

Case Example

John, a 6-year-old boy with ASD and IDD, is enrolled in a class with five other students. John can mand independently, follow two-step instructions, and engages in relatively frequent vocal stereotypy. His teachers report that John tends to leave his seat many times in the classroom, which interrupts the lesson. Even when the teacher manages to keep John in his seat, he is often off-task and distracts other students in the class when he becomes aggressive (hitting, throwing items). John also reportedly engages in some skin-picking behaviors causing redness on the surface of his skin by the end of the day. Teachers report that incidents of aggression happen primarily during work periods, compared to "unstructured play time" when John is left to play on his own. Four months ago, John was prescribed risperidone (0.5 milligrams) and lisdexamfetamine (40 milligrams [trade name Vyvanse®]), an oral administration route, by his psychiatrist. John's teachers

TABLE 23.1. Recommendations for Monitoring Medication Effects Summarized

Item	Description
Behavioral conceptualization and assessment	
1	Consider psychotropic medications as motivating operations, conditional or discriminative stimulus, or establishing new response–reinforcer relations.
2	Consider potential effects of psychotropic medications on behavioral programming.
3	Create ways to assess whether medications impact conditions under which problem behavior occurs.
Conducting behavioral assessments	
4	Conduct repeated assessments, including functional behavior assessment, reinforcer/preference assessments.
5	Determine when (and for how long) assessments identified with rationale should be conducted. For example, during current medication condition, as well as once steady state is reached pending medication adjustment, or continuously across attempts to titrate or discontinue medications.
Measurement of behavior	
6	Measure psychotropic medication impact on all behavior, including "non-target" behavior (e.g., stereotypical, adaptive behavior).
7	Identify important behavior characteristics: for example, how often the behavior occurs, the duration of problem behavior episode, the intensity, the context in which the behavior occurs, and corresponding states (e.g., fatigue, mood, hunger, illness).
8	Consider data collection on pain, including collecting qualitative data on pain state providing a rationale.
	Measurement of adverse side effects
9	In collaboration with caregivers and other relevant clinicians, consider what side effects may be likely, how they might manifest, when the best time to assess them may be, and so forth.
10	Consider the observability of suspected adverse side effects.
11	Collect data on presence of adverse side effects to determine potential impact on problem behavior.
12	Identify direct measurement of adverse side effects, including biological measures (e.g., blood glucose levels); clinical measures (e.g., weight, blood pressure, heart rate); as well as monitoring development and progression of movement-related adverse side effects (e.g., tardive dyskinesia).
Data collection	
13	Two factors impacting data collection by caregivers are understanding the need for data collection, and the complexity of data collection system. Neglecting either may compromise data collection.
14	Provide adequate training to caregivers on how to assess and collect data for target behavior and adverse side effects with sound rational. Or include data collection as staff performance evaluation component.
Working with prescribers	
15	Behavior analysts are infrequently involved in decisions regarding psychotropic medication use by their clients.
16	Behavior analysts' have expertise and qualifications to work with prescribers for the purpose of monitoring, and training others on data collection to assess behavior–environment interaction evolvement.

Note. Content summary from Valdovinos (2019). Psychotropic medication in intellectual and developmental disabilities: Patterns of use and recommendations for monitoring effects.

TABLE 23.2. Considerations for Developing Comprehensive Behavioral Assessments to Monitor Medication Effects on Behavior

Item	Description
Challenging behavior	
1	Three to five questions posed to caregivers to help prioritize their treatment goals for the client and target behaviors to address (e.g., What do you want this medication to do for client *X*? Will you be advocating for a decrease in concurrent psychotropic medications? What type of behavior would be evidence that suggests this medication is not benefiting your loved one? Which side effect are you most concerned about?)
2	Rationale for choice of target challenging behavior; clearly informed by medication properties, where applicable, and incorporated caregiver feedback
3	Defined data collection schedule/system: (a) clearly informed by medication property; (b) consider half-life, titration, administration route, and how this plays a role in when assessment should be done; (c) historical exposure to other drugs (how long might it take for you to see impact, based on historical medication metabolizing)
4	Overall feasibility of data collection schedule (i.e., likelihood of accurate data being collected, accurately reflect outcomes across environments, if applicable)
Adaptive behavior	
5	Medication half-life and/or steady state identified and clearly considered in choice of adaptive behavior to be monitored and data collection schedule (if different from challenging behavior mentioned earlier)
6	Overall feasibility of data collection schedule
7	Sleep data collection process
8	Identified common side effects
9	Data collection strategy for monitoring common ASE (how you might monitor for drugs withdrawal; weigh gain; increased hunger, latency to task completion, increased sleep or sleeplessness, reduction in overall skills acquisition, etc.)
Functional analysis	
10	Appropriate choice of FA variation with rationale
11	FA setting identified with rationale (in-home; designated assessment space)
12	Considerations of potential setting events (sleep deprivation; as-needed administration; disease states [e.g., flu])
13	Medication half-life/steady-state considerations in FA schedule
14	Description of a plan to streamline data collection system. For example, (a) a medication that could incite attentional problems (ASE)—side effects could be monitored during an FA's escape condition wherein data is collected on the clients' capacity to "attend" to all tasks (operationally define *attending*); (b) measure overall movement and/or instances of falling asleep during a low stimulation FA condition (i.e., alone)—Is there overall less/more movement on the part of the client? (e.g., percentage duration pacing)
15	Summarized data collection system in eight sentences or less, in a way that could be understood by a professional/caregiver without a BA degree

Note. Adapted from Cox et al. (2022). Copyright © 2022 American Psychological Association. Used with permission.
ASE = Adverse side effects; FA = functional analysis.

report that his behavior has improved. However, according to John's parents, he is having difficulty sleeping, has begun having urination accidents (despite being toilet trained since age 3), and has begun to engage in a *new* motor stereotypy, where he suddenly jerks his head left several consecutive times. His parents are also concerned about how much medication he is taking. However, his teachers are encouraged by what they are seeing from him in the classroom, even though no direct data collection currently takes place in either setting.

Possible Approaches to Monitoring Drug Effects

Behavior analysts may consider speaking with caregivers to gather information to guide goal development, that is, what they expect the medications may do for John, or perhaps what medication *success* looks like (e.g., sustained low rates of PB vs. no PB, limited notable ASEs). From here, the behavior analyst may engage with the prescriber (or relevant medical team member) to gather pertinent psychotropic drug characteristics that may inform ASE assessment, as well as assessment timelines (e.g., half-life, steady state). Importantly, when a medication is taken, ASEs are experienced immediately, while it may take days or weeks for a medication to impart its therapeutic effects. Augmenting direct ASE monitoring with caregiver input may alert the need for immediate consultation if ASEs appear alarming.

Following this, behavior analysts may help caregivers' narrow goals to target specific PB, and operationally define select target behaviors. In John's case, the team may consider collecting daily aggression data given that this behavior could result in more unfavorable outcomes (e.g., expulsion) compared to the self-injurious behavior described. If possible, data could be collected on self-injury and aggression. However, it will be important for behavior analysts to consider the feasibility of their plan given existing barriers to unlimited data collection (e.g., minimal access to collecting data in the school or at home, caregivers' capacity to collect accurate data, other clients the behavior analyst must support). During this time, adaptive behaviors should also be selected and operationally defined. In John's case, on-task behavior may be targeted. For example, behavior analysts may consider collecting partial-interval data for short periods of time across the day for a finite period (e.g., 3 days before a drug change and for 3 days once the drug had reached steady state). Behavior analysts should also select and develop an appropriate FA. In John's case, it may be appropriate to conduct a slightly modified FA protocol with shortened conditions (5 minutes; Wallace & Iwata, 1999). For example, they may conduct the FA in the classroom and implement standard demand and attention conditions, with unstructured playtime (as described in the scenario) as their control condition. They may also consider conducting a no-interaction (alone) condition to monitor reported *head jerking* that seems to be new in association with the most recent medication adjustment (possible ASE). Parents are also reporting sleep difficulties, and trouble sleeping has been listed as an ASE of Vyvanse. Therefore, collecting sleep data could be easily achieved by having John don wearable technology to monitor sleep. The behavior analyst may also consider assigning misurination data collection (a simple tally) to parents for a short period. The behavior analysts' final step may be generating a short paragraph to disseminate the assessment plan to the team in understandable language. For example, one might say:

> "In gathering feedback and information from everyone, it appears John's risperidone dosage is likely at its intended level in his system. Given that we should see an impact

of Vyvanse shortly after John has taken his medication, I will complete a *structured assessment* at 1:30 P.M. every week for 1 month during the current medication phase. These assessments will stop until the next medications change. During the structured assessments, I will also be collecting data on head jerking and on-task behavior. I am asking John's educational assistant (EA) to collect on-task behavior data for 3 days in the current medication phase, and again for 3 days following the next medication change. Observation periods will be 10 minutes long. During these periods, every 10 seconds, she will check off whether John was on-task (doing his work) or not. This will be done two times a day (once in the morning and afternoon). I ask that parents tally when he has *accidents* and support him in wearing a fitbit, so that we can monitor his sleep patterns. Finally, if possible, his EA will tally aggressive behavior instances. Perhaps this tally can be recorded in his communication book, so parents are up to date on how often these are occurring. Further research in applied behavioral pharmacology will be important to develop an established evidence base on the topic. However, the fact remains that behavior analysts play an important role in supporting caregivers and clients. Fortunately, our science provides behavior analysts with the tools to monitor treatment effectiveness and adverse side effects of psychotropic medication."

REFERENCES

Arenas, M. C., Vinader-Caerols, C., Monleón, S., Parra, A., & Simón, V. M. (1999). Dose dependency of sex differences in the effects of repeated haloperidol administration in avoidance conditioning in mice. *Pharmacology, Biochemistry and Behavior, 62*(4), 703–709.

Arnsten, A. F. T. (2009). Toward a new understanding of attention-deficit hyperactivity disorder pathophysiology: An important role for prefrontal cortex dysfunction. *CNS Drugs, 23*(Suppl. 1), 33–41.

Beaufour, C. C., Ballon, N., Le Bihan, C., Hamon, M., & Thiébot, M.-H. (1999). Effects of chronic antidepressants in an operant conflict procedure of anxiety in the rat. *Pharmacology, Biochemistry and Behavior, 62*(4), 591–599.

Beavers, G. A., Iwata, B. A., & Lerman, D. C. (2013). Thirty years of research on the functional analysis of problem behavior. *Journal of Applied Behavior Analysis, 46*(1), 1–21.

Bédard, A.-M., Maheux, J., Lévesque, D., & Samaha, A. (2011). Continuous, but not intermittent, antipsychotic drug delivery intensifies the pursuit of reward cues. *Neuropsychopharmacology, 36*(6), 1248–1259.

Behavior Analyst Certification Board. (2020). Professional and ethical compliance code for behavior analysts. Retrieved from *www.bacb.com/ethics-information/ethics-codes*.

Benvenga, M. J., & Leander, J. D. (1995). Olanzapine, an atypical antipsychotic, increases rates of punished responding in pigeons. *Psychopharmacology, 119*(2), 133–138.

Bowring, D. L., Totsika, V., Hastings, R. P., Toogood, S., & Griffith, G. M. (2017). Challenging behaviours in adults with an intellectual disability: A total population study and exploration of risk indices. *British Journal of Clinical Psychology, 56*(1), 16–32.

Branford, D., Gerrard, D., Saleem, N., Shaw, C., & Webster, A. (2019). Stopping over-medication of people with intellectual disability, Autism or both (STOMP) in England part 1—history and background of STOMP. *Advances in Mental Health and Intellectual Disabilities, 13*(1), 31–40.

Brunton, L. L., Hilal-Dandan, R., & Knollmann, B. C. (2018). *Goodman & Gilman's: The pharmacological basis of therapeutics.* McGraw-Hill Education.

Byrne, S., Walter, G., Hunt, G., Soh, N., Cleary, M., Duffy, P., . . . Malhi, G. (2010). Self-reported side effects in children and adolescents taking risperidone. *Australasian Psychiatry, 18*(1), 42–45.

Carlson, G., Pokrzywinski, J., Uran, K., & Valdovinos, M. (2012). The use of reinforcer assessments in evaluating psychotropic medication effects. *Journal of Developmental and Physical Disabilities, 24*(5), 515–528.

Charlot, L. R., Doerfler, L. A., & McLaren, J. L. (2020). Psychotropic medications use and side effects of individuals with intellectual and developmental disabilities. *Journal of Intellectual Disability Research, 64*(11), 852–863.

Cleary, A., Walsh, F., Connolly, H., Hays, V., Oluwole, B., Macken, E., & Dowling, M. (2012). Monitoring and documentation of side effects from depot antipsychotic medication: An interdisciplinary audit of practice in a regional mental health service. *Journal of Psychiatric and Mental Health Nursing, 19*(5), 395–401.

Conine, D. E., & Vollmer, T. R. (2019). Relative preferences for edible and leisure stimuli in children with autism. *Journal of Applied Behavior Analysis, 52*(2), 557–573.

Couppis, M. H., & Kennedy, C. H. (2008). The rewarding effect of aggression is reduced by nucleus accumbens dopamine receptor antagonism in mice. *Psychopharmacology, 197*(3), 449–456.

Courtemanche, A. B., Schroeder, S. R., & Sheldon, J. B. (2011). Designs and analyses of psychotropic and behavioral interventions for the treatment of problem behavior among people with intellectual and developmental disabilities. *American Journal on Intellectual and Developmental Disabilities, 116*(4), 315–328.

Cox, A. D., Davis, S., & Feldman, M. (2022). Medication training for behavior analysts: A brief report. *Behavior Analysis: Research and Practice, 22*(1), 130–142.

Cox, A. D., Pritchard, D., Penney, H., Eiri, L., & Dyer, T. J. (2022). Demonstrating an analyses of clinical data evaluating psychotropic medication reductions and the ACHIEVE! program in adolescents with severe problem behavior. *Perspectives on Behavior Science, 45*, 125–151.

Cox, A. D., & Virues-Ortega, J. (2016). Interactions between behavior function and psychotropic medication. *Journal of Applied Behavior Analysis, 49*(1), 85–104.

Cox, A. D., & Virues-Ortega, J. (2022). Long-term functional stability of problem behavior exposed to psychotropic medications. *Journal of Applied Behavior Analysis, 55*(1), 214–229.

Cox, A. D., Virues-Ortega, J., Julio, F., & Martin, T. L. (2017). Establishing motion control in children with autism and intellectual disability: Applications for anatomical and functional MRI. *Journal of Applied Behavior Analysis, 50*(1), 8–26.

Crosland, K. A., Zarcone, J. R., Lindauer, S. E.,

Valdovinos, M. G., Zarcone, T. J., Hellings, J. A., & Schroeder, S. R. (2003). Use of functional analysis methodology in the evaluation of medication effects. *Journal of Autism and Developmental Disorders, 33*(3), 271–279.

Deb, S., Unwin, G., & Deb, T. (2015). Characteristics and the trajectory of psychotropic medication use in general and antipsychotics in particular among adults with an intellectual disability who exhibit aggressive behaviour. *Journal of Intellectual Disability Research, 59*(1), 11–25.

Dekeyne, A., & Millan, M. (2003). Discriminative stimulus properties of antidepressant agents: A review. *Behavioural Pharmacology, 14*(5–6), 391–407.

de Kuijper, G. M., & Hoekstra, P. J. (2017). Physicians' reasons not to discontinue long-term used off-label antipsychotic drugs in people with intellectual disability: Physicians' reasons on long-term use of antipsychotics. *Journal of Intellectual Disability Research, 61*(10), 899–908.

DeLeon, I. G., Iwata, B. A., & Roscoe, E. M. (1997). Displacement of leisure reinforcers by food during preference assessments. *Journal of Applied Behavior Analysis, 30*(3), 475–484.

Dicesare, A., McAdam, D. B., Toner, A., & Varrell, J. (2005). The effects of methylphenidate on a functional analysis of disruptive behavior: A replication and extension. *Journal of Applied Behavior Analysis, 38*(1), 125–128.

Esbensen, A. J., Greenberg, J. S., Seltzer, M. M., & Aman, M. G. (2009). A longitudinal investigation of psychotropic and non-psychotropic medication use among adolescents and adults with autism spectrum disorders. *Journal of Autism and Developmental Disorders, 39*(9), 1339–1349.

Evenden, J., & Ko, T. (2005). The psychopharmacology of impulsive behavior in rats VIII: Effects of amphetamine, methylphenidate, and other drugs on responding maintained by a fixed consecutive number avoidance schedule. *Psychopharmacology, 180*(2), 294–305.

Garcia, D., & Smith, R. G. (1999). Using analog baselines to assess the effects of naltrexone on self-injurious behavior. *Research in Developmental Disabilities, 20*(1), 1–21.

Ginsburg, B. C., Koek, W., Javors, M. A., & Lamb, R. J. (2005). Effects of fluvoxamine on a multiple schedule of ethanol- and food-maintained behavior in two rat strains. *Psychopharmacology, 180*(2), 249–257.

Hess, J., Matson, J., Neal, D., Mahan, S., Fodstad, J., Bamburg, J., & Holloway, J. (2010). A comparison of psychotropic drug side effect profiles in adults diagnosed with intellectual disabilities and autism spectrum disorders. *Journal of Mental Health Research in Intellectual Disabilities, 3*(2), 85–96.

Huffman, L. C., Sutcliffe, T. L., Tanner, I. S. D., & Feldman, H. M. (2011). Management of symptoms in children with autism spectrum disorders: A comprehensive review of pharmacologic and complementary-alternative medicine treatments. *Journal of Developmental and Behavioral Pediatrics, 32*(1), 56–67.

Iwata, B. A., Dorsey, M. F., Slifer, K. J., Bauman, K. E., & Richman, G. S. (1994). Toward a functional analysis of self-injury. *Journal of Applied Behavior Analysis, 27*(2), 197–209. (Reprinted from 1982, *Analysis and Intervention in Developmental Disabilities, 2*(3), 3–20).

Ji, N. Y., & Findling, R. L. (2016). Pharmacotherapy for mental health problems in people with intellectual disability. *Current Opinion in Psychiatry, 29*(2), 103–125.

Jobski, K., Höfer, J., Hoffmann, F., & Bachmann, C. (2017). Use of psychotropic drugs in patients with autism spectrum disorders: A systematic review. *Acta Psychiatrica Scandinavica, 135*(1), 8–28.

Joel, D., Ben-Amir, E., Doljansky, J., & Flaisher, S. (2004). "Compulsive" lever-pressing in rats is attenuated by the serotonin re-uptake inhibitors paroxetine and fluvoxamine but not by the tricyclic antidepressant desipramine or the anxiolytic diazepam. *Behavioural Pharmacology, 15*(3), 241–252.

Kalachnik, J. E. (1999). "You tell me it's the institution, well, you know, you better free your mind instead." In N. A. Wieseler & R. H. Hanson (Eds.), *Challenging behavior of persons with mental health disorders and severe developmental disabilities* (pp. 151–203). American Association on Mental Retardation.

Lamy, M., Pedapati, E. V., Dominick, K. L., Wink, L. K., & Erickson, C. A. (2020). Recent advances in the pharmacological management of behavioral disturbances associated with autism spectrum disorder in children and adolescents. *Paediatric Drugs, 22*(5), 473–483.

Laraway, S., Snycerski, S., Michael, J., & Poling, A. (2003). Motivating operations and terms to describe them: Some further refinements. *Journal of Applied Behavior Analysis, 36*(3), 407–414.

Li, A., & Poling, A. (2018). Board certified be-havior analysts and psychotropic medications: Slipshod training, inconsistent involvement, and reason for hope. *Behavior Analysis in Practice, 11*(4), 350–357.

Lloyd, B. P., Torelli, J. N., & Symons, F. J. (2016). Issues in integrating psychotropic and intensive behavioral interventions for students with emotional and behavioral challenges in schools. *Journal of Emotional and Behavioral Disorders, 24*(3), 148–158.

Lunsky, Y., Khuu, W., Tadrous, M., Vigod, S., Cobigo, V., & Gomes, T. (2018). Antipsychotic use with and without comorbid psychiatric diagnosis among adults with intellectual and developmental disabilities. *Canadian Journal of Psychiatry, 63*(6), 361–369.

Martin, C. D., Bool, H. M., George, A. M., Carr, K. A., Epstein, L. H., Hawk, L. W., Jr., & Richards, J. B. (2018). Social reinforcement as alternative to sucrose reinforcement is increased by nicotine and methylphenidate in male Fischer-344 rats. *Psychopharmacology, 235*(7), 1981–1985.

Martin, T. L., Yu, C. T., Martin, G. L., & Fazzio, D. (2006). On choice, preference, and preference for choice. *Behavior Analyst Today, 7*(2), 234–241.

Matson, J. L., & Hess, J. A. (2011). Psychotropic drug efficacy and side effects for persons with autism spectrum disorders. *Research in Autism Spectrum Disorders, 5*(1), 230–236.

Matson, J. L., & Neal, D. (2009). Psychotropic medication use for challenging behaviors in persons with intellectual disabilities: An overview. *Research in Developmental Disabilities, 30*(3), 572–586.

Meyer, J. S., & Quenzer, L. F. (2019). *Psychopharmacology: Drugs, the brain, and behavior.* Oxford University Press.

Michael, J. (1982). Distinguishing between discriminative and motivational functions of stimuli. *Journal of the Experimental Analysis of Behavior, 37*(1), 149–155.

Molina-Ruiz, R. M., Martín-Carballeda, J., Asensio-Moreno, I., & Montañés-Rada, F. (2017). A guide to pharmacological treatment of patients with intellectual disability in psychiatry. *International Journal of Psychiatry in Medicine, 52*(2), 176–189.

Northup, J., Fusilier, I., Swanson, V., Huete, J., Bruce, T., Freeland, J., . . . Edwards, S. (1999). Further analysis of the separate and interactive effects of methylphenidate and common classroom contingencies. *Journal of Applied Behavior Analysis, 32*(1), 35–50.

Northup, J., Fusilier, I., Swanson, V., Roane, H., & Borrero, J. (1997a). An evaluation of methylphenidate as a potential establishing operation for some common classroom reinforcers. *Journal of Applied Behavior Analysis, 30*(4), 615–625.

Northup, J., Jones, K., Broussard, C., DiGiovanni, G., Herring, M., Fusilier, I., & Hanchey, A. (1997b). A preliminary analysis of interactive effects between common classroom contingencies and methylphenidate. *Journal of Applied Behavior Analysis, 30*(1), 121–125.

Pitts, R. C. (2014). Reconsidering the concept of behavioral mechanisms of drug action. *Journal of the Experimental Analysis of Behavior, 101*(3), 422–441.

Rasmussen, L., Pratt, N., Roughead, E., & Moffat, A. (2019). Prevalence of psychotropic medicine use in Australian children with autism spectrum disorder: A drug utilization study based on children enrolled in the longitudinal study of Australian children. *Journal of Autism and Developmental Disorders, 49*(1), 227–235.

Rodriguez, R. (1992). Effect of various psychotropic drugs on the performance of avoidance and escape behaviors in rats. *Pharmacology Biochemistry and Behavior, 43*(4), 1155–1159.

Scheifes, A., de Jong, D., Stolker, J. J., Nijman, H. L. I., Egberts, T. C. G., & Heerdink, E. R. (2013). Prevalence and characteristics of psychotropic drug use in institutionalized children and adolescents with mild intellectual disability. *Research in Developmental Disabilities, 34*(10), 3159–3167.

Scheifes, A., Walraven, S., Stolker, J. J., Nijman, H. L. I., Egberts, T. C. G., & Heerdink, E. R. (2016). Adverse events and the relation with quality of life in adults with intellectual disability and challenging behaviour using psychotropic drugs. *Research in Developmental Disabilities,49–50*, 13–21.

Shannon, H. E., Hart, J. C., Bymaster, F. P., Calligaro, D. O., DeLapp, N. W., Mitch, C. H., . . . Swedberg, M. D. B. (1999). Muscarinic receptor agonists, like dopamine receptor antagonist antipsychotics, inhibit conditioned avoidance response in rats. *Journal of Pharmacology and Experimental Therapeutics, 290*(2), 901–907.

Sheehan, R. (2018). Optimising psychotropic medication use. *Tizard Learning Disability Review, 23*(1), 22–26.

Sheehan, R., Hassiotis, A., Strydom, A., & Morant, N. (2019). Experiences of psychotropic medication use and decision-making for adults with intellectual disability: A multistakeholder qualitative study in the UK. *BMJ Open, 9*(11), Article e032861.

Sheehan, R., Hassiotis, A., Walters, K., Osborn, D., Strydom, A., & Horsfall, L. (2015). Mental illness, challenging behaviour, and psychotropic drug prescribing in people with intellectual disability: UK population based cohort study. *BMJ: British Medical Journal, 351*, Article h4326.

Sheehan, R., Horsfall, L., Strydom, A., Osborn, D., Walters, K., & Hassiotis, A. (2017). Movement side effects of antipsychotic drugs in adults with and without intellectual disability: UK population-based cohort study. *BMJ Open, 7*(8), Article e017406.

Sheehan, R., Lunsky, Y., & Hassiotis, A. (2018). Achieving better health for people with intellectual disability: The power of policy. *BJPsych Open, 4*(2), 47–48.

Simó-Pinatella, D., Font-Roura, J., Planella-Morató, J., McGill, P., Alomar-Kurz, E., & Giné, C. (2013). Types of motivating operations in interventions with problem behavior: A systematic review. *Behavior Modification, 37*(1), 3–38.

Sokolowski, J. D., & Seiden, L. S. (1999). The behavioral effects of sertraline, fluoxetine, and paroxetine differ on the differential-reinforcement-of-low-rate 72-second operant schedule in the rat. *Psychopharmacology, 147*(2), 153–161.

Sommi, R. W., Benefield, W. H., Curtis, J. L., Lott, R. S., Saklad, J. J., & Wilson, J. (1998). Drug interactions psychotropic drugs. In S. Reiss & M. G. Aman (Eds.), *Psychotropic medications and developmental disabilities: The international consensus handbook* (pp. 115–131). Ohio State University.

Song, M., Ware, R., Doan, T. N., & Harley, D. (2020). Psychotropic medication use in adults with intellectual disability in Queensland, Australia, from 1999 to 2015: A cohort study. *Journal of Intellectual Disability Research, 64*(1), 45–56.

Stahl, S. M. (2013). *Stahl's essential psychopharmacology: Neuroscientific basis and practical applications.* Cambridge University Press.

Torelli, J. N., Lambert, J. M., Francis, R. N., Picou, C. G., Mastel, M. A., O'Flaherty, C. A., & Vandelaar, E. M. (2019). Effects of dexmethylphenidate on targeted and non-targeted behaviours during functional analyses: A brief report. *Developmental Neurorehabilitation, 22*(8), 565–568.

Valdovinos, M. G. (2019). Psychotropic medication in intellectual and developmental disabilities: Patterns of use and recommendations for monitoring effects. *Current Developmental Disorders Reports, 6*(4), 195–201.

Valdovinos, M. G., Caruso, M., Roberts, C., Kim, G., & Kennedy, C. H. (2005). Medical and behavioral symptoms as potential medication side effects in adults with developmental disabilities. *American Journal of Mental Retardation, 110*(3), 164–170.

Valdovinos, M. G., Henninger-McMahon, M., Schieber, E., Beard, L., Conley, B., & Haas, A. (2016). Assessing the impact of psychotropic medication changes on challenging behavior of individuals with intellectual disabilities. *International Journal of Developmental Disabilities, 62*(3), 200–211.

Valdovinos, M. G., Nelson, S. M., Kuhle, J. L., & Dierks, A. M. (2009). Using analogue functional analysis to measure variations in problem behavior rate and function after psychotropic medication changes: A clinical demonstration. *Journal of Mental Health Research in Intellectual Disabilities, 2*(4), 279–293.

Valdovinos, M. G., Roberts, C., & Kennedy, C. H. (2005). Functional analysis of tardive dyskinesia: Implications for assessment and treatment. *Journal of Applied Behavior Analysis, 38*(2), 239–242.

Valdovinos, M. G., Schieber, E., McMahon, M., Beard, L., Wilkinson, A., & Carpenter, J. (2017). Adverse side effects of psychotropic medication and challenging behavior: Pilot work assessing impact. *Journal of Developmental and Physical Disabilities, 29*(6), 969–982.

van Haaren, F., & Weeden, M. (2013). Some guidelines for conducting research in applied behavioral pharmacology. *Journal of Applied Behavior Analysis, 46*(2), 498–506.

Varvel, S. A., Vann, R. E., Wise, L. E., Philibin, S. D., & Porter, J. H. (2002). Effects of antipsychotic drugs on operant responding after acute and repeated administration. *Psychopharmacology, 160*(2), 182–191.

Virues-Ortega, J., Pritchard, K., Grant, R. L., North, S., Hurtado-Parrado, C., Lee, M. S. H., . . . Yu, C. T. (2014). Clinical decision making and preference assessment for individuals with intellectual and developmental disabilities. *American Journal on Intellectual and Developmental Disabilities, 119*(2), 151–170.

Wallace, M. D., & Iwata, B. A. (1999). Effects of session data duration on functional analysis outcomes. *Journal of Applied Behavior Analysis, 32*(2), 175–183.

Willner, P. (2015). The neurobiology of aggression: implications for the pharmacotherapy of aggressive challenging behaviour by people with intellectual disabilities: Neurobiology of aggression. *Journal of Intellectual Disability Research, 59*(1), 82–92.

Zarcone, J. R., Lindauer, S. E., Morse, P. S., Crosland, K. A., Valdovinos, M. G., McKerchar, T. L., . . . Schroeder, S. R. (2004). Effects of risperidone on destructive behavior of persons with developmental disabilities: III. Functional analysis. *American Journal of Mental Retardation, 109*(4), 310–321.

CHAPTER 24

Relational Frame Theory and Acceptance and Commitment Therapy

Jordan Belisle
Jonathan Tarbox

We are at a crossroads in the field of applied behavior analysis (ABA). The broader field of behavior analysis, including the philosophy of radical behaviorism and the experimental analysis of behavior, has brought about a paradigm shift (Kuhn, 1962) with new and exciting models and technologies (Belisle, 2020). Advances in the study of neurobiological and environment interactions have coincided with a much more in-depth understanding of operant and respondent learning. Research in behavioral economics has extended our understanding of the dynamics between delay and probability, as well as the ongoing competition between reinforcers in a vastly complex social world. Most relevant to this chapter, our understanding of human language and cognition has moved beyond elementary operants that have been a primary focus of applied behavior-analytic practices for decades (Harte & Barnes-Holmes, 2021), opening up enormous applications within and outside of interventions for individuals across populations.

Whereas the experimental and philosophical work has become increasingly broad in scope without sacrificing precision and depth, the same growth is occurring more slowly and with potentially greater resistance within our applied subfield. How do we progress from theory and well-controlled experiments to impactful technologies that have the potential to change the lives of people? Likewise, when new technologies emerge that could radically transform the everyday practices of applied behavior analysts, are each of us willing to adapt even though old strategies have been successful in a relatively narrow field of application?

Acceptance and commitment therapy or training (both approaches hereafter referred to as ACT) represents an approach to intervention that applies advances in our understanding of human language and cognition to improve the lives of people. Over 400 randomized controlled trials have supported applications of ACT with a variety of clinical and nonclinical populations (Hayes, 2021). Early research supported the use of ACT-based interventions to improve quality of life and remediate symptoms of individuals with anxiety and major depressive symptoms—with and without medication. Later research both extended the use of ACT with military veterans experiencing posttraumatic stress and improved quality of life in patients with chronic pain. When applied with parents of children with disabilities and caregivers, short-term ACT-based interventions have been shown to decrease caregiver burnout and stress (e.g., Puolakanaho et al., 2020)—and early evidence supports the use of ACT-based strategies directly with children with and without disabilities (Fang & Ding, 2020; Szabo, 2019; Suarez, Moon, & Najdowski, 2021).

A common question we are asked is "How could one approach be so effective across so many populations?" It is for the same reason that strategies such as differential reinforcement or well-developed token systems can influence so many different behavior patterns and can be applied at the level of individual clients or within whole systems, such as a school or clinic. ACT is not a singular approach or strategy—it is the application of well-established behavior change principles that have been developed and refined in hundreds of research laboratories over the past 40 years. When we apply these principles, behavior changes. It is up to the behavior analyst to develop a functional-analytic model that is grounded in the basic theory and to translate the model in a way that is useful to consumers.

As with other topics presented in this book, translational research is necessary to cultivate a strong bridge between basic principles and practice. In this chapter, we review these basic principles grounded in relational frame theory (RFT) as they relate to ACT with clients. This chapter is not a technical manual on how to implement ACT; rather, it is designed to augment and support a growing library of training content available to behavior analysts by describing the basic underlying theory. We are hopeful that behavior analysts who read this chapter will feel more comfortable in the grounding of ACT within behavior-analytic theory and experimental analysis—and to explore the fruits of this technology with the clients and families they serve. Below, we discuss RFT as the experimental and theoretical foundation for ACT.

RFT: The Basic Model

RFT expands upon two prior models of human language and cognition, verbal behavior (Skinner, 1957) and stimulus equivalence theory (Sidman, 1994). A full-length review of these prior theories is outside the scope of this chapter, but it is important to note that their impact on the field of ABA was considerable in the areas of language training for individuals with disabilities and in educational settings. RFT models the apparent generativity of human language learning—that new verbal behavior can emerge in the absence of direct reinforcement. For example, if a person is presented with a picture of a dog (A) and is told that this is called a "dog" (B) (A-B), they may derive without direct training that the word *dog* (B) refers to a four-legged animal with a long snout and floppy ears (A) (B-A). This bidirectional relation is called *mutual entailment*. Bidirectional naming (BiN) is one example of mutual entailment that may be a pivotal cusp in the development of generative language. Once a person learns to name objects, any name-object entailed relation can develop through both speaker and listener behavior. If the same person is told that "dog" (B) is spelled *D-O-G* (C) (B-C), we might expect the mutually entailed C-B relation to emerge without direct training (i.e., "What does D-O-G spell?").

In addition, more complex combinatorial relations may emerge, such as when shown the picture of the dog (A) and asked, "What does this spell?" evoking the spelling response D-O-G (C) (A-C), or when shown the text D-O-G (C) and the person can select the picture of a dog from an array (A) (C-A). This is an example of a relatively simple, three-member coordinated class but it illustrates the importance of derived relations in the development of symbolic and referential language. Not only does this provide a basic model, it shows how private verbal behaviors can come to refer to real-world experiences, and evoke or elicit external behavior through the transformation of stimulus function.

Transformation of stimulus function is a process wherein the functions of stimuli are altered due to participation in relational frames. Consider a person who has had positive experiences with dogs, including playing, cuddling, and traveling. Not only does seeing dogs bring about positive affective (i.e., emotional) experiences, but hearing the word *dog* or seeing the D-O-G written in a book or magazine can also elicit this same private emotional responding. Moreover, a song coming on the radio on a long drive could evoke a string of thoughts that arrive at the private verbal behavior of "dog," producing a spontaneous positive feeling that is experienced privately. This same process can also lead to spontaneous suffering if, for example, a different person was bitten or attacked by a dog in the past. Suddenly, not only will seeing a dog in the natural environment elicit negative affective emotional responses, but so too will hearing the word *dog*, reading about a D-O-G, or engaging in a string of private verbal behavior that brings about memories of the time he was attacked by an angry dog.

Behavior analysts implementing ACT likely deal with much more pervasive private stimulus functions that contribute to psychological suffering. For example, the thought "I am not good enough" can be entailed with infinite events, such as performance in school, keeping contact with family and friends, health and fitness goals, and the list goes on. Because of the transformation of stimulus function, engaging in any of these events can evoke a stream of private verbal behavior that leads to negative affective experience and, as a function, to experientially avoidant behavior. Take, for example, a person with a substance use addiction and a history of trauma. Because of combinatorial entailment, any number of external or verbal stimuli can lead to reexperiencing trauma and elicit negative emotional arousal symptoms that operate as a motivating operation for escape. Consuming the substance not only alleviates withdrawal symptoms but can also attenuate unwanted thoughts and feelings by inhibiting executive functioning processes. It is for this reason that ACT-based processes such as acceptance and willingness, discussed later in the chapter, are so powerful—because change necessitates experiencing unwanted thoughts, feelings, and even withdrawal to begin the journey toward valued reinforcement.

We are seeing an exponentiation in research in major behavior analytic journals on RFT and transformations of stimulus functions (Belisle et al., 2020). Functional transfers described earlier are consistent with the most researched pattern of relating based on coordination or sameness. When two things are related based on coordination, functions simply transfer from the function-carrying class member to other class members. However, not all relations are based on sameness. Some other, common relations include distinction (i.e., A is different from B), opposition (i.e., A is the opposite of B), comparison (e.g., A is bigger than B), hierarchy (i.e., A contains B), and deictic (e.g., I am A and you are B).

The way that verbal events are related can impact corresponding transformations of stimulus function. In a basic experimental arrangement, Dougher et al. (2007) presented unfamiliar symbol combinations (A, B, and C) to consenting participants and collected skin conductance measures as a measure of momentary anxiety. When the symbol combination *B* was paired with shock, an increase in anxiety was observed when only the *B* combination was presented. The participants were then taught that *A* is *smaller* than *B* and *B* is *smaller* than *C*. The function did not simply transfer from *B* to *A* and *C*; rather, the participants experienced an even greater increase in anxiety given *C* and a weaker increase in anxiety given *A*. The functions did not simply transfer, they were transformed in terms of *B*.

Consider how a frame of opposition might operate in this same way. If *A* carries an aversive function, and if *B* is the same as *A* and *C* is the opposite of *B*, we may expect not only that the participant can derive *C* is the opposite of *A*, but *C* may acquire an appetitive function due to the frame of opposition (see Perez et al., 2015). As can be seen in this example, relational frames can be enormously complex at a molecular level, exerting considerable influence across a wide variety of stimuli and responses, after a relatively small amount of training or experience.

Private Events and Behavior–Behavior Relations

Discussing the influence of private events on overt behavior is still relatively uncommon in the science of behavior analysis, so some readers may be curious about how this can be done while remaining conceptually systematic within the science. RFT and ACT are built upon the philosophical foundation of *radical behaviorism,* which was defined by the full and equal inclusion of private events, alongside overt behavior and environmental events, as the subject matter of behavior analysis (Skinner, 1945; Moore, 2008). Put simply, private events are assumed to influence overt behavior in the same manner in which overt events do; as discriminative stimuli, rules, and so forth. This philosophical perspective allows us to examine how private events interact with socially meaningful overt behavior, not as hypothetical causes, but as part of the complex behavior–environment relations that comprise a person's repertoire.

Figure 24.1 provides a visual diagram of the complex interplay between relational framing, other behavior, and contextual variables. From the inside-out, Rel-B refers to relational framing behavior, which is described in this section of the chapter. Relational framing behavior is learned overtly in childhood but then later often occurs at the private level. From a radical behavioral perspective, there needn't be any functional difference between relational framing that occurs at the private versus public level. For example, a parent of an autistic child might say to herself, "I feel like a mad mother," and this verbal behavior, either covert or overt, can then influence other important behaviors in their life. Ext-B refers to external or public behavior that makes contact with the external context. These are the types of behaviors that we are more accustomed to dealing with in traditional behavior-analytic interventions, such as aggression, self-harm, substance use, among other socially relevant behaviors. Rel-B and Ext-B are constantly interacting and influencing one another, as indicated by the bidirectional arrow (i.e., a behavior–behavior relation).

As noted by Hayes and Brownstein (1986), behavior–behavior relations are insufficient in isolation to explain behavior. We must also consider the context within which behavior–behavior relations are likely to occur. At some point, private behavior must interact with public behavior that makes contact with the external environment in a way that strengthens or weakens both the public behavior (Ext-B) and the private behavior (Rel-B). Therefore, we must also examine the antecedent and consequence functions that surround these complex behavioral interactions.

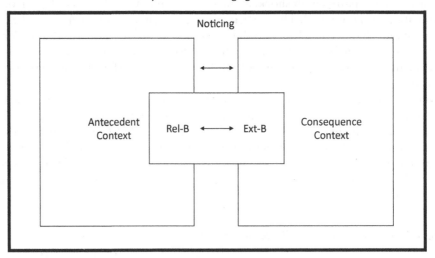

FIGURE 24.1. Dynamic interplay between behavior–behavior relations, antecedent and consequence context events, the act of noticing, and the temporally extended context within which all of this occurs. Used with permission from Dr. Jordan Belisle, HUB Research and Practice Laboratory.

Introduction to ACT

ACT is an approach to intervention that seeks to improve the lives of people by promoting psychological flexibility. Hayes and colleagues (Hayes et al., 2006; Hayes et al., 2011) have defined *psychological flexibility* as a complex behavioral phenomenon, consisting of "Contacting the present moment fully as a conscious human being, and based on what the situation affords, changing or persisting in behavior in the service of chosen values" (Hayes et al., 2006, p. 6). This definition can be effective when communicating with consumers but will require unpacking to translate in a manner that is conceptually systematic with behavioral principles. ACT implementers refer to less-technical terms as "middle-level" terms, which are often used when interacting with consumers. Because ACT is grounded in an account of human language and cognition, it is important that behavior analysts use words that already have meaning for the listener. Unpacking the definition of psychological flexibility behavior analytically, however, is something that behavior analysts should be able to do. We offer one interpretation below.

"Contacting the present moment . . ." delineates between attending (a behavior) to events occurring here and now (i.e., public and private stimuli) versus attending to our own verbal behavior about events occurring in the past or in the future (i.e., private verbal stimuli).

". . . as a conscious human being . . ." appreciates that we are observers of our own experience. Skinner (1957) described this as occurring when a person is both the speaker and the listener within the same skin (i.e., thinking). We contend that this goes beyond simply speaking and listening, to occurring when one is both the see-er and the seen—or the observer and the observed. How we observe our own behavior undoubtedly affects the way that we interact with our world, which can lead to success as well as suffering.

The phrase ". . . and based on what the situation affords, changing or persisting in behavior . . ." alludes to the importance of context in directing behavior and behavior change. When behavior is successful in contacting reinforcement and avoiding punishment, persisting in that behavior is necessary even when public and private barriers emerge. On the other hand, when behavior no longer contacts reinforcement or results in excessive experiences of punishment, adapting behavior in response to changing contingencies.

Finally, ". . . in the service of chosen values" appreciates that not all reinforcers are valued the same. Often, smaller-sooner negative reinforcers control our behavior. We avoid unwanted public and private experiences, and this pattern of escape and avoidance behavior is referred to as *experiential avoidance*. Because of our unique capacity for language learning, aversive private experiences can emerge without a clear external aversive event, such as when one starts to think of a long-lost relationship or starts to fixate on public speaking. This process is referred to as *cognitive fusion* that can even further exacerbate experiential avoidance.

Instead, ACT challenges us to contact larger-later and more verbally abstracted forms of reinforcement, such as improving relationships with loved ones, being a good father or mother, feeling and being physically healthy and fit, or any other broad category of meaningful reinforcement. Whereas our cognitive abilities can lead us to suffer, it is these same cognitive abilities that allow us to conceptualize what really matters and what we want our lives to be about. For behavior analysts using ACT-based technologies, the centralized question is "How can I help my client make their life be more about what they want it to be about?" and "How can my client make their life be less about simply escaping their life and those in it?"

One way to think about psychological flexibility from a translational perspective is as encompassing topographically broad and adaptive response classes that maximize valued reinforcement (Dixon et al., 2023). ACT-based interventions seek to broadly strengthen behaviors that maximize valued positive reinforcement and weaken avoidant and cognitively fused behaviors that have become rigid and stuck. Correlational research has shown that psychological flexibility is a behavioral process that likely leads people to suffer across a variety of diagnoses. For example, low levels of psychological flexibility are predictive of mood disorders such as anxiety and depression (e.g., Leahy et al., 2012; Fonseca et al., 2020), the probability that a person will develop a substance use disorder (Mallik et al., 2021), and the quality of life of chronic pain patients (Gentili et al., 2019), among other sources of suffering (Levin et al., 2014). According to an ACT-based approach, we suffer when we stop chasing valued positive reinforcers in our lives, choosing to instead withdraw and avoid those parts of our lives that bring us pain. Unfortunately, withdrawing and avoiding often brings us even further from those parts of our lives that we value the most, such as friends, family, and health. This problem may be a uniquely human experience that is not controlled exclusively by external contingencies but rather by our own rules about them.

Rule-Governed Behavior: A Barrier to Psychological Flexibility

Skinner (1969) distinguished between behavior that is contingency-governed versus behavior that is rule-governed, where the latter may be less sensitive to changing contingencies. Consider this finding that has been replicated in multiple studies on schedule insensitivity (e.g., Hayes et al., 1986). In the general arrangement, participants are given a computerized task in which they press a button at a specific rate to earn points in a mixed schedule. In the first schedule, they may be required to press the button as fast as possible to maximize points and, in the second schedule, to press the button slowly to maximize points. Participants are neither told when the schedule changes nor that it will change. A second manipulation is that only half of the participants are given a rule initially to press the button quickly—the other participants are given no instructions. The first outcome should not be surprising; people who are given the rule quickly adapt to the first schedule, and the no-rule group takes considerably longer. However, when the schedule changes, only participants who did not receive the rule adapt to the new contingency; the group operating under the rule in the first schedule continue to follow the rule into the second schedule, even though following the rule no longer maximizes access to high rates of reinforcement.

From a translational perspective, the results of this study should be concerning when most of our technologies rely on influencing behavior by altering direct contingencies; that is, if behavior is maintained by rules more than contingencies, then altering the contingencies may not change behavior in any meaningful way. Where behavior change does occur, the changes are likely nonfunctional and contrived, and may be likely to relapse or resurge when contrived sources of reinforcement and punishment are no longer forthcoming.

Moreover, greater influence of inaccurate rules over behavior may be predictive of greater psychological suffering. McAuliffe and colleagues (2014) explored the negative features of rule-governed behavior using the schedule insensitivity task. In their study, participants were divided into two groups based on levels of depression symptoms (high depression and low depression). Both groups completed a schedule insensitivity task similar to that described earlier, except that all participants were given rules. At the start of the experiment, the rules were accurate: Rules described the contingency. Given the accurate rule, participants in both groups adapted to the schedule quickly. At the midpoint of the experiment the schedule changed, such that the rule that was accurate in the prior phases was no longer accurate. The researchers observed that participants with high depression were more likely to continue to follow the inaccurate rule after the change in schedule than participants with low depression—suggesting that continued adherence to inaccurate rules (that may at one time have been accurate) could contribute to the behavior patterns observed in something like depression.

ACT is not intended to simply replace inaccurate rules with more accurate rules. Directly training every potentially adaptive rule would take a lifetime. Moreover, as contingencies change naturally as a person's life progresses or due to major life-altering events, such as the loss of a loved one or a change in profession, rules that were adaptive at one time may become maladaptive in the new context. Because the external context is dynamic and ever changing, we must instead change the way that clients interact with rules to influence behavior.

When rules emerge from a generalized pattern of rule following, regardless of the specific external contingencies, we refer to this pattern of rule following as *pliance*. Pliance is typical at younger developmental ages and can be adaptive when rules are accurate. However, persistent, rigid repertoires of pliance can lead to maintained patterns of responding when contingencies change, and behavior no longer contacts valued reinforcement. *Tracking,* on the other hand, occurs when rules are based on the observed internal and external contingencies. Tracking is typical at older developmental ages and when people become more proficient at tasks that were once novel. Tracking can also be problematic when self-generated rules inaccurately describe the external contingencies, again leading to schedule insensitivity.

ACT interventions attempt to foster a dynamic interplay between Rel-B and Ext-B that is sensitive to immediate and temporally extended external contingencies. The act of noticing plays a central role in this process, as one must attend to stimuli in order for those stimuli to influence behavior. Throughout ACT, the behavior analyst challenges the client to notice behavior–behavior relations ("What are you thinking?" or "What are you feeling?"), as well as the context within which certain patterns of thinking or feeling are likely to occur. In so doing, the goal is to promote sensitivity of behavior to externally occurring events and to notice patterns that encourage self-management of one's overt behavior. Essentially, "to make people aware of their experiences fully as a conscious human being," as is appreciated in our initial definition of psychological flexibility. The idea of "noticing" may come across as prescribing an internal controlling agent (i.e., those who notice), so it is important to consider that noticing, or consciously experiencing, also occurs within a dynamic and ever-changing process; that is, beyond simply encouraging clients to notice behavior–environment and behavior–behavior relations, ACT-based interventions also attempt to foster a context that is likely to reinforce and maintain the act of noticing, as doing so allows the client to chase larger-later and abstract reinforcers (i.e., valued reinforcers). Changing how these various features interact within a complex behavior stream is at the heart of all ACT models.

Core Processes and the ACT Hexaflex

ACT interventions attempt to promote psychological flexibility by augmenting and strengthening six complex behavioral repertoires, commonly referred to as "psychological flexibility processes" in the ACT literature. These six core behavioral repertoires are depicted as the ACT hexaflex model in Figure 24.2 (Hayes et al., 2011). The six repertoires on the left in Figure 24.2 shows patterns of responding that are likely to lead to psychological *inflexibility*—or chasing smaller-sooner negative reinforcers. For example, fixating on the past or ruminating on the future can introduce aversive functions that operate as motivating operations for escape-maintained behavior to make those thoughts and feelings go away. Consider, when your mind wanders, where does it go? We tend to fixate on events in the past that carry negative experience, such as a difficult conversation with a friend or loved one. We also tend to focus on future events that we are anxious about, such as a big exam or a performance. This mode of problem solving was evolutionarily adaptive, because attending to aversive public and private events enabled us to avoid external events that were physically harmful. However, modern life for most of us very rarely presents physically dangerous stimuli, yet we continue to respond to aversive private events as though they are dangerous. Focusing too rigidly on these events can not only lead us to suffer but also can set the occasion for negatively reinforced maladaptive behaviors, such as avoiding the event that brings about anxious feelings, or by drinking or using illicit substances as a self-medicating strategy against our own private experiences.

Without clarity about what we value, we might be tempted to treat those smaller-sooner negative sources of reinforcement (i.e., escape from aversive public and private experiences) as the valued outcome (i.e., "I just want to feel OK"). Now consider the question, "If your life could only be about one thing, what would it be about?" Surely,

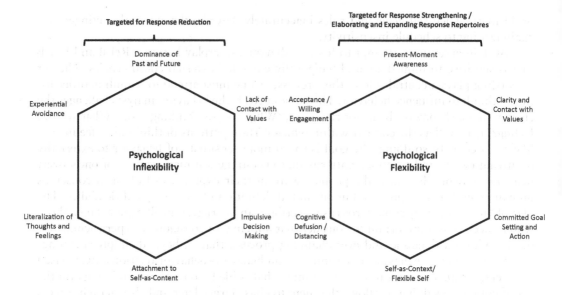

FIGURE 24.2. ACT hexaflex model, with less-flexible behavioral repertoires depicted on the left, and·more-flexible behavioral repertoires on the right. Broadly speaking, ACT seeks to establish the repertoires on the right as replacement behaviors for the repertoires on the left. Component images used with permission from Dr. Steven Hayes, University of Nevada, Reno.

the answer is not "to just feel OK." Rather, when we dig deeper, we can identify larger-later more abstract reinforcers (i.e., values) that matter more—when we can notice them. A lack of clarity or contact with these values can lead to a lack of engagement in behavior that contacts these values. Clarifying values is similar to tracking, or creating a rule specifying that when someone engages in specific patterns of behavior, they move closer to those things in life that they value. On the other hand, by failing to notice or consider these broader valued reinforcers, the same rule-governed process of tracking can lead to rules such as "There is no way I can be a good father," "They don't even want me at the party," or "I am not smart enough to take the challenging college courses." These rules then set the stage for the behavior–behavior relations of avoiding that is maintained by smaller-sooner negative reinforcers—at the expense of valued living.

We also construct stories around our actions and literalize the content of those stories (i.e., attachment to self-as-content). For example, imagine the single parent working two jobs and the narrative "I work hard and suffer, so that my children can have a better life." The literalized content is that she is a person who suffers and must suffer to satisfy this narrative. Altering behavior that may be more in line with her values, such as asking for help from friends and family or taking out loans to receive training for a higher paying job, could also be inconsistent with the self-rule of "one who suffers for family," and therefore these behaviors may be less likely to occur, despite how the natural consequences of engaging in those behaviors may be highly reinforcing, if only the person would contact them. Therefore, although the parent is engaging in high rates of behavior—the behavior may not be in line with obtaining those larger-later and abstract values and may compete with other values, such as time with their family or general health and psychological well-being. This is closely related to the process of cognitive fusion that interacts with experiential avoidance of unwanted thoughts and feelings that contributes to behavior patterns that are psychologically inflexible. We can become unwilling to attempt new behaviors that threaten the smaller-sooner negative forms of reinforcement that we have grown accustomed to experiencing. The psychological flexibility model of ACT provides a way forward, toward chasing rather than escaping, and these six core processes are depicted in the right half of Figure 24.2.

Present-Moment Awareness

Present-moment awareness is most closely related to the well-known behavioral process of stimulus control. Is your behavior under the influence of the external events that it contacts, here and now? Or is your behavior under the control of self-generated verbal stimuli about events happening at another place or at another point in time? Our behavior is more likely to be affected by the external environment when we attend to the external environment. For example, McHugh et al. (2012) conducted a version of the schedule sensitivity task described earlier, in which participants completed a 15-minute mindfulness induction task prior to the schedule change. Results suggested greater schedule sensitivity or adaptability when behavior was redirected to the present moment. Present-moment awareness provides a ready demonstration of a behavior–behavior relation, as the internal behavior of intentionally attending to present moment events that is typically directed by our own verbal behavior can affect how our external behavior responds to the external world.

Dixon et al. (2019) conducted a similar study evaluating the effect of a 5-minute present-moment awareness training session on momentary rates of impulsivity in a delay discounting task, where participants engaged in less impulsive response patterns following the mindfulness activity. These basic experiments provide insight as to the mechanisms that underlie the successes of mindfulness-based intervention, within and outside of the ACT context, in improving quality-of-life outcomes by bringing behavior more in line with external reinforcement and less under the control of inaccurate rules.

Values

Values are motivative augmental rules (Hebert et al., 2021; Paliliunas, 2021; Plumb et al., 2009) that are designed to strengthen behaviors that lead to larger-later abstract forms of reinforcement. What are those larger-later reinforcers that you want your life to be about? One way to consider values is as abstract categories of reinforcement. For example, a person who finds being with friends and family, going to parties, and working together in teams enjoyable likely values relationships more broadly. By noticing these abstract verbal categories of reinforcement, we can augment behavior that contacts this reinforcement (e.g., "What is one thing you can do that will move you closer in your relationships today?"). Identification of what really matters can also provide the verbal behavior needed to compare competing response options. For example, do I stay home and relax or attend a family event? Whereas staying home may serve negative reinforcement functions in terms of reduced response effort or potential discomfort of seeing family, stating the value in the form of "Which choice is in the service of building meaningful relationships?" may strengthen the probability of attending the family event. Values in the form of motivative augmental stimuli are insufficient, however, without considering the external context. Consider that if being with family is reinforcing, by attending the family event, the chance of contacting those social reinforcers is high, even further strengthening the operant of seeking valued relationships. However, if those social reinforcers are not sufficiently powerful, then building relationships may not be as valuable as initially believed. To aid in clarifying what really matters, consider the question "If your life could be about one thing, what would it be about?" This simple question can help to identify valued reinforcement to guide behavior change efforts.

Committed Action

Committed actions are those behaviors that contact the external environment and produce positive reinforcers that are values-consistent. From a matching-law perspective, psychological flexibility plays out in the ongoing competition between committed actions and avoidance behaviors maintained by negative reinforcement. Consider the example of the single parent who values spending more time with his children and improving his physical and psychological well-being. The broader values have been identified, but how do we start to move in a valued direction? When we think about committed actions, we want to consider the behavioral process of shaping—building successive approximations toward larger patterns of values-driven behavior. A first small step could be to research college loan options that are available for nontraditional students or to call a friend to help take care of their child while they complete work from home. These examples might be workable with some clients and not others—there is no one-size-fits-all solution. Rather, by identifying valued outcomes, we can develop small goals that can be accomplished in the short term (e.g., in the next few days) that are specific and measurable. As smaller goals are completed successfully, we can progress to larger behavior targets to build momentum. And although we are undoubtedly interested in increasing adaptive values-consistent behavior, perhaps more important is that chasing values through committed action becomes a generalized pattern of responding that is strong and resistant. We also want to foster variability when rigid behaviors fail to contact reinforcement, and to reinforce persistence when larger-later values are achievable through committed action and engagement.

Self-as-Context

Self-as-context is the opposite of self-as-content and seeks to deliteralize stories or verbal behavior that we attach to ourselves. The behavioral repertoires that self-as-context training seeks to strengthen may be among the most abstract of those contained in the ACT work, and they extend Skinner's account of the self as consisting of repertoires of behavior directed at oneself (Skinner, 1974). Self-awareness and self-discrimination are shaped by the verbal community as we learn to discriminate our own behavior from others in the service of predicting our own behavior and that of others. ACT extends this account by evaluating the functions of self-discriminations based on patterns, where self-as-context verbal discriminations are sensitive to external contextual variables. For example, if a student does poorly on a test, they may think "I am so stupid" or "I don't do tests well." These statements may be repetitive or rigid ("fused" in ACT jargon) and lack contextual control. Whereas the statements "I did poorly on this test because I did not study the material" or "I was not at my best today and did poorly on the test" serve to deliteralize the story of one's "intelligence" and "aptitude," instead placing control on external variables that may come and go. This approach not only creates distance between the event and stories about the event, but also noticing the context where behavior that we may want to change is occurring can help with identifying committed actions that may be more values-consistent, such as making time to study for the test. Self-as-context also appreciates the role of a transcendental or conscious self that exists across contexts. One metaphor that illustrates this idea can be developed by imagining the first house you grew up in and noticing the furniture inside the house and the colors of the walls. Then, walk through the house in a time warp where months are seconds. What changes in the house? What remains the same? The furniture is the stories or content with which we fill the house, and we are the house that experiences all of these changes. Therefore, part of the ACT processes is to bring greater noticing toward this transcendental and conscious experience.

Defusion

Defusion is the deliteralization of those momentary thoughts that are evoked as we progress through each day. The purpose of defusion is not to alter the form of the thoughts, because that would simply serve those same negative reinforcement functions; rather, the purpose of defusion is to alter the function and control thoughts, as private verbal stimuli, have within the behavior–behavior relations. Conceptually, consider that in our conceptualized model in Figure 24.1, the external behavior (Ext-B) is the product of two competing sources of control, the external contingencies and relational verbal behavior (Rel-B). If we can weaken the power of momentary relational verbal behavior when doing so is in the service of our values, then we necessarily strengthen the control of the external contingencies. Belisle et al. (2019) conducted a study with recreational gamblers in which they arranged the environment to support the rule that one color of slot machine was better than the other. For half of the participants, they also attempted to defuse this rule by offering multiple relations, such as "How is this color good?"; "How is this color bad?"; "How is this color like the other color?"—generating more context to weaken the power of any one rule about color that could affect slot machine play. The gamblers also were required to say the two colors over and over again as quickly as possible as a version of the Titchener repetition task. To illustrate, try saying your name over and over as fast as you can for 1 minute. You will also notice that the words start to blend together and lose their meaning. When the two groups of gamblers then completed a simulated gambling task with slot machines differing in color, the group that did not do the defusion activity showed a clear bias toward the slot machine with the color that cohered with the rule. The group that received defusion training, however, appeared to allocate their responding more based on wins and losses in the game (i.e., schedule matching). ACT contains a number of strategies to promote defusion, that is, to weaken rigid control by unhelpful rules. Some simple strategies include singing the anxiety-provoking thought as a birthday song to weaken its influence in the moment, or adding the verbal behavior "I am having the thought that . . ." prior to the thought. This latter strategy also serves to strengthen the act of noticing the thought, which can then create an opportunity to engage in behavior that weakens its influence.

Acceptance

Acceptance occurs when a person is willing to experience unwanted public or private events when doing so is in the service of their values. When behavior is stuck and rigid, that is, maintained by long patterns of negative reinforcement and is highly resistant to change, engaging in committed action necessitates the momentary experience of the aversive thoughts and emotions that one has a history of previously avoiding. Acceptance is not the same as surrender, such as "Well, I guess I will just always feel this way." Instead, acceptance is all about change: "I don't want to feel this way, and I am willing to feel this way more for now so I can feel better tomorrow." Behaviorally speaking, acceptance work consists of engaging in behavior that does not avoid, and sometimes even moves closer to, aversive stimuli, when doing so results in larger-later positive reinforcement.

Utilizing the motivative augmental functions of values can strengthen acceptance repertoires. For example, brief values clarification activities that are designed to bring larger-later abstract values to the psychological present have been shown to decrease social stress, as well as biological indicators of stress such as momentary blood cortisol levels (Gregg et al., 2014) that could impact people's willingness to approach stressful situations. The process of shaping can also be used to strengthen acceptance repertoires. As with systematic desensitization, we want to build-in exposure at a rate that is comfortable for the client and likely to contact success. As exposure to the aversive events contacts appetitive sources of external reinforcement, we can build on patterns of acceptance and willingness as a higher-order pattern of responding to stress and anxiety and the urge to escape and avoid.

The six complex behavioral repertoires (or "core ACT processes") described earlier are interconnected. You can engage in committed action at a higher rate when you are present and able to defuse challenging thoughts. Acceptance and willingness are easier when we can identify and experience values-consistent outcomes. For this reason, ACT interventions target each of these processes simultaneously, and in Figure 24.2, the processes are linked within the ACT hexaflex. Successful intervention involves building each of these processes as generalized operant repertoires and tailoring the intervention to address how these behaviors make contact with the external environment to foster the act of noticing and the development of a broader dynamic context that supports psychologically flexible responding.

As with all behavior-analytic approaches, we can do more with it if we know the basic principles that inform its development and use. In the case of ACT, each of the core processes described earlier extend directly from RFT as a contemporary operant approach to understanding human language and cognition (Hayes, 2004; Barnes-Holmes et al., 2004). Understanding how relational framing participates in psychological flexibility and inflexibility is important for at least two reasons. First, understanding the basic theory is necessary to inform translational research efforts that could change the way ACT is conducted in light of new experimental findings. Second, practitioners familiar with the basic theory may be better able to adapt or adjust ACT-based interventions by knowing more precisely the complex interplay between relational frames and the behavior they are targeting.

Translational research has begun to determine how these patterns of relational responding interact with the six core processes of the ACT hexaflex. For example, Paliliunas (2021), extending prior work (e.g., Plumb et al., 2009), describes values as motivative augmental rules that operate within hierarchical relational frames, wherein functions contained in the overarching value transfer to goals and committed actions contained within the value. A complete account may be forthcoming by assuming that each type of relation is evident within each of the six core processes, where working out the particulars is the task of translational research to inform ACT interventions. We provide a starting point in the following section.

ACT Processes and Relational Behavior

Table 24.1 provides a starting point to guide translational research related to each of the relational frames as they may participate in the core processes of the ACT hexaflex. Each of the major relational frame families are provided in the left column, and each of the core processes are listed at the top. Each cell provides an example of how the relational frame family participates in each core process. Readers will notice that the contribution of frames of coordination are identical across each of the core processes, highlighting a major limitation of an account based solely on coordinated or equivalence relations. That is to say, stimulus equivalence is a key foundational repertoire but cannot meaningfully distinguish the unique and complex differences between the various behavioral repertoires that ACT trains. Once we add relations other than sameness, the ACT model begins to take shape, opening considerable avenues for research and practice.

Values

Starting with values, frames of coordination allow us to label events and to begin to interact with our world verbally. Frames of distinction are necessary to discriminate between different events that are in the service of the same value, events that may be values-consistent but in the service of different values, and events that are values-consistent and values-inconsistent. This final discrimination likely involves frames of opposition. Not only are values-consistent and values-inconsistent outcomes different, they are the opposite. For example, if feeling close to family and friends is something you value, then feeling isolated and alone is the opposite. Noticing this opposition can help augment the functional properties of values statements (e.g., "Is staying home alone all weekend the same or the opposite of your value of feeling close and connected with friends and family?"). Values are also necessarily comparative, as not all values are held equal. For example, a person may value leisure and relaxation but value providing for their family even more. Noticing these comparisons can also help guide decision making when some choices are in the service of one value but momentarily detract from others. As noted earlier, the relationship between values, outcomes, and committed actions are hierarchical, because multiple events can be in the service of a single value. Finally, deictic relating is likely involved in empathetic responding that can extend from consideration of one's own values, as well as the values of others. For example, making sense of another's behavior may be easier by considering her values and how they may differ from our own. Furthermore, understanding how our own values here-now may differ from our own values there and then may contribute to self-kindness or self-compassion that is interconnected within ACT intervention (Marshall & Brockman, 2016).

Committed Action

As with values, discriminating between different actions that may be in the service of one's values, in the service of different values, or not in the service of any values is critical to directing behavior in the context of behavior–behavior relations; that is, two or more different actions could serve the same valued function, producing greater variability within values-consistent behavior. Committed actions are also the opposite of impulsive actions that serve experiential avoidance functions. For example, if engaging in one behavior leads to excessive suffering, what is the opposite of that behavior? Identifying actions that are in opposition to stuck patterns of experiential avoidance can be

TABLE 24.1. Examples of Potential Relational Frame Families Evident within the Six Core ACT Processes

	Values	Committed action	Present-moment awareness	Self-as-context	Defusion	Acceptance
Coordination	Appetitive and aversive events are coordinated with verbal descriptions and evaluations about the events.	Appetitive and aversive events are coordinated with verbal descriptions and evaluations about the events.	Appetitive and aversive events are coordinated with verbal descriptions and evaluations about the events.	Appetitive and aversive events are coordinated with verbal descriptions and evaluations about the events.	Appetitive and aversive events are coordinated with verbal descriptions and evaluations about the events.	Appetitive and aversive events are coordinated with verbal descriptions and evaluations about the events.
Distinction	Values-consistent and -inconsistent verbal descriptions and evaluations are different from other descriptions and evaluations, and values categories differ from other values categories.	Values-consistent and -inconsistent actions are different from other values-consistent actions that are coordinated with verbal descriptions and evaluations.	Events occurring in the past, present, and future are different from other events happening in the past, present, and future that are coordinated with verbal descriptions and evaluations.	Appetitive and aversive verbal descriptions and evaluations are different from other appetitive and aversive verbal descriptions and evaluations.	Verbal descriptions and evaluations are different from the public and private physical events that they refer to and are different from other verbal descriptions and evaluations.	Appetitive and aversive verbal descriptions and evaluations are different from other appetitive and aversive verbal descriptions and evaluations.
Opposition	Values-consistent verbal description and evaluations are the opposite of values-inconsistent verbal descriptions and evaluations.	Values-consistent actions are the opposite of values-inconsistent actions.	Events occurring in the present moment are the opposite of events occurring in the past and future, and publicly observable events are the opposite of privately observable events.	Appetitive and aversive verbal descriptions and evaluations that are fixed and rigid (i.e., self as content) are the opposite of verbal descriptions and evaluations that are dynamic and flexible (i.e., self-as-context).	Verbal descriptions and evaluations that are strongly coordinated with public and private physical events (i.e., fused) are the opposite of verbal descriptions and evaluations that are different from or weakly coordinated with public and private events (i.e., defused).	Appetitive private and public events (i.e., wanted) are the opposite of aversive events (i.e., unwanted), and approaching wanted and unwanted public and private events (i.e., acceptance) is the opposite of avoiding wanted and unwanted private events.
Comparison	Values-consistent verbal descriptions	Values-consistent actions are better	Attending to events in the present	Verbal descriptions that are dynamic	Verbal descriptions that are defused	Approaching wanted and unwanted public

and evaluations are better than neutral and values-inconsistent verbal descriptions and evaluations.	than neutral actions and values-inconsistent actions.	moment is better than attending to events in the past or future when doing so is values-consistent.	and flexible (i.e., self-as-context) are better than verbal descriptions that are fixed and rigid (i.e., self-as-content).	and flexible are better than verbal descriptions that are fused and rigid when doing so is values-consistent.	and private events is better than avoiding unwanted public and private events when doing so is values-consistent.
Hierarchical Different values-consistent verbal descriptions and evaluations can be contained in the same value or values-system in values-categories.	Sets of values-consistent actions can be contained in (in the service of) the same value or value system.	Sets of events are contained in the present moment, in the past, or in the future, where events in the present are ever-changing.	Different verbal descriptions and events are contained in a broad class of self-as-content and other verbal descriptions and events are contained in a broad class of self-as-context.	Sets of verbal relations that are strongly coordinated and rigid are contained in a broad class of fused evaluations and sets of verbal relations are weakly coordinated and flexible are contained in a broad class of defused evaluations.	Sets of values-consistent actions can be contained in the category of "approach" actions and other values-inconsistent actions can be contained in the category of "avoidance" actions.
Deictic Values-consistent and inconsistent descriptions are something "I-have-now" (i.e., my values today), but differ from other people's values here-now and there-then (i.e., perspective taking).	Values-consistent and inconsistent actions are something "I-do-now" (i.e., my actions today), but differ from other people's actions here-now and there-then, and may participate in a different values or value system.	Present-moment events are happening to "me-here-now" that differ from past and future events that are happening to "me-there-then," and differ from events happening to other people "here-now" and "there-then."	Verbal descriptions and evaluations consistent with self-as-content include coordinated relations with "I" or "you," but verbal descriptions and evaluations consistent with self-as-context include "here" versus "there" and "now" versus "then" descriptions and evaluations.	Fused verbal descriptions and evaluations strongly and rigidly participated in "I," "here," and "now" relational classes, and defused descriptions and evaluations weakly and flexibly participant in "I" or "you," "here" or "there," and "now" and "then" relational classes.	Acceptance of appetitive and aversive experienced events happening to "me-here-now" can strengthen values-consistent behavior "there-then" (i.e., later) or values-consistent behavior in others either now (you-there-now) or later (you-there-later).

immensely helpful in directing ACT-consistent behavior change. Committed actions are also inherently comparative. For example, texting a family member may be in the service of feeling more connected with family. This action may be better than isolating from family but not as fulfilling as making the time to visit one's family. Comparative relations also play a central role in shaping processes within ACT-based interventions. For example, following negative experiences with family, seeing family may be a step too far; however, texting a family member may be *more* tolerable as an initial step toward greater connectedness. Committed actions are hierarchically related to one's values, and part of ACT intervention is to strengthen this relationship. Deictic and hierarchical relations can also contribute to empathetic or compassionate responding by identifying that although the actions of the other may not be aligned with our personal values, greater compassion and understanding may be achieved by considering how one's actions align or fail to align with their own values or values system.

Present-Moment Awareness

The act of present-moment awareness requires noticing, and this often involves verbal behavior discriminating between observed events in the present environment. For example, when noticing objects in a room to direct present-moment attention, it is necessary to distinguish between external physical objects and internal private evaluations of them. Interaction with present-moment events is also distinct from interacting with thoughts about events occurring at another time or at another place. In addition, private experiences can be considered the opposite of pubic or external experiences. Contextual comparing is also a necessary feature of present-moment awareness in the sense that, in some contexts, intentional awareness of the present moment is *more* in the service of one's values than fixating on a future event. However, in other contexts, fixating on a future event momentarily may be *more* in the service of one's values (e.g., problem solving). The act of noticing and directing one's attention based on context undoubtedly involves moment-to-moment comparative relations. All of these relational patterns in the context of present-moment awareness necessarily extend from deictic relational framing, distinguishing events that are happening to me-here-now from events happening to me-there-then, others-here-now, or others-there-then.

Self-as-Context

As with the previous processes, self-as-context necessitates distinguishing between different evaluations and stories that we tell about ourselves and others. Part of the ACT process is building a frame of opposition between evaluations that extend from self-as-context and those that extend from self-as-content—or the conceptualized self. In this way, when we notice that our verbal behavior about ourselves appears fused and highly conceptualized, the functions of this event can be transformed through the frame of opposition (i.e., "do the opposite"), resulting in new verbal behavior that puts the content of our experience into context. We may also notice that because of the oppositional relationship between these two approaches to self, strengthening one process necessarily weakens the other. Therefore, if we strengthen and augment our behavioral repertoire labeled self-as-context, we will necessarily see a reduction in the behavior we allocate to our repertoire of rigid verbal rules about and evaluations of self (i.e., "self-as-content"). Not only are these competing processes the opposite, but they also exist in a comparative relation, because we assume that self-as-context is more likely to promote psychological flexibility and well-being than self-as-content. The descriptions of self-as-content, self-as-context, and even the transcendental self are hierarchical, because we want the functions of these evaluations about evaluations to transform all topographies of verbal self-descriptions that a person experiences.

Defusion

Defusion necessitates weakening the functional influence of all of the relational frame families as they exist within behavior–behavior interactions. As can be seen in the previous frame families, the way that we engage in distinction, opposition, comparison, hierarchical, and deictic framing can promote psychological flexibility or inflexibility as it operates within a complex stream of behavior. In general, if we can weaken the control of these relations more globally, greater control can be exerted by the external environment to promote greater sensitivity to the dynamic shifts in contingencies that happen throughout our lives. We also want to promote noticing fused (i.e., strong and highly connected) versus defused relations and promote defusion-consistent responding when we notice that relations are highly fused. Defusion strategies, such as the repetition task, singing the relation as a birthday song, or coloring the relation in a picture, all have the same effect on behavior–behavior relations of weakening the functional characteristics of the relational frame in the moment. Noticing these relations necessitates hierarchically relating to thoughts with specific characteristics as "fused" and others as "defused." Deictic relating may also play a central role in defusion, where relational frames that participate in "I-here-now" may be more fused than relational frames about ourselves at a different time or about others. Part of self-compassion training is to transfer functions of relational framing about others (that tend to be more contextualized) to relational framing about oneself. For example, when a person is suffering and engaging in highly fused self-evaluations (e.g., "I am so stupid"), an ACT trainer might ask if he would say or believe those same things about a friend in the same situation.

Acceptance

Noticing similarities (coordination) and differences (distinction) among events is also central to acceptance. In addition, oppositional frames are necessary to acceptance and operate on two streams. First, aversive and appetitive private experiences are the opposite, where aversive experiences operate as a motivating operation to escape or avoid, and appetitive private experience operate as a motivating operation to approach. Second, approaching is the opposite of avoiding. These two frames of opposition interact, because we want to encourage approaching of appetitive experiences even when this necessitates approaching of unwanted aversive experiences (i.e., willingness). Therefore, there may be multiple levels of comparative relations at play, where appetitive is better than aversive, approach is better than avoid, and the decision to approach or avoid is more important than simply seeking appetitive experiences and avoiding aversive experiences. This complex interplay between comparison and oppositional frames sets the stage to diminish experiential avoidance that occurs when we exclusively focus on the aversive–appetitive comparison frame, without consideration of approach–avoidance in relation to our values. Acceptance may therefore also play a role in the hierarchical relationship between values and committed action, where engaging in committed action may require (i.e., contains) acceptance-based processes. Deictic relations are also involved in this process, where acceptance is something that I-do-now in order to move toward my values later. Acceptance may also lead to committed action intended to improve the lives of others-here-now and others-there-later (i.e., altruistic responding or compassionate responding), that likely necessitates deictic framing of the other core processes as previously described.

Once again, by examining each of the core processes in turn, along with each of the relational frames, we arrive at the interconnectedness involved in complex patterns of relational framing that can foster flexible or inflexible patterns of responding. It is up to basic experimental and translational researchers to continue to examine these complex interactions with precision, scope, and depth, and in a way that can inform ACT-based approaches. For practicing behavior analysts, the previous breakdown provides a starting point to begin to interpret the functions of relational patterns evident within each of the six core processes. For those who are interested in further exploring the complex dynamics of relational verbal behavior and psychological flexibility, two new and compatible models are emerging to explore the dynamic interaction of relational frames: the hyper-dimensional and multilevel model (HDML; Barnes-Holmes et al., 2020) and relational density theory (RDT; Belisle & Dixon, 2020). We explore these two models briefly below.

Exploring Complexity: The HDML and RDT

Relational dynamics (Belisle, 2022) is concerned with how relational frames organize, or self-organize, in complex ways. The HDML and RDT both attempt to look at higher-order properties of relational frames and how complex interactions at lower levels can lead to orderly interactions at higher levels. The HDML provides a coherent multilevel and multidimensional framework to describe simple, as well as complex, patterns of relating. Levels of relational framing include mutual and combinatorial entailment that we described earlier, as well as more complex levels such as relational framing, relational networks, relations among relations, and relating of relational networks. Complex interactions at these higher levels are likely necessary to describe ACT approaches more fully, such as the use of analogy, metaphors, and storytelling. For example, given the metaphor of watching leaves on a stream (a commonly used present-moment and defusion training procedure), relational frames about the passage of time and movement away from oneself are transferred to the concept of thoughts in the present moment. The HDML also describes multiple dimensions across which relational frames might differ, including coherence (consistency between past and present relational responding), complexity (level of detail or relations), derivation (degree of practice), and flexibility (sensitivity to the environment). The result is 20 analytic units from which we can begin to interpret complex relational behavior. In theory, Table 24.1 could be superimposed on the more complex HDML framework, even further guiding research on relational frames as they relate to ACT.

RDT describes how higher-order properties consistent with Newtonian classical mechanics may describe how relational frames evolve over time and in response to the external context. According to Belisle and Dixon (2020), RDT represents a theoretical synthesis between behavior momentum theory and RFT. From an RDT perspective, we are interested in how relational frames change. For example, if a person is given a piece of new information, such as "The world is flat," how do they respond to this information? Relational resistance is a higher-order property that suggests larger and stronger relational frames are also more resistant to change. Therefore, if we have established multiple relations supporting that the earth is, in fact, round, then this new piece of information will be unlikely to influence other relational frames (i.e., we still believe the earth is round). However, a young child who is only starting to learn about the world may be more likely to believe that the earth is flat, because a large relational network has not taken shape around the idea that the earth is round.

A model of relational coherence (Belisle & Clayton, 2021) also extends off of a general theory of gravity in that relations that are closer together are more likely to merge. For example, a "flat earther" may have a history of relational framing around conspiracies and antiscientific beliefs that make it more likely that he will accept, rather than reject, the premise that the earth is flat. In the context of ACT, we may be interested in understanding how fused thoughts and beliefs emerge and self-organize, resulting in larger patterns of maladaptive rule-governed behavior that leads to greater suffering. As with the HDML, new findings in RDT may open up translational research opportunities that relate directly to applications of ACT.

Summary

We have seen an explosion in research and practice related to RFT and ACT in the field of behavior analysis, including developments in the underlying theory, basic and translational research on its core assumptions, and applications across multiple populations and behavioral challenges. We are embarking on a new frontier in our practice that will open up new applications and opportunities for practitioners and researchers. These developments in our field come with new opportunities for training, insight, and the adoption of innovative technologies that can make the world better for people. We are only now starting to put together the building blocks of human complexity that will change our field forever. We are creating new rules—a new playbook. It is up to every behavior analyst to decide whether the contents presented in this chapter and in other resources are simply too complex or diverge too greatly from practice as usual. But consider that inflexible responding to the status quo can only lead to narrow application and an inability to adapt to new challenges. When we are fused to the past, we experientially avoid the future. Once we can break free from the psychological chains of our own rigidity, we can begin to chase that which we truly value, affecting changes in the lives of our clients toward the lives that they value, and affecting change in our own lives that we value in turn. Our science has always been about exploring all aspects of human behavior. So, let's explore and be variable—remain persistent in our pursuit of innovation and discovery—and consistent with our value of serving the world with a science of human behavior.

REFERENCES

Barnes-Holmes, D., Barnes-Holmes, Y., & McEnteggart, C. (2020). Updating RFT (more field than frame) and its implications for process-based therapy. *Psychological Record, 70*, 605–624.

Barnes-Holmes, Y., Barnes-Holmes, D., McHugh, L., & Hayes, S. C. (2004). Relational frame theory: Some implications for understanding and treating human psychopathology. *International Journal of Psychology and Psychological Therapy, 4*, 355–375.

Belisle, J. (2020). Model dependent realism and the rule-governed behavior of behavior analysts: Applications to derived relational responding. *Perspectives on Behavior Science, 43*(2), 321–342.

Belisle, J., & Clayton, M. (2021). Coherence and the merging of relational classes in self-organizing networks: Extending relational density theory. *Journal of Contextual Behavioral Science, 20,* 118–128.

Belisle, J., & Dixon, M. R. (2020). Relational density theory: Nonlinearity of equivalence relating examined through higher-order volumetric-mass-density. *Perspectives on Behavior Science, 43,* 259–283.

Belisle, J., Paliliunas, D., Dixon, M. R., & Speelman, R. C. (2019). Decreasing influence of arbitrarily applicable verbal relations of recreational gamblers: A randomized controlled trial. *Journal of Applied Behavior Analysis, 52*(1), 60–72.

Belisle, J., Paliliunas, D., Lauer, T., Giamanco, A., Lee, B., & Sickman, E. (2020). Derived relational responding and transformations of function in children: A review of applied behavior-analytic journals. *Analysis of Verbal Behavior, 36,* 115–145.

Dixon, M. R., Hayes, S. C., & Belisle, J. (2023). *Acceptance and commitment for behavior analysts: A practice guide from theory to treatment.* Routledge/Taylor & Francis.

Dixon, M. R., Paliliunas, D., Belisle, J., Speelman, R. C., Gunnarsson, K. F., & Shaffer, J. L. (2019). The effect of brief mindfulness training on momentary impulsivity. *Journal of Contextual Behavioral Science, 11,* 15–20.

Dougher, M. J., Hamilton, D. A., Fink, B. C., & Harrington, J. (2007). Transformation of the discriminative and eliciting functions of generalized relational stimuli. *Journal of the Experimental Analysis of Behavior, 88*(2), 179–197.

Fang, S., & Ding, D. (2020). A meta-analysis of the efficacy of acceptance and commitment therapy for children. *Journal of Contextual Behavioral Science, 15,* 225–234.

Fonseca, S., Trindade, I. A., Mendes, A. L., & Ferreira, C. (2020). The buffer role of psychological flexibility against the impact of major life events on depression symptoms. *Clinical Psychologist, 24*(1), 82–90.

Gentili, C., Rickardsson, J., Zetterqvist, V., Simons, L. E., Lekander, M., & Wicksell, R. K. (2019). Psychological flexibility as a resilience factor in individuals with chronic pain. *Frontiers in Psychology, 10,* 1–11.

Gregg, J. A., Namekata, M. S., Louie, W. A., & Chancellor-Freeland, C. (2014). Impact of values clarification on cortisol reactivity to an acute stressor. *Journal of Contextual Behavioral Science, 3*(4), 299–304.

Harte, C., & Barnes-Holmes, D. (2021). A primer on relational frame theory (RFT). In M. P. Twohig, M. E., Levin, & J. M. Peterson (Eds.), *Oxford handbook of acceptance and commitment therapy* (pp. 77–108). Oxford University Press.

Hayes, S. C. (2004). Acceptance and commitment therapy, relational frame theory, and the third wave of behavioral and cognitive therapies. *Behavior Therapy, 35,* 639–665.

Hayes, S. C. (2021). ACT randomized controlled trials since 1986. Retrieved from *https://contextualscience.org/act_randomized_controlled_trials_since_1986.*

Hayes, S. C., & Brownstein, A. J. (1986). Mentalism, behavior–behavior relations, and a behavior-analytic view of the purposes of science. *The Behavior Analyst, 9*(2), 175–190.

Hayes, S. C., Brownstein, A. J., Haas, J. R., & Greenway, D. E. (1986). Instructions, multiple schedules, and extinction: Distinguishing rule-governed from schedule-controlled behavior. *Journal of the Experimental Analysis of Behavior, 46*(2), 137–147.

Hayes, S. C., Brownstein, A. J., Zettle, R. D., Rosenfarb, I., & Korn, Z. (1986). Rule-governed behavior and sensitivity to changing consequences of responding. *Journal of the Experimental Analysis of Behavior, 45*(3), 237–256.

Hayes, S. C., Luoma, J. B., Bond, F. W., Masuda, A., & Lillis, J. (2006). Acceptance and commitment therapy: Model, processes and outcomes. *Behaviour Research and Therapy, 44*(1), 1–25.

Hayes, S. C., Strosahl, K., & Wilson, K. G. (2011). *Acceptance and commitment therapy: The process and practice of mindful change* (2nd ed.). Guilford Press.

Hebert, E. R., Flynn, M. K., Wilson, K. G., & Kellum, K. K. (2021). Values intervention as an establishing operation for approach in the presence of aversive stimuli. *Journal of Contextual Behavioral Science, 20,* 144–154.

Kuhn, T. (1962). *The structure of scientific revolutions.* University of Chicago Press.

Leahy, R. L., Tirch, D. D., & Melwani, P. S. (2012). Processes underlying depression: Risk aversion, emotional schemas, and psychological flexibility. *International Journal of Cognitive Therapy, 5*(4), 362–379.

Levin, M. E., MacLane, C., Daflos, S., Seeley, J. R., Hayes, S. C., Biglan, A., & Pistorello, J.

(2014). Examining psychological inflexibility as a transdiagnostic process across psychological disorders. *Journal of Contextual Behavioral Science, 3*, 155–163.

Mallik, D., Kaplan, J., Somohano, V., Bergman, A., & Bowen, S. (2021). Examining the role of craving, mindfulness, and psychological flexibility in a sample of individuals with substance use disorder. *Substance Use and Misuse, 56*(6), 782–786.

Marshall, E. J., & Brockman, R. N. (2016). The relationships between psychological flexibility, self-compassion, and emotional well-being. *Journal of Cognitive Psychotherapy, 30*, 60–72.

McAuliffe, D., Hughes, S., & Barnes-Holmes, D. (2014). The dark-side of rule governed behavior: An experimental analysis of problematic rule-following in an adolescent population with depressive symptomatology. *Behavior Modification, 38*(4), 587–613.

McHugh, L., Procter, J., Herzog, M., Schock, A. K., & Reed, P. (2012). The effect of mindfulness on extinction and behavioral resurgence. *Learning and Behavior, 40*, 405–415.

Moore, J. (2008). *Conceptual foundations of radical behaviorism*. Sloane.

Paliliunas, D. (2021). Values: A core guiding principle for behavior-analytic intervention and research. *Behavior Analysis in Practice, 15*(1),115–125.

Perez, W. F., de Almeida, J. H., & de Rose, J. C. (2015). Transformation of meaning through relations of sameness and opposition. *Psychological Record, 65*, 679–689.

Plumb, J. C., Stewart, I., Dahl, J., & Lundgren, T. (2009). In search of meaning: Values in modern clinical behavior analysis. *Behavior Analyst, 32*(1), 85–103.

Puolakanaho, A., Tolvanen, A., Kinnunen, S. M., & Lappalainen, R. (2020). A psychological flexibility-based intervention for burnout: A randomized controlled trial. *Journal of Contextual Behavioral Science, 15*, 52–67.

Sidman, M. (1994). *Equivalence relations and behavior: A research story*. Authors Cooperative.

Skinner, B. F. (1945). The operational analysis of psychological terms. *Psychological Review, 52*, 268–277.

Skinner, B. F. (1957). *Verbal behavior*. Appleton-Century-Crofts.

Skinner, B. F. (1969). *Contingencies of reinforcement: A theoretical analysis*. Appleton-Century-Crofts.

Skinner, B. F. (1974). *About behaviorism*. Knopf.

Suarez, V. D., Moon, E. I., & Najdowski, A. C. (2021). Systematic review of acceptance and commitment training components in the behavioral intervention of individuals with autism and developmental disorders. *Behavior Analysis in Practice, 15*, 126–140.

Szabo, T. G. (2019). Acceptance and commitment training for reducing inflexible behaviors in children with autism. *Journal of Contextual Behavioral Science, 12*, 178–188.

CHAPTER 25

Ethical Considerations
of Translational Research

Alison M. Betz

Science without ethics is lame,
and ethics without science is blind.
—ALBERT EINSTEIN

Within the field of behavior analysis, the term *translational research* has been used more frequently in recent years (Kyonka & Subramaniam, 2018; McIlvane, 2009). Despite its popularity, behavior analysts have yet to come to a consensus as to what exactly falls under the umbrella of translational research. Let's assume there is a continuum or spectrum of research with "pure" basic laboratory research falling on one end and "pure" applied research on the other. If one defines *translational* as any research that falls between these two ends of this spectrum, the majority of those conducting research within behavior analysis would likely be considered translational researchers. In fact, Lerman (2003) suggested that *translational research* can be defined as a programmatic attempt to produce research that is informed by practice or vice versa. With this definition, any research with the purpose of evaluating the generality of a phenomena demonstrated in the basic laboratory to human populations, research attempting to evaluate basic findings to clinical settings, or research testing the results of applied research to the community setting would be considered translational in nature.

Vollmer (2011) offered three variations of translational research in behavior analysis, the first of which is applications of behavioral principles first studied in the basic research laboratory. According to Vollmer, this variation is likely the purest form of translational research and is accomplished when the researcher translates the logic of behavioral methodology by studying behavioral principles that were first demonstrated in the basic research laboratory. The importance of this type of translational research, particularly to applied behavior analysis, can be seen by examining the behavioral principles that are now commonplace in applied practice (reinforcement, discrimination training, shaping, etc.) (Vollmer, 2011). All such principles were initially studied in the basic laboratory, then translated to clinical application.

Translational research of this variation continues to hold a strong presence in many areas of study across behavior analysis, such as treatment relapse (e.g., Cohenour et al., 2018; Kimball et al., 2018; Podlesnik et al., 2019), behavioral economics (e.g., DeLeon et al., 2013; Leon, Wilder, & Saini, 2021), and effects of treatment integrity on learning (e.g., Bergmann et al., 2021). Take, for example, research evaluating demand curves to assess reinforcer efficacy under varying response requirements with nonhuman animals (e.g., hens). Basic research comparing demand curves constructed under across- and within-session increases in unit price has shown general correspondence across some response measures; however, metrics used to evaluate demand during across-session phases were not predictive of those used during within-session phases (Foster et al., 1997; Tan & Hackenberg, 2015). In a translational study, Leon et al. (2021) extended this area of research by conducting a similar comparison of within- and across-session increases of unit price with individuals with intellectual and developmental disabilities (IDDs). The authors used arbitrary responses (i.e., card touch, card sorting) as the target task across all phases and conditions. As in previous research, the authors constructed and compared reinforcer–demand functions for within- and across-session phases (see Leon et al., 2021, for a detailed description of how demand functions were constructed and data analysis). The results of Leon et al. also showed little convergence between the measures obtained by the different methods of increasing unit price, with participants often responding under higher unit prices during the within-session phase when compared to the across-session phase.

Vollmer (2011) describes the second variation of translational research as research that is meant to solve applied problems more systematically and with more methodological rigor than studies conducted directly within the community. It may be argued that this variation is most widely implemented and accepted within applied behavior analysis. It is common for researchers to evaluate the effects of a treatment, for example, in a highly controlled clinical setting prior to implementing such procedures within the natural environment. Take, for example, researchers who evaluate treatment for severe problem behavior in individuals with autism spectrum disorder (ASD) or IDDs in a highly controlled treatment room in which extraneous variables can be controlled. Betz et al. (2013) evaluated schedule-thinning procedures during functional communication training with four children who had been referred to a program for the assessment and treatment of several problem behavior. Although all participants were attending the program to address problem behavior that occurred in the natural environment (e.g., home and school), effects of treatment were first systematically evaluated in a controlled setting described by the authors as 3 × 3 meter therapy rooms that were equipped with observation panels, a table, and chairs, and only relevant session materials were present. Furthermore, the treatment was implemented in sessions of short duration (i.e., 10 minutes). Because the authors implemented highly systematic procedures with a great deal of experimental rigor, they were able to show proof of concept and show that problem behavior maintained at low rates following functional communication training without gradual schedule thinning. However, due to the methodological rigor, the authors were unable to draw conclusions regarding the effects of the treatment in a more naturalistic environment or when implemented for longer durations.

Finally, the third variation involves translating what we know about behavior analysis to other methodologies and perhaps disciplines to address a broader range of social problems. All these variations of translational research, particularly the second and third variations, involve a specialized skills set that may require the researcher to be more sensitive to the ethics of conducting this type of research.

Because there has yet to be an overwhelming consensus on what constitutes translational research and its definition within the context of behavior analysis, for the purposes of this chapter, we assume that translational research includes any research that systematically attempts to evaluate behavioral phenomena demonstrated in the basic laboratory under controlled conditions to improve or inform clinical practice (within-discipline translation) or to translate behavioral logic to other methodologies to address social problems (across-discipline translation). Due to the complexity of such processes, our purpose in this chapter is to highlight ethical considerations within the context of translational research and provide recommendations to ensure ethical standards are being met.

The Evolution of Ethical Codes Relevant to Translational Research

In 1973/2017, the American Psychological Association published a code of ethics entitled *Ethical Principles of Psychologists and Code of Conduct*. The code has eight sections that outline appropriate ethical conduct across areas, such as working in one's area of competence, confidentiality, and others. The eighth section outlines ethical guidelines for research and publication. This section includes 15 subsections detailing ethical standards for conducting and publishing research, with the primary purpose of protecting research participants, the community, and investigators. Although many behavior analysts do not identify as psychologists, many behavior-analytic training programs are housed in departments that follow the American Psychological Association code of conduct, particularly when it comes to research and publication.

As a result of the National Research Act of 1974, The *Belmont Report* was written by the National Commission for the Protection of Human Subjects of Biomedical and Behavioral Research (1979), which was created to outline basic ethical principles that underlie the conduct of biomedical and behavioral research involving human participants and included guidelines to ensure that such research is conducted in accordance with the specified principles. The basic principles were those that the authors of the report felt were particularly relevant to the ethics of research involving human subjects and include (1) respect for persons, (2) beneficence, and (3) justice.

According to the report, *respect for persons* incorporates two ethical beliefs: Individuals should be treated as autonomous agents, and individuals with diminished autonomy are entitled to protection. The principle of *beneficence* refers to treating individuals in an ethical manner by respecting their decisions and protecting them from harm. Additionally, it refers to making efforts to ensure the well-being of individuals. The authors provided two rules referred to as "complementary expressions of beneficent actions" (National Commission of the Protection of Human Subjects in Biomedical and Behavioral Research, 1979). These two rules are (1) do not harm and (2) maximize possible benefits and minimize possible harms. Finally, the principle of *justice* refers to ensuring that there is equal distribution of what is deserved. According to the Belmont Report, an injustice has occurred when a benefit to which a person is entitled is denied without a good reason. Specifically, the report states that "injustice arises from social, racial, sexual and cultural biases institutionalized in society" (p. 5). For example, many research subjects in the early to mid-20th century included poor ward patients, while the improved medical care was delivered primarily to the private patients. As written, the Belmont Report is concerned with what could be referred to as *distributive justice*, a call for fair allocation of society's benefits and burdens (Mastroianni et al., 1994). To this day, researchers are still held to the ethical standards described in the Belmont Report, and many field-specific ethical codes encompass these ethical principles.

The term *translational* did not appear in the scientific literature until the early 1990s and was used to describe basic research in genetics (Kyonka & Subramaniam, 2018). Since then, use of the term has increased. In fact, the National Institutes of Health (NIH; 1999) created a roadmap for biomedical sciences that was labeled the "bench to bedside and back" model, which focused on translating the results of basic research into clinical practice. Now it was the responsibility of both basic and applied researchers to address issues of the other domains and practice. Another initiative of this model was referred to as "to the community and back," which encouraged the implementation of the products from basic and applied research in the community. This initiative resulted in public health scientists being responsible as well. Throughout the next several decades, the biomedical field continues to refine the translational model, which has not been adopted and revised in many other fields, including behavior analysis. Although slightly unique in its characteristics, translational research is still considered research, thus requiring researchers to consider relevant ethical principles and standards, including the *Ethics Code for Behavior Analysts* (Behavior Analyst Certification Board, 2020).

Ethics Code for Behavior Analysts

In 2001, the Behavior Analyst Certification Board® (BACB) published its own version of ethical guidelines specifically for behavior analysts who are board certified, including Board Certified Behavior Analysts (BCBAs) and Board Certified Associate Behavior Analysts (BCaBAs). Like the American Psychological Association's ethical code, the BACB's *Guidelines for Responsible Conduct for Behavior Analysts* (Behavior Analyst Certification Board, 2021) outlined principles that were developed to guide behavior analysts' ethical behavior. According to the initial published document, the guidelines were developed to address ethical concerns particular to BCBAs and BCaBAs, and referenced existing codes such as the Belmont Report, the American Psychological Association, the American Educational Research Association, as well as several others (BACB, 2001). Like previous codes, the BACB ethical guidelines addressed issues such as responsible conduct for a behavior analyst, responsibility to the client, ethical guidelines for assessment and treatment, and responsibilities to the field and colleagues. Additionally, the BACB's guidelines included a section targeting scholarship and research (Section 7; BACB, 2001).

Since the publication of the original document, the BACB has revised the guidelines multiple times to ensure it remains relevant and continues to address modern-day ethical issues. Most recently, the BACB published the *Ethics Code for Behavior Analysts*, which includes a section (Section 6) entitled, Responsibility in Research (BACB, 2020). In terms of research ethics, the current code provided by the BACB is similar to the previous code and those provided by the Americal Psychological Association, including guidelines on informed consent, confidentiality, reviewing research, and research in service delivery, to name a few. Furthermore, the BACB's ethics code provides definitions relevant to research for which behavior analysts can refer (BACB, 2020, pp. 7–8). Specifically, the BACB defines *research* as "any data-based activity, including analysis of preexisting data, designed to generate generalizable knowledge for the discipline. The use of an experimental design does not by itself constitute research" (p. 8). They also define a research participant as, "any individual participating in a defined research study for whom informed consent has been obtained" (p. 8).

Because of the nature of research conducted by behavior analysts, particularly the use of single-case experimental designs, it is common for behavior analysts to conduct research within the context of service delivery. For example, a clinician may be attempting to solve a clinical problem by implementing a new or modified intervention. Thus, they design systematic evaluation to closely monitor the effects with the intent to disseminate the results to the broader behavior-analytic community. In this case, the clinician is now playing the role of a researcher as well. Because there may be competing contingencies controlling clinical and research behaviors, behavior analysts may find themselves in situations in which ethical decision making may be difficult. To assist with such decisions, the BACB included ethical guidelines surrounding research in service delivery (Code 6.03), which specifies that when behavior analysts conduct research in the context of service delivery, they must arrange such research in a way that "client services and the welfare are prioritized" (BACB, 2022, p. 17). Additionally, the BACB specifies that when research is conducted in the context of service delivery, the behavior analyst must comply with the ethics requirements for both service delivery and research.

Ethics for Animal Research

It is important to note that translational research can include studies using animals as subjects as well. For example, Brown et al. (2020) used a reverse-translational preparation to test predictions of quantitative theories of resurgence (e.g., behavioral momentum theory) by examining resurgence following two conditions of differential reinforcement of alternative behavior (DRA). The authors conducted the study first in the applied setting with children receiving treatment for destructive behavior (Experiment 1) followed by a similar experiment conducted in a laboratory setting using rats (Experiment 2). Thus, translational researchers using a reverse-translational or similar model must also be aware of the ethical guidelines for using nonhuman animals in research.

In 2012, the American Psychological Association developed guidelines for psychologists working with nonhuman animals, specifying that "the acquisitions, care, housing, use, and disposition of nonhuman animals in research must be in compliance with applicable federal, state, and local laws and regulations, institutional policies." This document provides ethical guidelines in areas including (I) Justification of the Research; (II) Personnel; (III) Care and Housing of Laboratory Animals; (IV) Acquisition of Laboratory Animals; (V) Experimental Procedures; (VI) Field Research; and (VII) Educational Use of Nonhuman Animals. The American Psychological Association notes that it recognizes the document as "guidelines" rather than "standards," as it serves a different purpose. Unlike standards, guidelines are "meant to be aspirational in intent and provide recommendations for the professional conduct of specified activities" (p. 10). The committee goes on to note that the guidelines are not meant to be exhaustive. Thus, researchers using nonhuman animals should ensure they are familiar with local, state, and institutional regulations and laws, which most likely are overseen by an Institutional Animal Care and Use Committee (IACUC). As the name implies, an IACUC is a committee developed by a research institution to oversee the use of nonhuman animals in research. These committees often include veterinarians, scientists, and nonscientist members.

IACUC guidelines are critical in ensuring laws about animal research in the United States and are followed. Because most animal research is funded by the NIH or other federal agencies, The NIH Office of Laboratory Animal Welfare (OLAW) has been directed to develop policies that describe the role of IACUC. Thus, every institution that uses certain animals for research must have a local IACUC, which reviews research protocols and conducts evaluations of the institution's animal care and use. IACUC's primary responsibilities are to ensure that procedures with animals avoid or minimize discomfort, distress, and pain to the animals; that consistent with sound research design, animals have appropriate living conditions and medical care; that personnel are adequately trained; and that methods of euthanasia are consistent with American Veterinary Medical Association Panel on Euthanasia. Another important function of the IACUC is to ensure that scientists who use nonhuman animals in their research seek out appropriate alternatives to animal use when possible. For example, cell cultures may be used instead of living animals for some cellular-level research. For more details on policy and laws regarding the use of laboratory animals in research, please refer to the OLAW website (*www.olaw. nih.gov*).

Ethics for Translational Research

While all the previously described ethical codes and guidelines specific to research are applicable to behavior-analytic researchers, they may not be sufficient when it comes to conducting translational research. It can be argued that ethical considerations are greater in translational research compared to pure basic or clinical research when using human participants, as the purpose may not be of clinical importance. This is particularly true when conducting translational research that focuses on testing basic principles developed in laboratory studies or when attempting to solve applied studies within the context of the laboratory, as the certainty of the outcome is unknown.

As previously noted, translational research involves extending results of basic research by evaluating the same behavioral processes with clinical populations, some of which may be identified as vulnerable populations, such as children, individuals with developmental or intellectual disabilities, or both. Furthermore, it is often the case that, at least in the initial phases of moving from basic to applied research, one or more key components of applied behavior analysis is missing, such as addressing socially significant problems. For example, a researcher may use an arbitrary response such as a card touch or button press, or entering hypothetical data into a computer. In such instances, the target response is not likely socially significant. Additionally, researchers may choose to conduct sessions in highly controlled environments, such as a sterile therapy room or empty office, rather than in the natural environment, to minimize the likelihood of extraneous variables that may make it more difficult to attribute the results to the behavioral process being studied. Such research components may limit generality and can better be described as translational in nature rather than applied.

Results of translational research are not any less meaningful than those of applied studies, but additional considerations may be needed. For example, Milo, Mace, and Nevin (2010) evaluated preference of constant versus varied reinforcer delivery in children with autism. To evaluate preference, the authors presented the participant with two Big Red® switches, where pressing one switch resulted in access to one constant reinforcer and pressing the other resulted in access to one of three randomly chosen reinforcers that varied across responses. The results of the study showed that all participants showed preference for varied reinforcers and, when compared to constant reinforcer delivery, varied reinforcers resulted in higher rates of responding under maintenance conditions and were more resistant to distraction.

Although the results may help inform practitioners when designing and implementing interventions for the natural environment, the results should be taken with caution, as the target response was not similar to those targeted in the natural environment.

Furthermore, when conducting translational research such as this, there will also likely be specific ethical considerations that arise while conducting the research.

We describe in the following sections of this chapter ethical issues that are particularly relevant when conducting translational research. Some of these issues have been clearly outlined in the ethical codes mentioned earlier; however, this chapter focuses on providing guidelines for translational researchers specifically to ensure that their research is ethically sound.

Ethical Guidelines for Translational Research

When conducting translational research, special ethical considerations must be made. Translational researchers must be particularly sensitive to the ethical and societal implications of their research. In other words, translational researchers must take the time to fully consider and appreciate the implications of their work, the extent to which the outcomes can benefit the scientific community, and the risks involved in conducting such research.

Deception

When using humans as participants in translational research, deception may be necessary. This is particularly true when the participants are verbally competent human beings, because simply knowing the purpose of the study or the behavior of interest may influence the participant's responding. A well-known example of the use of deception is the Milgram (1974) study. The purpose of the study was to evaluate the conflict between obedience to authority and personal conscience. In this study, participants were deceived by first being told they would be paired with another participant, when in fact they were actually paired with a research assistant pretending to be a participant. During the study, the participant was asked to test the "learner" on previously learned word pairs by naming a word and asking the learner to recall its partner. The teacher was told to deliver an electric shock to the learner every time he made a mistake, increasing the level of the shock each time. The learner primarily gave wrong answers (on purpose), requiring the teacher to administer a shock. Of course, the participant was not actually delivering an electric shock; rather, deception was used by making the participant believe the learner was in pain. Because the purpose of the study was to evaluate obedience to authority, if the participant refused the experimenter, who wore a white lab coat, the experimenter then gave a series of orders and prods to ensure they continued. The results showed that all participants continued to deliver shocks up to 300 volts, and 65% of participants continued to the highest level of 450 volts. One may argue that participants' behavior would have likely been affected if the participants knew the true purpose of the study.

It is not uncommon for translational researchers, including behavior analysts, to use deception. Thus, it is critical that researchers know how to minimize the possible unwanted side effects of deception. Such safeguards include (1) using deception only when necessary, (2) not using deception if it will cause physical harm or emotional distress, and (3) debriefing those who were deceived following participation.

Use Deception Only When Necessary

As specified in the American Psychological Association's Code of Conduct (2017), researchers should not conduct studies including deception unless it is determined that such techniques are justified given the potential value of the results. If, however, deception is deemed necessary (which may be more likely in translational research), there are ethical guidelines that researchers should follow.

Do Not Deceive Participants about Research
That May Cause Physical Pain or Severe Emotional Distress

If the researcher anticipates there is a chance of a participant being emotionally or physically harmed while participating in the study, it is the researcher's responsibility to ensure this is discussed and the participant is aware of such possibilities prior to giving consent. Thus, deception can still be used about the general purpose of the study or other aspects of participation, but the researcher must disclose the possibility of physical pain or emotional distress.

Inform Participants about Any Deception

The researcher should divulge this information as early as possible, such as immediately following the individual's participation. If by explaining the deception to one or more participants prior to end of data collection for the entire study could impact the results (e.g., the participant informed of deception may discuss the deceptive techniques with other participants), the researcher may wish to inform all participants of the deception at the conclusion of data collection. It is up to the researcher to determine when is the best time to explain deception. Additionally, once participants are informed of the deception, the researcher should allow the opportunity for the participants to withdraw their data from the study. If a participant chooses to do so, the researcher should respect that choice, avoid convincing the participant otherwise, and ensure that such a choice does not result in adverse outcomes for the individual (e.g., it will not impact current services).

Behavior analysts conducting research should not necessarily avoid using deception. In some cases, it is necessary to conduct a valid study that can produce meaningful results. For example, Matey et al. (2019) evaluated whether being required to deliver feedback following an observation would affect accuracy of data collection during observations. Prior to the study, the researchers told participants they were randomly assigned to be an observer and their role was to observe and collect data on another participant's posture during completion of a work task. What participants were not told was that they were actually observing confederates trained to perform with specific accuracies, nor were they aware that the true primary dependent variables were the accuracy of their observation data across various feedback conditions (i.e., observation only, required-feedback). It was argued that deception was necessary because if the participants knew the true purpose of this study prior to participating, they may have intentionally or unintentionally altered the feedback they provided.

Given that deception was deemed necessary, unlike Milgram (1974), Matey et al. (2019) used the previously described safeguards to minimize potential negative effects, First, prior to the start of the study, the researchers obtained approval, including the use of deception, from their institutional review board. Objective and unbiased reviews of the study's procedures ensured that deception was necessary, and the likelihood of physical harm or emotional distress was minimal. Second, to avoid possible emotional distress or retaliation that might occur if the study was conducted in an actual work environment, the researchers chose to conduct a translational study mimicking a work environment. By using a translational approach, researchers likely minimized any possible side effects of deception that may have tarnished an established working relationship. Finally, researchers debriefed (i.e., informed participants of the true nature of the study) following their last session.

Clinical Priorities

Translational researchers must, first and foremost, remember that the purpose of research is to ask and answer important questions and improve the quality of clinical treatment. Keeping this purpose in mind is particularly important, as more and more translational research is occurring with sensitive populations and in clinical settings. For example, translational researchers may choose to evaluate a basic principle within a clinical population such as individuals with autism, adults with dementia, or those with traumatic brain injuries.

Be Sensitive to Participants from Vulnerable Populations

When including human participants in research, it is critical to ensure that they freely choose to participate and are informed of any consequences involved for declining to participate or to withdraw from participation. Thus, a researcher who is recruiting individuals who are limited in their ability to voluntarily participate must do so with sensitivity and caution. Researchers should ensure that such individuals are able to understand the potential risks and benefits, as well as the consequences of their decision to participate. If potential participants are unable to independently make this decision, the researcher obtains consent from a legal guardian or person responsible for decision making, and assent when possible.

Treat All Participants with Dignity and Respect

As with any researcher who includes humans as participants, translational researchers should make every effort to prevent those participating from being harmed or suffering. Researchers follow applicable ethical principles, guidelines, and codes to ensure minimal and unnecessary pain or discomfort. It is particularly important for translational researchers to keep in mind any possibly harmful or negative outcomes that may occur as a result of participating, as the outcomes are unknown. In applied research, it may be the case that the potential for harm or other risks is outweighed by the possible therapeutic benefits. For example, intentionally reinforcing severe problem behavior during a functional analysis while conducting applied research is often justified, as the benefits of a function-based treatment likely outweigh the potential risks of participating (assuming the researcher includes precautions that minimize harm during such assessments). Within translational research, the possible benefits may be too uncertain to justify potential harm.

Because of this uncertainty, the translational researcher may choose to modify one or more variables in the study to minimize the probability of inflicting harm on participants. For example, rather than targeting severe problem behavior to evaluate a basic principle, the translational researcher may decide to use an arbitrary response (e.g., card touch). For example, St. Peter Pipkin et al. (2010) conducted a translational evaluation of the effects of treatment integrity failures while implementing DRA. In Experiment 1, the authors evaluated two types of integrity failures, reinforcing problem behavior and failing to reinforce appropriate behavior during DRA in a human operant arrangement using undergraduate research students and arbitrary responses of clicking a black circle on a computer screen (representing problem behavior).

The results of the St. Peter Pipkin et al. (2010) study showed that in the human operant experiment, reinforcing problem behavior during DRA was more detrimental to outcomes than failing to reinforce the alternative response. The authors were then able to replicate the results during actual DRA implementation as a treatment for problem behavior. The authors noted that by conducting a translational evaluation prior to an applied study, they were able to more precisely isolate and evaluate the effects of specific variables before attempting to evaluate such procedures in an applied setting with actual problem behavior. Furthermore, the authors suggested that using a translational to applied approach allowed them to quickly determine the potentially most influential variables in the human operant experiment, which they used to inform the procedures they evaluated in the applied setting.

Prioritize Clinical Outcomes

As more research is being conducted in applied settings such as university-based clinics, schools, hospitals, and even clinical organizations, it is critical that translational researchers keep in mind the clinical priorities of the participant. To prioritize clinical treatment, translational researchers should keep in mind those variables that contribute to positive treatment outcomes, including treatment goals. Specifically, translational researchers should consider whether current or future treatment goals or behaviors can be targeted during treatment to benefit the client. On the other hand, researchers must be also cautious of using treatment goals as target responses during research. Extreme caution should be used when the possible outcomes of the research are not reversible, as it may have detrimental effects on clinical treatment, client progress toward goals, and/or effectiveness of future treatment.

If the researcher chooses to use a current treatment goal or target behavior as the dependent variable within a translational study, and the intervention that is being evaluated is not evidence-based, the research must consider whether there is a more efficient treatment that can be implemented. If there is a more efficacious treatment, the researcher must determine whether implementing an intervention that may not be as effective is appropriate. Will the outcomes and knowledge acquired by conducting the study significantly contribute to the scientific community so much that it justifies implementing a less efficient procedure? Ultimately, the translational researcher must keep in mind that when targeting treatment goals, clinical work must come first.

Recognizing One's Limitations

Translational research often includes taking what has been learned from basic research and extending it to clinical populations to solve practical problems. As these extensions begin to show promising results, additional research is conducted to further identify the underlying behavioral principles and processes in effect with the attempt to further refine the procedures to improve its effectiveness. Thus, as noted by Lerman (2003), basic research will play a direct role in the development of the procedures, interventions, and data analysis within the clinical context. Therefore, to conduct translational research, one must be aware of and understand both basic and applied research.

Gain Exposure to Both Applied and Basic Research

To ensure an understanding of complementary disciplines and improve dissemination, as well as potential impact of the research, translational researchers must expose themselves to both basic and applied research. Behavior analysts who have primarily trained in basic laboratory research need to learn the process of clinical practice. This will allow the basic researcher to understand how to incorporate processes into clinical practice and determine how what one has learned from basic research can be translated into clinical practice. Similarly, those trained in applied research and/or clinical practice must be knowledgeable about basic research processes and principles.

Create a Team of Experts

It may be difficult for a researcher to acquire the expertise in both basic and applied research, as well as clinical practice. Thus, creating a team of experts who can collaborate on translational research projects may be more practical. When creating a team of researchers, basic researchers should consider identifying applied researchers who are experts in the area they would like to study. Furthermore, bringing on someone who may not have research expertise, but rather experience working with the target population in the clinical setting, may improve the social acceptability of the project, as they are aware of the day-to-day issues and concerns that arise in clinical treatment.

As translational research within behavior analysis becomes more and more prevalent, many researchers are collaborating across basic and applied disciplines, resulting in significant collaborations to the field. For example, Kelley et al. (2015) discussed strategies for improving treatment outcomes using a translational approach. One strategy the authors noted is to conduct research on the basic processes that contribute to treatment failures. They also stated that linking the methods of applied researchers to concepts based on basic science can be an effective strategy for solving clinical problems.

To demonstrate this translational approach, Kelley et al. (2015) conducted two experiments to evaluate the renewal paradigm in the context of both basic and translational research to begin to bridge the gap between basic and applied literature and in the conceptualization of the causes of treatment relapse. In Experiment 1, the authors evaluated applied behavior analysis (ABA) renewal with pigeons using procedures commonly used in basic behavioral research. Experiment 2 was a translational replication of Experiment 1 in which children with autism participated. Results showed that for both species, returning to the previously reinforced stimulus context produced immediate increases of the extinguished response.

Brown et al. (2020) also used a translational approach by combining basic and applied research to evaluate resurgence of problem behavior. In this study, however, the authors conducted a reverse-translation sequence of studies in which they tested the quantitative theories of resurgence (i.e., behavior momentum theory and resurgence as choice) in the treatment of problem behavior when using DRA. The authors first tested their predictions with participants who engaged in destructive behavior (Experiment 1), followed by testing the same conditions in the laboratory setting with rats (Experiment 2). The authors reported they observed proportionally lower levels of the target behavior during and following DRA with extinction for the target response. It should be noted, however, that the levels of resurgence were similar following both arrangements. By conducting this study in a translational nature, particularly by conducting Experiment 2 with nonhuman animals, the authors noted they were able to better isolate the contingencies.

Both of the previously mentioned studies were conducted by research groups including those that had been expertly trained in the area of basic behavioral research and applied research. By collaborating with researchers from areas outside of their own expertise, they were able to produce valuable research that has greatly contributed to what behavior analysts know about resurgence and can be used to better treat those with destructive behavior. Furthermore, by including experts in both basic and applied research, the researchers were able to conduct ethically sound studies, keeping in mind both research and clinical ethical issues that may have surfaced.

Conclusions

It is evident that translational research results in valuable findings that can be used by behavior analysts to inform treatment and likely improve the outcomes of behavioral interventions. However, it is also apparent that translational research requires one to take into consideration unique ethical issues. Therefore, one must think critically about their approach and determine whether the knowledge and benefits that may be a result of their study outweighs the possible risks and unknown outcomes. Throughout this process of evaluation, researchers should keep in mind that the risks associated with translational work can be quite subjective, as the researchers are often unaware of possible risks, especially when it is the first time humans are exposed to the independent variable.

As with all research, translational research is a process during which one evaluates whether a novel or understudied intervention is effective, often while using a clinically sensitive population. Thus, those involved must recognize that it is not equivalent to treatment and that there may not be an additional benefit for those participating. This must be clearly explained to potential participants to ensure informed consent. And, with this in mind, translational researchers must be willing to take full responsibility for their work, its integrity, and the outcomes.

To ensure that ethically sound translational research is being conducted by behavior analysts, translational researchers can establish an ethical framework for their research and take the lead in creating additional guidelines to ensure ethical and responsible conduct. Furthermore, to optimize the benefits of their research, translational researchers must ensure they are disseminating their work in a way that can have the greatest impact on the application of our science.

REFERENCES

American Psychological Association. (2012). Guidelines for ethical conduct in the care and use of nonhuman animals in research. Retrieved from *www.apa.org/science/leadership/care/care-animal-guidelines.pdf*.

American Psychological Association. (2017). Ethical principles of psychologist and code of conduct (2002, amended effective June 1, 2010, and January 1, 2017). (Original work published 1973). Retrieved from *www.apa.org/ethics/code*.

Behavior Analyst Certification Board. (2020). Ethics code for behavior analysts. Retrieved from *https://bacb.com/wp-content/ethics-code-for-behavior-analysts*.

Bergmann, S., Kodak, T., & Harman, M. J. (2021). When do errors in reinforcer delivery affect learning?: A parametric analysis of treatment integrity. *Journal of Experimental Analysis of Behavior, 115,* 561–577.

Betz, A. M., Fisher, W. W., Roane, H. S., Mintz, J. C., & Owen, T. M. (2013). A component analysis of schedule thinning during functional communication training. *Journal of Applied Behavior Analysis, 46,* 291–241.

Brown, K. R., Greer, B. D., Craig, A. R., Sullivan, W. E., Fisher, W. W., & Roane, H. S. (2020). Resurgence following differential reinforcement of alternative behavior implemented with and without extinction. *Journal of Experimental Analysis of Behavior, 113,* 449–467.

Cohenour, J. M., Volkert, V. M., & Allen, K. D. (2018). An experimental demonstration of AAB renewal in children with autism spectrum disorder. *Journal of the Experimental Analysis of Behavior, 110,* 63–73.

DeLeon, I. G., Gregory, M. K., Frank-Crawford, M. A., Allman, M. J., Wilke, A. E., Carreau-Webster, A. B., & Triggs, M. M. (2013). Examination of the influence of contingency on changes in reinforcer value. *Journal of Applied Behavior Analysis, 44,* 543–558.

Foster, T. M., Template, W., Cameron, B., & Poling A. (1997). Demand curves for food in hens: Similarity under fixed-ratio and progressive ratio schedules. *Behavioral Processes, 39,* 177–185.

Kelley, M. E., Liddon, C. E., Ribeiro, A. Greif, A. E., & Podlesnik, C. A. (2015). Basic and translational evaluation of renewal of operant responding. *Journal of Applied Behavior Analysis, 48,* 390–401.

Kimball, R. T., Kelley, M. E., Podlesnik, C. A., Forton, A., & Hinkle, B. (2018). Resurgence with and without an alternative response. *Journal of Applied Behavior Analysis, 51,* 854–865.

Kyonka, E. G., & Subramaniam, S. (2018). Translating behavior analysis: A spectrum rather than a road map. *Perspectives in Behavioral Science, 41,* 591–613.

Leon, Y., Wilder, D., & Saini, V. (2021). Within- and across-session increases in work requirement do not produce similar response output. *Journal of Applied Behavior Analysis, 54,* 966–983.

Lerman, D. C. (2003). From the laboratory to community application: Translational research in behavior analysis. *Journal of Applied Behavior Analysis, 36,* 415–419.

Mastroianni, A. C., Faden, R., & Federman, D. (1994). *Ethical and legal issues including women in clinical studies* (Vol. 1). National Academy Press.

Matey, N., Gravina, N., Rajagopal, S., & Betz, A. (2019). Effects of feedback delivery requirements on accuracy of observations. *Journal of Organizational Behavior Management, 39,* 247–256.

McIlvane, W. J. (2009). Translational behavior analysis: From laboratory science in stimulus control to intervention with persons with neurodevelopmental disabilities. *Behavior Analysis, 32*(2), 273–280.

Milgram, S. (1974). *Obedience to authority: An experimental view.* Harper & Row.

Milo, J. S., Mace, C. F., & Nevin, J. A. (2010). The effects of constant versus varied reinforcers on preference and resistance to change. *Journal of Experimental Analysis of Behavior, 93,* 385–394.

National Commission of the Protection of Human Subjects in Biomedical and Behavioral Research. (1979). The Belmont Report: Ethical principles and guidelines for protection of human subjects of research. Retrieved from *www.hhs.gov/ohrp/regulations-and-policy/belmont-report/read-the-belmont-report/index.html.*

National Institutes of Health Office of Clinical Research Education and Collaboration Outreach. (1999). Bench-to-bedside and back Program (BtB). Retrieved from *https://ocreco.od.nih.gov/btb/btb_program.html.*

National Institutes of Health Office of Laboratory Animal Welfare. (2015). PHS Policy on Humane Care and Use of Laboratory Animals. Retrieved from *https://olaw.nih.gov/policies-laws/phs-policy.htm.*

Podlesnik, C. A., Duroda, T., Jimenez-Gomez, C., Abreu-Rodrigues, J., Cancado, C. R., Blackman, A. L., . . . Teixeira, S. C., (2019). Resurgence is greater following a return to the training context than remaining in the extinction context. *Journal of the Experimental Analysis of Behavior, 111,* 416–435.

St. Peter Pipkin, C., Vollmer, T. R., & Sloman, K. N. (2010). Effects of treatment integrity failures during differential reinforcement of alternative behavior: A translational model. *Journal of Applied Behavior Analysis, 43,* 47–70.

Tan, L., & Hackenberg, T. D. (2015). Pigeons' demand and preference for specific and generalized conditioned reinforcers in a token economy. *Journal of the Experimental Analysis of the Behavior, 104,* 296–314.

Vollmer, T. R. (2011). The variations of translational research: Comments on Critchfield (2011). *Behavior Analyst, 34,* 31–35.

Index